To Ed with many thanks
for his contributions —
[signature]

Gut–Brain Peptides in the New Millennium

*A Tribute to John Walsh
by his Collaborators*

Gut–Brain Peptides in the New Millennium

*A Tribute to John Walsh
by his Collaborators*

Editor
YVETTE TACHÉ

Associate Editors
YOSHIAKI GOTO
GORDON OHNING
TADATAKA YAMADA

Managing Editor
LORI ENNIS

CURE Foundation

Library of Congress Cataloging-in-Publication Data
Gut-brain peptides in the new millennium : a tribute to John Walsh by his collaborators / Editor, Yvette Taché ; associate editors, Yoshiaki Goto, Gordon Ohning, Tadataka Yamada ; managing editor, Lori Ennis.
     p. cm.
   Includes bibliographic references and index.
   ISBN 0-9721054-0-9
    1. Gastrointestinal hormones. 2. Peptic ulcer--Pathophysiology. I. Taché, Yvette. II. Walsh, John H.

QP572.G35 G86 2002
612.3'2—dc21

2002071496

In Memoriam

JOHN H. WALSH, M.D.
1938–2000

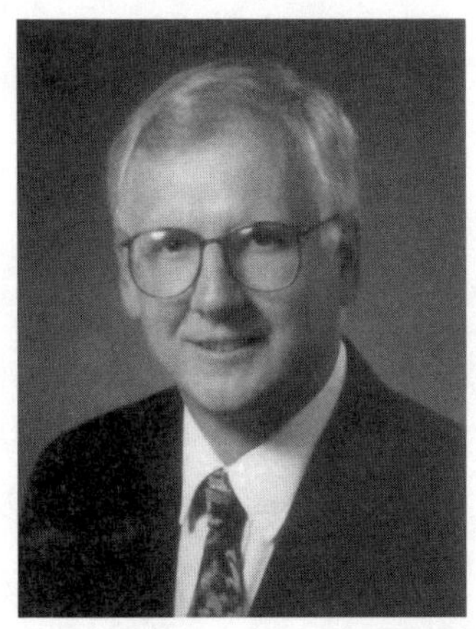

Preface

This book, written in memory of John Harley Walsh, M.D., is a tribute to a man whose influence in the field of gastrointestinal physiology was both profound and worldwide. He was a superb clinician-scientist, a dedicated mentor and a wonderful friend. His untimely death left a large void in the lives of his friends, colleagues and trainees. In this book, they have come together to honor him by their scientific contributions, which characterize the breadth of John's own interest in the field covering topics ranging from molecular and cell biology to human disease. Scientific rigor combined with a style that was easy, comfortable and low key, intellectual generosity and an uncommon spirit of collaboration endeared him to generations of trainees, scientists and clinicians.

John was handpicked by the late Morton I. Grossman to be his key scientific partner. In the early 1970s, together, they ran arguably the best and most productive gastrointestinal laboratory sought after by postdoctoral fellows from all over the United States and the world. In 1975, Morton Grossman and John Walsh founded the Center for Ulcer Research and Education (CURE), an NIH-funded UCLA center for gastrointestinal research. From the beginning until his death, John provided, officially and unofficially, the "glue" that made CURE a nurturing family of investigators. In 1987, John became Director of CURE and expanded the research vision of the Center. The traditional strengths in cell biology, integrative physiology and neurosciences, as well as clinical research in peptic ulcer and esophageal diseases were to continue. But the focus of research was expanded to include the entire gastrointestinal tract with new programs in inflammatory, malignant, genetic and functional diseases. He brought a major emphasis on molecular biology and cell "signaling" by recruiting Enrique Rozengurt. Characteristically, as he built up the research portfolio of CURE, and his stature rose nationally and internationally, John never lost "the common touch" and the warmth, generosity and kindness with which he treated all around him.

This book, which contains a broad collection of papers from friends and trainees, is written in loving memory of John Harley Walsh, a leading gastrointestinal investigator of the 20th century.

Haile T. Debas, M.D.

Acknowledgments

"I believe that man will not merely endure; he will prevail. He is immortal, not because he alone among creatures has an inexhaustible voice, but because he has a soul, a spirit capable of compassion and sacrifice and endurance."

—William Faulkner, 1950

Dr. John Walsh was a renowned and respected leader in gastroenterology at the time of his passing on June 14, 2000. We all mourn his loss as a valued colleague, mentor, and friend. His voice may have been silenced, but his spirit will live on through the work of his collaborators and trainees. It is, therefore, fitting that this compendium of work was produced in his memory as it was written by the very colleagues, trainees, and friends who held him so dear. Even the largest redwood tree begins as but a seed. We are indebted to Dr. Yoshi Goto for his determined efforts to gather a group on the first anniversary of Dr. Walsh's passing in Honolulu, Hawaii in June 2001. Although small in number, this meeting initiated the sequence of events that led to this memorial publication. The initial expectations were to receive 20–25 short chapters written by Dr. Walsh's former fellows and collaborators. The editors are deeply grateful for the magnitude of the response and thank each and every author for their contribution. The final version includes over 40 chapters written by 50 authors and co-authors and covers the breadth and depth of Dr. Walsh's influence as well as his interest in both basic and clinical research.

Of course such an undertaking would have been impossible without the generous support of Eisai Inc./Janssen Pharmaceutica in the form of an educational grant to cover the expenses incurred in the initial gathering and producing this volume. The editors are deeply grateful of their recognition of Dr. Walsh as a long time collaborator and advisor. Last, but certainly not least, the editors are extremely indebted to Ms. Lori Ennis for her tireless efforts, dedication and infinite patience in bringing this project to fruition. Her competence and efficiency were essential components of this finished product within less than a year of its initial conceptualization.

Although it is still difficult at times to comprehend that Dr. John Walsh is no longer among us, we sincerely hope that his spirit will perdure through the compassion, sacrifice, and endurance of those who will follow in his steps.

Contributors

Yasutada Akiba, M.D., Ph.D.
Keio University School of Medicine
35 Shinanomachi
Shinjuku-ku, Tokyo 150
Japan

Diane L. Barber, Ph.D.
Department of Stomatology
University of California
San Francisco, CA 94143

Izäk Biemond, Ph.D.
Leiden University Medical Centre
Leiden, The Netherlands

Nicholas C. Brecha, Ph.D.
CURE: Digestive Diseases Research Center
VA Greater Los Angeles Healthcare System
Digestive Diseases Division; and
Departments of Medicine and Neurobiology
University of California–Los Angeles
Los Angeles, CA 90073

F. Charles Brunicardi, M.D.
Michael E. DeBakey Department of Surgery
Baylor College of Medicine
Houston, TX 77030

Alison M.J. Buchan, Ph.D.
Department of Physiology
University of British Columbia
2146 Health Sciences Mall
Vancouver, BC V6T 1Z3
Canada

Nigel W. Bunnett, Ph.D.
University of California–San Francisco
521 Parnassus Avenue, Box 0660
San Francisco, CA 94143-0660

Monica C. Chen, Ph.D.
CURE: Digestive Diseases Research Center
VA Greater Los Angeles Healthcare System
Digestive Diseases Division
Medical and Research Services
University of California–Los Angeles
Los Angeles, CA 90073

James Croom, Ph.D., FACN
Department of Poultry Science
North Carolina State University
Raleigh, NC 27695

Sebastian G. de la Fuente, M.D.
Department of Surgery
Duke University Medical Center
Durham, NC 27710

Haile Debas, M.D.
Dean's Office
University of California–San Francisco
513 Parnassus Ave., S-224
San Francisco, CA 94143-0410

Rod Dimaline, Ph.D.
Physiological Laboratory
University of Liverpool
Crown Street
Liverpool L69 3BX
United Kingdom

Graham Dockray, Ph.D.
Department of Physiology
University of Liverpool
Crown Street, P.O. Box 147
Liverpool L69 3BX
United Kingdom

Misako Ebata, M.A.
Department of Applied Pharmacology
Kyoto Pharmaceutical University
Misasagi, Yamashina
Kyoto 607-8414
Japan

Viktor E. Eysselein, M.D.
Division of Gastroenterology
Harbor/UCLA Medical Center
Torrance, CA 90509

John B. Furness, Ph.D.
Department of Anatomy and Cell Biology
University of Melbourne
Parkville, Victoria 3052
Australia

Andrew S. Giraud, Ph.D.
Department of Medicine
Western Hospital
Footscray, Victoria 3011
Australia

Yoshiaki Goto, Ph.D.
Clinical Research Division
AT Company
Nippon Colin Co., Ltd.
2700-1 Hayashi
Komaki 485-8501
Japan

David Y. Graham, M.D.
Department of Medicine
Veterans Affairs Medical Center and
Division of Molecular Virology
Baylor College of Medicine
Houston, TX 77030

John R. Grider, Ph.D.
Medical College of Virginia
Division of Gastroenterology
P.O. Box 980711
Richmond, VA 23298

Herbert F. Helander, M.D.
AstraZeneca AB
SE-431 83 Mölndal
Sweden

Peter Holzer, Ph.D.
Department of Experimental and Clinical
    Pharmacology
University of Graz
Universitätsplatz 4, A-8010 Graz
Austria

Dennis M. Jensen, M.D.
CURE: Digestive Diseases Research Center
VA Greater Los Angeles Healthcare System
Digestive Diseases Division
University of California-Los Angeles
Los Angeles, CA 90073

Ji-Guang Jin, M.D., Ph.D.
Medical College of Virginia
Division of Gastroenterology
P.O. Box 980711
Richmond, VA 23298

Sophie Julien, D.E.A.
Department of Medicine
University of Sherbrooke
Sherbrooke, Quebec
Canada J1H 5N4

Neil Kaplowitz, M.D.
Keck School of Medicine of the University
    of Southern California
USC Research Center for Liver Diseases
2011 Zonal Avenue, HMR101
Los Angeles, CA 90033

Jonathan D. Kaunitz, M.D.
CURE: Digestive Diseases Research Center
VA Greater Los Angeles Healthcare System
Digestive Diseases Division
University of California–Los Angeles
Los Angeles, CA 90073

David A. Keire, Ph.D.
CURE: Digestive Diseases Research Center
VA Greater Los Angeles Healthcare System
Digestive Diseases Division
University of California–Los Angeles
Los Angeles, CA 90073

Yoshihiro Keto, Ph.D.
Department of Applied Pharmacology
Kyoto Pharmaceutical University
Misasagi, Yamashina
Kyoto 607-8414
Japan

Thomas O.G. Kovacs, Ph.D.
CURE: Digestive Diseases Research Center
VA Greater Los Angeles Healthcare System
Digestive Diseases Division
University of California–Los Angeles
Los Angeles, CA 90073

Jean Lainé, M.Sc.
Department of Medicine
University of Sherbrooke
Sherbrooke, Quebec
Canada J1H 5N4

Cornelis B.H.W. Lamers, M.D., Ph.D.
Leiden University Medical Centre
Leiden, The Netherlands

Chin-Yu Lin, D.D.S.
Department of Stomatology
University of California
San Francisco, CA 94143

Kevin C. Kent Lloyd, D.V.M., Ph.D.
Center for Comparative Medicine
School of Veterinary Medicine
One Shields Avenue
University of California–Davis
Davis, CA 95616

Atsushi Maeda, M.D.
Institute of Geriatrics
Tokyo Women's Medical College
2-15 Shibuya
Shibuya-ku, Tokyo 150-0002
Japan

Gabriel M. Makhlouf, M.D., Ph.D.
Medical College of Virginia
Division of Gastroenterology
P.O. Box 980711
Richmond, VA 23298

Vicente Martínez, D.V.M., Ph.D.
Nervous System Research
Novartis Pharma AG
WSJ-386.109
Basel, Switzerland CH-4002

Emeran A. Mayer, M.D.
CURE: Neuroenteric Disease Program
VA Greater Los Angeles Healthcare System
University of California–Los Angeles
Los Angeles, CA 90073

James E. McGuigan, M.D.
Department of Medicine
University of Florida College of Medicine
Gainesville, FL 32610-0421

Douglas C. McVey, B.S., M.S.
Departments of Cell Biology and Medicine
Duke University Medical Center; and
Durham VA Medical Center
Durham, NC 27710

Stefan Moldovan, M.D.
Michael E. DeBakey Department of Surgery
Baylor College of Medicine
Houston, TX 77030

Jean Morisset, Ph.D.
Department of Medicine
University of Sherbrooke
Sherbrooke, Quebec
Canada J1H 5N4

John E. Morley, M.B., B.Ch.
Division of Geriatric Medicine
Saint Louis University School of Medicine
1402 S. Grand Blvd.
St. Louis, MO 63104

Karnam S. Murthy, Ph.D.
Medical College of Virginia
Division of Gastroenterology
P.O. Box 980711
Richmond, VA 23298

Elke Niebergall-Roth, M.D.
Department of Medicine II
Gastroenterology and Hepatology
University Hospital of Heidelberg–
    Mannheim
Mannheim, Germany

Michael Norman, M.D.
Michael E. DeBakey Department of
   Surgery
Baylor College of Medicine
Houston, TX 77030

G. Johan A. Offerhaus, M.D., Ph.D.
University Medical Centre
Amsterdam, The Netherlands

Gordon V. Ohning, M.D., Ph.D.
CURE: Digestive Diseases Research Center
VA Greater Los Angeles Healthcare System
Digestive Diseases Division
University of California–Los Angeles
Los Angeles, CA 90073

Susumu Okabe, Ph.D.
Department of Applied Pharmacology
Kyoto Pharmaceutical University
Misasagi, Yamashina
Kyoto 607-8414
Japan

Theodore N. Pappas, M.D.
Department of Surgery
Duke University Medical Center
Durham, NC 27710

Joseph R. Pisegna, M.D.
CURE: Digestive Diseases Research Center
VA Greater Los Angeles Healthcare System
Division of Gastroenterology and Hepatology
University of California–Los Angeles
Los Angeles, CA 90073

Pierre Poitras, M.D.
Department of Medicine and Physiology
Université de Montréal
Montréal, Canada

Daniel P. Poole, M.Sc.
Department of Anatomy and Cell Biology
University of Melbourne
Parkville 3010
Victoria, Australia

Helen E. Raybould, Ph,D.
Department of Anatomy, Physiology and
   Cell Biology
University of California–Davis
School of Veterinary Medicine
Davis, CA 95616

Joseph R. Reeve, Jr., Ph.D.
CURE: Digestive Diseases Research Center
VA Greater Los Angeles Healthcare System
Digestive Diseases Division
University of California–Los Angeles
Los Angeles, CA 90095

Jens F. Rehfeld, Ph.D.
Department of Clinical Biochemistry
Rigshospitalet
University of Copenhagen
Copenhagen, Denmark

**Enrique Rozengurt, M.V., Ph.D.,
   FRC. Path.**
School of Medicine and Molecular Biology
   Institute
Department of Medicine
University of California–Los Angeles
Los Angeles, CA 90095

George Sachs, M.B., Ch.B., D.Sc., M.D.
Departments of Physiology and Medicine
VA Greater Los Angeles Healthcare System
University of California–Los Angeles
Los Angeles, CA 90073

Mohamed Sagar, M.D., Ph.D.
Department of Medicine
Division of Gastroenterology
McMaster University
Hamilton, Ontario
Canada; and
Huddinge University Hospital
Karolinska Institute
Stockholm, Sweden

Rein Seensalu, M.D., Ph.D.
St Görans Hospital; and
Huddinge University Hospital
Karolinska Institute
Stockholm, Sweden

Arthur Shulkes, Ph.D.
Department of Surgery
University of Melbourne
Austin and Repatriation Medical Centre
Heidelberg, Victoria
Australia, 3084

Manfred V. Singer, M.D.
Department of Medicine II
Gastroenterology and Hepatology
University Hospital of Heidelberg–
 Mannheim
Mannheim, Germany

Lee W. Slice, Ph.D.
CURE: Digestive Diseases Research Center
VA Greater Los Angeles Healthcare System
Digestive Diseases Division
University of California–Los Angeles
Los Angeles, CA 90073

Andrew H. Soll, M.D.
CURE: Digestive Diseases Research Center
VA Greater Los Angeles Healthcare System
Digestive Diseases Division
Medical and Research Services
University of California–Los Angeles
Los Angeles, CA 90073

Travis E. Solomon, M.D., Ph.D.
CURE: Digestive Diseases Research Center
VA Greater Los Angeles Healthcare System
Digestive Diseases Division
University of California–Los Angeles
Los Angeles, CA 90073

Paul E. Squires, Ph.D.
Molecular Physiology
University of Warwick
England

Catia Sternini, M.D.
CURE: Digestive Diseases Research Center
VA Greater Los Angeles Healthcare System
Digestive Diseases Division; and
Departments of Medicine and Neurobiology
University of California–Los Angeles
Los Angeles, CA 90073

Yvette Taché, Ph.D.
CURE: Digestive Diseases Research Center
VA Greater Los Angeles Healthcare System
Digestive Diseases Division
Department of Medicine and Brain
 Research Institute
University of California–Los Angeles
Los Angeles, CA 90073

Toku Takahashi, M.D., Ph.D.
Department of Surgery
Duke University Medical Center
Durham, NC 27710

Chengwei Tang, M.D., Ph.D.
West China Hospital
Sichuan University
Sichuan
People's Republic of China

Ian L. Taylor, M.D., Ph.D.
Dean's Office
Tulane University School of Medicine
1430 Tulane Avenue
New Orleans, LA 70112

Baiqin Teng, M.D.
Medical College of Virginia
Division of Gastroenterology
P.O. Box 980711
Richmond, VA 23298

Steven R. Vigna, Ph.D.
Departments of Cell Biology and Medicine
Duke University Medical Center; and
Durham VA Medical Center
Durham, NC 27710

Yu Hua Wang
CURE: Digestive Diseases Research Center
Division of Digestive Diseases; and
Department of Medicine and Brain
 Research Institute
University of California–Los Angeles
Los Angeles, CA 90095

Jen Yu Wei, Ph.D.
CURE: Digestive Diseases Research Center
Division of Digestive Diseases
Department of Medicine and Brain
    Research Institute
University of California–Los Angeles
Los Angeles, CA 90095

Helen C. Wong, M.S., M.T.
CURE: Digestive Diseases Research Center
VA Greater Los Angeles Healthcare System;
Digestive Diseases Division
University of California–Los Angeles
Los Angeles, CA 90073

Ruud A. Woutersen, Ph.D.
TNO Nutrition and Food Research
    Institute
Zeist, The Netherlands

Tadataka Yamada, M.D.
GlaxoSmithKline
709 Swedeland Road
King of Prussia, PA 19406-0939

Katsuko Yamashita, M.D.
Institute of Geriatrics
Tokyo Women's Medical College
2-15 Shibuya, Shibuya-ku, Tokyo 150-0002
Japan

Hong Yang, M.D., Ph.D.
CURE: Digestive Diseases Research Center
VA Greater Los Angeles Healthcare System;
and Digestive Diseases Division
Department of Medicine and Brain
    Research Institute
University of California–Los Angeles
Los Angeles, CA 90073

Ningxin Zeng
Department of Medicine
School of Medicine
Texas Tech University–El Paso
El Paso, TX

Table of Contents

INTRODUCTION

**I. GASTRIN, ECL AND D CELLS:
REGULATION AND FUNCTION**

III. PATHOPHYSIOLOGY OF NERVE-GUT INTERACTIONS

IV. PROCESSES OF GASTROINTESTINAL INJURY AND REPAIR

V. PANCREATIC REGULATION

Introduction

Gut-Brain Peptides in the New Millennium, edited by Y. Taché
CURE Foundation, Los Angeles, CA. © 2002

In Memoriam
John H. Walsh

Address to the 13th International Congress
on Gastrointestinal Hormones

October 24, 2000

Tadataka Yamada
Research and Development, GlaxoSmithKline
King of Prussia, PA

This, the 13th International Congress on Gastrointestinal Hormones, REG-PEP 2000, will no doubt be an outstanding meeting under the expert organization of our Australian colleagues led by Arthur Shulkes. But for many of us who have a long history of attendance at these meetings, we cannot help but feel a sense of incompleteness by the absence of John Walsh who was, in many ways, the major intellectual, social, and spiritual leader of this biennial congregation. John was at once my teacher, my mentor, my colleague, my competitor, and my friend. It is difficult to remember that we won't look up tomorrow and see him at the podium making an incisive and salient point as he thinks on his feet, looking up at a screen inside his head to tap the vast sum of knowledge that he stored there for such occasions.

For this audience, there is no need to re-visit the countless contributions that John made to medical science. Suffice it to say that he was a master working at the interface between basic cellular and molecular science and human physiology and pathology. He never looked at technical data without thinking of the big picture in man. Some of you are keenly aware of his cutting edge research interests in the structure and function of receptors, but did you know that more than 15 years ago, he was already recognized as among the 250 most cited scientists in the world for the preceding decade? Did you know also that, aside from his devotion to science, he was a wonderful clinician who treated his patients with intelligence and compassion and imparted that style of caring to his medical trainees?

John always worked in an environment at CURE made exciting by the presence of a combination of renowned colleagues, impressionable and ambitious trainees, and a steady stream of international visitors. Indeed, I wouldn't be surprised if more than half of the people in this room have collaborated with John in one way or another.

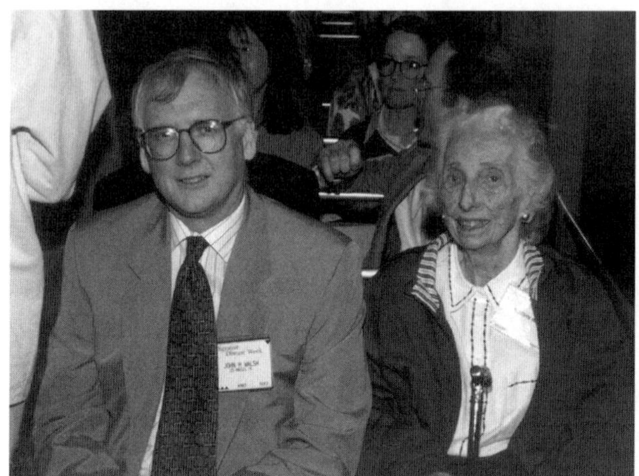

FIGURE 1. *John with his Mother, Aimee Walsh.*

To provide a description of what it was like to work in his laboratory, I quote from a biography of John written for *Gastroenterology*. "Grossman was in a laboratory one floor below and was the father figure for us all. In the laboratory next door, Andrew Soll had just developed the isolated canine gastric parietal cell preparation, the first system to permit investigators in gastrointestinal research the opportunity to work at the cellular level. A group of investigators, including Travis Solomon, Gordon Kauffman, Haile Debas, and Yvette Tache, were working with in vivo experiments on hormone biology and exploring the concept of the brain–gut axis. Pioneering human studies were being conducted by Jon Isenberg, Andrew Ippoliti, and

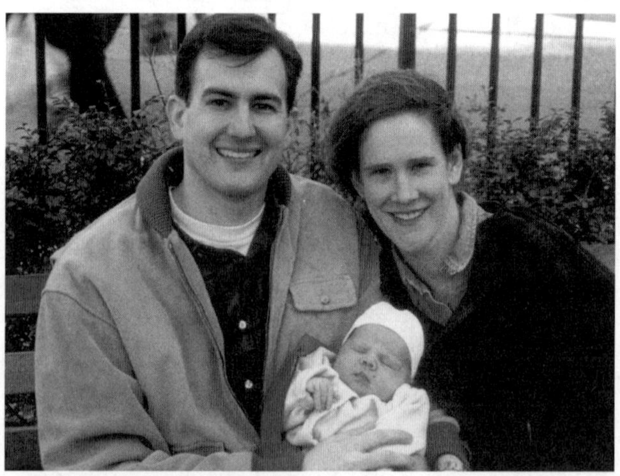

FIGURE 2. *Harley, Lindsay and Lily Walsh.*

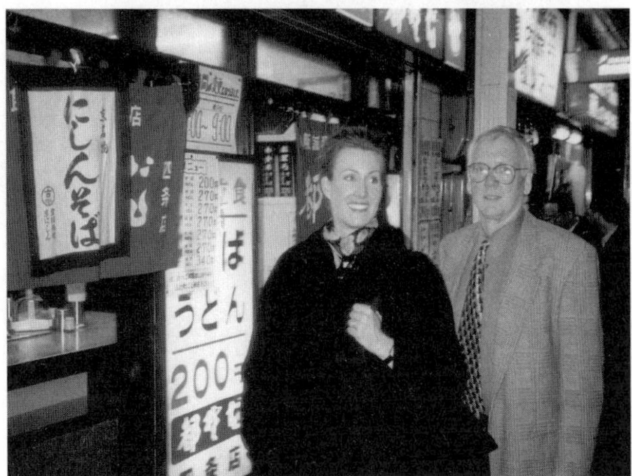

FIGURE 3. *Courtney Shands Phleger and John.*

Dennis Jensen. Studies of mucosal blood flow by in vivo microscopy were being conducted by Paul Guth and his visiting scientists Andre Robert and Brendan Whittle. Charles Code maintained an active laboratory on gastrointestinal motility. Neil Kaplowitz was the odd man out as a liver biochemical pharmacologist but greatly enhanced the intellectual vigor and vitality of the Center. In the middle of all this was placed the Walsh laboratory. At the

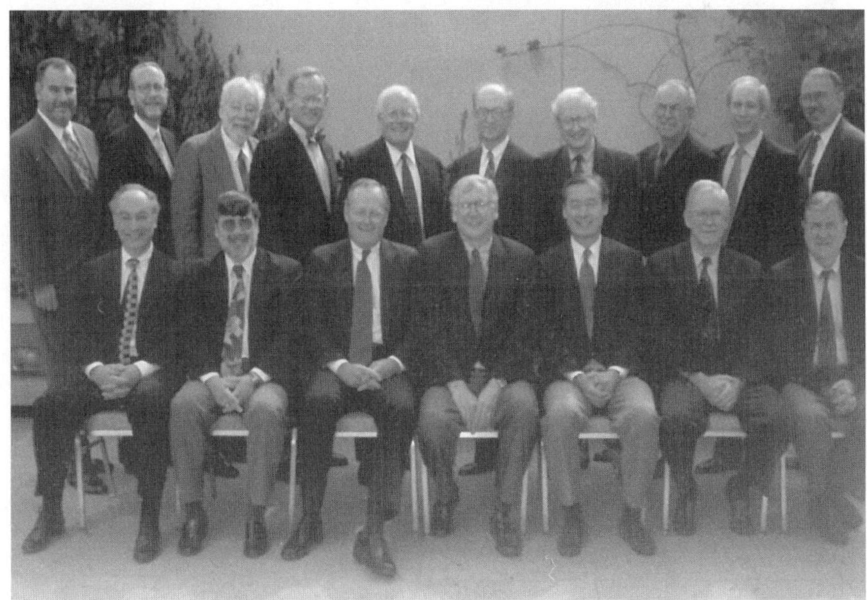

FIGURE 4. *AGA governing Board, 1994.*

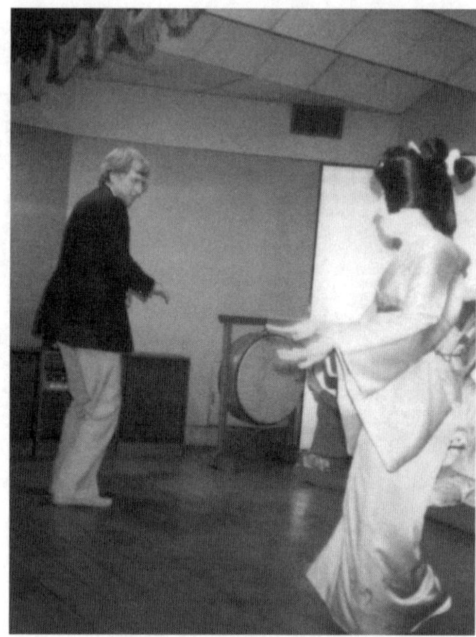

FIGURE 5. *John and a dancing friend.*

time I was a fellow, an incredible array of coworkers was laboring side by side with their thousand tube assays. Ian Taylor and I were in the clinical training program. Joe Reeve and Steve Vigna came as Ph.D. postdoctoral fellows. Visiting foreign scholars included Cornelis Lamers from Belgium, Arthur Shulkes from Australia, Pierre Poitras from Canada, Jan Kleibeuker from The Netherlands, Nigel Bunnett from England, Viktor Eysselein from Germany, Irvin Modlin from South Africa by way of England, and Emeran Mayer from Germany by way of Canada. Two prominent scientists, Jack Hansky from Australia and S.K. Lam from Hong Kong, were conducting their sabbaticals with us as well. I remember it as a time of incredible productivity. The competition to get our samples on the two gamma counters in the laboratory was intense, requiring us to return at all hours of the night to change our tubes. John orchestrated our activities in the manner of a virtuoso conductor."

John had many loves. He loved his family above all. He was devoted to his mother who had an abiding influence on his life and she is said to have been every bit as memorable as he was (Figure 1).

He had two handsome and accomplished children—Harley, shown in this picture with his family (Figure 2), and Courtney Shands (Figure 3).

Courtney Shands revealed that every Sunday of her adult life she received a bouquet of flowers from her father.

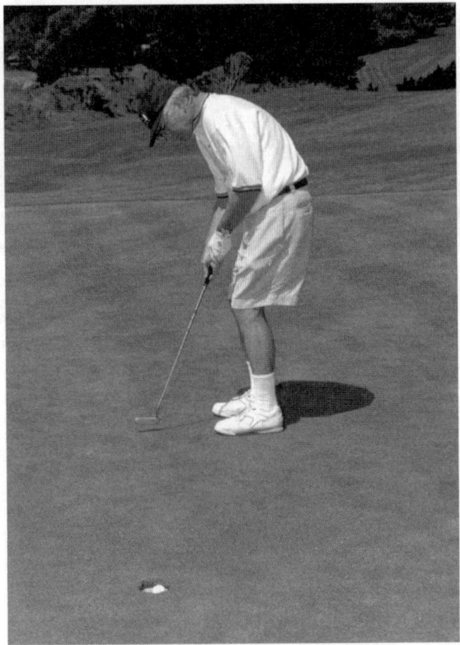

FIGURE 6. *John at his favorite pastime*

Professionally his first love was CURE, of which he was the Co-director or Director since its inception over 25 years ago. His entire professional life after training was spent at UCLA, an institution for which he remained passionately loyal and committed to the end. No small amount of UCLA's luster resulted from John's many accomplishments. He was devoted to the American Gastroenterological Association and to its journal, Gastroenterology. He served with great distinction as the AGA President in 1994 (Figure 4). He was a loyal servant of the NIH and represented the gastroenterology community there on both the Digestive Disease Study Section and the Advisory Council of the NIDDK. And, of course, he maintained a true commitment to this meeting, having organized the 10th Congress in Santa Barbara and served on the International Steering Committee from the beginning.

John always had fun wherever he went and he went to every corner of the world. A true bon vivant, he was as at home in a fancy restaurant in Paris, or at a tuxedo ball, or dancing with a geisha(Figure 5), or partying at home. Although he would never consider himself a great athlete, he loved the outdoors and sports and he was a willing participant in all manner of fun. I am eternally grateful for the fact that just a few days before he died, John and I stole a morning away from the DDW meeting in San Diego to have an early morning round of golf together (Figure 6). That is how I will always remember him, outdoors in a beautiful setting, playing a game that he loved, chatting about people, politics and science, and above all engaging in friendly but real competition.

I close with the words of Milton, a poet beloved by John:

> Yet once more, O ye Laurels and once more
> Ye Myrtles brown, with Ivy never-sear
> I com to pluck your Berries harsh and crude,
> And with forc'd fingers rude,
> Shatter your leaves before the mellowing year.
> Bitter constraint and sad occasion dear,
> Compels me to disturb your season due:
> For Lycidas is dead, dead ere his prime
> Young Lycidas, and hath not left his peer:
> Who would not sing for Lycidas? he knew
> Himself to sing, and build the lofty rhyme.
> He must not flote upon his watry bear
> Unwept, and welter to the parching wind
> Without the meed of som melodious tear.

I.

Gastrin, ECL and D Cells:
Regulation and Function

Gut-Brain Peptides in the New Millennium, edited by Y. Taché
CURE Foundation, Los Angeles, CA. © 2002

1

To Study the Molecular Nature of Gastrin—and to Know John Walsh: A Flashback to the Seventies

Jens F. Rehfeld
Department of Clinical Biochemistry, Rigshospitalet, University of Copenhagen, Denmark

INTRODUCTION

Scientifically and socially the nineteen seventies was a fascinating and bubbling decade. Young scientists in the western world had in many ways larger opportunities than before and after. The seventies was the period in which gastrointestinal endocrinology exploded from a narrow discipline cultivated in a few laboratories mainly in Europe and North America to an issue that dominated the research in basic and clinical gastroenterology worldwide. The master and model hormone in this development was gastrin. And with his devoted and productive gastrin research, John Walsh became a central person in an international gang of impetuous young scientists.

In the following I have tried to describe my perception of the attempts to define the nature of bioactive gastrin molecules, a central issue in gut endocrinology in the seventies. Part of the perception came through the interaction with John. Therefore, I hope that the story that follows will contribute to the multifaceted picture of John.

LONDON, July 1972

I first met John on a hot summer day in London in 1972. A small gastrin-meeting for Anglo Scandinavian gastroenterologists and physiologists was attended also by a few Americans. Among them John. The venue was an auditorium in an old physiology-institute without air-conditioning. The subtropical temperature necessitated open air channels, which turned out to interfere with the organizers plan to immortalize the meeting by taping presentations and discussion for a book. Unfortunately, they had placed the tape recorder in front of an air channel leading to the dog section of the local animal house. The tape turned out to contain nothing but barking dogs.

The meeting was otherwise timely and topical. After Rod Gregory's and Hilda Tracy's purification of gastrin in 1964 (1), and the subsequent establishment of reliable radioimmunoassays in the States and Australia in 1968–70 by McGuigan and others (2–5), the interest for gastrin boomed worldwide in the early seventies. Not only was and is gastrin the master hormone of the gut, but it was also the first gastrointestinal hormone to be measured in plasma.

Since 1968, I had struggled to establish a sensitive radioimmunoassay for gastrin. Flemming Stadil joined the fight in early 1970, and just before Christmas that year, the assay started to work. By then, we had immunized several series of rabbits and guinea pigs, had a host of promising gastrin antisera (6), and during 1971, we improved the technique for radioiodination to achieve an unusual high specific activity of the gastrin tracer (7). The assay papers were still "in press" at the London-meeting. But our oral presentations were well received by John and the remaining audience, which included Rod Gregory himself.

John joined Flemming and me for lunch. We knew his name from a paper about tissue degradation of tetragastrin (8) and for his development of a hepatitis-B antibody radioimmunoassay with Berson and Yalow (9). John told us that he recently had left the Berson-Yalow laboratory in Bronx to move to Morton Grossman in California, where he wished to concentrate his research on gastrin. We took it for granted that he already had brought gastrin antisera from Bronx (4) to set up the assay in Los Angeles. But John didn't tell us then that Rosalyn Yalow would not let collaborators have antisera, when they moved to other laboratories. Perhaps John was also too shy or too proud to ask beginners like us for help. Anyway, it was a pleasure to meet him and to establish a lasting contact. I still recall John's boyish and gentle smile on that particular London-day. In the evening Flemming and I visited some interesting Soho-bars to celebrate what we took for acceptance in the gastrin club.

COPENHAGEN, September 1972

What John couldn't or wouldn't do, Mort Grossman didn't mind. So in early September 1972 Mort visited my lab, and on top of his agenda was a request to send a useful gastrin antiserum to John. I was pleased and honored to comply, and sent a sample of our best antiserum to Los Angeles, while Mort the next day continued his Europe-tour. The antiserum (no. 2604) is unique in the sense that it happens to measure all the carboxyamidated (i.e., bioactive) forms of gastrin equally well without cross-reactivity with any cholecystokinin peptide. In other words, it binds gastrin-17, gastrin-34 and gastrin-71 equally irrespective of degree of sulfation and irrespective of mammalian species differences (6). The antiserum was, therefore, perfectly suited to what was to be John's major project in the years to come! Studies of the biological activity and metabolism of the new molecular forms of gastrin in man and dog (10–12). I was (and John and Morton were also, I presume) happy that the antiserum worked well in Los Angeles. Later John raised a multitude of excellent gastrin antisera for himself and many other researchers—including me. By the way, antiserum no. 2604 still serves as a reference antiserum here and elsewhere.

The next point on Mort's Copenhagen-agenda was the new molecular forms of gastrin. It was a large issue, that would continue to be a main point on gastrin meetings in the following decade. Yalow and Berson (13) had in 1970 set the gastrin-world on fire by showing that the predominant hormonal form of gastrin in plasma was not the heptadecapeptide amide (gastrin-17) so carefully purified as the antral gastrin by Gregory and Tracy (1), but clearly a larger form. The new observation was a challenge for any serious gastroenterologist. And not surprisingly, the experienced Liverpool-pair, Gregory and Tracy, met the challenge by showing in October 1972 that the "big"-gastrin of Yalow and Berson was a 34-amino acid peptide corresponding to gastrin-17 extended at its N-terminus (14). They knew the amino acid composition, but didn't know the N-terminal sequence yet.

The background for the discussion with Mort in Copenhagen was that I earlier had worked with insulin in plasma, and had been captivated by Steiner's discovery of proinsulin (15), which turned out to circulate in plasma (16). Accordingly, I found it necessary to examine whether our gastrin assay in addition to gastrin-17 would measure also gastrin-34, and— second—whether gastrin-34 might be a biosynthetic precursor in analogy with proinsulin. Therefore, I set out in late 1970 to examine the molecular pattern of gastrin in plasma from hypergastrinemic patients using long high-resolution gel columns and ion exchange chromatography. The results were surprising (Figure 1). In addition to "big" gastrin-34 and "little" gastrin-17, human plasma also contained a somewhat larger gastrin, which I called component I (17) but John and Mort "Rehfeld's component" (18). Moreover, I also found a smaller new form of gastrin (19), which I named component IV (Figure 1), whereas John, Mort and Rod would call it "mini"-gastrin (11, 20). Years later, Anders Johnsen and I identified component I as gastrin-71, the "biggest" possible bioactive gastrin (21), and component IV or "mini"-gastrin was shown by Gregory, et al. to be gastrin-14 (22). On top of these findings Mort and I also discussed the phenomenon of "big big"-gastrin (23). We didn't run short of topics that day.

LIVERPOOL, May 1973

I had not yet met Rod Gregory face to face. After his and Hilda Tracy's publication of the amino acid composition of gastrin-34 in October 1972 (14), Flemming Stadil and I sent Lancet a "Letter to the Editor" (24), in which we

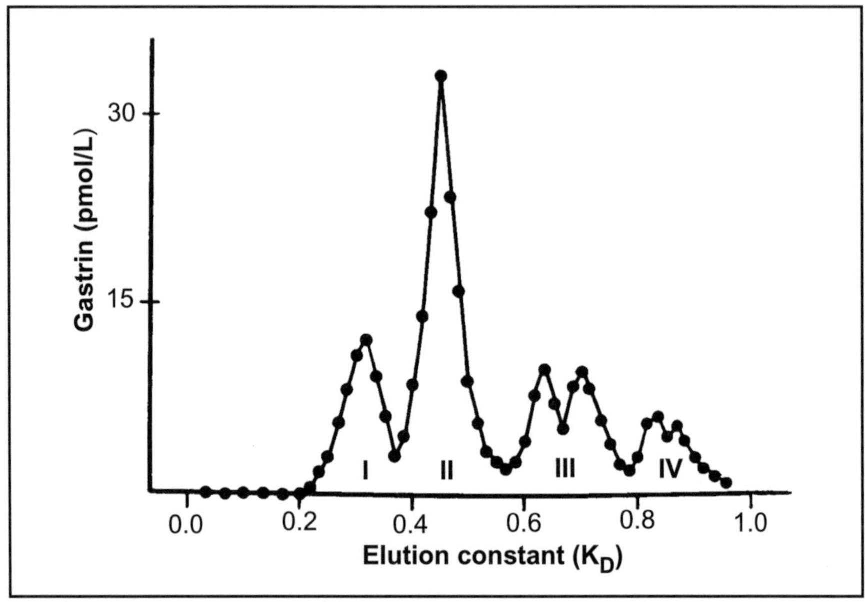

FIGURE 1. *Gel chromatographic elution pattern of bioactive (i.e., carboxyamidated) gastrins in plasma from a patient with hypergastrinemia due to pernicious anemia (ref. 25). The components numbered I–IV correspond to gastrin-71, -34, -17 and -14, respectively. The double-peaks of gastrin-17 and -14 are due to the occurrence of both sulfated and non-sulfated gastrins.*

discussed the nature of component I in relation to gastrin-34 and to Yalow's "big big"-gastrin (23). That discussion was continued in a long personal letter from Rod Gregory in which he invited me to Liverpool. Soon after, I got a letter from John about the rapid progress in his bioactivity studies of gastrin-34 and gastrin-14 (10, 11). John also mentioned, that he and Mort would go to Liverpool in early May 1973 for further discussion of the significance of the new molecular forms of gastrin. What a splendid opportunity I thought, and called Rod Gregory to suggest that my visit to Liverpool coincided with that of Mort's and John's.

It was a very stimulating and friendly meeting in spite of an awkward entrance into the inner gastrin circles. In Copenhagen airport, I realized that I had forgotten my passport, and therefore reached Liverpool with half a days delay. As a humble excuse, I brought a sizable bottle of Danish snaps of which Rod would take a large beer-glass after dinner, and soon after fall asleep. This unusual way of snaps-drinking became a tradition during my subsequent visits to Liverpool in the years to come.

The scientific content of the meeting was also superb. Rod Gregory had provided John with pure human gastrin-34 for infusion studies, that surprisingly revealed a near tenfold slower metabolism of gastrin-34 in comparison with that of gastrin-17. John could, therefore, offer a solid explanation for the discrepant gastrin-17/gastrin-34 ratios in antral extracts and peripheral plasma (10, 12). Rod had also provided me with gastrins for chromatographic calibration so that we could show that the circulating "big"- and "mini"-gastrins indeed resembled gastrin-34 and -14, although at that time, we thought that "mini"-gastrin was a tridecapeptide (20, 22). Moreover, as emphasized by Mort, the chromatographic plasma studies showed for the first time, that the partial tyrosyl-sulfation that Rod and Hilda had found in antral and gastrinoma tissue (1, 14, 20, 22) wasn't an extraction artifact, since the circulating gastrins displayed the same partial sulfation without extraction (19, 24, 25, see also Figure 1). Later we have shown that the specific sulfation pattern for gastrin is due to the sequence immediately N-terminal to the tyrosyl-residue to be O-sulfated (26). Thus, by the end of the Liverpool visit, consensus regarding the nature of most hormonal gastrins in tissue and plasma was reached. The open questions concerned the molecular nature of "big big"-gastrin (23, 27) and component I (17). In Copenhagen, however, we had a gastrinoma patient with sky-high gastrin concentrations. And both Hilda and Rod were keen to try to isolate component I from plasmapheretic pools of that patient. So with plasmapheresis in mind (and the passport safely in the pocket) I returned from an exciting first-meeting with Rod Gregory and Hilda Tracy, chaperoned by John and Mort.

LOS ANGELES, October 1974

Gastrointestinal hormones were—mildly spoken—topical in the seventies. The combination of pure peptides, new hormones, specific antibodies, and sensitive radioimmunoassays opened endless gates for biochemical, clinical, histological, pharmacological, and physiological studies. Also, it was not difficult to publish gut hormone and brain-gut papers in high-impact journals. In the early seventies, gastrin was the gut hormone of choice that attracted most interest. It was, therefore, a timely effort of Jim Thompson to organize a symposium on gastrointestinal hormones in October 1974 (28) with emphasis on the growing number of gastrins. Two days before the symposium opened in Texas, some of us met informally with John and Mort in Los Angeles to discuss the state of affairs. The guest of honor was Rod Gregory, who was going to present the sequence of "big"- and "mini"-gastrins in Galveston, but several other gastrin news would also be presented. In Los Angeles we agreed that a foreseeable problem would be "big big"-gastrin, which Ros Yalow then reported to be the predominant gastrin in normal plasma of man, pig and dog (27, 29, 30). In other words, "big big"-gastrin was according to Yalow now *the* gastrin.

The problem was difficult. On one hand "big big"-gastrin looked more and more like a simple chromatographic artifact caused by interference in the antigen-antibody binding of radioimmunoassays by plasma proteins concentrated in the void volume of Sephadex G-50 columns. On the other hand, it is not easy to prove non-existence from neither a practical nor a theoretical point of view. Moreover, Ros Yalow was an international celebrity due to her and Sol Berson's invention of the radioimmunoassay technique, and accordingly, she was an expert on radioimmunoassays. We also knew that she was on the shortlist for a Nobel prize.

To complicate the matter further, after Berson's death in 1972 she had published some strange papers on "big big"-hormones ("big big"-ACTH, "big big"-insulin, "big big"-glucagon, and now "big big"-gastrin). And she was known to be sensitive to criticism, in particular when her use of radioimmunoassays was questioned. Now we knew that Rod Gregory would give the first presentation in the gastrin session at Jim Thompson's symposium, followed by Ros Yalow on "big big"-gastrin, and then I should present some evidence for the artifactual nature of "big big"-gastrin. As we sat in Mort's office and discussed the plan for the debate in Texas in the name of sound science, Mort's secretary suddenly announced that Ros Yalow unexpectedly had arrived to meet Mort and John. An angel walked through the room, and the meeting stopped.

GALVESTON, October 1974

Jim Thompson's symposium was very well organized and scientifically on the cutting edge. I recall it as one of the best and most important symposia I have attended. The proceedings are still a useful textbook (28). As predicted, however, the gastrin session turned after Rod's shining opening with the publication of the gastrin-34 sequence into a tough battle about "big big"-gastrin.

Ros Yalow stood up in anger and protested violently when Mort, Norman Track and I questioned the nature of "big big"-gastrin. The chairman, Jim Thompson, could hardly control the discussion, and soon after Yalow left the symposium. As apparent in the proceedings (28), Ros Yalow is the only speaker not present on the photo. After the dramatic overture, the symposium continued in a quiet and friendly atmosphere. By the end of the meeting, however, John, Graham Dockray, and I agreed that it would be expedient to have the gastrin laboratories in Los Angeles, Liverpool and Copenhagen independently study the "big big"-phenomenon, and then to have the results published simultaneously in order to settle the issue.

Back in Copenhagen with samples from Flemming Stadil and with Thue Schwartz' green fingers doing immunosorption, we had after almost a year, results that provided solid evidence that "big big"-gastrin indeed was a reproducible chromatographic artifact. I sent the manuscript to John, but neither he nor Graham wanted—after further thought—to join the "big big" showdown. Perhaps John found it inappropriate to challenge his former supervisor. And perhaps it was difficult to have Ros Yalow as an antagonist living in the States. So as a lonely cowboy I submitted the manuscript to Gastroenterology. Ros Yalow was the reviewer, and tried to shoot it down with endless protests and invectives. She called it "the worst pontifical verbiage" she had ever seen. She managed to delay publication for one and a half years. But in 1977, the paper was eventually published (31) just before the announcement that the Nobel prize in medicine and physiology that year would go to Roger Guillemin, Andrew Schally and—Rosalyn Yalow.

The paper, nevertheless, contributed to end the debate about "big big"-gastrin and other "big big"-hormone phenomena. And with the cloning of gastrin cDNA a few years later (32, 33) it became obvious that the gastrin gene could not encode a protein of a size proposed for "big big"-gastrin (Figure 2). The largest possible gastrin would be gastrin-71, the previous component I (Ref. 21, Figures 1 and 2).

AARHUS, August 1978

Gastrin has an unusually well defined and well studied active site (34, 35), the tetrapeptide amide (-Trp-Met-Asp-Phe-NH_2) common for the C-terminus of all bioactive gastrins (Figures 1 and 2). Therefore, when Rod Gregory reported that antral extracts contained a tridecapeptide corresponding to the N-terminal sequence of gastrin-17, both he, Hilda Tracy and others thought that perhaps the antral G-cells also produced the complementary C-terminal tetrapeptide amide (for review, see ref. 36). The idea gained support when John and Graham Dockray developed a radioimmunoassay specific for the N-terminal sequence of gastrin-17, and showed that a peptide corresponding to the N-terminal fragment of gastrin-17 circulated in human plasma (37).

Simultaneously with the interest in the molecular nature of gastrin, I also wanted to study cholecystokinin (CCK), the other member of the gastrin family. The homologous C-terminus of the two hormones was, however, a major obstacle for the production of CCK-specific antibodies (for review, see refs. 38 and 39). So in the effort to develop a CCK radioimmunoassay, a number of cross reacting antisera specific for the common C-terminal tetrapeptide epitope was inevitably raised (40, 41). Using such antisera we saw that CCK and gastrin producing tissues, in addition, to known CCK and gastrin peptides contained a short peptide, which by chromatography eluted like the common C-terminal tetrapeptide amide. As reported first at the gastrin symposium in Aarhus (42) we believed initially, with reference to the

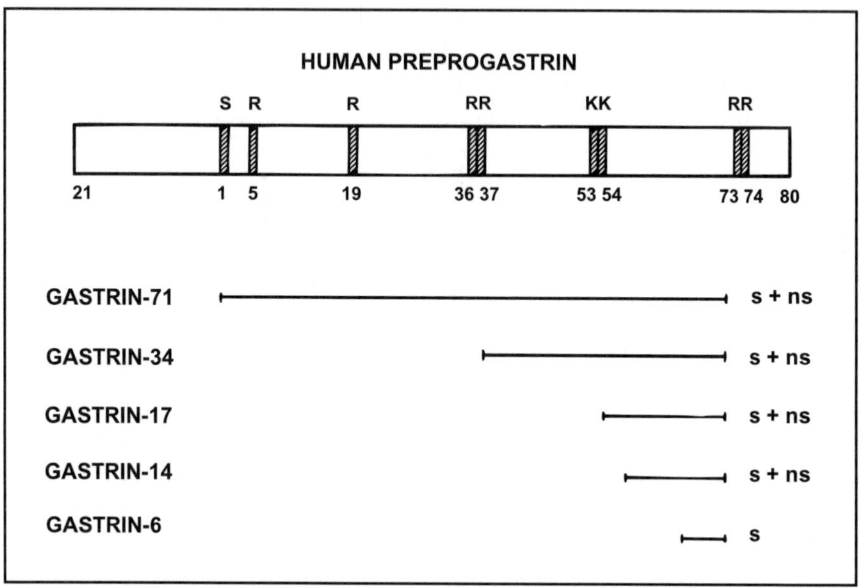

FIGURE 2. *Schematic presentation of structurally identified carboxyamidated products of human preprogastrin. The cleavage sites at basic amino acid residues (R and K) are indicated on preprogastrin. s and ns mean "sulfated" and "non-sulfated."*

complementary 1–13 fragment of gastrin-17 identified in Liverpool (36, 37), that we had found the long sought tetrapeptide in substantial amounts (43, 44). But the final structure identifications showed that the small peak from brain and intestinal extracts was mainly CCK-5, the C-terminal tetrapeptide amide equipped with a glycyl residue at the N-terminus (45, 46), whereas antral extracts contained mainly a tyrosyl-sulfated hexapeptide (47, 48). But trace amounts of the free tetrapeptide amide were nevertheless present in all the tissues examined. The chemical identification of the small peptides terminated a long debate with Graham Dockray, and settled the number and structure of bioactive gastrins as shown in Figure 2. John never revealed his position in this debate to me. He could be rather diplomatic.

AFTERWORD

In parallel with the research on the molecular structure and biology of gastrin peptides in the seventies, John and I broadened our interests to related fields after some years. John and his coworkers studied the regulation of gastric acid secretion in a wide physiological and clinical context. He also got involved with several new gut hormones and their neurotransmitter function, whereas I tried to stick to CCK peptides in the brain and elsewhere.

In the eighties and nineties our ways separated even more, although we still would meet at gut peptide symposia all over the world. It was always a pleasure to see John. I enjoyed his friendly companionship and our talks between the scientific sessions of the meetings, where John would drop the reserved and formal sides of his character to become open and close—also about the personal and social aspects of our occasionally turbulent lives (Figure 3).

I guess that we—in spite of sporadic competitive projects—were tied together of a feeling, that we and a few other contemporaries were pioneers in a development, that changed gut endocrinology from a narrow physiological discipline to an area of broad interest for clinical gastroenterologists, diabetologists, neuro- and molecular biologists. The starting platform for both of us were the highly specific antibodies that we developed for sensitive radioimmunoassays.

In the development that began in the late nineteen sixties, we always knew that we stood on the shoulders of older impressive pioneers like Solomon Berson, Roderick Gregory, Morton Grossman, Erik Jorpes, Viktor Mutt, and Rosalyn Yalow. We also knew that we would have to pass on the torch to the next generation in due course. Sad that John died too early to watch what the new generation does to gut endocrinology in the name of molecular and cell biology in the beginning of this millennium. He would have enjoyed it!

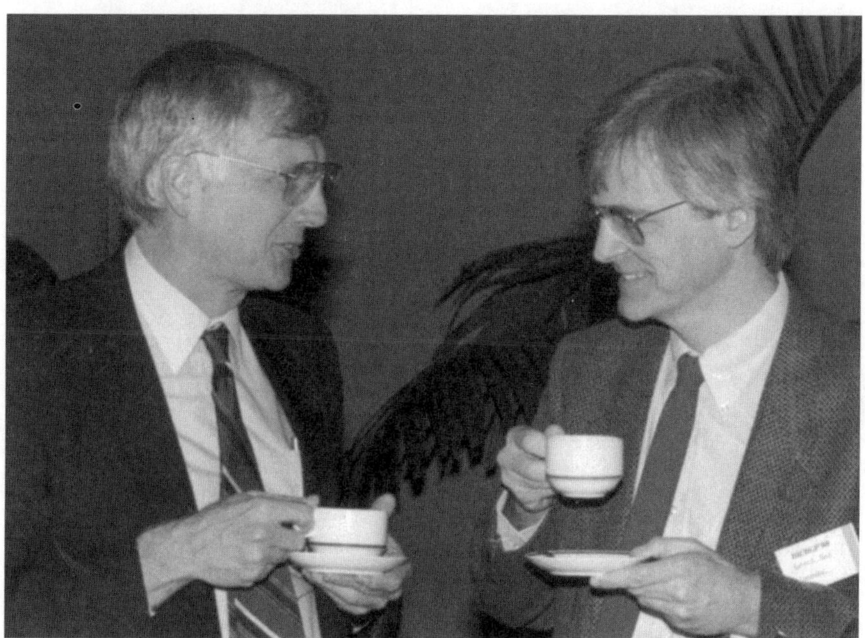

John and I in a coffee break during an international gut hormone symposium in Beijing, China, in November 1988.

REFERENCES

1. Gregory RA, Tracy HJ. The constitution and properties of two gastrins extracted from hog antral mucosa. *Gut* 1964;5:103–17.

2. McGuigan JE. Immunochemical studies with synthetic human gastrin. *Gastroenterology* 1968;54:1005–11.

3. Hansky J, Cain MD. Radioimmunoassay of gastrin in human serum. *Lancet* 1969;2:1388–90.

4. Yalow RS, Berson SA. Radioimmunoassay of gastrin. *Gastroenterology* 1970; 58: 1–14.

5. McGuigan JE, Trudeau WL. Studies with antibodies to gastrin: Radioimmunoassay in human serum and physiological studies. *Gastroenterology* 1970; 58:139–50.

6. Rehfeld JF, Stadil F, Rubin B. Production and evaluation of antibodies for the radioimmunoassay of gastrin. *Scand J Clin Lab Invest* 1972; 30:221–32.

7. Stadil F, Rehfeld JF. Preparation of ^{125}I-labelled synthetic human gastrin for radioimmunoanalysis. *Scand J Clin Lab Invest* 1972; 30:361–8.

8. Laster L, Walsh JH. Enzymatic degradation of C-terminal tetrapeptide amide of gastrin by mammalian tissue extracts. *Fed Proc* 1968;27:1328–30.

9. Walsh JH, Yalow RS, Berson SA. Detection of Australia antigen antibody by means of radioimmunoassay technique. *J Infect Dis* 1970;121:550–4.

10. Walsh JH, Debas HT, Grossman MI. Pure human big gastrin. Immunochemical properties, disappearance halftime, and acid-stimulating action in dogs. *J Clin Invest* 1974; 54:477–85.

11. Debas HT, Walsh JH, Grossman MI. Pure human minigastrin: secretory potency, and disappearance rate. *Gut* 1974; 15:686–9.

12. Walsh JH, Isenberg JI, Ansfield J, Maxwell V. Clearance and acid-stimulating action of human big and little gastrins in duodenal ulcer subjects. *J Clin Invest* 1976;57:1125–31.

13. Yalow RS, Berson SA. Size and charge distinctions between endogenous human plasma gastrin in peripheral blood and heptadecapeptide gastrins. *Gastroenterology* 1970;58:609–15.

14. Gregory RA, Tracy HJ. Isolation of two "big gastrins" from Zollinger-Ellison tumor tissue. *Lancet* 1972;2:797–9.

15. Steiner DF, Oyer PE. The biosynthesis of insulin and probable precursor of insulin by a human islet cell carcinoma. *Proc Natl Acad Sci USA* 1967;57:473–80.

16. Sherman BM, Gorden P, Roth J, Freychet P. Circulating insulin: the proinsulin-like properties of "big" insulin in patients without islet cell tumors. *J Clin Invest* 1971;50:849–58.

17. Rehfeld JF. Three components of gastrin in human serum: Gel filtration studies on the molecular size of immunoreactive gastrin in serum. *Biochim Biophys Acta* 1972; 285:364–72.

18. Walsh JH, Grossman MI. Gastrin. *N Engl J Med* 1975;292:1324–32.

19. Rehfeld JF, Stadil F. Gel filtration studies on immunoreactive gastrin in serum from Zollinger-Ellison patients. *Gut* 1973;14:369–73.

20. Gregory RA, Tracy HJ. Isolation of two minigastrins from Zollinger-Ellison tumor tissue. *Gut* 1974; 15:683–5.

21. Rehfeld JF, Johnsen AH. Identification of gastrin component I as gastrin-71, the largest possible bioactive progastrin product. *Eur J Biochem* 1994;223:765–73.

22. Gregory RA, Tracy HJ, Harris JI, Runswick MJ, Moore S, Kenner GW, Ramage R. Minigastrin, corrected structure and synthesis. *Hoppe-Seylers Z Physiol Chem* 1979;360:73–80.

23. Yalow RS, Berson SA. And now "big big" gastrin. *Biochem Biophys Res Comm* 1972;48:391–5.

24. Rehfeld JF, Stadil F. "Big gastrins" in the Zollinger-Ellison syndrome. *Lancet* 1972;2:1200.

25. Rehfeld JF, Stadil F, Vikelsöe J. Immunoreactive gastrin components in human serum. *Gut* 1974; 15:102–11.

26. Bundgaard JR, Vuust J, Rehfeld JF. Tyrosine O-sulfation promotes the proteolytic processing of progastrin. *EMBO J* 1995;14:3073–9.

27. Yalow RS, Wu N. Additional studies on the nature of "big big" gastrin. *Gastroenterology* 1973; 65:19–27.

28. Thompson JC, Ed. *Gastrointestinal Hormones.* Austin & London: University of Texas Press, 1975.

29. Straus E, Yalow RS. Studies on the distribution and degradation of heptadecapeptide, "big" and "big big" gastrin. *Gastroenterology* 1974;66:936–43.

30. Yalow RS. Heterogeneity of peptide hormones with relation to gastrin. In *Gastrointestinal Hormones* (Thompson JC, Ed.). Austin & London: University of Texas Press, 1975, pp. 25–41.

31. Rehfeld JF, Schwartz TW, Stadil F. Immunochemical studies on macromolecular gastrins: Evidence that "big big" gastrins in blood and mucosa are artifacts. *Gastroenterology* 1977;73:469–77.

32. Yoo OH, Powell CT, Agarwal KL. Molecular cloning and nucleotide sequence of full-length cDNA coding for porcine gastrin. *Proc Natl Acad Sci USA* 1982;79:1049–53.

33. Boel E, Vuust J, Norris F, Norris K. Wind A, Rehfeld JF, Marcker KA. Molecular cloning of human gastrin cDNA: Evidence for evolution of gastrin by gene duplication. *Proc Natl Acad Sci USA* 1983; 80:2866–9.

34. Tracy HJ, Gregory RA. Physiological properties of a series of synthetic peptides structurally related to gastrin. *Nature* 1964;204:931–3.

35. Morley JS, Tracy HJ, Gregory RA. Structure-function relationships in the active C-terminal tetrapeptide sequence of gastrin. *Nature* 1965;207:1356–9.

36. Gregory RA. Some aspects of the structure of gastrin and gastrin-like forms and fragments in gut and brain. In *Gastrins and the Vagus* (Rehfeld JF, Amdrup E, Eds.). London, New York, San Francisco: Academic Press, 1979; pp.47–55.

37. Dockray GJ, Walsh JH. Aminoterminal gastrin fragment in serum of Zollinger-Ellison syndrome patients. *Gastroenterology* 1975;68:222–30.

38. Rehfeld JF. How to measure cholecystokinin in plasma? *Gastroenterology* 1984;87:34–8.

39. Rehfeld JF. How to measure cholecystokinin in tissue, plasma and cerebrospinal fluid? *Regul Pept* 1998;78:31–9.

40. Rehfeld JF. Immunochemical studies on cholecystokinin. I. Development of sequence-specific radioimmunoassays for porcine triacontatriapeptide cholecystokinin. *J Biol Chem* 1978;253:4016–21.

41. Rehfeld JF. Accurate measurement of cholecystokinin in plasma. *Clin Chem* 1998;44:991–1001.

42. Rehfeld JF, Amdrup E, Eds. *Gastrins and the Vagus.* London, New York, San Francisco: Academic Press, 1979.

43. Rehfeld JF, Larsson LI. The predominating molacular form of gastrin and cholecystokinin in the gut is a small peptide corresponding to the C-terminal tetrapeptide amide. *Acta Physiol Scand* 1979; 105:117–9.

44. Rehfeld JF, Goltermann N. Immunochemical evidence of cholecystokinin tetrapeptides in hog brain. *J Neurochem* 1979;32:1339–41.

45. Rehfeld JF, Hansen HF. Characterization of procholecystokinin products in the porcine cerebral cortex: Evidence of different processing pathways. *J Biol Chem* 1986;261:5832–40.

46. Shively J, Reeve JR, Eysselein VE, Ben-Avram CN, Vigna SR, Walsh JH. CCK–5: sequence analysis of a small cholecystokinin from canine brain and intestine. *Amer J Physiol* 1987;252:G272–5.

47. Gregory RA, Dockray GJ, Reeve JR, Shively J, Miller C. Isolation from porcine antral mucosa of a hexapeptide corresponding to the C-terminal sequence of gastrin. *Peptides* 1983;4:319–23.

48. Rehfeld JF, Hansen CP, Johnsen AH. Post-poly(Glu) cleavage and degradation modified by O-sulfated tyrosine: A novel posttranslational processing mechanism. *EMBO J* 1995;14:389–96.

Gut-Brain Peptides in the New Millennium, edited by Y. Taché
CURE Foundation, Los Angeles, CA. © 2002

2

The Gastrins: Their Identities and Functions as Gastric Paracrine Organizers

Graham J. Dockray
Department of Physiology, University of Liverpool, Liverpool, UK

INTRODUCTION

Following the isolation and chemical characterization of the heptadecapeptide gastrins (G17) by Gregory and Tracy in the 1960s (1), it became clear that other active gastrins could be identified by bioassay of tissue extracts, or by radioimmunoassay of plasma after separation by gel filtration. Subsequently, Gregory and Tracy isolated the 34-amino acid residue big gastrins, or G34 (2). These shared the primary sequence of G17 at their C-terminus and like G17 existed in tyrosine-sulfated and unsulfated forms. By the mid-1970s it had become important to know the biosynthetic, metabolic and biological relationships of different gastrins. John Walsh had already made seminal observations on gastrin-degrading enzymes in tissue extracts (3). He then showed G17 was cleared about 5-times more rapidly than G34 in both man and dog; interestingly, similar plasma concentrations of G17 and G34 produced similar rates of gastric acid secretion (4–6). It seemed then, that secretion of G34 would lead to proportionately higher and more prolonged increases in plasma concentrations compared to the release of corresponding amounts of G17. The relevant control mechanisms are interesting because G34 predominates in plasma after a meal in normal subjects although it makes only a modest contribution to the gastrin stores in the G-cell. G34 is also the main form in the plasma of hypergastrinemia subjects (7, 8). Recent studies in genetically modified mice have raised two other general issues regarding the biology of the gastrins. First, it seems that in addition to their effects on acid secretion, amidated gastrins such as G17 and G34 may also influence the organization of the gastric mucosa (9). Second, products of *gastrin* gene other than the amidated gastrins may exert their own biological activities (10–12). In particular some precursor peptides appear to be growth factors. The present chapter focuses on mechanisms that determine the production of different gastrins, and possible downstream mediators by which the amidated gastrins may influence epithelial organization.

Gastrin Processing

The *gastrin* gene encodes a precursor peptide which, depending on the species, consists of 101 (man) or 104 (rat) residues. There is a single copy of the primary sequence of G34. The antibodies first used in gastrin radioimmunoassay showed high specificity for the amidated COOH-terminal sequence of G17. These antibodies typically reacted with G34 (due to the shared sequence) but did not react with biosynthetic intermediates or precursors that lack the COOH-terminal amide, or were extended beyond it. For the most part such antibodies also exhibit low affinity for the structurally related cholecystokinin group of peptides. In the early 1970s Walsh found it was possible to generate gastrin-specific antibodies which did not require the COOH-terminal amide group, and which identified novel naturally occurring peptides (13). In the following years, his group and many others then raised antibodies to different parts of progastrin and used these to assay various biosynthetic intermediates (14–17). This approach has provided valuable insight into the identity of different progastrin-derived peptides, although it does not provide rigorous evidence of the kinetic relationships between them. For the latter purpose it is necessary to carry out pulse-chase labelling studies with HPLC separation of the labelled products (18, 19).

Direct studies of gastrin biosynthesis using pulse-chase labeling, immunoprecipitation of labeled peptides by panels of antibodies reacting with all major precursors, intermediates and products, together with on-line scintillation counting after HPLC, have provided a powerful approach to dissect biosynthetic mechanisms (18). This type of approach coupled with electron microscopic immunogold localization of different peptides has also allowed identification of the sub-cellular sites of post-translational processing of progastrin. The data indicate that the signal peptide is rapidly removed from preprogastrin at the endoplasmic reticulum; thereafter, progastrin moves through the Golgi complex to the *trans*Golgi network (TGN) where it is phosphorylated and sulfated (18). In endocrine cells, progastrin is then sequestered in secretory vesicles following which there is relatively rapid cleavage at two pairs of Arg residues. Prior phosphorylation of Ser at position 96 may delay cleavage at one of these sites (Arg-94-95) (20). Carboxypeptidase removal of COOH-terminal basic residues from the products of cleavage yields G34 extended at the COOH-terminus by Gly (ie G34-Gly). The latter yields G34 through the action of peptidyl α-amidating mono-oxygenase. Both G34 and G34-Gly may be cleaved at a pair of Lys residues generating G17 and G17Gly, respectively (19). (Figure 1)

Cleavage of G34 and G34-Gly at Lys-57-58 is critically dependent on secretory vesicle pH. Studies using a pH sensitive form of green fluorescent

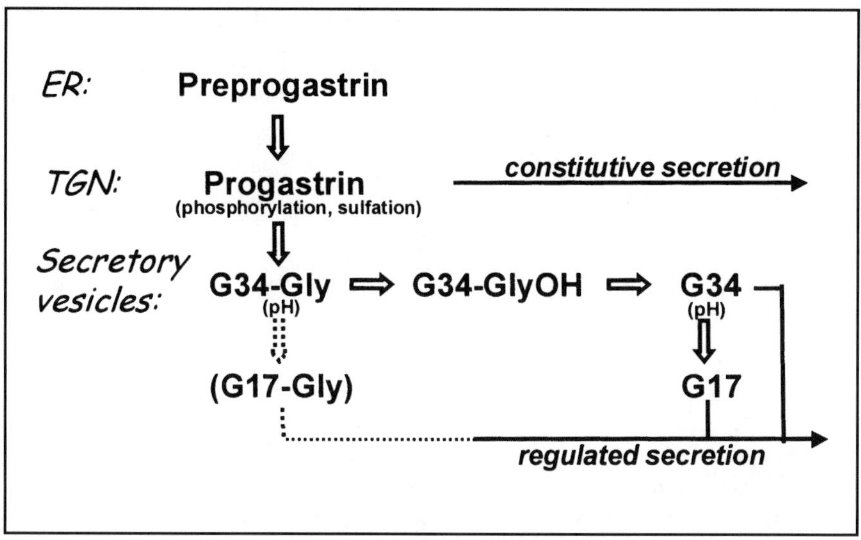

FIGURE 1. *Schematic representation of preprogastrin processing pathways showing the major biosynthetic intermediates and products secreted via the constitutive or regulated routes of exocytosis. Possible control mechanisms are indicated in parentheses; the relevant sub-cellular compartment is shown to the left, and common variations between species are shown broken lines. ER, endoplasmic reticulum, TGN, tran-Golgi network, see text for description of different forms of gastrin.*

protein (GFP) targeted to secretory vesicles in a hamster insulinoma cell line (HIT cells) reveal a pH of about 5.5 (21). It has long been known that endocrine cell secretory vesicles also store biogenic amines. This capacity depends on the activity of the vesicular monoamine transporters, VMAT1 or VMAT2, which act as proton-amine exchangers in concentrating biogenic amines in secretory vesicules. Expression of VMAT2 in HIT cells raises secretory vesicle pH to 6.5, and inhibits cleavage of G34. The VMAT inhibitor reserpine, lowers secretory vesicle pH and increases rates of G34 cleavage. In normal rat G-cells, reserpine slightly increased rates of G34 cleavage suggesting that amine transport activity is physiologically modulated, and providing a way to regulate G34:G17 ratios (21).

Over the last few years, there has been growing interest in the expression of the *gastrin* gene in non-endocrine cells, and in particular in colon cancer cells (22–24). These cells lack secretory vesicles of the so-called regulated pathway of secretion. As a consequence, progastrin is largely secreted by the constitutive route, i.e., from TGN to cell surface. This occurs in colorectal cancer cells, and in transgenic mice expressing the gene in liver (12). It seems that both progastrin, and the Gly-gastrins are growth factors for the colon (12). In addition, the Gly-gastrins may potentiate the effects of amidated gastrins on gastric epithelial maturation (10, 25–27).

Gastric Acid and Control of G-cell Function

Modern views of the way that gastric acid inhibits gastrin release are based on careful quantitative studies by Walsh and colleagues in the 1970s (28, 29). Release of somatostatin from D-cells mediates the inhibitory effects of acid on G-cell secretion. In *H. pylori* infected individuals, antral D-cell function is depressed, and G-cell function is accordingly upregulated, suggesting a basis for the moderate hypergastrinemia that may be found in these subjects (30).

It appears that gastric acid also controls many other aspects of G-cell function, including G-cell abundance and gastrin synthesis (31–33). Thus, studies in rats in which acid-inhibition of the G-cell has been removed by administration of the $H^+/K^+ATPase$ inhibitor omeprazole, exhibit increased gastrin mRNA abundance due to increased transcription (29, 34). In addition, there are increased rates of progastrin mRNA translation; these are not just secondary to increased mRNA abundance, because they occur before changes in gastrin mRNA (31). There are also increased rates of G34 cleavage (32), and increased abundance of the mRNA species encoding the prohormone convertases PC1/3 and PC2 (35). Taken together these data emphasise the integrated nature of G-cell responses to gastric acid. It is not yet clear that all these responses are attributable to somatostatin, but it would not be surprising if they were.

Paracrine Networks in the Corpus

Enterochromaffin-like (ECL) cells

Gastrin acts at gastrin-CCK_B receptors on ECL cells to release histamine which stimulates acid secretion. In addition, there are increased ECL cell numbers in hypergastrinemic rats and patients (36, 37), and stimulation of the expression of several genes required for histamine synthesis and secretion (see Chapter by Dimaline).

Recent studies indicate, gastrin also increases expression of regenerating gene (Reg), Reg1α in rat ECL cells and in the AR4-2J cell line (38, 39) (Figure 2). There is increased Reg1α in gastric biopsies of hypergastrinemic patients which is probably attributable to expression in both ECL and chief cells. Mutations of Reg1α that prevent the secretion of peptide (due to loss of signal peptide function) are associated with ECL cell tumors in hypergastrinemic patients (39). This suggests that Reg might normally play a restraining role in ECL cell proliferation. At first sight this is difficult to link to evidence that Reg is a growth factor (38). Interestingly, however, recent studies have identified a putative receptor (EXTL3); it appears that Reg acts via EXTL3 to increase proliferation at relatively low concentrations, but at high concentrations it produces apoptosis (40). The latter observation would be compatible with a role for Reg1α in limiting ECL cell numbers, since there are presumably high concentrations locally in the vicinity of ECL cells (Figure 2).

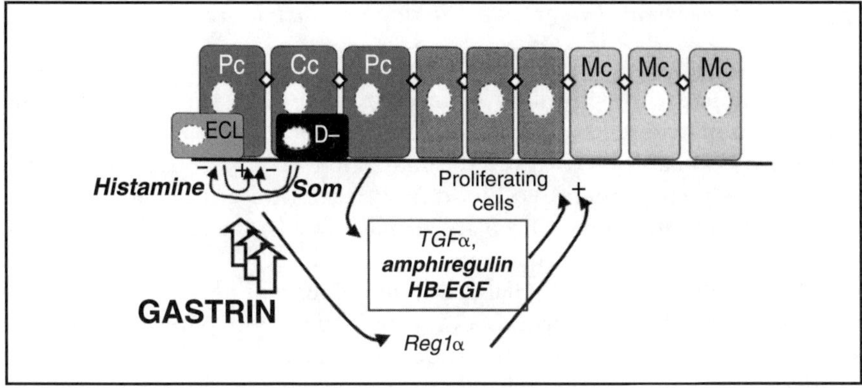

FIGURE 2. *Schematic representation of different paracrine mediators of gastrin in the gastric corpus. Gastrin stimulates histamine release from enterochromaffin like (ECL) cells, Reg1α from ECL and chief cells (Cc), somatostatin from D-cells, and transforming growth factor-α (TGFα), amiphiregulin and heparin binding epidermal growth factor (HB-EGF) from parietal cells (Pc). Histamine stimulates acid secretion, somatostatin inhibits it, and TGFα, aphiregulin and HB-EGF stimulate proliferation; so does Reg1α, although it may also stimulate apoptosis in high concentrations. Mucus cells (MC) of the neck and surface do not normally respond to gastrin, but may be targets for paracrine mediators.*

Parietal Cells

It is well established that parietal cells express the gastrin-CCK$_B$ receptor, but the physiological significance of this is less clear given the importance ascribed to release of histamine in gastrin-stimulated acid secretion. One possibility is that gastrin directly acts on parietal cells to control activities other than acid secretion. In this context it is interesting to note that gastrin-CCK$_B$ receptor stimulation increases production of transforming growth factor (TGF)α, amphiregulin and heparin binding (HB)-epithelial growth factor (EGF) (9) (Figure 2). In addition, stimulation of this receptor, like others coupled to G$\alpha_{q/11}$, increases shedding of the membrane bound precursor of these growth factors via proteolysis to liberate their extracellular domains (41, 42). EGF-family peptides act on parietal cells to either stimulate or inhibit acid secretion (depending on the duration and experimental model) (43). These peptides are also plausible mediators of the proliferative effects of gastrin. The increase in proliferation in response to gastrin is well known (44), but expression of the gastrin-CCK$_B$ receptor by proliferating cells has been controversial. In a cell model, we recently co-cultured AGS-cells expressing the gastrin-CCK$_B$ receptor, with cells not expressing the receptor but labelled by stable expression of green flourescent protein (GFP) (42). In this model, gastrin inhibits proliferation of the cells expressing the receptor (analogous to parietal cells), but stimulates proliferation of cells not expressing the receptor through release of HB-EGF which in turn acts via EGF receptor and activation of MAPkinase pathways.

Overview: Integrative Biology of Gastrin-regulated Paracrine Networks

The maintenance of a healthy stomach requires a balance between the stimulation of acid secretion i.e., an aggressive force, and the stimulation of protective mechanisms to resist the damaging effects of acid. Protective mechanisms include increased blood flow, inhibition of acid secretion, increased cell proliferation (to replace damaged cells), increased cell migration to cover damaged areas, and increased secretion of mucus and bicarbonate by surface epithelial cells. One emerging idea is that the multiple products of progastrin processing by acting both directly and indirectly through activation of paracrine networks together balance aggressive and protective mechanisms. For example, it is thought that the Gly-Gastrins potentiate amidated gastrins in stimulating acid secretion (26). However, the Gly-extended gastrins also stimulate gastric epithelial cell migration which is protective (27). Similarly, the amidated gastrins stimulate acid secretion, histamine secretion and histamine synthesis: all of which are aggressive. But they also increase somatostatin release, as well as production and release of members of the EGF family which are generally protective. The extent to which disruption of the balance between aggressive and defensive actions contributes to gastrointestinal pathology now needs to be determined.

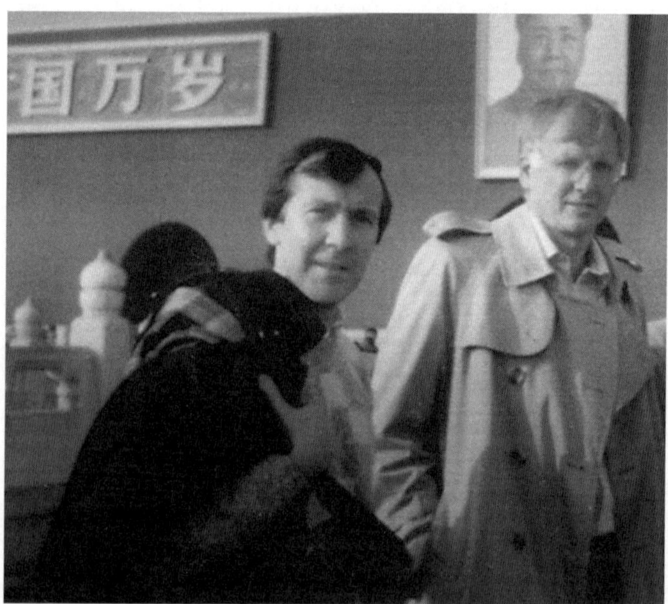

Drs. Graham Dockray and John Walsh in Beijing, 1988.

REFERENCES

1. Gregory RA, Tracy HJ. The constitution and properties of two gastrins extracted from hog antral mucosa. *Gut* 1964;5:103–14.
2. Gregory RA, Tracy HJ. Isolation of two "big gastrins" from Zollinger-Ellison tumor tissue. *Lancet* 1972;2:797–9.
3. Laster L, Walsh JH. Enzymatic degradation of C-terminal tetrapeptide amide of gastrin by mammalian tissue extracts. *Fed Proc* 1968;27:1328–30.
4. Walsh JH, Debas HT, Grossman MI. Pure human big gastrin: immunochemical properties, disappearance half time and acid stimulating action in dogs. *J Clin Invest* 1974;54:477–85.
5. Walsh JH, Isenberg JI, Ansfield J, Maxwell V. Clearance and acid-stimulating action of human big and little gastrins in duodenal ulcer subjects. *J Clin Invest* 1976;57:1125–31.
6. Eysselein VE, Maxwell V, Reedy TJ, Wunsch E, Walsh JH. Similar acid stimulatory potencies of synthetic human big and little gastrins in man. *J Clin Invest* 1984;73:1284–90.
7. Dockray GJ, Taylor IL. Heptadecapeptide gastrin: measurement in blood by specific radioimmunoassay. *Gastroenterology* 1976;71:971–7.
8. Dockray GJ, Varro A, Dimaline R, Wang TC. The gastrins: their production and biological activities. *Ann Rev Physiol* 2001;63:119–39.
9. Wang TC, Dangler CA, Chen D, Goldenring JR, Koh TJ, Raychowdhury R, Coffey RJ, Ito S, Varro A, Dockray GJ, Fox JG. Synergistic interaction between hypergastrinemia and *Helicobacter* infection in a mouse model of gastric cancer. *Gastroenterology* 2000;118:36–47.
10. Seva C, Dickinson CJ, Yamada T. Growth-promoting effects of glycine-extended progastrin. *Science* 1994;265:410–2.
11. Singh P, Owlia A, Varro A, Dai B, Rajaraman S, Wood T. Gastrin gene expression is required for the proliferation and tumorigenicity of human colon cancer cells. *Cancer Research* 1996;56:4111–5.
12. Wang TC, Koh TJ, Varro A, Cahill RJ, Dangler CA, Fox JG, Dockray GJ. Processing and proliferative effects of human progastrin in transgenic mice. *J Clin Invest* 1996;98:1918–29.
13. Dockray GJ, Walsh JH. Amino terminal gastrin fragment in serum of Zollinger-Ellison syndrome patients. *Gastroenterology* 1975;68:222–30.
14. Sugano K, Aponte GW, Yamada T. Identification and characterization of glycine-extended post-translational processing intermediates of progastrin in porcine stomach. *J Biol Chem* 1985;260:11724–9.
15. Pauwels S, Desmond H, Dimaline R, Dockray GJ. Identification of progastrin in gastrinomas, antrum, and duodenum by a novel radioimmunoassay. *J Clin Invest* 1986;77:376–81.
16. Azuma T, Taggart RT, Walsh JH. Effects of bombesin on the release of glycine-extended progastrin (gastrin G) in rat antral tissue culture. *Gastroenterology* 1987;93:322–9.
17. Rehfeld JF, Johnsen AH. Identification of gastrin component I as gastrin-71. The largest possible bioactive progastrin product. *Eur J Biochem* 1994;223:765–73.
18. Varro A, Henry J, Vaillant C, Dockray GJ. Discrimination between temperature- and brefeldin A-sensitive steps in the sulfation, phosphorylation, and cleavage of progastrin and its derivatives. *J Biol Chem* 1994;269:20764–70.
19. Varro A, Voronina S, Dockray GJ. Pathways of processing of the gastrin precursor in rat antral mucosa. *J Clin Invest* 1995;95:1642–9.
20. Bishop L, Dimaline R, Blackmore C, Deavall D, Dockray GJ, Varro A. Modulation of the cleavage of the gastrin precursor by phosphorylation. *Gastroenterology* 1998;115:1154–62.
21. Blackmore CG, Varro A, Dimaline R, Bishop L, Gallacher DV, Dockray GJ. Measurement of secretory vesicle pH reveals intravesicular alkalinization by vesicular monoamine transporter type 2 resulting in inhibition of prohormone cleavage. *J Physiol* 2001;531:605–17.
22. Nemeth J, Taylor B, Pauwels S, Varro A, Dockray GJ. Identification of progastrin derived peptides in colorectal carcinoma extracts. *Gut* 1993;34:90–5.
23. Kochman ML, Delvalle J, Dickinson CJ, Boland CR. Post-translational processing of gastrin in neoplastic human colonic tissue. *Biochem Biophys Res Comm* 1992;189:1165–9.
24. Ciccotosto GD, McLeish A, Hardy KJ, Shulkes A. Expression, processing, and secretion of gastrin in patients with colorectal carcinoma. *Gastroenterology* 1995;109:1142–53.

25. Koh TJ, Dockray GJ, Varro A, Cahill RJ, Dangler CA, Fox JG, Wang TC. Overexpression of glycine-extended gastrin in transgenic mice results in increased colonic proliferation. *J Clin Invest* 1999;103:1119–26.

26. Chen D, Zhao CM, Dockray GJ, Varro A, Van Hoek A, Sinclair NF, Wang TC, Koh TJ. Glycine-extended gastrin synergizes with gastrin 17 to stimulate acid secretion in gastrin-deficient mice. *Gastroenterology* 2000;119:756–65.

27. Hollande F, Choquet A, Blanc EM, Lee DJ, Bali JP, Baldwin GS. Involvement of phosphatidylinositol 3-Kinase and mitogen-activated protein kinases in glycine-extended gastrin-induced dissociation and migration of gastric epithelial cells. *J Biol Chem* 2001;276:40402–10.

28. Walsh JH, Richardson CT, Fordtran JS. pH Dependence of acid secretion and gastrin release in normal and ulcer subjects. *J Clin Invest* 1975;55:462–8.

29. Wu SV, Giraud A, Mogard M, Sunii K, Walsh JH. Effects of inhibition of gastric secretion on antral gastrin and somatostatin gene expression in rats. *Am J Physiol* 1990;258:G788–G793.

30. Moss SF, Legon S, Bishop AE, Polak JM, Calam J. Effect of Helicobacter pylori on gastric somatostatin in duodenal ulcer disease. *Lancet* 1992;340:930–2.

31. Bate GW, Varro A, Dimaline R, Dockray GJ. Control of preprogastrin messenger RNA translation by gastric acid in the rat. *Gastroenterology* 1996;111:1224–9.

32. Macro JA, Bate GW, Varro A, Vaillant C, Seidah NG, Dimaline R, Dockray GJ. Regulation by gastric acid of the processing of progastrin- derived peptides in rat antral mucosa. *J Physiol* 1997;502:409–19.

33. Dockray GJ, Dimaline R, Forster ER, Evans D, Sandvik AK, Varro A. Gastrin cell responses to acidification of the achlorhydric rat stomach. *Am J Physiol* 1993;265:G440–G444.

34. Dimaline R, Evans D, Varro A, Dockray GJ. Reversal by omeprazole of the depression of gastrin cell function by fasting in the rat. *J Physiol* 1991;433:483–93.

35. Macro JA, Dimaline R, Dockray GJ. Identification and expression of prohormone-converting enzymes in the rat stomach. *Am J Physiol* 1996;279:G87–G93.

36. Larsson H, Carlsson E, Mattsson H, Lundell L, Sundler F, Sundell G, Wallmark B, Watanabe T, Hakanson R. Plasma gastrin and gastric enterochromaffinlike cell activation and proliferation: studies with omeprazole and randitidine in intact and antrectomized rats. *Gastroenterology* 1986;90:391–9.

37. Bordi C, D'Adda T, Azzoni C, Pilato FP, Carbuana P. Hypergastrinemia and gastric enterochromaffin-like cells. *Am J Surg Path* 1995;19:S8–S19.

38. Fukui H, Kinoshita Y, Maekawa T, Okada A, Waki S, Hassan MDS, Okamato H, Chiba T. Regenerating gene protein may mediate gastric mucosal proliferation induced by hypergastrinemia in rats. *Gastroenterology* 1998;115:1483–93.

39. Higham AD, Bishop LA, Dimaline R, Blackmore CG, Dobbins AC, Varro A, Thompson DG, Dockray GJ. Mutations of RegIalpha are associated with enterochromaffin-like cell tumor development in patients with hypergastrinemia. *Gastroenterology* 1999;116:1310–8.

40. Kobayashi S, Akiyama T, Nata K, Abe M, Tajima M, Shervani NJ, Unno M, Matsuno S, Sasaki H, Takasawa S, Okamoto H. Identification of a receptor for Reg (regenerating gene) protein, a pancreatic beta-cell regeneration factor. *J Biol Chem* 2000;275:10723–6.

41. Prenzel N, Zwick E, Daub H, Leserer M, Abraham R, Wallasch C, Ullrich A. EGF receptor transactivation by G-protein-coupled receptors requires metalloproteinase cleavage of proHB-EGF. *Nature* 1999;402:884–8.

42. Varro A, Noble P-J, Wroblewski L, Bishop L, and Dockray GJ. Gastrin-cholecystokininB receptor expression in AGS cells is associated with direct inhibition and indirect stimulation of cell proliferation via paracrine activation of the EGF-receptor. *Gut* 2002, in press.

43. Takeuchi Y, Yamada J, Yamada T, Todisco A. Functional role of extracellular signal-regulated protein kinases in gastric acid secretion. *Am J Physiol* 1997;273:G1263-G1272.

44. Ohning GV, Wong HC, LLoyd KCK, Walsh JH. Gastrin mediates the gastric mucosal proliferative response to feeding. *Am J Physiol* 1996;271:G470–G476.

Gut-Brain Peptides in the New Millennium, edited by Y. Taché
CURE Foundation, Los Angeles, CA. © 2002

3

Gastrin–Somatostatin Interactions: From Ontogeny to Pathology

Arthur Shulkes

Department of Surgery, University of Melbourne, Austin and Repatriation Medical Centre, Heidelberg, Victoria, Australia

INTRODUCTION

My career in regulatory peptides began in 1978 with a postdoctoral fellowship at CURE under the supervision of John Walsh. This was a time of great expansion and excitement in the regulatory peptide field and fellows from around the world were drawn to CURE like a magnet, all eager to work with and learn from John. Other fellows at this time included Cor Lamers, Irvin Modlin, Pierre Poitras, Steve Vigna, and Tachi Yamada. My project was on developing radioimmunoassays for Gastric Inhibitory Peptide (GIP) and Vasoactive Intestinal Polypeptide (VIP) in order to determine their biological roles. I continued this work back in Australia, but it was inevitable with John's outstanding work on the regulation of gastrin and gastric secretion plus the emerging interest in somatostatin, that one of the first projects in my new laboratory in Melbourne was to study gastrin-somatostatin interactions. Developmental aspects were examined initially as my colleague, Ken Hardy, had previously established a neonatal sheep model that enabled blood and gastric juice samples to be taken over a 6 week period. In this chapter, I review the role of gastrin-somatostatin interactions in development, in the adult and in disease.

GASTRIN–ACID–SOMATOSTATIN REGULATORY LOOP

The major secretagogues controlling gastric acid secretion are gastrin (hormone stored in G cells of the antrum), histamine (paracrine agent stored in enterochromaffin like (ECL) cells of the corpus) and acetylcholine (vagal cholinergic mediator) (1). The gastrin–acid feedback loop, whereby increased gastric acidity inhibits gastrin secretion and decreased acidity stimulates gastrin release, is central to the regulation of gastric acid secretion (2). Somatostatin synthesized in D cells of the stomach is one of the more important components of this system as it inhibits both gastrin and gastric acid secretion and has appropriate morphological localization in both corpus and antrum (3). Acid is a stimulant of somatostatin but the feedback loop can also be modulated by a direct effect of gastrin on somatostatin secretion (2, 4, 5). The function of this paracrine pathway is to restore somatostatin secretion thereby attenuating the gastrin response. Acute immunoneutralization with somatostatin antisera results in an increase in plasma gastrin and gastric acidity indicating a continuous inhibitory role for somatostatin (6). Many of the inhibitors of gastric acid secretion, such as calcitonin gene related peptide and cholecystokinin (CCK), probably function by releasing somatostatin (3, 7). Taken together with the reports of somatostatin receptors on parietal and gastrin cells, and gastrin receptors on both somatostatin and parietal cells, there is strong evidence for a close interrelationship between gastrin, acid and somatostatin (1, 3).

Gastrin has a dual stimulatory effect on parietal cell function. The direct effect is by gastrin receptors on the parietal cell, while probably the more important pathway is by gastrin stimulating histamine release from ECL cells which in turn activates the parietal cell (8). This latter proposal that gastrin stimulates acid via the release of histamine is supported by the finding that gastrin increases the synthesis of histidine decarboxylase, the enzyme responsible for histamine production (9). Somatostatin inhibits the effects of gastrin both at parietal and ECL cells and inhibits histamine release by ECL cells (9). Histamine is therefore important in the interaction between gastrin and somatostatin.

ONTOGENY OF GASTRIN–SOMATOSTATIN INTERACTIONS

Progressive hypergastrinemia is observed in ovine, and human fetuses and in the neonatal rat (10), yet expected increases in the secretion of gastric acid are small indicating that feedback regulatory mechanisms governing fetal acid secretion are either not present, underdeveloped or inhibited (10). Nevertheless, gastric acid can be stimulated in the immature sheep and rat by exogenous infusions of gastrin and histamine (11, 12) and somatostatin has also been reported to inhibit ovine fetal gastrin secretion (13) suggesting that gastrin, histamine and somatostatin receptors are functional. The regulation of gastrin acidity in the immature animal is different to the adult. For instance, in both the neonatal rat and sheep, the secretory response to pentagastrin precedes that of histamine (11, 12) and infusion of acid does not inhibit gastrin secretion (10). Similarly, gastrin stimulated somatostatin secretion is histamine independent in the fetus and histamine dependent in the adult (14).

The relative achlorhydria in the fetus may be the result of an excess tonic inhibitory effect of somatostatin. Yee, et al. (15) have reported that the fall in the ratio of antral somatostatin to gastrin coincides with the onset of fetal gastric secretion in the fetal rabbit. In the neonatal sheep, although antral and fundic somatostatin increases more rapidly than antral gastrin, the onset of endogenous gastric acidity coincides with a fall in somatostatin type 2 receptor expression (16). Rao, et al. (12) demonstrated a tonic inhibitory role for CCK and opioid peptides on gastric acid secretion in the neonatal rat but did not examine the contribution of somatostatin. The Walsh group using an anti-somatostatin antibody showed that somatostatin had a direct inhibitory role on gastrin secretion in the suckling rat as administration of the antibody produced a two fold increase in circulating gastrin (17). Taken together, these findings suggest that there is a regulatory pathway linking gastrin and somatostatin in the neonate which serves to modulate gastrin secretion and gastric acidity. However, there are significant differences in the fetus such as the non-essential role for histamine and that gastric acidity has no direct effect on gastrin secretion.

GASTRIN–SOMATOSTATIN INTERACTIONS IN THE ADULT

Determining particular roles for gastrin and somatostatin in the regulation of gastrointestinal function is particularly difficult because of the multiple receptor subtypes for both these peptides and that somatostatin is not only released into the circulation but also functions as a paracrine agent (1, 2, 3). A major advance, led by John Walsh and magnificently supported by Helen Wong who generated the antisera, was the use *in vivo* of acute and chronic immunoneutralization against gastrin, somatostatin and other regulatory peptides. Using a monoclonal antibody against gastrin, the CURE group were able to show that gastrin mediated the gastric mucosal proliferative response to feeding (18), the acid stimulatory response to bombesin (19) and that gastrin was the principal mediator of the cephalic and gastric phases of acid secretion (20, 21, 22). Studies with a somatostatin monoclonal antibody demonstrated that the inhibitory effect of CCK on gastric acid secretion was through release of endogenous somatostatin (23) and that the low gastric acid secretion in the urethane anesthetized rat was via increased output of somatostatin and inhibition of gastrin secretion (24). Other groups have shown that acute immunoneutralization (6) with somatostatin antisera results in an increase in plasma gastrin and gastric acidity indicating a continuous inhibitory role for somatostatin. However, long term immunization against somatostatin has no effect on basal gastrin or gastric acidity implying a reset of regulatory mechanisms (5). More recently the Walsh group demonstrated using a combination of somatostatin receptor subtype 2 knockout mice with gastrin and somatostatin immunization that this receptor subtype plays a major role in mediating endogenous somatostatin suppression of gastric acid secretion. This suppression is predominantly through inhibition of gastrin's action probably on the ECL cells (25).

The pivotal role of gastrin in the regulation of gastric function has been confirmed with the use of transgenic mice lacking either the gastrin gene or the gastrin/CCK-B receptor gene. These mice have elevated gastric pH, decreased parietal and D cells and are unresponsive to acute histaminergic, cholinergic and gastrinergic stimulation. Thus, gastrin is required both for maturation and function of the gastric secretory system (26, 27)

In general, antral gastrin and somatostatin synthesis are reciprocally regulated by gastric lumenal contents. Rats rendered achlorhydric by treatment with the H/K ATPase inhibitor omeprazole have decreased abundance of antral SOM mRNA and increased amounts of gastrin mRNA (28). Fasting increases antral SOM mRNA within 12 hours (29) and SOM peptide within two days (30); refeeding or inhibiting acid secretion of the food deprived animals returns SOM mRNA to the non-fasting state within 2 hours (29, 31). An increase in antral SOM synthesis is parallelled by a decrease in antral gastrin mRNA suggesting an inhibitory role for gastric antral SOM upon gastrin synthesis (29). In contrast to the antrum, lumenal contents have little effect on fundic SOM gene expression or peptide content (31, 30) illustrating separate regulatory mechanisms for SOM in the acid and non-acid secretory regions of the stomach.

An increase in gastric acidity inhibits gastrin secretion (1) and studies, predominantly *in vitro* using isolated perfused stomachs, suggest that this inhibition is mediated by the release of somatostatin (2, 6). However, somatostatin does not have an obligatory role since varying gastric pH in sheep and in humans alters gastrin release without affecting somatostatin secretion (5, 32, 33).

DISORDERS OF GASTRIN–SOMATOSTATIN INTERACTIONS

More than a quarter of century ago, John Walsh and his colleagues demonstrated that patients with duodenal ulcer disease have decreased inhibitory reflexes to control gastric acid secretion resulting in elevated and sustained gastric acidity (34). The finding that *Helicobacter pylori* infection of the antrum is necessary for most cases of duodenal ulcer disease and that the infection alters the balance between gastrin and somatostatin synthesis, storage and secretion have provided an explanation for the dysregulation of gastric acidity

(35). Treatment is now directed to eradication of *Helicobacter pylori* and consequent normalization of the somatostatin–acid–gastrin regulatory loop.

Subjects with predominantly antral *Helicobacter pylori* infection have increased gastric acidity and an increased acid secretion in response to gastrin releasing peptide (GRP) or gastrin stimulation (36). This hyperchlorhydria is associated with increased gastrin and diminished somatostatin expression (35) and is consistent with impaired inhibitory control. In addition, an increased parietal cell mass may also be involved in *Helicobacter pylori* infected duodenal ulcer subjects (36). Furthermore, the post-translational processing of gastrin is abnormal with infected patients having a greater proportion of bioactive amidated gastrin (37). Eradication of *Helicobacter pylori* returns the levels of gastrin and somatostatin to normal and reverses the hyperacidity. Bacterial products and inflammatory cytokines such as tumor necrosis factor (TNF) TNFα and interleukin 1 may be the effectors for the hormonal and secretory changes (35, 38). It is interesting that in the absence of treatment the hyperacidity and hypergastrinemia and low somatostatin can be self perpetuating because it restricts the infection to the antrum leaving a healthy corpus to continue secreting acid.

In contrast, colonization of the corpus results in gastritis and a low acid secretion, decreased corpus somatostatin content (39) and in some instances a consequential increase in gastrin secretion (40), which in turn, may accelerate the progression to gastric cancer (41). However, little is known of the characteristics of the gastrin–acid somatostatin regulatory loop in gastric cancer and interpretation is complicated by the autocrine production of gastrin by the tumor itself (40, 42).

It is apparent that a better understanding of the functions and regulatory control of the gastrin–somatostatin feedback loop including the distinct regulatory mechanisms between antrum and corpus is required when assessing potential treatment regimens for patients with duodenal ulcers and patients at risk of developing gastric cancer. Similarly the controversy of whether to eradicate *Helicobacter pylori* in subjects with non-ulcer dyspepsia or with gastroesophageal reflux (43) should also be viewed in the context of how the gastrin–acid somatostatin feedback loop has been altered.

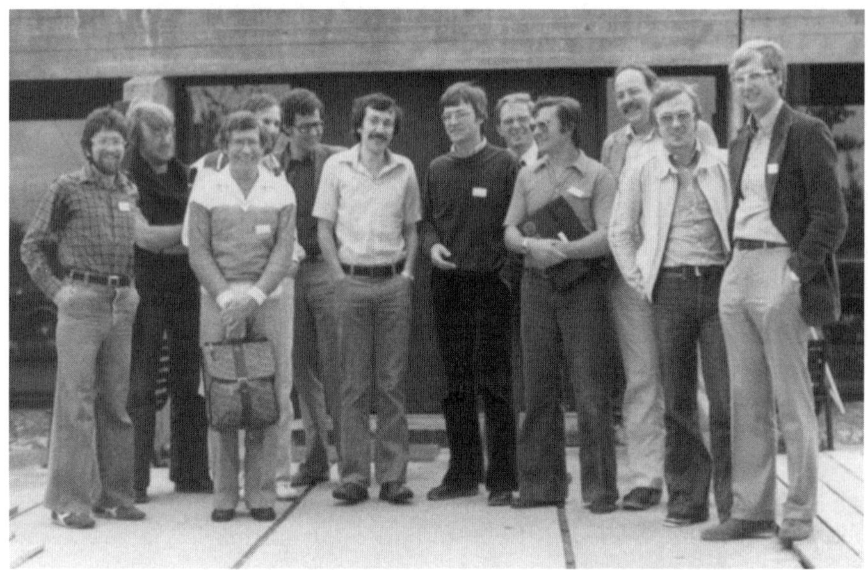

Some of the delegates at the Gastrins and the Vagus workshop organized by Jens Rehfeld and held in Aarhus, Denmark August 25–27, 1978. The author is the one in the flares on the left and J.H. Walsh is on the right.

ACKNOWLEDGMENTS

Arthur Shulkes is a Senior Principal Research Fellow of the National Health and Medical Research Council of Australia.

REFERENCES

1. Walsh JH. Gastrin. In: *Gut Peptides: Biochemistry and Physiology.* Walsh JH, Dockray GJ, ed. New York: Raven Press, 1994;75–121.
2. Schubert ML, Makhlouf GM. Neural, hormonal, and paracrine regulation of gastrin and acid secretion. *Yale J Biol Med* 1992;65:553–60.
3. Shulkes A. Somatostatin: physiology and clinical applications. *Baillieres Clin Endocrinol Metab* 1994;8: 215–36.
4. Shulkes A, Read M. Regulation of somatostatin secretion by gastrin- and acid-dependent mechanisms. *Endocrinology* 1991;129:2329–2334.
5. Westbrook SL, McDowell GH, Hardy KJ, Shulkes A. Active immunization against somatostatin alters the regulation of gastrin in response to gastric acid secretagogues. *Am J Physiol* 1998;274:G751-G756.
6. Holst J, Jørgensen PN, Rasmussen TN, Schmidt P. Somatostatin restraint of gastrin secretion in pigs revealed by monoclonal antibody immunoneutralization. *Am J Physiol* 1992;263:G908–912.
7. Zavros Y, Fleming WR, Hardy KJ, Shulkes A. Regulation of fundic and antral somatostatin secretion by cholecystokinin and gastrin. *Am J Physiol* 1998;274:G742-G750.
8. Dockray GJ, Varro A, Dimaline R. Gastric endocrine cells; gene expression, processing and targeting of active products. *Physiol Rev* 1996;76:767–798.
9. Prinz C, Zanner R, Gerhard M, Mahr S, Neumayer N, Hohne-Zell B, Gratzl M. The mechanism of histamine secretion from gastric enterochromaffin-like cells. *Am J Physiol* 1999;277:C845–C855.

10. Shulkes A. Ontogeny of gastrointestinal regulatory peptides and their function. Thorburn G, Harding R, Ed. In: *Textbook of Fetal Physiology*. Oxford, Oxford University Press, 1994;236–244.
11. Shulkes A, Chick P, Hardy KJ, Robinson P, Trahair J. Ontogeny of gastric acidity in the ovine fetus. *J Dev Physiol* 1985;7:195–206.
12. Rao RK, Pepperl S, Porreca F. Tonic suppression of gastric acid secretion by endogenous peptides in neonatal rats. *Am J Physiol* 1995;269:G721-G728.
13. Shulkes A, Hardy KJ. Effect of somatostatin on basal concentrations of gastrin and pancreatic polypeptide in the fetal sheep. *Biol Neonate* 1982;42:249–256.
14. Grabau BJ, Zavros Y, Hardy KJ, Shulkes A. Developmental regulation of gastric somatostatin in the sheep. *Endocrinology* 1999;140:603–608.
15. Yee LF, Wong HC, Calaustro EQ, Mulvihill SJ. Roles of gastrin and somatostatin in the regulation of gastric acid secretion in the fetal rabbit. *J Surg Res* 1996;63:364–368.
16. Kolivas S, Volombello T, Shulkes A. Expression of receptors regulating gastric acidity in the developing sheep stomach. *Regul Pept* 2001;101:93–100.
17. Martin MG, Wu SV, Ohning G, Wong H, Walsh JH. Parenterally or enterally administered anti-somatostatin antibody induces increased gastrin in suckling rats. *Am J Physiol* 1994;266:G417–424.
18. Ohning GV, Wong HC, Lloyd KC, Walsh JH. Gastrin mediates the gastric mucosal proliferative response to feeding. *Am J Physiol* 1996;271:G470–476.
19. Kovacs TO, Lloyd KC, Wong H, Walsh JH. Inhibition of bombesin-stimulated acid secretion by immunoneutralization of gastrin in dogs. *Am J Physiol* 1995;268:G54–58.
20. Kovacs TO, Lloyd KC, Lawson DC, Pappas TN, Walsh JH. Inhibition of sham feeding-stimulated acid secretion in dogs by immunoneutralization of gastrin. *Am J Physiol* 1997;273:G399–403.
21. Kovacs TO, Walsh JH, Maxwell V, Wong HC, Azuma T, Katt E. Gastrin is a major mediator of the gastric phase of acid secretion in dogs: proof by monoclonal antibody neutralization. *Gastroenterology* 1989;97:1406–1413.
22. Lloyd KC, Raybould HE, Taché Y, Walsh JH. Role of gastrin, histamine, and acetylcholine in the gastric phase of acid secretion in anesthetized rats. *Am J Physiol* 1992;262:G747–755.
23. Lloyd KC, Raybould HE, Walsh JH. Cholecystokinin inhibits gastric acid secretion through type "A" cholecystokinin receptors and somatostatin in rats. *Am J Physiol* 1992;263:G287–292.
24. Yang H, Wong H, Wu V, Walsh JH, Taché Y. Somatostatin monoclonal antibody immunoneutralization increases gastrin and gastric acid secretion in urethane-anesthetized rats. *Gastroenterology* 1990;99:659–665.
25. Martínez V, Curi AP, Torkian B, Schaeffer JM, Wilkinson HA, Walsh JH, Taché Y. High basal gastric acid secretion in somatostatin receptor subtype 2 knockout mice. *Gastroenterology* 1998;114:1125–1132.
26. Wang TC, Dockray GJ. Lessons from genetically engineered animal models I. Physiological studies with gastrin in transgenic mice. *Am J Physiol* 1999;277:G6–G11.
27. Hinkle KL, Samuelson LC. Lessons from genetically engineered animal models III. Lessons learned from gastrin gene deletion in mice. *Am J Physiol* 1999;277:G500–G505.
28. Brand SJ, Stone D. Reciprocal regulation of antral gastrin and somatostatin gene expression in omeprazole induced achlorhydria. *J Clin Invest* 1988;82:1059–1066.
29. Wu SV, Giraud A, Mogard M, Sumii K, Walsh JH. Effects of inhibition of gastric secretion on antral gastrin and somatostatin gene expression in rats. *Am J Physiol* 1990;258:G788–793.
30. Shulkes A, Caussignac Y, Lamers CB, Solomon TE, Yamada T, Walsh JH. Starvation in the rat: effect on peptides of the gut and brain. *Aust J Exp Biol Med* 1983;61:581–587.
31. Sandvik AK, Dimaline R, Forster ER, Evans D, Dockray GJ. Differential control of somatostatin messenger RNA in rat gastric corpus and antrum. *J Clin Invest* 1993;91:244–250.
32. Ferahköse Z, Hüseyin A, Mentes B. Effect of systemic gastric acid stimulation and intragastric pH changes on synchronous antral gastrin and somatostatin release in anesthetized, nonatropinized duodenal ulcer patients and controls. *Dig Dis Sci* 1994;39:2143–2148.
33. Jensen SL, Holst JJ, Christiansen LA, Shokouh-Amiri, MH, Lorentsen M, Beck H, Jensen HE. Effect of intragastric pH on antral gastrin and somatostatin release in anaesthetised, atropinized, duodenal ulcer patients and controls. *Gut* 1987;28:206–209.
34. Walsh JH, Richardson CT, Fordtran JS. pH dependence of acid secretion and gastrin release in normal and ulcer subjects. *J Clin Invest* 1975;55:462–468.

35. Calam J, Gibbons A, Healey ZV, Bliss P, Arebi N. How does Helicobacter pylori cause mucosal damage? Its effect on acid and gastrin physiology. *Gastroenterology* 1997;113 (Suppl):S43–49.
36. McColl KE, El-Omar E, Gillen D. Helicobacter pylori gastritis and gastric physiology. *Gastroenterol Clin North Am* 2000;29:687–703.
37. Zavros Y, Paterson A, Lambert J, Shulkes A. Expression of progastrin-derived peptides and somatostatin in fundus and antrum of nonulcer dyspepsia subjects with and without Helicobacter pylori infection. *Dig Dis Sci* 2000;45:2058–2064.
38. El-Omar EM, Chow WH, Rabkin CS. Gastric cancer and H. pylori: Host genetics open the way. *Gastroenterology* 2001;121:1002–1005.
39. Gotz JM, Veenendaal RA, Biemond I, Muller ES, Veselic M, Lamers CB. Serum gastrin and mucosal somatostatin in Helicobacter pylori-associated gastritis. *Scand J Gastroenterol* 1995;30:1064–1068.
40. Konturek PC, Konturek SJ, Sulekova Z, Meixner H, Bielanski W, Starzynska T, Karczewska E, Marlicz K, Stachura J, Hahn EG. Expression of hepatocyte growth factor, transforming growth factor alpha, apoptosis related proteins Bax and Bcl-2, and gastrin in human gastric cancer. *Aliment Pharmacol Ther* 2001;15:989–999.
41. Wang TC, Dangler CA, Chen D, Goldenring JR, Koh T, Raychowdhury R, Coffey RJ, Ito S, Varro A, Dockray GJ, Fox JG. Synergistic interaction between hypergastrinemia and Helicobacter infection in a mouse model of gastric cancer. *Gastroenterology* 2000;118:36–47.
42. Henwood M, Clarke PA, Smith AM, Watson SA. Expression of gastrin in developing gastric adenocarcinoma. *Br J Surg* 2001;88:564–568.
43. Fox JG, Wang TC. *Helicobacter pylori*—not a good bug after all. *New Engl J Med* 2001;345:784–789.

Gut-Brain Peptides in the New Millennium, edited by Y. Taché
CURE Foundation, Los Angeles, CA. © 2002

4

The Role of Amino Acids and Calcium in the Regulation of Human Gastrin Cell Function

P. E. Squires
Molecular Physiology, University of Warwick, England

A. M. J. Buchan
Department of Physiology, University of British Columbia, Vancouver, Canada

Gastrin release from human antral G cells is well known to be regulated by multiple stimuli, including hormones, neurotransmitters, amino acids (AA) and ions such as calcium (1). Information concerning the regulation of human G cell function has come from a number of different experimental paradigms ranging from clinical studies to *in vitro* studies with isolated epithelial cell cultures (1, 2). These studies have indicated that the majority of stimuli act directly on the G cell interacting with cell surface receptors to activate intracellular signaling pathways, however, an exception to this is AAs.

For many years there has been considerable debate concerning the mechanism of action of AAs that results in the stimulation of gastrin release. In experimental animal models uptake of the AA and intracellular conversion to amines has been shown to alter the intra-vesicular pH of gastrin granules influencing both secretion and post-translational processing of the peptide (3–5). Alternatively, in the isolated canine G cell model both AAs and amines stimulated gastrin release but by different mechanisms (6). Gastrin release in response to AAs was inhibited by addition of somatostatin, while the response to amines was unaffected.

The newly identified calcium-sensing, or perhaps more properly, the divalent cation sensing receptor (CaSR) is a member of the third family of G protein coupled receptors showing the greatest structural similarity to the metabatropic glutamate receptors (7). All the members of this family share a long N-terminal extracellular region required for ion/ligand binding. The CaSR receptor is expressed on numerous cell types both epithelial (e.g. kidney) and endocrine (calcitonin and parathyroid hormone) and was originally isolated due to effects on the regulation of plasma calcium levels with several known human disorders being caused by either activating or inactivating mutations (8). However, more recently the receptor has been identified on cell types without any known action on calcium homeostasis. Not

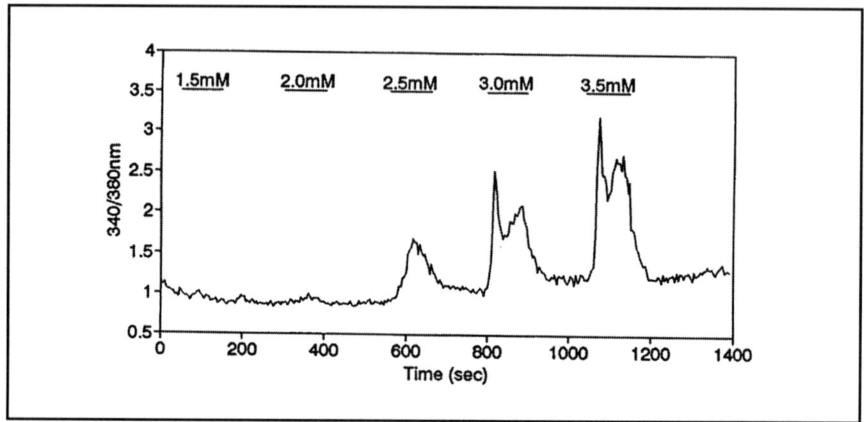

FIGURE 1. *A typical intracellular response profile of a G cell stimulated with increasing concentrations of extracellular calcium. Note that below 2mM there is no significant increase in intracellular calcium levels. In addition, at 3.0 and 3.5mM the increase in intracellular calcium levels remains elevated until removal of the high external calcium stimulus.*

only is the CaSR expressed on multiple cell types but the intracellular signaling pathways activated by receptor stimulation are varied and dependent on the cell phenotype. In parathyroid hormone (PTH) cells the predominant coupling is to the inhibitory Gi complex resulting in the inhibition of PTH release, however in the majority of other endocrine cells the receptor activates either the Gs (calcitonin) or Gq/11 (gastrin and insulin) pathways resulting in the stimulation of hormone release (9–12).

Recently, we identified the presence of the CaSR on human antral G cells by both molecular biological and functional studies (13). Increasing extracellular calcium results in a stimulation of hormone release, with prolonged activation of the receptor causing inhibition of insulin but not gastrin release (14, 12). The primary cell cultures used to study the regulation of gastrin release were generated from human antrum obtained through a collaboration with the British Columbia. Transplant Society. While this culture preparation is not pure, over 30% of the cells are gastrin-immunoreactive and the precise response of these cells can be monitored using intracellular Ca^{2+} imaging systems. A hallmark of the effect of Ca^{2+} on the gastrin cells is an immediate increase in intracellular calcium consistent with the release of calcium from intracellular stores through activation of IP3 receptors known to be expressed in the G cells (Figure 1, Ref. 15). The intial peak of intracellular calcium is followed by a sustained plateau level that, unlike other endocrine cells expressing the receptor, is maintained until extracellular Ca^{2+} is returned to basal levels (Figure 1).

In the gastrin cells while increasing extracellular Ca^{2+} resulted in significant increases in gastrin release the sensitivity of the cells is significantly lower

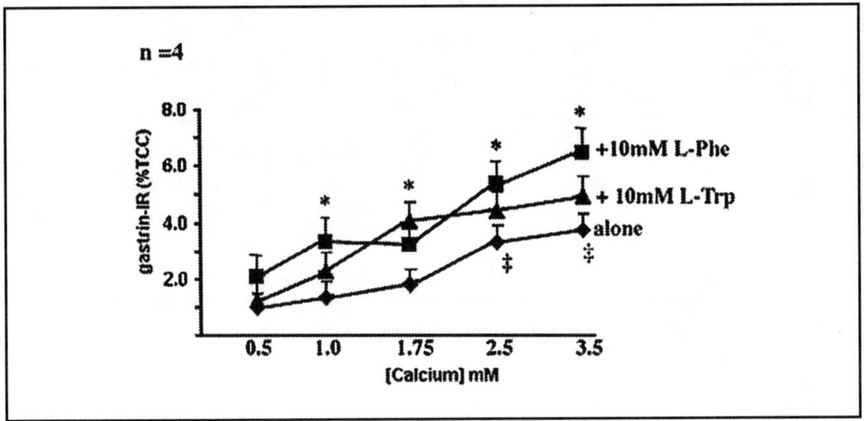

FIGURE 2. *Increasing extracellular calcium levels results in a significant increase in gastrin release at 2.5 and 3.5mM (alone, n = 4, mean ± SEM, t-test ‡p < 0.05). Increasing extracellular calcium in the presence of 10mM Phe or Trp shifted the concentration response curve to the left resulting in a significant increase in gastrin release at 1.0mM calcium, indicating that AA were altering the sensitivity of the CaSR (n = 4, mean ± SEM, t-test ★ p < 0.05).*

than that previously reported for calcitonin and PTH cells. The latter cells respond to Ca^{2+} concentrations above 1mM while the G cells require >1.75mM to obtain a significant elevation of basal gastrin release (Figure 2). We have sequenced the mRNA encoding the CaSR expressed by the human antral G cells and there is no evidence for differential exon splicing, therefore, the change in sensitivity of the receptor is unlikely to be caused by modifications to the structure of the receptor (12). However, these data do not rule out the possibility that there is differential glycosylation of the N-terminal ion binding region that affects the sensitivity to ambient Ca^{2+} levels.

An alternative possibility is that the intracellular signaling pathways activated by the CaSR in the G cells are differentially regulated such that hormone release is only achieved at higher concentrations of extracellular Ca^{2+}. The finding that the intracellular Ca^{2+} profile obtained in Ca^{2+} stimulated G cells differs from that of all other CaSR expressing cells investigated to-date would support this suggestion.

A common mechanism utilized by the CaSR is activation of Store Operated capacitative Calcium channels (SOCs) rather than voltage gated calcium channels as the source of calcium to maintain increased cytosolic levels. We are currently determining whether the sustained intracellular Ca^{2+} plateau in stimulated G cells is the result of activation of one of the human transient receptor potential (Trp) family of non-selective cation channels (16). The Trp1 channel in the plasma membrane has been demonstrated to couple directly to IP3RII in the endoplasmic reticulum (ER) of platelets and mediate the

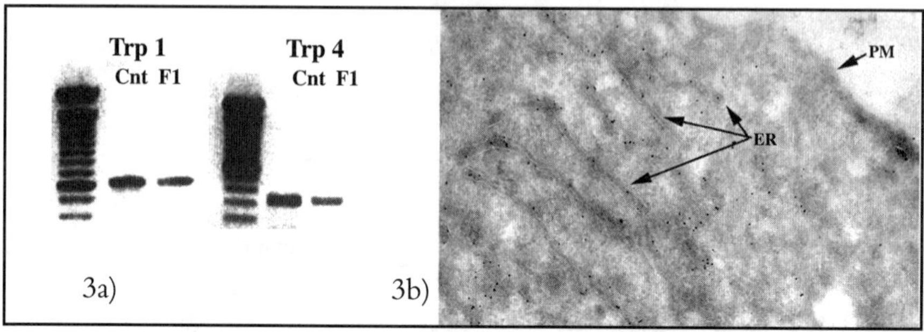

FIGURE 3. *(a) The products obtained by RT-PCR for the Trp-1 and -4 channels showed high levels of mRNA expression. (b) Cryoelectron microscopy of a section of human antrum immunostained with antibodies to human pro-gastrin (a kind gift from Dr. G. Dockray). Note that the ER stained using these antibodies was present in the cortical region of the cell. × 10,000.*

store operated calcium entry (17). It is possible that activation of the IP$_3$R in the G cell by CaSR results in a similar coupling between plasma membrane Trp channels in G cells and the IP$_3$Rs. Of the 6 known members of the Trp family the F1 fraction of human antral epithelial cells used for the gastrin studies contains mRNA encoding TRps 1, 4, 5 and 6 with the highest mRNA levels being detected for Trps 1 and 4 (Figure 3a). We are currently determining the precise Trp channels expressed by the G cells using channel specific antibodies. The coupling of the Trp channels in the plasma membrane to the IP$_3$Rs requires that ER be located in the cortical region of the G cells. Earlier studies of the ultrastructure of G cells demonstrated the presence of ER (located using the presence of unprocessed pro-gastrin-IR) lying directly under the plasma membrane (Figure 3b) indicating that proximity of the two proteins would not be an issue.

While the majority of stimuli of the G cell act through cell surface receptors, the mechanism of action of AAs remain uncertain. Recent studies with the CaSR in transfected HEK cells have demonstrated that the receptor can be activated by the extracellular addition of aromatic AAs such as phenylalanine and tryptophan (18).

The possibility that AAs regulate endocrine cell function through activation of the CaSR led us to complete release studies using the primary gastrin cell cultures. The original work on the interaction between CaSR and aromatic AAs indicated that the L isomers increased intracellular calcium levels only above a threshold level of extracellular calcium (>1mM) and resulted in a leftward shift in the concentration response curve to increasing extracellular calcium levels. While these data indicate that calcium signaling through CaSR activation can be modulated by concomitant increases in AA, it does not address whether this is translated into changes to the overall function of the cell, in the case of an endocrine cell such as gastrin, an increase in hormone release. To determine if ambient AA concentrations affected the sensitivity of the G cell CaSR, we completed experiments in the presence or absence of 10 mM phenylanaline or tryptophane AAs known to stimulate gastrin release *in vivo* (19). The results were similar to those obtained with the transfected HEK cells, with elevated AAs resulting in a significant increase in gastrin release in response to increasing extracellular calcium (Figure 2). These data indicated that at least in human G cells expressing the CaSR, a significant proportion of AA-stimulated gastrin release may be due to interactions with the cell surface CaSR. The exact contribution of this interaction to the resulting secretion cannot be determined in the absence of CaSR antagonists.

ACKNOWLEDGMENTS

I would like to take this opportunity to recognize the help and encouragement I received from John Walsh during my career. John was always supportive of our work with the isolated G cell model and recognized the complexities and challenges in working with the human cell preparation. He will be greatly missed by all those who knew and worked with him. These studies were supported by a grant from the Canadian Institutes of Health Research.

REFERENCES

1. Walsh JH. Physiology and pathophysiology of gastrin. *Mt Sinai J Med* 1992;59:117–24.
2. Campos RV, Buchan, AMJ , Meloche RM, et. al. Gastrin secretion from human antral G cells in culture. *Gastroenterology* 1990; 99:36–40.
3. Dial EJ, Cooper LC, Lichtenberger LM. Amino acid- and amine-induced gastrin release from isolated rat endocrine granules. *Am J Physiol* 1991;260:G175–81.
4. Lichtenberger LM, Delansorne R, Graziani LA. Importance of amino acid uptake and decarboxylation in gastrin release from isolated G cells. *Nature* 1982;295:698–700.
5. Voronina S, Henry J, Vaillant C, Dockray GJ, Varro A. Amine precursor uptake and decarboxylation: significance for processing of the rat gastrin precursor. *J Physiol* 1997;501 :363–74.
6. DelValle J, Yamada T. Amino acids and amines stimulate gastrin release from canine antral G-cells via different pathways. *J Clin Invest* 1990;85:139–43
7. Brown EM. G protein-coupled, extracellular Ca^{2+} (Ca^{2+}(o))-sensing receptor enables Ca^{2+}(o) to function as a versatile extracellular first messenger. *Cell Biochem Biophys* 2000;33:63–95.
8. Brown EM, MacLeod RJ. Extracellular calcium sensing and extracellular calcium signaling. *Physiol Rev* 2001;81:239–297.
9. Chang W, Pratt S, Chen TH, Chen TH, Bourguignon L, Shoback D. Amino acids in the cytoplasmic C terminus of the parathyroid Ca^{2+}-sensing receptor mediate efficient cell-surface expression and phospholipase C activation. *J Biol Chem* 2001;276:44129–36.
10. Malaisse WJ, Louchami K, Laghmich A, Ladriere L, Morales M, Villaneuva-Penacarrillo ML, Valverde I, Rasschaert J. Possible participation of an islet B-cell calcium-sensing receptor in insulin release. *Endocrine* 1999;11:293–300.

11. Squires PE. Non-Ca^{2+}-homeostatic functions of the extracellular Ca^{2+}-sensing receptor (CaR) in endocrine tissues. *J Endocrinol* 2000;165:173–7.
12. Buchan AMJ, Squires PE, Ring M, Meloche MR. Mechanism of action of the calcium-sensing receptor in human antral gastrin cells. *Gastroenterology* 2001;120:1128–39.
13. Ray JM, PE Squires, SB Curtis, RM, Meloche MR, Buchan AN. Expression of the calcium-sensing receptor on human antral gastrin cells in culture. *J Clin Invest* 1997;99: 2328–2333.
14. Squires PE, Harris TE, Persaud SJ, Curtis SB, Buchan AM, Jones PM. The extracellular calcium-sensing receptor on human beta-cells negatively modulates insulin secretion. *Diabetes* 2000;49:409–17.
15. Squires PE, Meloche RM, Buchan AMJ. Bombesin-evoked gastrin release and calcium-signaling in human antral G-cells in culture. *Am J Physiol* 1999;276:G227–237.
16. Clapham DE, Runnels LW, Strubing C. The TRP ion channel family. *Nat Rev Neurosci* 2001;2:387–96.
17. Rosado JA, Sage SO. Activation of store-mediated calcium entry by secretion-like coupling between the inositol 1,4,5-trisphosphate receptor type II and human transient receptor potential (hTrp1) channels in human platelets. *Biochem J* 2001;356–359.
18. Conigrave AD, Quinn SJ, Brown EM. L-amino acid sensing by the extracellular Ca^{2+}-sensing receptor. *Proc Natl Acad Sci USA*. 2000;97:4814–9.
19. McCallum RW, Kuljian B, Holloway RH, Walsh JH. Effect of intragastric amino acids on lower esophageal sphincter pressure and serum gastrin in man. *Am J Gastroenterology* 1986;81:168–71.

Gut-Brain Peptides in the New Millennium, edited by Y. Taché
CURE Foundation, Los Angeles, CA. © 2002

5

Molecular Regulation of ECL Cell Function

Rod Dimaline
Physiological Laboratory, University of Liverpool, Liverpool, UK

INTRODUCTION

The discovery by Edkins of gastrin almost a century ago (1) suggested a hormonal regulation of gastric acid secretion, analogous to the acid-secretin-pancreas mechanism outlined by Bayliss & Starling three years earlier (2). However, the role of gastrin and indeed its very existence remained controversial for many years, not least because the histamine that was almost always present in the tissue extracts of the time, was found to be a powerful acid secretagogue itself (3). In fact it was almost 60 years after Edkins' initial report that gastrin was finally isolated and characterized (4). Even then, the relative importance of gastrin and histamine, and their mechanisms of interaction in stimulating acid secretion from the parietal cell were hotly contested. The eventual resolution of the problem depended on progress in a number of areas. These included the development of histamine H2 antagonists by Black and colleagues and of immunological probes for gastrin by Walsh and colleagues in the 1970's (5, 6), and the realization in the 1980's that the enterochromaffin-like (ECL) cell was the source of gastric histamine, and a target for gastrin (7). The currently prevailing view is that acid secretion is acutely regulated physiologically by histamine released from the ECL cell in response to gastrin. With the recognition of the ECL cell as a pivotal integrator of acid secretion, attention has focused in recent years on molecular mechanisms of ECL cell responses to circulating gastrin in physiological, pharmacological and clinical circumstances.

GASTRIN AND PHYSIOLOGICAL REGULATION
OF THE ECL CELL

In the gastric acid secreting mucosa, gastrin was shown to increase both the activity, and mRNA abundance of the key enzyme, histidine decarboxylase (HDC), which converts histidine to histamine (8–10). The mRNA response was rapid (within 15 minutes) and was elicited by physiological circulating

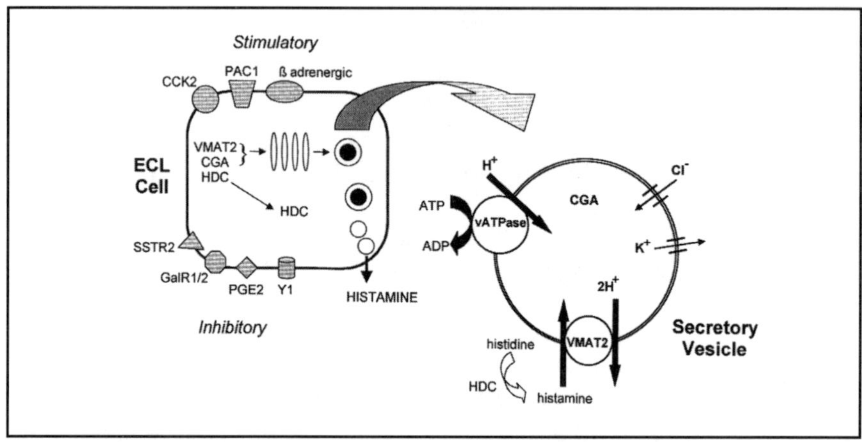

FIGURE 1. *Schematic representation of the ECL cell showing entry of VMAT2 and CGA into the secretory pathway, and cytoplasmic location of HDC. Stimulatory receptors shown are for Gastrin/CCK (CCK2), PACAP (PAC1), and catecholamines (β adrenergic). Inhibitory receptors shown are for somatostatin (SSTR2), galanin (GalR1/2), PYY (Y1) and prostaglandin E2 (PGE2). Inset shows secretory granule with membrane resident transporters VMAT2 and v-type ATPase. Putative chloride and potassium channels are also illustrated.*

concentrations of gastrin. This suggested that alterations in HDC gene expression might be important in underpinning changes in ECL cell function over the time taken to digest a single meal (11). A further protein recognized to be of potential importance for ECL cell function is chromogranin A (CGA). The chromogranins are considered to be indicators of neuroendocrine cell function; in the gastric acid–secreting mucosa CGA occurs predominantly, although not exclusively in ECL cells, and has been regarded as a marker for distribution of this cell type (12). Chromogranins are believed to play a role in secretory granule formation and stabilization (13). Consistent with this idea, CGA mRNA abundance in gastric corpus was shown to change, in parallel with that of HDC in response to changes in circulating gastrin concentrations (14).

Histamine is synthesized enzymatically by HDC in the cytosol, so that enhanced production and secretion in response to circulating gastrin requires an augmented sequestration of the amine into secretory vesicles. Two vesicular transporters VMAT1 and VMAT2, have been characterized that transfer monoamines from cytosol to vesicle in exchange for intravesicular protons, although their affinities for histamine are only about 1% and 10%, respectively, that for other monoamines such as dopamine and serotonin. Nevertheless, because VMAT2 is localized exclusively in ECL cells within the corpus, where histamine is essentially the only abundant substrate, and since VMAT2 is upregulated by gastrin, it is now generally accepted that this molecule serves as the ECL cell histamine transporter (15, 16) (Figure 1).

TRANSCRIPTIONAL REGULATION OF ECL CELL GENES

Following exposure to increasing concentrations of gastrin, the ECL cell exhibits a progressive, coordinated response to upregulate expression of the genes encoding the three proteins, HDC, VMAT2 and CGA, that are intimately associated with increased synthesis, storage and secretion of histamine (15). The mechanisms by which gastrin activates transcription of these genes has been investigated in detail, primarily in gastric cancer cell lines permanently transfected with the gastrin/CCKB receptor. In the case of HDC, Wang and colleagues have identified two overlapping gastrin response elements, just downstream of the transcriptional start site of the human HDC gene. Two separate and apparently novel proteins that bind to these response elements were identified; these are distinct from previously known transcription factors (17). The gastrin-stimulated transcription is mediated mainly through activation of ERK-related pathways, in a Raf-dependent, Ras-independent manner (18). In contrast, gastrin-stimulated transcription of the CGA promoter appears to be mediated by cooperative interaction of the well-defined transcription factors SP1 and CREB, acting through classical upstream SP1/Egr-1 and CRE response elements, respectively (19). In an extension of these studies, Hocker, et al. were able to demonstrate that approximately 5kb of the 5' flanking region of the CGA gene could direct ECL cell specific expression in the gastric corpus of transgenic animals, and that gastrin-responsiveness of the gene was retained (20). Transcriptional regulation of VMAT2 by gastrin seems to share features with, but is distinct from, that of both HDC and CGA. Thus gastrin activates the VMAT2 promoter through two canonical *cis*-regulatory elements, CRE and overlapping SP1/AP2 sites. The presence of both elements is required for full gastrin-responsiveness. However, while the CRE site is activated by phosphorylated CREB, the SP1/AP2 site is bound by a novel, relatively small nuclear factor that is clearly distinguishable from the AP or SP families of transcription factor. This gastrin response element binding protein (GREBP) is also different from those shown to regulate the HDC promoter (17, 21). Studies using the adenoviral oncoprotein, E1A, suggest that the cooperative interactions of CREB and the GREBP in activating VMAT2 may be coordinated by p300/CBP (21) (Figure 2).

CLINICAL ASPECTS OF ECL CELL FUNCTION

As well as upregulation of genes important for histamine biosynthesis and secretion, gastrin is well known to stimulate ECL cell growth. Thus rats treated chronically (lifelong) with high doses of potent inhibitors of gastric acid secretion develop ECL cell hyperplasia that progresses through dysplasia to

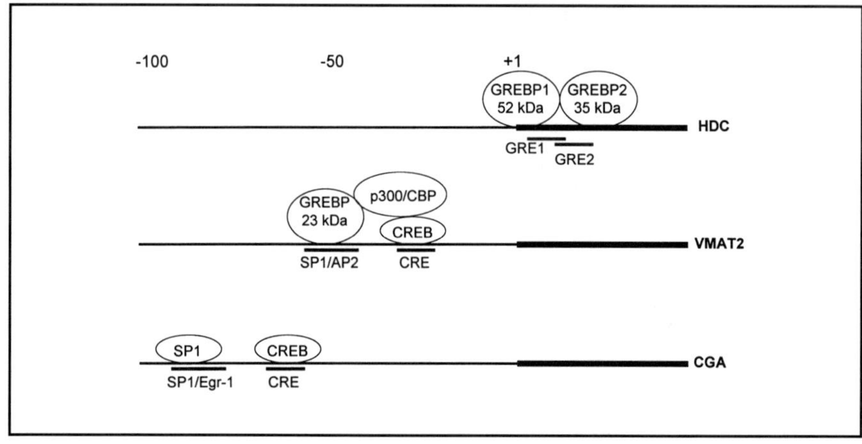

FIGURE 2. *Schematic representation of 5′-flanking regions of HDC, VMAT2 and CGA. Thin horizontal lines represents the promoter, thicker lines are downstream of the transcriptional start site (= +1). Response elements are underlined. Ellipses represent nuclear binding proteins involved in gastrin-mediated transcriptional activation. GREBP, gastrin response element binding protein.*

frank gastric carcinoid tumors (22). The concern that this tumor progression may emerge in patients undergoing long term, profound acid inhibitory therapy has not so far materialized. ECL cell hyperplasia is, however, commonly seen in chronic atrophic gastritis (CAG), and in a small proportion of CAG patients there is a progression to carcinoid tumors (23, 24). Small carcinoid nodules are often managed conservatively, but for larger tumors with metastatic potential, surgical intervention such as antrectromy or total gastrectomy may be indicated. Antrectomy (by far the least radical of the surgical procedures), to remove the source of circulating gastrin, is only appropriate where tumor growth remains gastrin-dependent and has not become autonomous. In an attempt to establish the gastrin-responsiveness of ECL cell tumors, Higham, et al. monitored expression of HDC, CGA and VMAT2 in carcinoid tumors of a CAG patient, before and after a 72h infusion of a potent somatostatin analogue (25). Dramatic down-regulation of circulating gastrin concentrations, and of expression of all three genes in the tumors as well as in normal gastric corpus mucosa suggested that this "octreotide suppression test" may be of some value in identifying patients that would benefit from antrectomy. The development of ECL cell tumors is almost certainly multifactorial, and for example in patients where hypergastrinaemia is one aspect of the multiple endocrine neoplasia syndrome, mutations of the menin gene lead to ECL cell carcinoid tumors (26). Another candidate tumor suppresser for ECL cells is the product of the *Reg1α* gene. Unlike menin, reg is found in the ECL cell (although not exclusively so) in a number of species (27, 28). Higham, et al., demonstrated upregula-

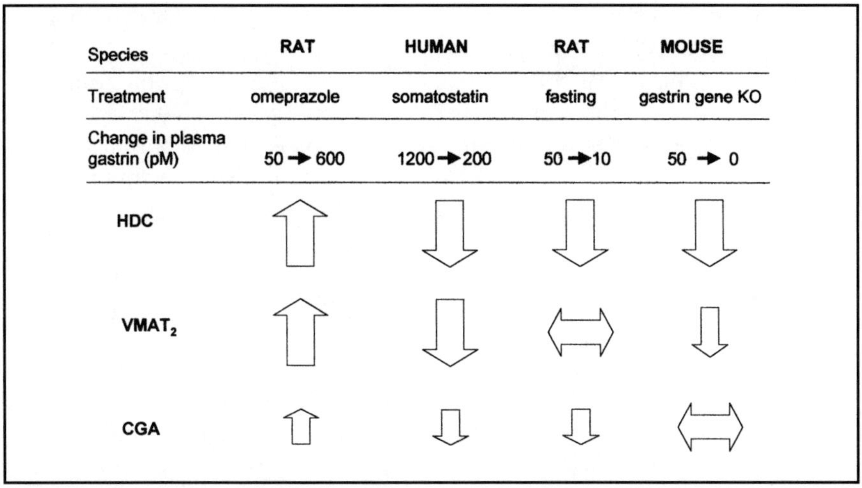

Species	RAT	HUMAN	RAT	MOUSE
Treatment	omeprazole	somatostatin	fasting	gastrin gene KO
Change in plasma gastrin (pM)	50 → 600	1200 → 200	50 → 10	50 → 0
HDC	⇧	⇩	⇩	⇩
VMAT$_2$	⇧	⇩	⇔	⇩
CGA	⇧	⇩	⇩	⇔

FIGURE 3. *Changes in ECL cell gene expression in four experimental models. Size and orientation of vertical arrows indicate relative magnitude and direction of response, respectively. Horizontal arrows signify no change. Column 1, rats treated with omeprazole for 5 days; column 2, chronic atrophic gastritis patients treated with the somatostatin agonist octreotide (25 μg. h^{-1}) for 72h to reverse hypergastrinaemia; column 3, rats fasted for 48h; column 4, gastrin deficient mice (29). Data is taken from published and unpublished studies.*

tion of reg by gastrin, and found mutations of reg in 3 out of 5 hypergastrinaemic patients with ECL cell carcinoid tumors (28). These observations raise the possibility that reg might normally act in a partly autocrine fashion, to limit the actions of hypergastrinaemia in promoting ECL cell growth. If so, then inactivating mutations of reg would expose the ECL cell to the unrestrained growth-promoting effects of gastrin.

OTHER REGULATORS OF THE ECL CELL

The striking, co-ordinated upregulation of HDC, VMAT2 and CGA in response to increased concentrations of gastrin, and reversal of the effect on return to normogastrinaemia (15, 25), might imply that these genes are always regulated in parallel. However, studies across a range of model systems indicate that this is clearly not the case (Figure 3).

For example, it is clear that HDC is particularly sensitive to both acute and chronic changes in circulating gastrin concentrations, whereas the expression of VMAT2 and CGA is not always compromised during hypogastrinaemia. Plainly this reflects, at least in part, the contribution of non-gastrin regulators of ECL cell function in maintaining expression of the latter genes. In this context it is interesting to note the range of stimulatory and inhibitory receptors identified *in vitro* using a variety of techniques including purified ECL cell preparations (Figure 1).

The neuropeptide PACAP is a potent stimulus of ECL cell histamine release, and activates both intracellular calcium and adenylate cyclase through the PAC1 receptor (30), moreover, like gastrin, it is able to stimulate ECL cell growth (31). It is now generally agreed that cholinergic receptors are of little or no significance in directly regulating the ECL cell (30, 32), and it seems possible therefore that PACAP, which is present in gastric nerve fibers (33), is a major physiological neural stimulant of this cell. It is not yet clear if PACAP upregulates expression of the genes essential for histamine biosynthesis and secretion. However, transcriptional responses of VMAT2 and CGA to gastrin and other stimuli are mediated at least in part by phosphorylation and binding of CREB to CRE (19, 21, 34), and PACAP has been shown to activate this cascade in a number of systems, including gut endocrine-type cells (35, 36).

It is well established that somatostatin is an important paracrine inhibitor of a number of gastrointestinal cell types, including G–cells, parietal cells and ECL cells (37). It is also becoming apparent that there are likely to be other physiologically important inhibitors of ECL cell function. Thus both galanin and PYY can potently inhibit histamine release from purified preparations of ECL cells (38), and *in vivo* would most likely operate in neurocrine and endocrine modes, respectively. At least part of the inhibitory actions of these three agents seems likely to be mediated through inhibition of calcium signalling (38, 39). It remains to be established if the physiological inhibitors of ECL cell activity also directly downregulate expression of key genes, and if so, what molecular mechanisms are involved.

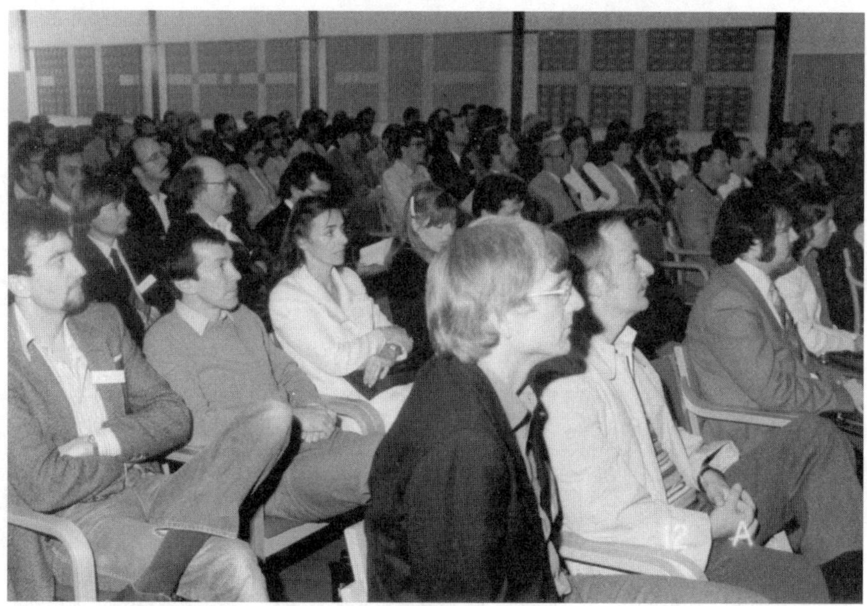

From left to right, first row: Drs. J.H. Walsh and J. Reeve; 2nd row: Dr. R. Dimaline, G. Dockray and Y. Taché. Gut Hormone Meeting, Stockholm Sweden, 1981.

REFERENCES

1. Edkins JS. On the chemical mechanism of gastric secretion. *Proc Roy Soc Ser B* 1905;76:376–76.
2. Bayliss WM, Starling EH. The mechanism of pancreatic secretion. *J Physiol* 1902;28:325–53.
3. Popielski L. β–imidazolylathylamin und die organextrakte. β–imidazolylathylamin als machtiger erreger der magendrusen. *Pflugers Arch* 1920;178:214–36.
4. Gregory RA, Tracy HJ. The constitution and properties of two gastrins extracted from hog antral mucosa. *Gut* 1964;5:103–14.
5. Black JW, Duncan WAM, Durant CJ, Ganellin CR, Parsons E. Definition and antagonism of histamine H2-receptors. *Nature* 1972;236:385–90.
6. Walsh JH, Debas HT, Grossman MI. Pure human big gastrin: immunochemical properties, disappearance half time and acid stimulating action in dogs. *J Clin Invest* 1974;54:477–85.
7. Hakanson R, Bottcher G, Ekblad E, Panula P, Simonsson M, Dohlsten M, Hallberg T, Sundler F. Histamine in endocrine cells in the stomach: a survey of several species using a panel of histamine antibodies. *Histochemistry* 1986;86:5–17.
8. Dimaline R, Sandvik AK. Histidine decarboxylase gene expression in rat fundus is regulated by gastrin. *FEBS Lett* 1991;281:20–22.
9. Sandvik AK, Dimaline R, Marvik R, Brenna E, Waldum HL. Gastrin regulates histidine decarboxylase activity and mRNA abundance in rat oxyntic mucosa. *Am J Physiol* 1994;267:G254–G258.
10. Chen D, Monstein HJ, Nylander AG, Zhao CM, Sundler F, Hakanson R. Acute responses of rat stomach enterochromaffinlike cells to gastrin:secretory activation and adaptation. *Gastroenterology* 1994;107:18–27.
11. Dimaline R, Sandvik AK, Evans D, Forster ER, Dockray GJ. Food stimulation of histidine decarboxylase messenger RNA abundance in rat gastric fundus. *J Physiol* 1993;465:449–58.
12. Simon J-P, Aunis D. Biochemistry of the chromogranin A protein family. *Biochem J* 1989;262:1–13.

13. Wiedenmann B, Huttner WB. Synaptophysin and chromogranins/secretogranins—widespread constituents of distinct types of neuroendocrine vesicles, and new tool in tumor dianosis. *Virchows Arch Cell Pathol* 1989;58:95–121.

14. Dimaline R, Evans D, Forster ER, Sandvik AK, Dockray GJ. Control of gastric corpus chromogranin A messenger RNA abundance in the rat. *Am J Physiol* 1993;264:G583–G588.

15. Dimaline R, Struthers J. Expression and regulation of a vesicular monoamine transporter (VMAT2) in rat stomach: a putative histamine transporter. *J Physiol* 1996;490:249–56.

16. Weihe E, Schafer MKH, Erickson JD, Eiden LE. Localization of vesicular monoamine transporter isoforms (VMAT1 and VMAT2) to endocrine cells and neurons in rat. *J Mol Neur* 1994;5:149–64.

17. Raychowdhury R, Zhang Z, Hocker M, Wang TC. Activation of human histidine decarboxylase gene promoter activity by gastrin is mediated by two distinct nuclear factors. *J Biol Chem* 1999;274: 20961–69.

18. Hocker M, Henihan RJ, Rosewicz S, Riecken EO, Zhang Z, Koh TJ, Wang TC. Gastrin and phorbol 12-myristate 13-acetate regulate the human histidine decarboxylase promoter through Raf-dependent activation of extracellular signal-regulated kinase-related signaling pathways in gastric cancer cells. *J Biol Chem* 1997;272:27015–24.

19. Hocker M, Raychowdhury R, Plath T, Wu H, O'Connor DT, Wiedenmann B, Rosewicz S, Wang TC. Sp 1 and CREB mediate gastrin-dependent regulation of chromogranin A promoter activity in gastric carcinoma cells. *J Biol Chem* 1998;273:34000–07.

20. Hocker M, Cramer T, O'Connor DT, Rosewicz S, Wiedenmann B, Wang TC. Neuroendocrine-specific and gastrin-dependent expression of a chromogranin A-luciferase fusion gene in transgenic mice. *Gastroenterology* 2001;121:43–55.

21. Watson F, Kiernan RS, Deavall DG, Varro A, Dimaline R. Transcriptional activation of the rat vesicular monoamine transporter 2 promoter in gastric epithelial cells: regulation by gastrin. *J Biol Chem* 2001;276:7661–71.

22. Betton GR, Dormer CS, Wells T, Pert P, Price CA, Buckley P. Gastric ECL-cell hyperplasia and carcinoids in rodents following chronic administration of H2-antagonists SK&F 93479 and oxmetidine and omeprazole. *Toxicol Pathol* 1988;16:288–98.

23. Borch K, Renvall H, Liedberg G. Gastric endocrine cell hyperplasia and carcinoid tumors in pernicious anemia. *Gastroenterology* 1985;88:638–48.

24. Bordi C, Yu JY, Baggi MT, Davoli C, Pilato FP, Baruzzi G, Gardini G, Zamboni G, Franzin G, Papotti M. Gastric carcinoids and their precursor lesions. A histologic and immunohistochemical study of 23 cases. *Cancer* 1991;67:663–72.

25. Higham A, Dimaline R, Varro A, Attwood S, Armstrong G, Dockray GJ, Thompson DG. Octreotide suppression test predicts beneficial outcome from antrectomy in a patient with gastric carcinoid tumor. *Gastroenterology* 1998;114:817–22.

26. Debelenko LV, Emmert-Buck MR, Zhuang Z, Epshteyn E, Moskaluk CA, Jensen RT, Liotta LA, Lubensky IA. The multiple endocrine neoplasia type I gene locus is involved in the pathogenesis of type II gastric carcinoids. *Gastroenterology* 1997;113:773–81.

27. Asahara M, Mushiake S, Shimada S, Fukui H, Kinoshita Y, Kawanami C, Watanabe T, Tanaka S, Ichikawa A, Uchiyama Y, Narushima Y, Takasawa S, Okamoto H, Tohyama M, Chiba T. Reg gene expression is increased in rat gastric enterochromaffin-like cells following water immersion stress. *Gastroenterology* 1996;111:45–55.

28. Higham AD, Bishop LA, Dimaline R, Blackmore CG, Dobbins AC, Varro A, Thompson DG, Dockray GJ. Mutations of Reglalpha are associated with enterochromaffin-like cell tumor development in patients with hypergastrinemia. *Gastroenterology* 1999;116:1310–18.

29. Koh TJ, Goldenring JR, Ito S, Mashimo H, Kopin AS, Varro A, Dockray GJ, Wang TC. Gastrin deficiency results in altered gastric differentiation and decreased colonic proliferation in mice. *Gastroenterology* 1997;113:1015–25.

30. Zeng N, Athmann C, Kang T, Lyu RM, Walsh JH, Ohning GV, Sachs G, Pisegna JR . PACAP type I receptor activation regulates ECL cells and gastric acid secretion. *J Clin Invest* 1999;104:1383–91.

31. Pisegna JR, Ohning GV, Athmann C, Zeng N, Walsh JH, Sachs G. Role of PACAP1 receptor in regulation of ECL cells and gastric acid secretion by pituitary adenylate cyclase activating peptide. *Ann NY Acad Sci* 2000;921:233–41.

32. Sandvik AK, Marvik R, Dimaline R, Waldum HL. Carbachol stimulation of gastric acid secretion and its effects on the parietal cell. *Br J Pharmacol* 1998;124:69–74.

33. Sundler F, Ekblad E, Absood A, Hakanson R, Koves K, Arimura A. Pituitary adenylate cyclase activating peptide: a novel vasoactive intestinal peptide-like neuropeptide in the gut. *Neuroscience* 1992;46:439–54.

34. Watson F, Deavall DG, Macro JA, Kiernan R, Dimaline R. Transcriptional activation of vesicular monoamine transporter 2 in the pre-B cell line Ea3.123. *Biochem J* 1999;337:193–99.

35. Delgado M, Munoz-Elias EJ, Kan Y, Gozes I, Fridkin M, Brenneman DE, Gomariz RP, Ganea D. Vasoactive intestinal peptide and pituitary adenylate cyclase-activating polypeptide inhibit tumor necrosis factor alpha transcriptional activation by regulating nuclear factor-kB and cAMP response element-binding protein/c-Jun. *J Biol Chem* 1998;273:31427–36.

36. Deavall, D. G., Raychowdhury, R., Dockray, G. J., and Dimaline, R. Control of CCK gene transcription by PACAP in STC-1 cells. *Am J Physiol* 2000;279:G605–12.

37. Walsh JH. Gastrointestinal Hormones, In: Johnson LR, editor. *Physiology of the Gastrointestinal Tract,* 3 ed. New York: Raven Press; 1994. p. 1–128.

38. Zeng N, Kang T, Wen Y, Wong H, Walsh J, Sachs G. Galanin inhibition of enterochromaffin-like cell function. *Gastroenterology* 1998;115:330–39.

39. Zeng N, Athmann C, Kang T, Walsh JH, Sachs G. Role of neuropeptide-sensitive L-type $Ca^{(2+)}$ channels in histamine release in gastric enterochromaffin-like cells. *Am J Physiol* 1999;277:G1268–G1280.

Gut-Brain Peptides in the New Millennium, edited by Y. Taché
CURE Foundation, Los Angeles, CA. © 2002

6

Neural Regulation of Gastric Endocrine Cells

Ningxin Zeng
Department of Medicine, School of Medicine, Texas Tech University at El Paso, El Paso, TX

George Sachs
*Departments of Physiology and Medicine, VA Greater Los Angeles Healthcare System
University of California–Los Angeles, Los Angeles, CA*

INTRODUCTION

John H. Walsh was a friend, first and foremost, and also a trusted colleague and collaborator. With his untimely death, we lost a gentle, empathetic, hospitable and loving human being. He had an uncanny ability to integrate concepts from many different areas and bring together individuals of disparate interests and temperament. With this, he produced much of significance and contributed greatly to the understanding of gastric physiology. Here we present the last chapter in many of our interactions with him, as a small tribute to his presence.

Gastric acid secretion is the net result of stimulatory and inhibitory mechanisms and is highly regulated (1, 2). Classically, gastric acid secretion is separated into cephalic and peripheral phases of regulation (1, 2). The central nervous system particularly via the vagus is responsible for initiation of gastric acid secretion (1–3). The neural transmitters involved in the cephalic phase present in efferent nerves from the enteric nervous system are less clear. The ability of the non-selective muscarinic antagonist, atropine, to effectively inhibit acid secretion implied that acetylcholine is a major neural mediator of secretion at the level of both endocrine and parietal cells (2–4). However, recent data show that only <10% of the isolated purified ECL cells respond to acetylcholine and H_2 antagonists have no inhibitory effect on carbachol stimulation of parietal cells from rabbits gland arguing that acetylcholine is less involved in transmission from the enteric nervous system than previously thought. However, the parietal cell has a muscarinic M_3 receptor capable of direct stimulation of this acid secreting cell (2, 5, 6). About 60% of centrally stimulated acid secretion in the rat is blocked by H_2 antagonism (3, 4), suggesting that neural mediation of ECL cell histamine release must be present to explain this effect of H_2 antagonists.

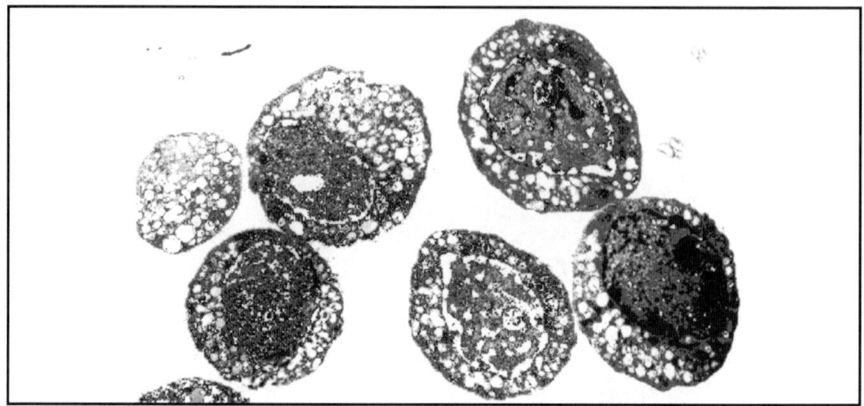

FIGURE 1. *The structure of ECL cells. Electron microscopic images of purified ECL cell preparation (original magnification 4000×).*

The gastric mucosa is extrinsically innervated by vagal afferent and efferent nerve fibers, by sympathetic fibers from the celiac ganglion, and by sensory fibers from the dorsal root of the spinal cord and is intrinsically innervated by neurons originating in the myenteric plexus (7). There are three major types of intrinsic neurons in the rat oxyntic mucosa containing different neuropeptides (7). The first class contains dominantly vasoactive intestinal polypeptide (VIP), gastrin releasing peptide (GRP) and pituitary adenylate cyclase activating peptide (PACAP). The second class contains neuropeptide Y (NPY) and VIP (7, 8). The third class contains galanin (9). In animal studies, almost all the above neuropeptides seem involved in the regulation of gastric acid secretion, but their targets cannot be defined in the intact animal. Thus, neural regulation of gastric acid secretion could be directly via receptors on parietal cell or indirectly via gastric endocrine cells. This paper focuses on the role of gastric endocrine cell as a link in neural mediation of regulation of gastric acid secretion.

Certainly, some of the data determined on isolated cell systems came as a surprise to John. Once convinced of their relevance, he encouraged us to pursue this topic with multiple suggestions and always constructive criticism of our reductionist approach that contrasted with his integrative organ instincts. The combinations of our talents, we hope, served to further the field of regulation of gastric acid secretion.

ISOLATION OF GASTRIC ENDOCRINE CELLS

Peripheral regulation of acid secretion depends on the functional status of at least 3 endocrine cells present in the gastric epithelium, the fundic enterochromaffin-like (ECL) cell, the antral gastrin (G) cell and the fundic and antral somatostatin (D) cells (2, 10). The interplay between the endocrine cells of the stomach has been elucidated by studies of response to injection of substances *in vivo* and by studies of the response of isolated cells either in terms of calcium signaling or release of ligand (2, 11).

The ECL cells produce and store histamine (12, 13). This biogenic amine is stored in vesicles to give a total content of 2.8–4.3 pg/cell of histamine, which is a relatively low amount compared to mast cells (12–20 pg/cell). As for other gastric endocrine cells, this is a small, ca. 10μ diameter cell found mostly towards the base of the fundic gastric gland. It contains acidic vacuoles with an eccentric electron dense spot (12). The ECL cell has been found to play a key stimulatory role by releasing histamine that stimulates acid secretion from fundic gland parietal cells (14). The major stimulatory endocrine peptide for histamine release from ECL cells is gastrin released from antral G cells. Both ligand-stimulus coupling in antral G cell and fundic ECL cell are inhibited by somatostatin released from antral and fundic D cells acting at a type 2 SST receptor subtype.

There are various means of identifying these cell types. Fluorescence microscopy can visualize the vacuoles of ECL cell accumulating acridine orange due to their acidity, resulting in a red fluorescence characteristic of acid spaces. Because ECL cell contain vacuoles rather than granules (such as G and D cells) they are somewhat less dense and can be purified almost to homogeneity from a gastric epithelial cell suspension. A combination of elutriation (to select a small cell population) and Nykodenz gradient centrifugation produces an ECL enriched population (>65%) (15). 48 hr culture in growth medium results in a cell population containing about 90% ECL cells (Figure 1). This model enables extensive studies of Ca^{2+} signaling and histamine release stimulated or inhibited by different ligands (16–20). A large number of receptors present on the ECL cell have been identified directly, by video imaging of calcium signaling, by PCR of a ECL cell cDNA library or RT/PCR of RNA isolated from ECL cells and also by measurements of histamine release from the ~90% pure population of these cells (15–22).

Compared to the ECL cell, the isolation of the D cell and G cell has been more difficult because of cell number, similar density and/or antral location. A relative high D cell yield was achieved by modifying the density gradient (7–12%) after elutriation, followed by cell culture (20–41%). The highest yield of antral G cells (20–30%) was achieved by elutriation and FACS followed by culture. Studies of the cells that have been enriched are also difficult since there are multiple ligands producing different end effects. Many of these ligands can also be released into the medium bathing a mixed endocrine cell population generating secondary effects. In order to identify explicitly each receptor present on a single cell type, we use a single cell approach by Ca^{2+} imaging system with constant superfusion. This system not only enables identification of specific types of endocrine cells by their characteristic Ca^{2+} signaling response to different ligands, but also helps identify new ligands, especially neuropeptides, that may play a role in the functional regulation of these endocrine cells (21).

PACAP AS A CANDIDATE NEUROPEPTIDE IN NEURAL STIMULATION OF GASTRIC ACID SECRETION BY MODULATING GASTRIC ENDOCRINE CELL FUNCTIONS

PACAP was first isolated from ovine hypothalamus and named on the basis of its ability to stimulate adenylate cyclase in primary anterior pituitary cells by Miyata, et al. in 1989 (23). This peptide is structurally related to the secretin family and has a 67% sequence homology with VIP. PACAP has two bioactive forms, PACAP-38 and PACAP-27. The amino acid sequence of PACAP has been conserved during evolution which may be related to its important physiological role. PACAP is widely distributed in neurons, including those of the gastrointestinal tract. PACAP-immunoreactive fibers were seen in the gastric mucosa of mouse, rat, hamster, and man, but not in the other species examined (8). PACAP immunoreactive cells appeared in the developing glands of the stomach starting in 18- and 20-week old fetuses. Neonatal treatment with capsaicin significantly reduced the concentration of PACAP-38 in the esophagus, stomach, and colon (24). Extrinsic denervation decreased the PACAP-38 concentration in the stomach indicating that PACAP- immunoreactive nerve fibers in the stomach originate from both intrinsic (enteric) and extrinsic (presumably sensory) sources suggesting that PACAP may have diverse actions on gastric physiology (24).

ECL Cells

Histamine release from ECL cells is a major mechanism for stimulation of acid secretion from parietal cells. Presumably, the histamine released has a privileged diffusion pathway to the parietal cells that are largely superficial to the ECL cells which are at the base of the fundic gastric gland. Releasing histamine from ECL cell is the major pathway of gastrin stimulation of gastric acid secretion.

The discovery of a stimulating PACAP receptor on ECL cells was serendipitous when we initially applied PACAP to identify D cells from a mixed gastric fundic endocrine cell population that included only 20–30% D cell. Based on the initial animal data that showed PACAP could inhibit gastric secretion via a possible pathway of inhibition of somatostatin release

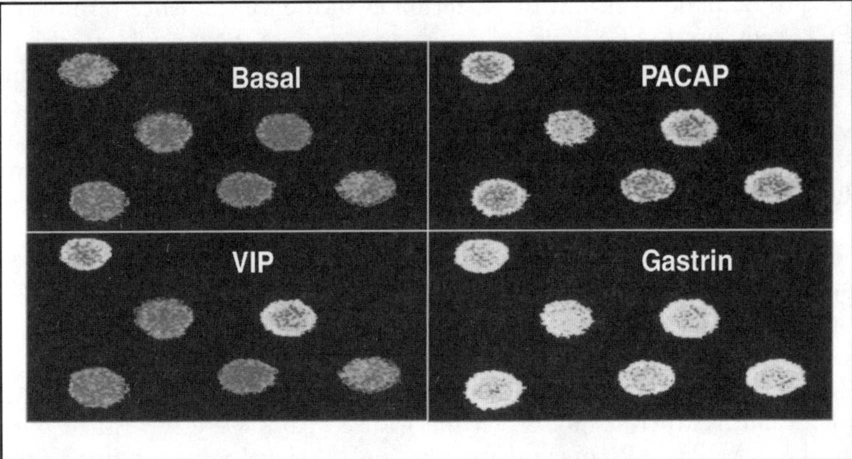

FIGURE 2. *Ca^{2+} signaling induced by PACAP, VIP and gastrin in ECL and D cells. Cells were loaded with 2 (M Fura-2AM for 30 min at 37°C, and then washed with growth medium and placed in a heated chamber (Medical Systems, Greenvale, NY). The temperature was maintained constant at 37°C. The cover slip was perfused with Ringer's buffer without or with the indicated peptides (PACAP-38, VIP or gastrin) at a rate of 5 ml/min, and there was constant superfusion with a peristaltic pump. Fura-2 fluorescence was measured by using a Nikon Fluo X40 objective with a Zeiss Axiovert 100TV microscope (Zeiss, Thornwood, NY) connected to a PC-XT computer programmed to rapidly alternate between the excitation wavelengths of 340 and 380 nm. Image pairs were captured under the control of Image-1/FL software (Universal Imaging, West Chester, PA) and expressed as the ratio of brightness level in the chosen field. PACAP and gastrin raise Ca^{2+} both in ECL cells and D cells, but VIP only raised Ca^{2+} signal in D cells. The data in the figures are averages of at least four experiments.*

from D cells, we expected that PACAP might elicit Ca^{2+} signals from D cells which would allow us to differentiate D cells from ECL cells in this mixed cell population. Surprisingly, PACAP-38 elicited a Ca^{2+} spike in more than 70–80% cells in this cell population that contained only 20–30% D cells (Figure 2). The interpretation of this was that ECL cells also have a PACAP receptor because 40–50% of cells in this population were ECL cells. Then, we applied PACAP to a population of about 85–90% pure ECL cells and found that essentially all the ECL cells in the preparation responded to PACAP with a peak of released intracellular Ca^{2+} of about 1.3 µM (25, 26) followed by a steady sustained Ca^{2+} influx.

PACAP binds to the VIP type 1 and 2 (VPAC1 and VPAC2) receptor subtypes but with higher affinity to the PACAP type 1 (PAC1) receptor. PAC1 has been cloned and exists as four major splice variants that are functionally coupled to both adenylate cyclase and phospholipase C (27).

A typical G7 biphasic calcium signal is obtained in the ECL cell. This implies that the PACAP G7 receptor is coupled to a G$_q$ or G$_{11}$ trimeric protein in the gastric ECL cell. Immunohistochemical staining using anti-PACAP receptor antibodies against the C terminus showed its presence on isolated ECL cells or in ECL cells of rat gastric mucosa. Western blot analysis showed that it was present as a 48 kDa protein on membrane preparations of 85% pure ECL cells (28). RT/PCR confirmed the presence of all splice variants of the receptor in the ECL cell preparation but no VIP1/PACAP or VIP2/PACAP receptors were found. Paralleling the Ca^{2+} signal response, PACAP-27 and PACAP-38 (EC_{50} 0.1nM) also dose dependently increased histamine release with an EC_{50} of 1 nM (26, 28).

The isolated rabbit gastric fundic gland is probably the simplest integrated secretory component that has been studied to elucidate mechanisms of stimulation of acid secretion as well as mechanisms of acid secretion per se (29). The advent of confocal microscopy has now enabled direct studies of signaling pathways in the ECL and parietal cells in this three-dimensional multicellular structure (6). When the gastric glands were superfused with 10–100 nM PACAP containing media, a Ca^{2+} signal was seen first in the ECL cell followed by a signal in adjacent parietal cells. In the presence of ranitidine, although the Ca^{2+} signal was retained in the ECL cell, the calcium signal was abolished in the parietal cell, indicating that the effect of PACAP on parietal cell Ca^{2+} signaling was secondary to histamine release from the ECL cell (6, 26). This result suggests that PACAP, rather than acetylcholine (since there was no carbachol stimulated signal in the ECL cell, only the parietal cell), is the neural mediator for ECL cell activation. PACAP links neural to paracrine stimulation of acid secretion (26).

PACAP also showed dose dependent stimulation of ECL cell growth *in vivo* (29). Chronic administration of PACAP (10 pmol/h for seven days) via an osmotic pump resulted in a more than twofold increase in bromo-deoxyuridine (BrdU) incorporation into ECL cells (31). It seems that PACAP effects resemble those of gastrin on ECL cell function. It stimulates histamine release and, can also stimulate ECL cell proliferation.

D Cells

As mentioned above, PACAP raises Ca^{2+} in D cells indicating functional PACAP receptor expression on D cells as well as ECL cells. VIP application resulted in a biphasic signal of Ca^{2+} only in D cells, whereas PACAP produced a signal in both cell types (Figure 2). Both VIP and PACAP induced dose dependent somatostatin release suggesting D cell may express VPAC rather than PAC1 whereas ECL cells express only PAC1 (25).

Early studies had shown that the effect of PACAP on acid secretion when given *in vivo* appears to be that of inhibition. These results are inconsistent with the effects observed on the isolated ECL cell. A possible explanation is that at these high doses intravenously, not only is the PACAP receptor stimulated on the ECL cell but a PACAP/VIP receptor is stimulated on the fundic D cell. In the isolated D cell population, PACAP and VIP induced somatostatin release equally. The somatostatin released acting at the SST2 receptor could then overwhelm the stimulation by PACAP at the PAC1 receptor on the ECL cell. Accordingly, rats were treated with both PACAP and neutralizing somatostatin antibody and this treatment converted the inhibitory action of IV PACAP to that of gastric stimulation (26). Recently Sandvik, et al. reported that vagally stimulated acid secretion was found to be inhibited partially by a PACAP antagonist, suggesting that PACAP play an important role in the neural regulation of gastric acid secretion (32).

From these data, it would seem likely that PACAP is acting as a neural mediator of gastric acid secretion by stimulation of the ECL cell and histamine release but at higher concentrations is also able to stimulate the fundic D cell to release somatostatin and inhibit ECL cell histamine release. Somatostatin may also have a direct effect on the parietal cell (26).

A possibility is that there are privileged pathways for PACAP release, locally in the vicinity of the ECL cell and at higher levels in the vicinity of fundic or antral D cells. Alternatively, VIP may be the mediator released in the vicinity of the D cell and PACAP may never achieve the concentration required to activate the VIP receptor on the D cell.

G Cells

Neuropeptides such as GRP stimulate gastric acid secretion indirectly via gastrin release from antral G cells (33). To determine whether PACAP could modulate antral G cell function, a relative high yield isolated rat antral G cell population by FACS was used for Ca^{2+} imaging and gastrin release studies. PACAP over a wide range of concentrations (100 pM to 100 nM) showed no Ca^{2+} stimulating or inhibiting signals in G cells that were identified by Ca^{2+} spikes induced by GRP but not CCK-8 (21). Further, PACAP-27 nor PACAP-38 showed an increased gastrin release from this population. However, PACAP showed a moderate but significant inhibition of GRP-induced gastrin release, reflecting the release of somatostin from contaminating D cells in this preparation since neutralizing somatostatin–antibody completely blocked the inhibitory effect of PACAP.

GALANIN AS A MAJOR NEUROPEPTIDE IN NEURAL INHIBITION OF GASTRIC ACID SECRETION TARGETING AT GASTRIC ENDOCRINE CELLS

Galanin is a 29-amino acid neuropeptide initially identified in the porcine intestine and now known to be widely distributed in central and peripheral neurons (9). Galanin has several functions in the central nervous system. In

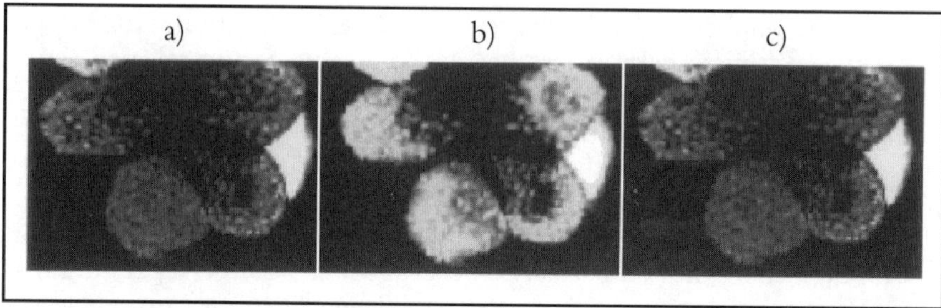

FIGURE 3. *Galanin inhibited PACAP induced Ca^{2+} signaling in the rabbit gland. The experiments were conducted on a Zeiss LSM 410 confocal microscope using a 63× objective and a 10× eyepiece. A 100× objective was used to observe the origin of the $[Ca^{2+}]_{in}$ signal using Fluo-4AM as the Ca^{2+} dye. The glands were excited at 488 nm and emission fluorescence, reflecting changes of $[Ca^{2+}]_{in}$ monitored at 510–525nm. Subsequent images were followed over the same area at 2 sec intervals and stored on a hard disc. At baseline, the ECL cell has a larger $[Ca^{2+}]_{in}$ signal than parietal cells (lane a). PACAP (10 nM) stimulates an increase of intracellular calcium in ECL cells followed by elevation of intracellular calcium in parietal cells adjacent to ECL cells (lane b). In the presence of ranitidine, although the calcium signal was retained in the ECL cell, the calcium signal was abolished in the parietal cell, indicating that the effect of PACAP on parietal cell calcium signaling was secondary to histamine release from the ECL cell (data not shown) (6). This effect has suggested that PACAP is the neural mediator for ECL cell activation and PACAP links neural to paracrine stimulation of acid secretion. When 100 nM galanin was introduced, the $[Ca^{2+}]_{in}$ signals in both ECL and parietal cells superfused with 10nM PACAP were completely inhibited (lane c). Each experiment is representative of at least 4 such experiments.*

addition, galanin has also been reported to have an inhibitory effect on insulin secretion in man and in the canine pancreas. Galanin has been shown to be present in high abundance in the neural elements of mucosal, submucosal and muscle layers of the stomach. Human gastric mucosa expresses galanin receptor mRNA suggesting that this peptide may be important in neurally-mediated inhibition of acid secretion. In rats, galanin inhibits basal and pentagastrin stimulated gastric secretion, as well as bombesin stimulated gastric secretion. Galanin has no effect on gastric acid secretion stimulated by bethanechol. Similarly, in dogs, galanin inhibits gastric secretion stimulated by bombesin but not that stimulated by ether bethanechol or histamine suggesting that galanin may target gastric endocrine cells (34, 35).

G Cells

An inhibitory effect of galanin on isolated rat antral G cells was initially reported by Wolfgang, et al. (36). Galanin was found to inhibit bombesin-stimulated gastrin release from isolated rat G cells in primary culture (36). In addition, galanin also inhibited basal and GRP-stimulated gastrin release in isolated stomachs.

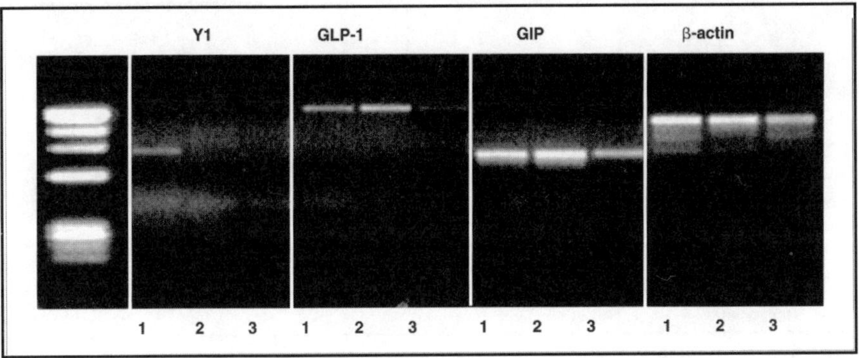

FIGURE 4. *Multiple neuropeptides expressed on gastric isolated cells. RNA was extracted from 1 gram of purified ECL cells (lane 1) parietal cells (lane 2) and chief cells (lane 3) using the Fast Track RNA Purification® kit (Invitrogen. La Jolla, CA). Total RNA (5 μg) from enriched rat ECL cells was used to synthesize cDNA by reverse transcriptase with oligo dT primers (Boehringer-Mannheim). PCR was performed in low salt Taq+ DNA polymerase buffer and 5 units Taq+ DNA polymerase (Stratagene, La Jolla, CA) in the presence of oligonucleotide primers under the following conditions: initial step (one cycle): 94°C for 2 min, 57°C for 1 min and 72°C for 2 min; followed by 94°C for 1 min, 57°C for 1 min, and 72°C for 2 min (30 cycles); and a final extension step (one cycle) at 94°C for 1 min, 57°C for 1 min, and 72° for 15 min. Amplified products were purified from 0.7% agarose gels using the Quiex Gel Extraction Kit®, subcloned into plasmid pCR-Script Amp SK(+) (Stratagene, La Jolla, CA). DNA sequence analysis was performed with 500 fmol of extracted DNA product using a DNA Autoanalyzer (ABT).*

Using an enriched rat G cell preparation, by combining elutriation and FACS, we found galanin inhibited basal and GRP induced Ca^{2+} signaling, indicating a direct effect of galanin on the G cell (unpublished observations).

ECL Cells

However, this direct action of galanin on antral G cells can not explain all the *in vivo* results. Galanin also inhibits pentagastrin-stimulated acid secretion (32) and high abundance galanin-immunoreactive neuronal fibers are present in the gastric fundus, indicating a possible direct action of galanin on fundic endocrine or exocrine cells (9). The effect of galanin on the isolated ECL cell was determined again by measuring the Ca^{2+} signaling and histamine release. Galanin dose-dependently inhibited gastrin-stimulated histamine release with an IC_{50} of 10^{-10} M as did the N terminal (1–13) fragment of galanin with tenfold lower affinity. PTX partially blocked this inhibitory effect as did a galanin inhibitor, galantide. Other galanin inhibitors such as galanin spantide I or galanin (1–13)-pro-pro-(ala-leu)2-ala had no effect. Both Ca^{2+} release and elevation of Ca^{2+} entry due to gastrin stimulation of the CCK-B receptor were inhibited by equimolar concentrations of

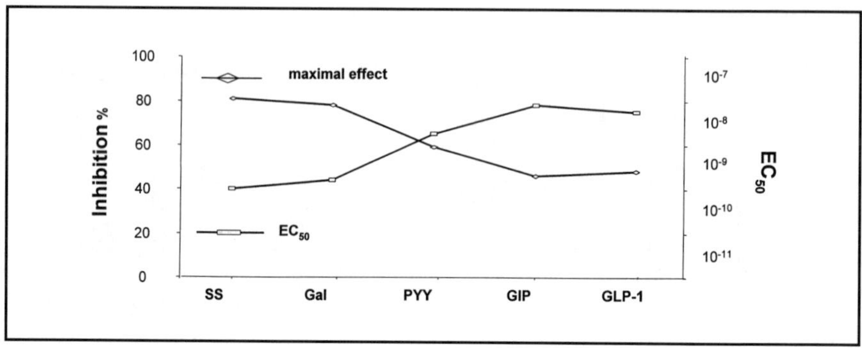

FIGURE 5. *Peptides and ECL cell function. This figure provides a summary of various neuropeptides we have found that are able to inhibit ECL cell function in terms of histamine release and Ca^{2+} signals showing equipotency of somatostatin and galanin. The high concentrations required for GIP and GLP query their physiological role in regulation of this cell type.*

galanin. This pharmacology of the galanin receptor on the ECL cell distinguishes it from the brain receptor (37). Compared to 60% of maximal inhibition of histamine release induced by gastrin, galanin almost completely inhibited PACAP stimulated histamine release (38, 39).

D Cells

No effect of galanin on isolated D cells was observed in terms of either Ca^{2+} signaling or somatostatin release. The inhibitory effect of galanin on ECL cell function was not affected by pretreatment with somatostatin-neutralizing antibody indicating the action is not indirect by release of somatostatin (32, 40).

In the perfused rabbit fundic gastric gland model, galanin also significantly inhibited PACAP induced Ca^{2+} signals in ECL cell and parietal cells (Figure 3) but had no effect on carbachol induced signals in parietal cells (data not shown). Inhibition of GRP-stimulated gastrin release and gastrin-stimulated histamine release from the ECL cell are the likely mechanism of acid secretion inhibition by galanin *in vivo*.

Besides the galanin receptor expressed on ECL cells, many other neuropeptide receptors are also found to be expressed in ECL cell, including receptors for PYY/NPY, GIP and GLP (Figure 4). PYY inhibited gastrin induced Ca^{2+} influx but had no effect on basal Ca or peak Ca^{2+} release. Compared with galanin and somatostatin, PYY required relatively high concentrations for inhibitory effects.

The inhibitory effects of these various peptides on ECL cell function are summarized in Figure 5. As we see from the figure, galanin is almost equipotent to somatotatin in inhibition of ECL cell function. Galanin is thus a

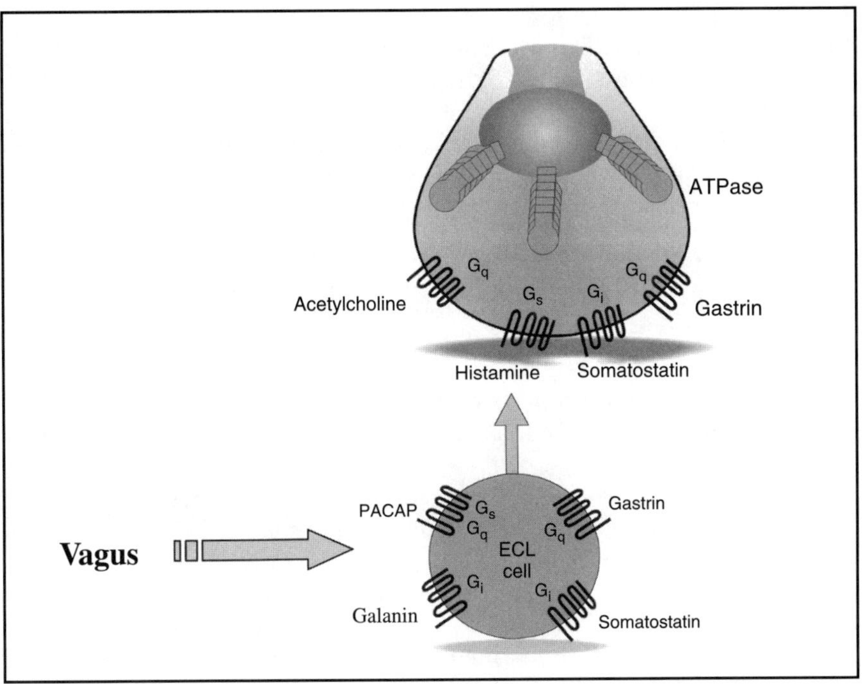

FIGURE 6. *A model of the role of gastric ECL cell as an important link in neural mediation of regulation of gastric acid secretion by modulation of histamine release by both endocrine and neuropeptide receptors.*

neuropeptide that may be involved in the neural regulation of gastric acid secretion by inhibiting both histamine release from fundic ECL cell and gastrin release from antral G cell.

CONCLUSION

The peripheral regulation of gastric acid secretion is achieved by interplay among at least three major gastric endocrine cells: the fundic enterochromaffin-like (ECL) cell, the antral gastrin (G) cell, and the fundic and antral somatostatin (D) cells. Receptor mapping showed that several neuropeptide receptors are expressed on gastric endocrine cells indicating their role as an important link in neural and endocrine mediation of regulation of gastric acid secretion. The effect of neuropeptides on the gastric ECL-like cell, D cell, and antral G cell has been studied in a purified cell preparation by video imaging of calcium signaling and measurements of histamine, somatostatin and gastrin release, respectively. The interaction between endocrine and parietal cells has been studied in gastric fundic glands by confocal microscopy.

Isolated ECL cells express PAC1 as shown by RT-PCR and anti–PAC1 AB staining. PACAP-27 and –38 dose-dependently raise Ca^{2+} in ECL cell and stimulate histamine release. PACAP and VIP are equipotent for release of somatostatin from D cells via a receptor subtype that is different from the PAC1 on ECL cells. Confocal studies of isolated fundic rabbit glands showed that PACAP induced histamine dependent stimulation of parietal cell. *In vivo*, vagal stimulation induced gastric acid secretion that is partially inhibited by PACAP antagonists indicating that central stimulation of acid secretion by alteration of ECL cell function is mediated, in part, by PACAP receptors on the ECL cell which activate calcium signaling and histamine release. PACAP-27 also dose dependently stimulated ECL cell proliferation. Chronic administration of PACAP (10 pmol/h for seven days) via osmotic pump resulted in a more than twofold increase in BrdU incorporation into ECL cells. PACAP has no effect on Ca^{2+} signaling and gastrin release from antral G cells.

RT-PCR of ECL cell RNA showed a galanin type I receptor subtype. Galanin significantly inhibited basal and gastrin induced Ca^{2+} mobilization and histamine release. Galanin has no effects on somatostatin release from D cells. Galanin also inhibits GRP induced Ca^{2+} signaling and gastrin release from isolated antral G cells.

Therefore, the gastric endocrine cells play a key role in neural regulation of gastric acid secretion with PACAP and galanin being candidate neuropeptides for positive and negative neural mediation of the regulation of gastric acid secretion (Figure 6).

ACKNOWLEDGMENTS

Supported in part by USVA and NIH grant #'s DK46917, 53462, 41301 and 17294.

REFERENCES

1. Walsh JH. Gastrointestinal Hormones. In: *Physiology of the Gastrointestinal Tract*. Ed. by Johnson LR, Raven Press, New York, 1994;1–129.

2. Sachs G. Regulation of gastric acid secretion. In: *Acid Related Diseases.* ed by Modlin IM and Sachs G. Schneztor-Verlag GmbH Konstanz, 1998;37–110.

3. Taché Y. Central nervous system regulation of acid secretion. In: *Physiology of the Gastrointestinal Tract,* Ed. Johnson LR, 2nd ed., Vol. 2, Raven Press, New York, 1987;911

4. Yanagisawa K, Yang H, Walsh JH, and Taché Y. Role of acetylcholine, histamine and gastrin in the acid response to intracisternal injection of the TRH analog, RX 77368, in the rat. *Regul Pept* 1990; 27:161–170.

5. Zeng N, Walsh JH, Kang T, Helander K, Helander HF and Sachs G. Selective ligand induced intracellular calcium changes in a population of isolated gastric endocrine cells. *Gastroenterology* 1996;110:1833–1846

6. Athmann C, Zeng N, Scott DR, Sachs G. Regulation of parietal cell calcium signaling in gastric glands. *Am J Physiol Gastrointest Liver Physiol* 2000;279:G1048–58.

7. Sundler F, Ekblad E, Hakanson R. The neuroendocrine system of the gut—an update. *Acta Oncol* 1991;30:419–27.

8. Sundler F, Erblad E, Absood A, Hakanson R, Koves K and Armura A. Pituitary Adenylate Cyclase-Activating Polypeptide: A novel vasoactive intestinal peptide-like neuropeptide in the gut. *Neuroscience* 1992;46:439–454.

9. Ekblad E, Rokaeus A, Hakanson R, Sundler F. Galanin nerve fibers in the rat gut: distribution, origin and projections. *Neuroscience* 1985;16:355–63.

10. Sachs G, Zeng N, Prinz C. Physiology of isolated gastric endocrine cells. *Ann Rev Physiol* 1997;59: 243–56.

11. Hakanson R and Owman C. Concomitant histochemical demonstration of histamine and catecholamines in enterochromaffin-like cells of gastric mucosa. *Life Sci* 1967;6:759–766.

12. Solcia E., Capella C, Buffa R, Usellini L, Fiocca R, Sessa F. Endocrine cells of the digestive system. In: *Physiology of the Gastrointestinal Tract,* Ed. by Johnson, LR, 2nd ed. 1987;111–130.

13. Andersson K, Mattson H and Larsson H. The role of gastric mucosal histamine in acid secretion and experimentally induced lesions in the rat. *Digestion* 1990;46:1–9.

14. Soll AH, Lewin KJ, Beaven MA. Isolation of histamine-containing cells from rat gastric mucosa: Biochemical and morphological differences from mast cells. *Gastroenterology* 1980;80:717–727.

15. Prinz C, Kajimura M, Scott DR, Mercier F, Helander HF, and Sachs G. Histamine secretion from rat enterochromaffinlike cells. *Gastroenterology* 1993;105:449–461.

16. Prinz C, Sachs G, Walsh JH, Coy DH and Wu SV. The somatostatin receptor subtype on rat enterochromaffin-like cells. *Gastroenterology* 1994;107:1067–1074.

17. Prinz C, Scott DR, Hurwitz D, Helander HF and Sachs G. Gastrin effects on isolated rat enterochromaffin-like cells in primary culture. *Am J Physiol* 1994;267:G663-G675.

18. Sandor A, Kidd M, Lawton GP, Miu K, Tang LH and Modlin IM. Neurohormonal modulation of rat enterochromaffin-like cell histamine secretion. *Gastroenterology* 1996;110:1084–92.

19. Zeng N, Walsh JH, Kang T, Wu SV, Sachs G. Peptide YY inhibition of rat gastric enterochromaffin-like cell function. *Gastroenterology* 1997;112:127–35.

20. Lindstrom E, Bjorkqvist M, Boketoft A, Chen D, Zhao CM, Kimura K, Hakanson R. Neurohormonal regulation of histamine and pancreastatin secretion from isolated rat stomach ECL cells. *Regul Pept* 1997;15:71:73–86.

21. Zeng N and Sachs G. Properties of Gastric Enterchromaffin-like Cells. *Yale J Biol Med* 1998;71: 161–172.

22. Lindstrom E, Hakanson R. Neurohormonal regulation of secretion from isolated rat stomach ECL cells: a critical reappraisal. *Regul Pept* 2001;2;97:169–80.

23. Miyata A, Arimura A, Dahl RR, Minamino N, Uehara A, Jiang L, Culler MD, Coy DH. Isolation of a novel 38 residue-hypothalamic polypeptide which stimulates adenylate cyclase in pituitary cells. *Biochem Biophys Res Commun* 989;164:567–74, 1.

24. Hannibal J, Ekblad E, Mulder H, Sundler F, Fahrenkrug J. Pituitary adenylate cyclase activating polypeptide (PACAP) in the gastrointestinal tract of the rat: distribution and effects of capsaicin or denervation. *Cell Tissue Res* 1998;291:65–79.

25. Zeng N, Bayle DB, Walsh, JH, Kang T, Sachs G. Localization of PACAP receptor on rat fundic ECL cell and D cells. *Gastroenterology* 1996;110:A1136.

26. Zeng N, Athmann C, Kang T, Lyu RM, Walsh JH, Ohning GV, Sachs G and Pisegna JR. PACAP type 1 receptor activation regulates ECL cells and gastric acid secretion. *J Clin Invest* 1999;104: 1383–91.

27. Pisegna JR, Wank SA. Cloning and characterization of the signal transduction of four splice variants of the human pituitary adenylate cyclase activating polypeptide receptor. Evidence for dual coupling to adenylate cyclase and phospholipase C. *J Biol Chem* 1996;271:17267–74.

28. Zeng N, Kang T, Lyu RM, Wong H, Wen Y, Walsh JH, Sachs G, Pisegna JR. The pituitary adenylate cyclase activating polypeptide type 1 receptor (PAC1-R) is expressed on gastric ECL cells: evidence by immunocytochemistry and RT-PCR. *Ann NY Acad Sci* 1998;11;865:147–56.

29. Berglindh T, Helander HF, and Obrink KJ. Effects of secretagogues on oxygen consumption, aminopyrine accumulation and morphology in isolated gastric glands. *Acta Physiol Scand* 1976;97: 401–414.

30. Lauffer JM, Modlin IM, Hinoue T, Kidd M, Zhang T, Schmid SW and Tang LH. Pituitary adenylate cyclase-activating polypeptide modulates gastric enterochromaffin-like cell proliferation in rats. *Gastroenterology* 1999;116:623–35.

31. Pisegna JR, Ohning GV, Athmann C, Zeng N, Walsh JH, Sachs G. Role of PACAP1 receptor in regulation of ECL cells and gastric acid secretion by pituitary adenylate cyclase activating peptide. *Ann NY Acad Sci* 2000;921:233–41.

32. Sandvik AK, Cui G, Bakke I, Munkvold B, Waldum HL. PACAP stimulates gastric acid secretion in the rat by inducing histamine release. *Am J Physiol* 2001;281:G997–G1003.

33. Schubert ML, Makhlouf GM. Neural regulation of gastrin and somatostatin secretion in rat gastric antral mucosa. *Am J Physiol* 1987;253:G721-G725.

34. Kato S, Korolkiewicz R, Rekowski P, Szyk A, Sugawa Y, Takeuchi K. Inhibition of gastric acid secretion by galanin in rats. Relation to endogenous histamine release. *Regul Pept* 1998;24;74:53–9.

35. Kisfalvi I Jr, Burghardt B, Balint A, Zelles T, Vizi ES, Varga G. Antisecretory effects of galanin and its putative antagonists M15, M35 and C7 in the rat stomach. *J Physiol Paris* 2000;94:37–42.

36. Schepp W, Prinz C, Tatge C, Hakanson R, Schusdziarra V, Classen M. Galanin inhibits gastrin release from isolated rat gastric G-cells. *Am J Physiol* 1990;258:G596–602.

37. Zeng N, Kang T, Wen Y, Wong H, Walsh J, Sachs G. Galanin inhibition of enterochromaffin-like cell function. *Gastroenterology* 1998;115:330–9.

38. Zeng N, Athmann C, Kang T, Walsh JH, Sachs G. Role of neuropeptide-sensitive L-type Ca^{2+} channels in histamine release in gastric enterochromaffin-like cells. *Am J Physiol* 1999;277:G1268–80.

39. Lindstrom E, Eliasson L, Bjorkqvist M, Hakanson R. Gastrin and the neuropeptide PACAP evoke secretion from rat stomach histamine-containing (ECL) cells by stimulating influx of Ca^{2+} through different $Ca^{(2+)}$ channels. *J Physiol* 2001;15;535:663–77.

40. Zeng N, Sachs G. Properties of isolated gastric enterochromaffin-like cells. *Yale J Biol Med* 1998;71:233–46.

Gut-Brain Peptides in the New Millennium, edited by Y. Taché
CURE Foundation, Los Angeles, CA. © 2002

7

Enterogastric Regulation of Gastric Acid Secretion

Kevin C. Kent Lloyd
*Center for Comparative Medicine, School of Veterinary Medicine
University of California, Davis, CA*

INTRODUCTION

While John Harley Walsh probably is most famous for his seminal scientific contributions to our understanding of the physiological role of gastrin in the stimulation of gastric acid secretion, his research investigations into the study of acid inhibition are no less significant. In the latter half of his career, John published more than 100 papers of original primary and collaborative research focusing on inhibitory pathways and mechanisms that directly or indirectly turn-off parietal cell secretory activity. His contributions included new discoveries and novel hypotheses that have culminated in a substantial advancement in our understanding of the regulation of gastric acid secretion.

PHYSIOLOGY OF THE MAMMALIAN STOMACH

Gastric Function

The function of the stomach is to receive and to accommodate food in preparation for digestion into their constitutive elements. Acid and pepsin secreted by the stomach mix with luminal contents and hydrolyze proteins into peptides and amino acids. These products, plus dietary fat and partially hydrolyzed sugars, are emptied into the duodenum where further processing occurs before absorption by the intestinal epithelium. The mechanisms controlling acid secretion and emptying are coordinated at three levels (brain, stomach, and bowel) and are capable of responding to changes in content and volume of a meal.

Regulation of Gastric Acid Secretion

Gastric acid secretion is regulated by both stimulatory and inhibitory mechanisms during three phases of digestion of a meal: cephalic, gastric, and intestinal (26). The cephalic phase is elicited by the thought, smell, taste, and swallowing of food. This effect is mediated by vagal reflex pathways and can account for up to 40% of maximum acid output. The gastric phase begins once the swallowed meal enters the stomach. Distention of the stomach stimulates acid secretion by vagal (cholinergic) reflex stimulation of parietal cells and to a lesser extent by gastrin. Cephalic phase inhibitory mechanisms have been demonstrated by central injection of bombesin and corticotropin releasing factor. Further, vagal regulation of an inhibitor of gastrin-stimulated secretion in the gastric fundus may exist.

By far, the gastric phase is predominated by the activation of acid stimulatory pathways, principally through meal-stimulated release of gastrin. Partially digested proteins, peptides, and amino acids cause antral "G" cells to release gastrin into the circulation. Gastrin stimulates parietal cell secretion directly and indirectly through release of histamine from enterochromaffin-like cells in the gastric fundus. Acidification of the antrum suppresses gastrin release and is the principal mechanism of gastric phase inhibition of acid secretion.

In contrast, acid secretion stimulated during the intestinal phase represents a relatively modest fraction of maximal acid output. Lumenal distention and partially digested proteins emptied from the stomach enhance acid secretion, mediated probably through vagal and/or splanchnic reflexes. On the other hand, as gastric contents enter the duodenum and the need for gastric acid-assisted digestion wanes, several mechanisms elicit profound inhibition of acid output. Physiological "feedback inhibition" of acid secretion in response to dietary nutrients (and distention) of the intestine and colon is often referred to as the enterogastric "reflex", although the pathways are not all neural, as suggested by the name.

ENTEROGASTRIC INHIBITION OF GASTRIC ACID SECRETION

The Enterogastric "Reflex"

Inhibition of gastric acid secretion and delayed gastric emptying are two well-known physiological responses to fat perfusion of the upper intestine. In 1886, Ewald and Boas (6) showed that fat perfusion of the small intestine inhibited gastric acid secretion and delayed gastric emptying. In 1930, Kosaka and Lim (7) hypothesized that dietary fat inhibits gastric function by causing the release of one or more substances, known as enterogastrones, from the upper small intestine of dogs. The intraluminal contents that lead to inhibition of gastric acid secretion and emptying are acid, hyperosmolar solutions, and fat. Of these three factors, intraluminal fat is the most potent inhibitor of gastric acid secretion and emptying.

The Elusive "Enterogastrone"

Three requirements must be fulfilled to characterize a substance as an enterogastrone: first, it should be released in response to the presence of fat in the intestine and circulating concentrations should be increased over basal levels; second, exogenous administration in a dose that attains the plasma concentration achieved physiologically should inhibit gastric acid secretion to an extent similar to that produced by intestinal fat; third, *in vivo* immunoneutralization or receptor antagonism should block the inhibitory effect of intestinal fat. It may be impossible to satisfy the first two requirements for candidates that act as neurotransmitters or that are active locally because plasma levels do not reflect tissue concentrations. Further, lack of selective and specific chemical blockers and antisera has hampered efforts to fulfill the third requirement.

In Vitro *and* In Vivo *Findings*

Isolated perfused organ preparations, mucosal sheets mounted in Ussing chambers, isolated glands, dispersed cells, and membrane vesicles have been used to examine the cellular events regulating gastric acid secretion. These techniques and methods have been especially useful in discerning how the parietal cell is eventually deactivated to stop pumping hydrogen ion.

Parietal cell secretion of acid secretion can be deactivated directly by switching on inhibitory pathways and indirectly by switching off stimulatory pathways (21). Separate receptors exist for gastrin, acetylcholine, and histamine on parietal cells, and for gastrin receptors on enterochromaffin-like cells that contain histamine. Thus, inhibition of gastrin, acetylcholine, and/or histamine release reduces the level of stimulation of the parietal cell. On the other hand, secretin, somatostatin, and neurotensin produce potent inhibition of acid secretion. Of these, somatostatin directly inhibits parietal cell secretion by binding to somatostatin receptors located on parietal cells and indirectly by inhibiting histamine release from ECL cells and acetylcholine release from cholinergic nerves.

On the other hand, although *in vitro* and *ex vivo* preparations have provided substantial information regarding the cellular level of integration of signals separated from external influences, the physiological significance of these findings is often inconclusive. *In vivo* models are essential to study extragastric influences on gastric acid secretion and emptying. For example, systemic administration of many substances, including secretin, peptide YY, neurotensin, vasoactive intestinal peptide, gastric inhibitory peptide, enteroglucagon, and somatostatin have been shown, either physiologically and/or pharmacologically, to inhibit gastric acid secretion, as reviewed earlier (25). One of the foremost methods used to study physiological inhibition of gastric acid secretion

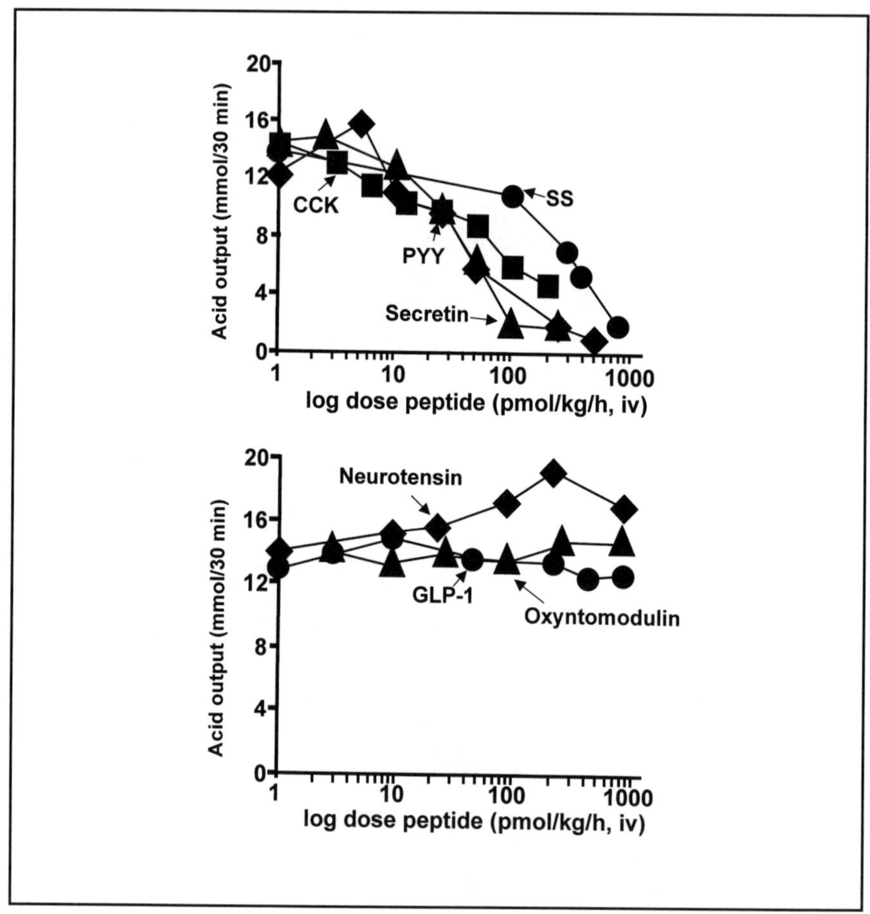

FIGURE 1. *Survey of gastrointestinal peptides in conscious dogs. The relative effect of increasing doses of gastrointestinal peptides infused intravenously on meal-stimulated gastric acid secretion as measured by intragastric titration to pH 5.5 of 8% peptone in conscious dogs (CCK = cholecystokinin-8, SST = somatostatin-14, PYY = peptide YY, GLP-1 = glucagon-like peptide I).*

during the intestinal phase of digestion utilized the technique of intragastric titration of a (peptone) meal, developed by Fordtran and Walsh (9).

Intragastric Titration

Once set-up and validated, intragastric titration is a simple and accurate method to measure meal-stimulated gastric acid secretion in mice (unpublished data, Lloyd, et al.), rats (17), dogs (8), non-human primates (unpublished data, Solnick & Lloyd), and humans (9). In essence, a test meal (e.g., 8% peptone), is first adjusted to a pH between 2.5 and 5.5 and is administered through a nasogastric tube or an indwelling gastric cannula. The meal is mixed in the stomach gently to avoid gastric distention using an oscillating pump which continuously draws a sample of the meal across the connecting tubes where they passed a pH probe monitoring intragastric acidity. An automatic titrator, set to a pre-determined pH "end-point", infuses through a separate tube into the stomach an amount of a dilute buffer, usually sodium hydroxide, to maintain intragastric pH at the fixed "end-point." After a period of time (15 to 30 min), the total amount of monovalent base infused into the stomach equals the amount of acid secreted by the stomach during that same time.

While the intragastric titration method bypasses the cephalic phase component, it does include the stimulatory components of both gastric and intestinal phases of total acid output (stimulatory only, because intragastric pH is maintained constant, thus blocking activation of intragastric acid–induced inhibitory pathways). However, because the intestinal phase contributes little to the gastric acid response to a meal, and because gastrin is the primary stimulant of acid secretion in response to a meal, intragastric titration can be considered a useful and accurate measurement of gastrin-mediated acid secretion during the gastric phase of digestion.

PATHWAYS AND MEDIATORS OF ENTEROGASTRIC INHIBITION OF ACID OUTPUT

The remainder of this chapter shall focus on enterogastric pathways and mediators that were of particular interest to John Harley Walsh. Each of the next several sections shall highlight very briefly the salient features of work conducted directly by, or in collaboration with, John from the early 1990's until his untimely death in 2000. The text shall be supported by summary figures and/or tables and appropriate citations.

A Survey of Gastrointestinal Peptides (Figure 1)

The relative effect of potential enterogastrones was studied by measuring peptone-stimulated gastric acid secretion during intragastric titration in dogs given increasing doses intravenously of several gastrointestinal-derived peptides (11). In this survey of gastrointestinal peptides, peptide YY (PYY) and secretin were more potent and efficacious than cholecystokinin and somatostatin as inhibitors of acid secretion, while all three were far more active than glucagon–like peptide (GLP)-1, neurotensin, and oxyntomodulin. Because the maximum acid inhibition was caused by supraphysiological if not pharmacological doses of individual peptides, though, no single peptide could be concluded to be an enterogastrone. A surprising result from this

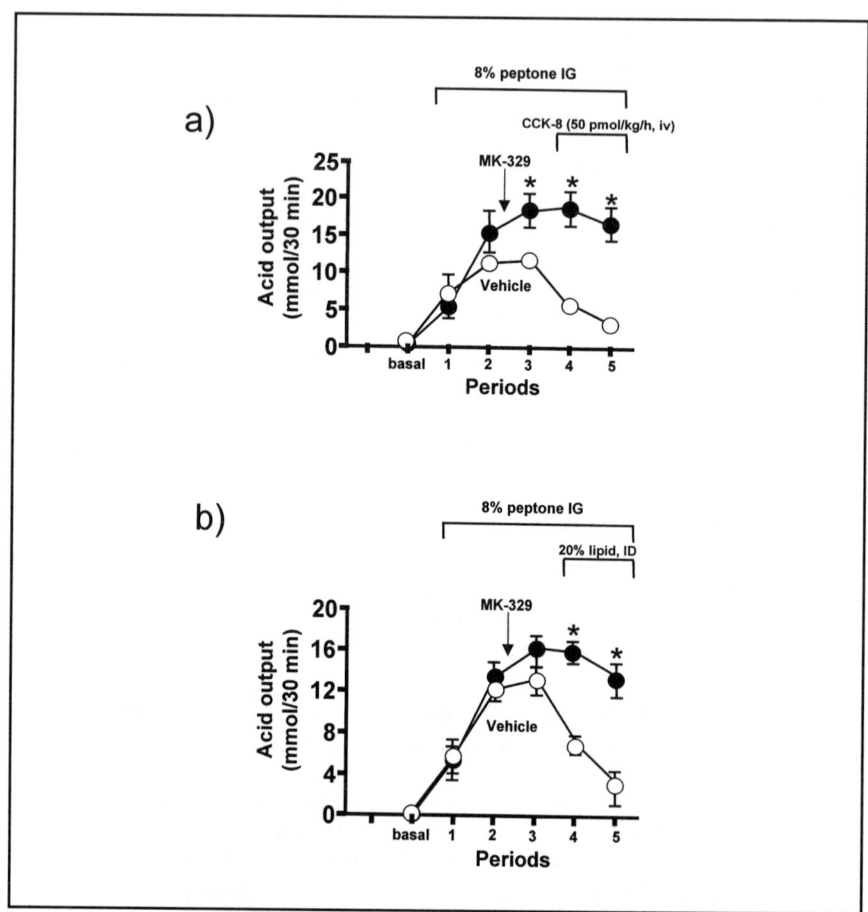

FIGURE 2. *Cholecystokinin and intestinal lipid inhibit gastric acid secretion by activation of CCK$_A$ receptors. The effect of a systemic dose (1 mg/kg) orally of the CCK$_A$ receptor antagonist, MK-329 (devazepide), on the inhibitory effect of (a) an intravenous infusion of a single dose (50 pmol/kg/h) of cholecystokinin-8 and (b) duodenal infusion of 20% lipid, on meal-stimulated gastric acid secretion as measured by intragastric titration to pH 5.5 of 8% peptone in conscious dogs. Black circles: devazepide + CCK; open circles = vehicle + CCK. ★ = P<0.05*

study was that an intravenous dose of cholecystokinin elicited acid inhibition. While provocative, establishing a physiologic role for cholecystokinin as an enterogastrone would prove to be difficult.

Cholecystokinin, Lipid, and CCK Receptors

The controversial hypothesis that endogenous cholecystokinin may be a physiologic inhibitor of gastric acid secretion has been difficult to test, not the least of which is its effect on gastric acid secretion which is highly variable and dependent on the species and conditions studied. About the time that John Walsh's studies were focusing on acid inhibitory mechanisms, the following observations on cholecystokinin activity had been demonstrated; full gastrin agonist activity in cats (28), rats (5), and mice (19), weak partial agonist activity in man (30) and dogs (22), and potent antagonism of gastrin-stimulated secretion in man (1) and dogs (23).

A fundamental explanation for these observations is the close C-terminus amino acid sequence homology between gastrin and cholecystokinin, and the existence of two receptor types, gastrin/CCK_B and CCK_A, that bind gastrin and cholecystokinin often expressed in the same cell. Characterization and availability (3, 4) of relatively selective, orally effective, and long-acting chemical antagonists of these receptor types provided tools to elucidate the mechanism of cholecystokinin's effects. In one study (15) using the CCK_A receptor antagonist MK-329 (devazepide), cholecystokinin was shown to be a full gastrin-agonist in dogs, by activation of gastrin/CCK_B receptors, and to be a potent inhibitor of meal-stimulated gastric acid secretion, by activation of CCK_A receptors (Figure 2a). The physiological implication of this latter observation was demonstrated in later experiments (15) when chemical antagonism of CCK_A receptors using MK-329 completely reversed the acid inhibitory effect of intestinal perfusion with lipid (Figure 2b). These findings provided significant evidence for cholecystokinin as a physiological regulator of gastric acid secretion in dogs, later confirmed also in man (2).

Cholecystokinin: Physiological or Pharmacological Acid Inhibitor? (Table 1)

The principle question that arose from the findings that cholecystokinin was a physiological mediator of intestinal fat-induced inhibition of gastric acid secretion was, "Where were the CCK_A receptors activating this phenomenon expressed?"…if the stomach, then cholecystokinin must be acting as a hormone, because gastric cholecystokinin expression is minimal to none; if peripherally (in the intestine) or centrally (across the blood brain barrier), then cholecystokinin must be acting as a paracrine and/or a neurotransmitter. In regards to these divergent hypotheses, circulating levels of CCK sometimes increase in response to intestinal nutrients, however, doses of exogenous CCK required to elicit known physiological actions of CCK produced much higher circulating levels (14). Because of this, circulating blood concentrations of CCK may not accurately reflect interstitial levels of the peptide. In fact, a recent study (13) indicates that acid inhibition caused by intestinal nutrients, including fat, is mediated by CCK_A receptors that are not activated by circulating cholecystokinin.

TABLE 1. *Cholecystokinin does not act as a humoral regulator of gastric acid secretion. The effect of various intraduodenal and intravenous treatments on 8% peptone meal-stimulated gastric acid secretion, plasma cholecystokinin, and plasma gastrin levels in conscious rats.*

	Parameters measured (vs IG peptone alone*)		
Intraduodenal Treatment	*Acid*	*Cholecystokinin*	*Gastrin*
Saline	↑	↔	↑
Complete Liquid Diet	↓	↑	↓
5% Lipid	↓	↑	↓
6% Casein	↔	↔	↔
20% Dextrose	↓	↔	↓
Soybean Trypsin Inhibitor	↔	↑	↔
Intravenous Treatment			
Cholecystokinin (pharmacological dose)	↓	↑	(n/d)
Cholecystokinin (physiological dose)	↔	↔	(n/d)

* vs basal during intraduodenal treatment with saline
n/d = not done.

Vagal Inhibition

Instead of an endocrine pathway, cholecystokinin is more likely acting in a paracrine and/or neural mechanism to elicit enterogastric acid inhibition. Cholecystokinin is a neuropeptide distributed throughout the enteric nervous system and binds to receptors on subdiaphragmatic vagal branches and in the brain. Capsaicin-sensitive sensory innervation of the intestine appears to transduce the afferent limb of the enterogastric reflex (12), likely mediated through a central vagal reflex (27). Further, intravenously-administered cholecystokinin as well as intestinal lipid-induced inhibition of gastric acid secretion was reduced, but not eliminated, by highly-selective vagotomy (11), indicating that enterogastric inhibition of acid secretion in large part is mediated through a vagal pathway to the gastric fundus (Figure 3).

Somatostatin Mediates Cholecystokinin-induced Acid Inhibition

Although a physiological role was beginning to emerge for cholecystokinin as a principal enterogastrone activating the afferent arm of a neural reflex from

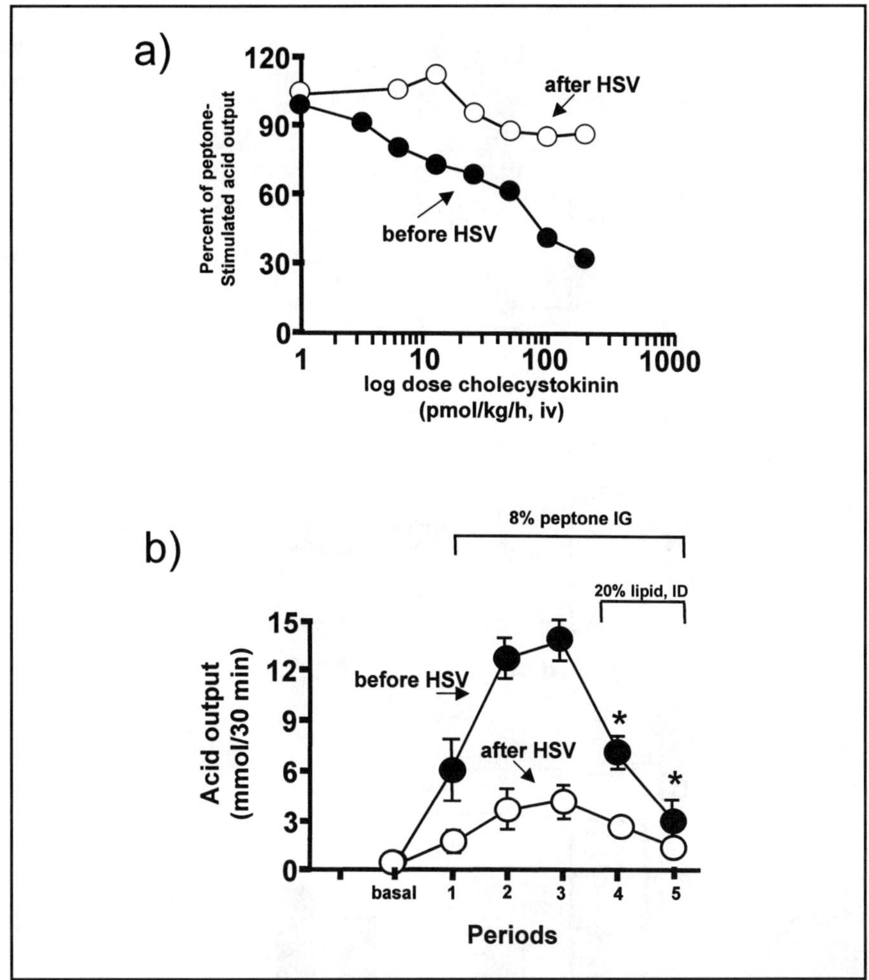

FIGURE 3. *CCK$_A$ receptors mediate acid inhibition through a gastric vagal pathway. The effect of highly-selective vagotomy (HSV) on the inhibitory effect of (a) increasing doses of cholecystokinin-8 intravenously infused and (b) intraduodenal infusion of 20% lipid, on meal-stimulated gastric acid secretion as measured by intragastric titration to pH 5.5 of 8% peptone in conscious dogs. $\star$ = P < 0.05*

the intestine, the effector of the efferent arm remained unknown. Numerous reports from *in vitro* studies using isolated populations of gastric mucosal cells elutriated from the dog stomach revealed an interaction between somatostatin-containing "D" cells and gastrin-containing "G" cells, histamine-containing "ECL" cells, and the acid pumping parietal cells. In fact, a direct link between cholecystokinin and somatostatin release in the gastric mucosa has been shown (14), but this interaction is more likely to represent

Lloyd

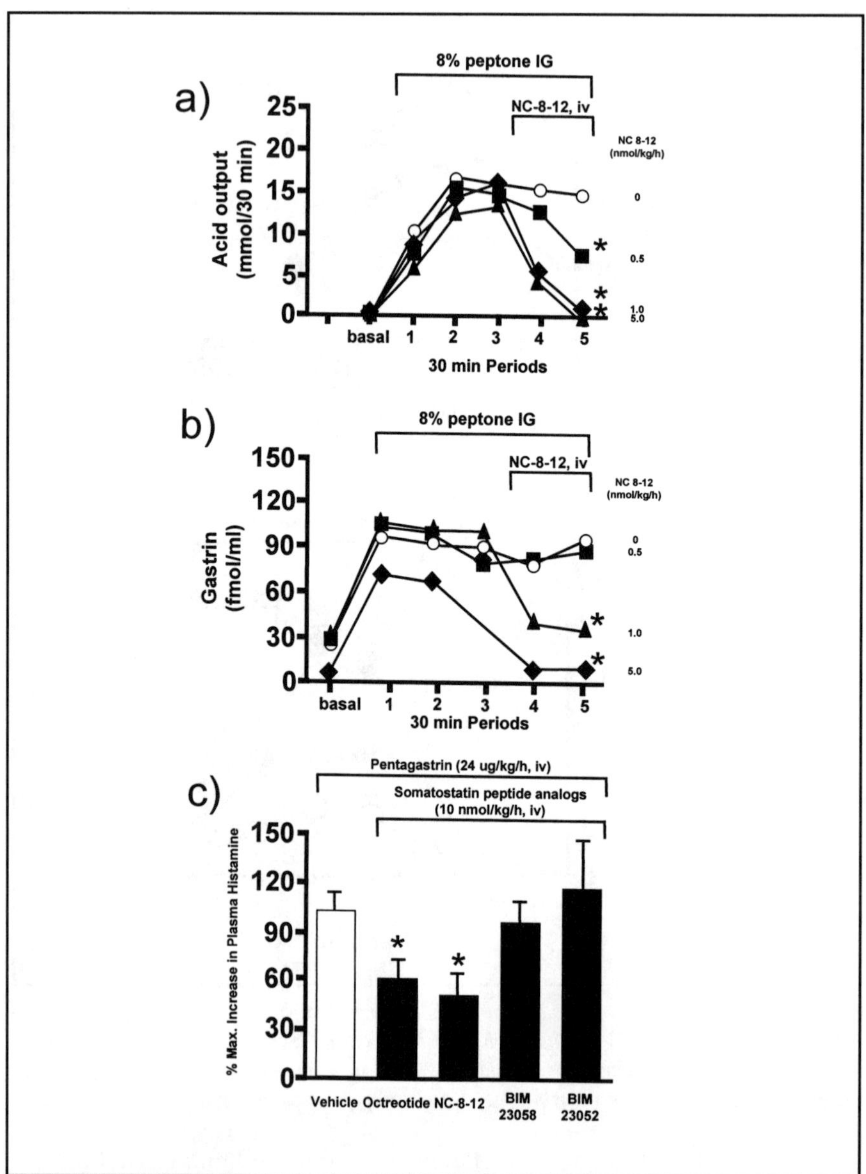

FIGURE 4. *sst_2 receptors mediate somatostatin inhibition of gastric acid secretion. The effect of increasing doses of the relatively selective sst_2 receptor agonist, NC 8-12, administered by intravenous infusion on meal-stimulated (a) gastric acid secretion as measured by, and (b) circulating gastrin in response to, intragastric titration to pH 5.5 of 8% peptone in conscious dogs; (c) The effect of single intravenous doses (10 nmol/kg/h) of either octeotride, the sst_2 chemical agonist (NC 8-12), the sst_3 chemical agonist (BIM-23058), and the sst_4 chemical agonist on portal venous histamine concentration in response to intravenous infusion of a single dose (24 μg/kg/h) of pentagastrin in conscious rats. ★ = P < 0.05*

a pharmacologic rather than a physiologic relationship. More intriguing are *in vivo* studies (16) which showed that cholecystokinin-induced inhibition of meal-stimulated acid secretion was reversed by immunoneutralizing somatostatin by intravenous administration of somatostatin monoclonal antibody Fab fragments.

Somatostatin Receptor Subtype 2

Somatostatin has long been known as a physiological peripheral and central regulator of gastric acid secretion; *in vivo* immunoneutralization using a somatostatin monoclonal antibody (29) enhances gastric acid secretion in urethane-anesthetized rats (31), most likely through a paracrine rather than an endocrine fashion (16) from somatostatin released in the gastric mucosa from "D" cells. The target of somatostatin, the somatostatin receptor, was found to be expressed as five distinct subtypes throughout the mammalian stomach. Utilizing receptor agonists relatively selective for a specific receptor subtype, it was found that activation of the somatostatin receptor subtype 2 (sst_2) was most effective at inhibiting secretagogue (18) as well as meal-stimulated (10) gastric acid secretion. Acid inhibition was inhibited in response to activation of sst_2 receptors expressed on mucosal "G" and "ECL" cells that regulate gastrin and histamine synthesis and release, respectively (Figure 4a, 4b, 4c).

Enterogastric Inhibition and sst_2 Receptors

The recent availability of mutant mice which have been genetically-altered using gene-targeting approaches have substantially increased the resolution of findings from physiological experiments: for example, studies using a "knockout" mouse for a particular gene are more definitive than those in which the gene product itself is either inhibited using a competitive chemical antagonist or immunoneutralized using circulating antibodies with relatively greater affinity for its ligand than the endogenous receptor. Physiological models of gastric acid secretion using mice have been developed (24) in which basal acid output was found to be significantly higher in sst_2 knockout mice than in wild-type control mice (20). Recent data (unpublished data, Lloyd, et al.) have also demonstrated that intestinal lipid-induced inhibition of meal-stimulated acid secretion is blocked in these same mice.

SUMMARY AND CONCLUSIONS

Enterogastric inhibition of gastric acid secretion was as interesting a focus of investigation to John Harley Walsh as was the role of gastrin in the stimulation of gastric acid secretion. This chapter has summarized only a small but important subset of research activities in which John Walsh was either directly or collaboratively involved. The hypothesis that cholecystokinin may be a major enterogastrone mediating intestinal phase regulation of gastric acid secretion was one of the first topics of conversation I had with John Walsh when I visited with him initially in 1987 to begin my academic research career. Since then, we showed that cholecystokinin was a potent inhibitor of pentagastrin- and meal-induced acid secretion, mediated by activation of CCK_A receptors through a central vagal reflex that elicits a somatostatin efferent mechanism effected by sst_2 receptors on gastric mucosal cells. These results indicate that CCK is a major physiologic enterogastrone released in response to dietary nutrients when in contact with the intestinal mucosa.

REFERENCES

1. Brooks AM, Grossman MI. Effect of secretin and cholecystokinin on pentagastrin-stimulated gastric secretion in man. *Gastroenterology* 1970;59:114–119.
2. Burckhardt B, Delco F, Ensinck JW, Meier R, Bauerfeind P, Aufderhaar U, Ketterer S, Gyr K, Beglinger C. Cholecystokinin is a physiological regulator of gastric acid secretion in man. *Eur J Clin Invest* 1994;24: 370–376.
3. Chang RS, Lotti VJ. Biochemical and pharmacological characterization of an extremely potent and selective nonpeptide cholecystokinin antagonist. *Proc Natl Acad Sci USA* 1986;83:4923–4926.
4. Chang RS, Lotti VJ, Monaghan RL, Birnbaum J, Stapley EO, Goetz MA, Albers-Schonberg G, Patchett AA, Liesch JM, Hensens OD, Springer JP. A potent nonpeptide cholecystokinin antagonist selective for peripheral tissues isolated from Aspergillus Alliaceus. *Science* 1985;230:177–179.
5. Chey WY, Sivasomboon B, Hendricks J. Actions and interactions of gut hormones and histamine on gastric secretion of acid in the rat. *Am J Physiol* 1973;224:852–856.
6. Ewald C, Boas J. Beitrage zur physiologie und pathologie der verdauung. *Virchows Arch Path Anat Physiol Klin Med* 1886;104:271–305.
7. Kosaka T, Lim RKS. On the mechanism of the inhibition of gastric secretion by fat. The role of bile and cystokinin. *Chinese Journal Physiology* 1930;4:213–220.
8. Kovacs TO, Walsh JH, Maxwell V, Wong HC, Azuma T, and Katt E. Gastrin is a major mediator of the gastric phase of acid secretion in dogs: proof by monoclonal antibody neutralization. *Gastroenterology* 1989;97:1406–1413.
9. Kovacs TOG, JH Walsh. Standard secretory tests: methodology. In Rozen, P., Ed. *Frontiers in Gastrointestinal Research*. Switzerland, S. Karger, Basel. 1990; 2–12.
10. Lloyd KC, Amirmoazzami S, Friedik F, Chew P, Walsh JH. Somatostatin inhibits gastrin release and acid secretion by activating sst_2 in dogs. *Am J Physiol* 1997;272:G1481-G1488.
11. Lloyd KC, Amirmoazzami S, Friedik F, Heynio A, Solomon TE, Walsh JH. Candidate canine enterogastrones: acid inhibition before and after vagotomy. *Am J Physiol* 1997;272:G1236–G1242.
12. Lloyd KC, Holzer HH, Zittel TT, Raybould HE. Duodenal lipid inhibits gastric acid secretion by vagal, capsaicin- sensitive afferent pathways in rats. *Am J Physiol* 1993;264:G659–G663.
13. Lloyd KC, Wang J, Solomon TE. Acid inhibition by intestinal nutrients mediated by CCKA receptors but not plasma CCK. *Am J Physiol* 2001;281:G924–G930.
14. Lloyd KCK, Maxwell KV, Chuang C-N, Wong HC, Soll AH, Walsh JH. Somatostatin is released in response to cholecystokinin by activation of type A CCK receptors. *Peptides* 1994;15: 223–227.
15. Lloyd KCK, Maxwell KV, Kovacs TOG, Miller J, Walsh JH. Cholecystokinin receptor antagonist MK-329 blocks intestinal fat-induced inhibition of meal-stimulated gastric acid secretion. *Gastroenterology* 1992;102:131–138.

16. Lloyd KCK, Maxwell KV, OhningG, Walsh JH. Intestinal fat does not inhibit gastric function through a hormonal somatostatin mechanism in dogs. *Gastroenterology* 1992;103:1221–1228.

17. Lloyd KCK, Raybould HE, Taché Y, Walsh JH. Role of gastrin, histamine, and acetylcholine in the gastric phase of acid secretion in anesthetized rats. *Am J Physiol* 1992;262:G747–G755.

18. Lloyd KCK, Wang J, Aurang K, Grönhed P, Coy DH, Walsh JH. Activation of somatostatin receptor subtype 2 inhibits acid secretion in rats. *Am J Physiol* 1995;268:G102-G106.

19. Lotti VJ, Chang RS, Kling PJ, Cerino DJ. Evidence that cholecystokinin octapeptide (CCK$_8$) acts as a potent, full agonist on gastrin receptors for acid secretion in the isolated mouse stomach: lack of antagonism by the specific CCK antagonist asperlicin. *Digestion* 1986;35:170–174.

20. Martinez V, Curi AP, Torkian B, Schaeffer JM, Wilkinson HA, Walsh JH, Taché Y. High basal gastric acid secretion in somatostatin receptor subtype 2 knockout mice. *Gastroenterology* 1998;114:1125–1132.

21. Soll AH, Walsh JH. Regulation of gastric acid secretion. *Ann Rev Physiol* 1979;41:35–53.

22. Stening FG, Grossman MI. Gastrin-related peptides as stimulants of pancreatic and gastric secretion. *Am J Physiol* 1969;217:262–266.

23. Stening GF, Johnson LR, Grossman MI. Effect of cholecystokinin and caerulein on gastrin- and histamine-evoked gastric secretion. *Gastroenterology* 1969;57:44–50.

24. Torkian B, Martinez V, Walsh JH, Taché Y. Model to study gastric acid secretion in mice: Effect of secretagogues and inhibitors on basal gastric acid secretion. *Gastroenterology* 1998;114(4),A1185.

25. Walsh JH. Gastrointestinal hormones. In: Johnson LR, Christensen J, Jacobson MJ, and Walsh JH, Eds. *Physiology of the Gastrointestinal Tract.* New York, Raven. 1987;181–253.

26. Walsh JH. Gastric secretion. In: Kelley WN, Ed. *Textbook of Internal Medicine.* Philadelphia, J.B. Lippincott Co. 1989;437–442.

27. Wang L, Cardin S, Martinez V, Taché Y, Lloyd KC. Duodenal loading with glucose induces fos expression in rat brain: selective blockade by devazepide. *Am J Physiol* 1999;277:R667–R674.

28. Way L. W. Effect of cholecystokinin and caerulein on gastrin secretion in cats. *Gastroenterology* 1971;60:560–565.

29. Wong HC, Walsh JH, Yang H, Taché Y, Buchan AM. A monoclonal antibody to somatostatin with potent *in vivo* immunoneutralizing activity. *Peptides* 1990;11:707–712.

30. Wormsley KG. Gastric response to secretin and pancreozymin in man. *Scand J Gastroenterol* 1968;3: 632–636.

31. Yang H, Wong HC, Wu V, Walsh JH, Taché Y. Somatostatin monoclonal antibody immunoneutralization increases gastrin and gastric acid secretion in urethane-anesthetized rats. *Gastroenterology* 1990; 99:659–665.

Gut-Brain Peptides in the New Millennium, edited by Y. Taché
CURE Foundation, Los Angeles, CA. © 2002

8

Interactions between Gastrin, Gastric Secretion, and *Helicobacter pylori* in Health and Disease

David Y. Graham
Department of Medicine, Veterans Affairs Medical Center and Division of Molecular Virology, Baylor College of Medicine, Houston, TX.

James E. McGuigan
Department of Medicine, University of Florida College of Medicine Gainesville, FL

INTRODUCTION

Fascination with the stomach and with gastric function has continued unabated for more than 150 years (1). Over time the focus has changed from what is secreted to how secretion is controlled (2). The advent of the H2-receptor antagonists, proton pump inhibitors, radioimmunoassay, molecular techniques, and the ability to measure meal-stimulated acid secretion *in situ* have combined to provide increasingly detailed understandings of the regulation of acid secretion. Relationships between ECL (enterochromaffin-like) cells, G-cells, D-cells, and parietal cells continue to be explored. Currently there is a large amount of information related to neuro-humoral interactions between nerves, G, D, ECL cells, secretory targets and various peptide messengers (3). While new factors will undoubtedly enter the drama, present understanding of the regulation of gastric physiology in the normal stomach has reached a high level of sophistication (3).

PERTURBATIONS IN GASTRODUODENAL PHYSIOLOGY IN DUODENAL ULCER

Until recently, peptic ulcer was a major cause of morbidity among humans. It was known that ulcers healed and tended not to recur if acid secretion was suppressed by drugs or surgery such that the old dictum "no acid–no ulcer" was literally true. The Holy Grail of physiologic studies in acid secretion was aimed at identification of a specific abnormality in gastroduodenal physiology which was responsible for development of duodenal ulcer disease. Despite decades of increasingly sophisticated study, one was not forthcoming. Nonetheless, many perturbations in gastric function were identified to be associated with duodenal ulcer in patients. These have included an increased parietal cell mass with its attendant increased maximal acid output, elevated basal acid output, prolonged acid and gastrin release responses to food, exaggerated acid and gastrin responses to meals, to infusion of bombesin or gastric releasing peptide, as well as defective pH feedback inhibition of gastrin release and acid secretion, rapid gastric emptying, and reduced duodenal bicarbonate secretion in response to instillation of acid (4). Studies have been performed in man, in experimental animals, and in isolated cell preparations. Experiments in animals and *in vitro* are, by their nature, designed to minimize confounding factors to permit analysis of an individual factor and thus clarify interactions between two or more components. Integration of the data obtained comes later. Our understanding of the interplay among various receptors, the endocrine, autocrine, and paracrine influences on gastric secretion has expanded greatly, but there is still much more to be known since data derived from animal studies have yet to be fully translated to humans.

GASTRITIS

A feature that was generally ignored in the pathogenesis of peptic ulcer was gastritis. Early in the past century it was recognized that peptic ulcer disease was almost invariably associated with gastric inflammation, (i.e., histologic gastritis) (5). It was also recognized that the distribution and pattern of gastritis differed between those with duodenal ulcer and gastric ulcer and those with gastritis without ulcer. Cross-sectional and follow-up studies showed that gastritis in patients with duodenal ulcer remained localized primarily to the antrum with little tendency to progress into the gastric corpus. This behavior differed from the pattern of gastritis in those with or without gastric ulcer, which also involved the antrum but in addition involved the gastric corpus, appearing to progress into the gastric corpus over time (6). This gradual increase in the amount and extent of gastritis resulted in decreasing gastric acid secretion with age. Corpus gastritis was also shown to be associated with a reduction in acid secretion which was out of proportion to the loss of parietal cells, suggesting the presence of an inhibitor of acid secretion which was associated with the inflammation (7, 8). These observations proved prophetic for what we have learned in the last decade regarding relationships between *H. pylori* and gastric acid secretion.

HELICOBACTER PYLORI

Despite the recognized association of gastritis with peptic ulcer for decades, the etiology of the gastritis remained a mystery. Most studies focused on diet and environmental factors as potential causes for the gastritis. In addition, because rapid advancements were being made in understanding the regulation of acid secretion, there was little impetus for the scientific community studying ulcer disease to incorporate gastritis into their investigations of peptic ulcer (9). Nevertheless, gastritis remained a topic of interest because of the strong association with gastric cancer which, until recently, was one of the most common cancers in humans. Interest in gastritis in ulcer disease began to change in the mid-1970's, when Steer, from a series of elegant studies, proposed bacterial infection as a possible cause of gastritis (10–13). In the early 1980's, Warren and Marshall, who were apparently unaware of the ongoing work by Steer, observed and cultured a bacterium associated with gastric inflammation and suggested that this bacterium was the cause of the gastritis and of the gastritis-associated diseases, duodenal ulcer, and gastric cancer (14). Self inoculation experiments by Barry Marshall and Arthur Morris proved that the bacterium was able to cause gastric inflammation and was not simply a secondary invader of inflamed gastric tissue (15–17). Treatment of the infection by McNulty, et al. showed that reduction in the bacterial load led to improvement in gastritis (18). From those studies it was logical to conclude that if the infection could be treated successfully, and the gastritis healed, it might be possible to prevent or cure the gastritis-related diseases, peptic ulcer and gastric cancer (19). The ability to grow *H. pylori* and to work with it in the laboratory produced a revolution in concepts regarding ulcer therapy and the natural history of the disease.

Progress of new and revolutionary ideas often requires new investigators to enter the field. The study of gastric physiology was no exception. Many major laboratories involved in studies of gastric physiology continued to study interactions at both the cellular and subcellular levels and were slow to integrate questions concerning the possible effects of *H. pylori* infection on gastric function (20). This reticence was possibly related to the need to retreat temporarily from sophisticated modern techniques and to return to relative crude techniques used to study gastric secretion in man. John Walsh had no such reticence in relation to his interest in gastrin and its role in health and disease and was one of the early players in this unfolding drama.

H. Pylori-*related Perturbations in Gastric Function and Gastrin Secretion*

One place that the story of gastrin and *H. pylori* might begin would be in 1971 when McGuigan and Trudeau reported that patients with duodenal ulcer produced an exaggerated gastrin release response to meals when compared with controls (21). They suggested that the trophic effect of gastrin might be responsible for the known increased parietal cell mass which was

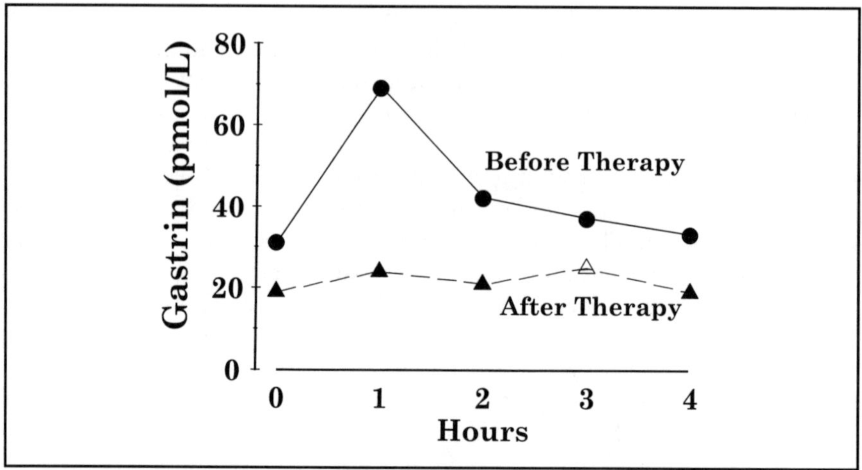

FIGURE 1. *A typical example of the effect of anti-*H. pylori *therapy on meal stimulated gastrin release is shown. The data show the plasma gastrin response of one of the authors (DYG) before and after anti-*H. pylori *therapy (22).*

characteristic of duodenal ulcer disease. This hypothesis remained controversial and it was only later that it became clear why.

In the late 1980s, a number of investigators began to examine meal–stimulated gastrin release in relation to *H. pylori* infection (22–27). It became apparent that *H. pylori* infection was associated with a slight increase in fasting serum gastrin levels compared to uninfected controls and with a marked increase in serum gastrin levels in response to meals. Exaggerated meal–stimulated gastrin release was not specific to patients with duodenal ulcer but rather was a one of a number of reversible phenomena related to the presence of an *H. pylori* infection (28). The differences in response of gastrin release among those with and without *H. pylori* infection also resolved the apparently opposite results obtained in different laboratories in relation to the observation of an exaggerated gastrin release response to meals among duodenal ulcer patients (29).

Details of how *H. pylori* infection enhances stimulation of gastrin release are still not clear despite the many experiments that have been conducted to define the parameters surrounding and responsible for the phenomenon. For example, we asked whether the changes in gastrin release was related to a nonspecific effect(s) of the antimicrobial agents used in the treatment of *H. pylori* infection on antral G cells (22). We, therefore, compared the effects bismuth subsalicylate and metronidazole had on fasting or meal stimulated gastrin release in *H. pylori* infected and in uninfected individuals and showed that the antibiotic therapy was associated with a reduction in gastrin release only among those with *H. pylori* infection (Figure 1).

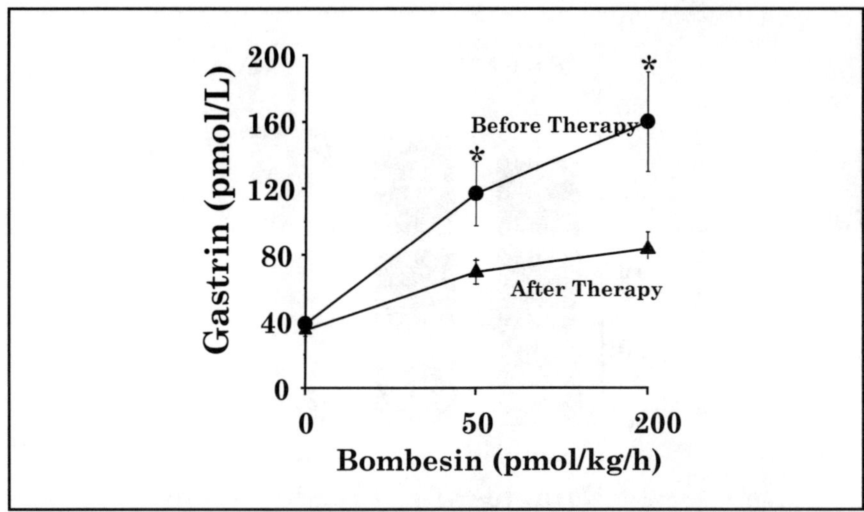

FIGURE 2. *The effect of anti-*H. pylori *therapy on the gastrin-releasing peptide (bombesin) induced gastrin release. Anti-*H. pylori *therapy resulted in a significant (*$*p = 0.01$*) blunting of the stimulated increase in plasma gastrin concentration among 11 duodenal ulcer patients. In contrast, antimicrobial therapy had not effect on bombesin-stimulated gastrin concentration among healthy subjects without* H. pylori *infection (30).*

We also examined the effect(s) of gastrin releasing peptide (using two 30 minute periods of bombesin infusion at 50 pmol/kg/hr followed by 200 pmol/kg/h) on *H. pylori* infected and uninfected individuals (30). Bombesin-stimulated gastrin release was studied because, unlike meal stimulated gastrin release, it is not sensitive to luminal factors such as pH. We confirmed that plasma gastrin concentration among fasting duodenal ulcer patients was significantly greater than among uninfected control subjects (38 ± 3 vs. 22 ± 1 pg/mL, $p < 0.001$) and that bombesin infusion significantly increased the plasma gastrin before and after therapy to eradicate *H. pylori*. The increase in bombesin-stimulated gastrin release was blunted following antimicrobial therapy in duodenal ulcer patients (Figure 2). In contrast, in the uninfected controls, the increase in bombesin-stimulated plasma gastrin concentrations remain similar before and after antimicrobial therapy.

In our early experiments we showed that eradication of the *H. pylori* infection reversed the exaggerated meal-stimulated gastrin release without affecting bulk intragastric pH (22). *H. pylori* urease hydrolyzes urea into ammonia and carbon dioxide and we, therefore, examined the possibility that the ammonia produced might increase the local pH in, or on, the gastric mucosa and therefore, limit the availability of hydrogen ions to pH sensitive sites controlling gastrin release. For that experiment we fed urea to *H. pylori* infected volunteers and found no significant change in serum gastrin

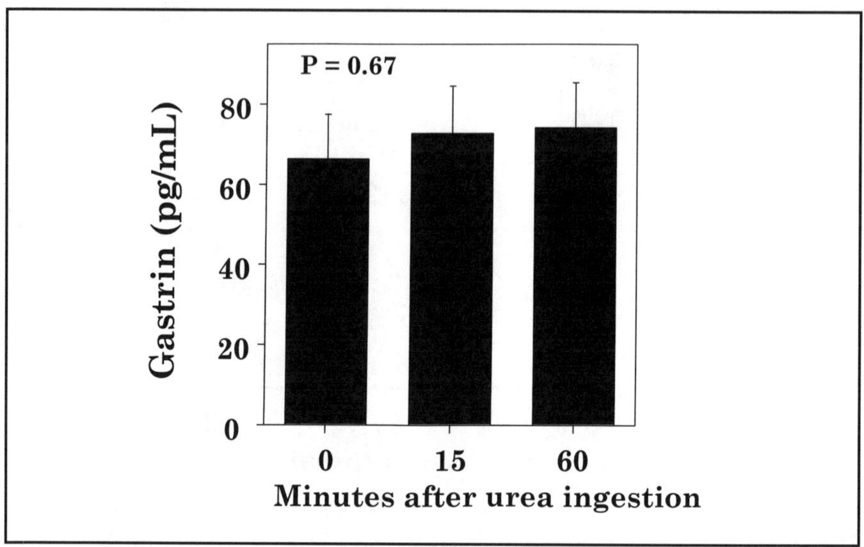

FIGURE 3. *Feeding 500 mg of urea in 120 mL of water 10 minutes after administration of 249 mL of a 25% glucose polymer solution had no significant effect on the serum gastrin concentration among 5 asymptomatic* H. pylori-*infected subjects. Serum gastrin was measured before and 15 and 60 minutes after urea administration (30).*

concentrations suggesting that local ammonia production was not a major factor in *H. pylori*-associated exaggerated gastrin release (median 62 pg/mL prior and 56 and 65 pg/mL at 15 and 60 min post oral administration of 500 mg of urea in 120 mL of water (Figure 3) (30).

We examined the early time course of the abatement of meal-stimulated gastrin release following therapy of *H. pylori* infection in relation to the changes in gastric histology, *H. pylori* density, as well as on the presence of luminal products related to the presence of *H. pylori* (31). In that study *H. pylori*-infected volunteers underwent upper endoscopy four times: baseline and at days 3, 14, and 42 post initiation of therapy. Gastric mucosal specimens were obtained with jumbo forceps to ensure that we could examine changes from the surface epithelium to the muscularis mucosae. Serum gastrin levels were measured before therapy, after 2 and 14 days therapy, and 4 weeks after completion of antibiotic therapy. The fasting serum gastrin levels were unchanged throughout the course of the experiments. Our expectations had been that 2 days of antibiotic therapy would eliminate *H. pylori* and any bacterial products as well as reduce the density of polymorphonuclear cells in the mucosa. After 14 days of therapy we expected that in addition to the absence of bacteria, and polymorphonuclear cells, there would also be a reduction in the density of mucosal mononuclear cells. These expectations were only partially achieved. The treatment-related decrease in

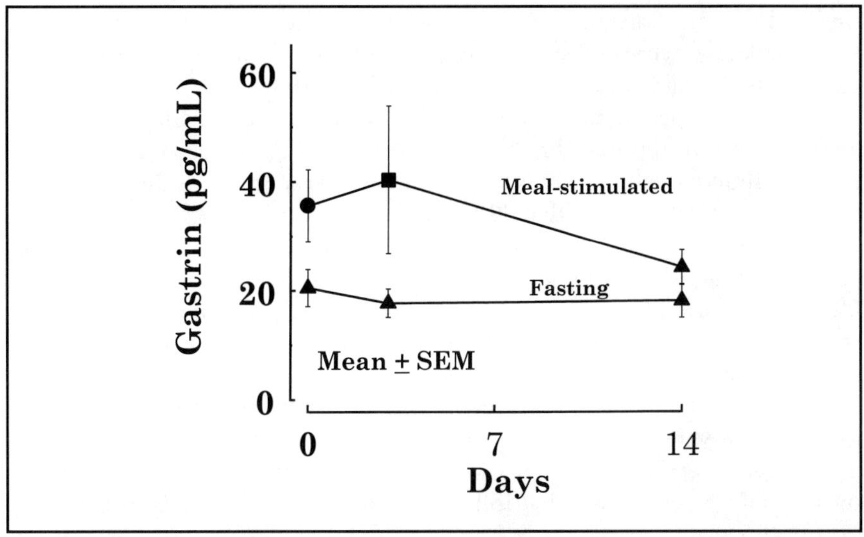

FIGURE 4. *The effect of anti-*H. pylori *therapy on the meal stimulated gastrin-release in 10* H. pylori *infected individuals. The gastrin concentration was unchanged after two days of antimicrobial therapy despite disappearance of both* H. pylori *and polymorphonuclear infiltration in the gastric mucosa. Meal-stimulated gastrin concentration was similar to the fasting level 2 weeks after starting therapy (31).*

meal-stimulated gastrin was observed but it was not immediate (Figure 4). After 2 days of therapy meal-stimulated gastrin release was unchanged compared to baseline despite histologic confirmation of a disappearance of both *H. pylori* and mucosal polymorphonuclear cell infiltration, as well as normalization of the gastric luminal ammonium concentration and the ammonium to urea ratio (32). The fact that meal-stimulated gastrin release remained exaggerated despite clearance of bacteria and disappearance of polymorphonuclear cells from the antral and corpus mucosa, suggested that neither the *H. pylori* nor *H. pylori* products, such as ammonium, were directly responsible for the *H. pylori*-associated exaggerated gastrin release. In addition, these experiments appeared to exonerate polymorphonuclear cells and polymorphonuclear cell–bacterial interactions as candidates for provocation of gastrin release. The observation that correlated best with the reversal of the exaggerated gastrin release was the reduction in density of the mucosal mononuclear cell infiltration. Of interest, that observation was consistent with reports of stimulation of gastrin release by co-cultivation of canine G-cells and mononuclear cells (33) and with other studies relating gastrin secretion and cytokines (34, 35). It is also consistent with the notion that *H. pylori*-associated exaggeration in gastrin secretion is most likely related, directly or indirectly, to local stimulation or release in inhibition of G-cells. We have subsequently studied mucosal interleukin (IL) IL-1 and IL-8 levels one and two days after beginning therapy and found that by one day they were markedly decreased suggesting that neither are directly involved in the exaggerated meal stimulation release (unpublished).

Studies in experimental animals have shown that gastrin and somatostatin are regulated in opposite directions but it is not clear which product of the *H. pylori* mucosal interaction is responsible for this complex interaction (36). Kaneko, et al. (37) noted that *H. pylori* infection was associated with a decrease in immunoreactive somatostatin in the human stomach and the decrease correlated with the grade of chronic inflammation. Domschke, et al. (38), had reported previously that the ratio of antral gastrin and somatostatin was higher in patients with duodenal ulcer (and presumably *H. pylori* infection) than in controls. Gastrin and somatostatin genes are regulated in opposite directions in a coordinated manner such that those stimuli that increase gastrin release are also associated with low somatostatin concentrations (36). This regulation was originally demonstrated in animal experiments. It has subsequently been shown that inflammation associated with *H. pylori* infection both stimulated gastrin release and inhibited somatostatin but remains unclear which product of the *H. pylori* mucosal interaction is responsible for this complex interaction.

While ammonia has been shown to stimulate gastrin release from G-cells in rats (39), the fact that neither ingestion of urea nor infusion of urea into the stomachs of *H. pylori*-infected individuals increased gastrin secretion suggests that ammonia does not have a role in stimulating gastrin release in humans (30, 40). In addition, for various physical and chemical reasons, lipid-soluble ammonia, the form which would be able to enter the mucosa and stimulate gastrin release is not likely to be present in gastric contents rather it is likely present as charged ammonium (32). The pK for the ammonia-ammonium buffer system is approximately 9.1 (41), and the low pH of the gastric contents favors retention of ammonia in gastric juice, where it is trapped as the positively charged ammonium. The products of urease, ammonia and carbon dioxide, take different paths in the stomach; ammonia predominantly remains in the gastric lumen, whereas the product carbon dioxide appears predominantly in the blood (42–44).

We also evaluated the effects of *H. pylori* therapy on the density and localization of antral G-cells and D-cells in normal volunteers and patients with duodenal ulcer before and after eradication of *H. pylori* (45). Because the interpretation of histological studies is critically dependent on the size and the embedding of the tissue used, jumbo gastric biopsy specimens were obtained. For gastrin immunocytochemistry, the tissues were incubated overnight with a monoclonal antibody raised against synthetic 1–16 gastrin proved by John Walsh. For somatostatin immunocytochemistry, tissues were incubated with a polyclonal antibody raised against synthetic somatostatin (Biogenex, San Ramon, CA). For observation and quantitation, five random fields of the glandular compartment, measuring approximately 780 mm^2, were selected and examined under a dry 40× objective, from each of two well-oriented antral mucosal samples. The number of gastrin and somatostatin-positive cells, including the nucleus in the plane of section, and of complete glandular profiles (defined as complete antral gland with a clearly visible lumen and totally within the microscopic field) were counted and recorded. The G-cell-per-gland ratio was determined for each observed field.

Immunohistochemical analysis of the G cells and D cells and the gastric antral glands in the biopsy specimens from normal volunteers and patients with duodenal ulcer before and after eradication of *H. pylori* showed no significant difference in the number of complete antral gastric gland profiles counted per field among the different groups (45). This observation supports the conclusion that the variable degrees of nonatrophic gastritis present in infected patients did not affect the glandular compartment. Likewise, no significant degrees of intestinal metaplasia or other modifications were present in the tissues examined. The mean number of G cells per antral gland profile was similar in volunteers without *H. pylori* and in volunteers with asymptomatic *H. pylori* infection (p > 0.35). By contrast, the number of G cells per gastric gland profile was significantly lower in duodenal ulcer patients than in control uninfected (p = 0.016) or asymptomatic *H. pylori* infected (p = 0.001) patients. Eradication of *H. pylori* infection in patients with duodenal ulcer did not result in an increase (normalization) in numbers of G-cells per gastric gland profiles (Figure 5).

The number of D cells per antral gland profile was numerically less in patients with *H. pylori* infection, either with duodenal ulcer or asymptomatic *H. pylori* gastritis, than in uninfected individuals (9.8 ± 1.4, 9.3 ± 1.6, and 13.2 ± 2.3, respectively), but differences were not statistically significant (p > 0.18). The number of D cells per complete antral gland was also not statistically different between groups for infected duodenal ulcer and uninfected controls, respectively (Figure 5). We also examined the ratio of G cells to D cells for patients with duodenal ulcer compared with uninfected controls and this was also similar (2.3 vs. 2.0, respectively). There were no statistical differences in the numbers of D cells, nor did G-cell/D-cell ratios increase after *H. pylori* eradication. For example, the median number of G or D cells per complete gland did not change statistically on follow-up of 6 months.

Our observation that the number of G cells per complete antral gland was less in infected patients than in normals was consistent with results of previous studies. There are several possibilities to explain the lack of, or slow recovery of G-cell numbers after successful eradication of the infection. For example, the numbers of G cells per gland counted may not reflect the actual number of gastrin-producing cells present if very actively secreting gastrin-producing cells become degranulated to the point where they can no longer be recognized by immunocytochemistry. For example,

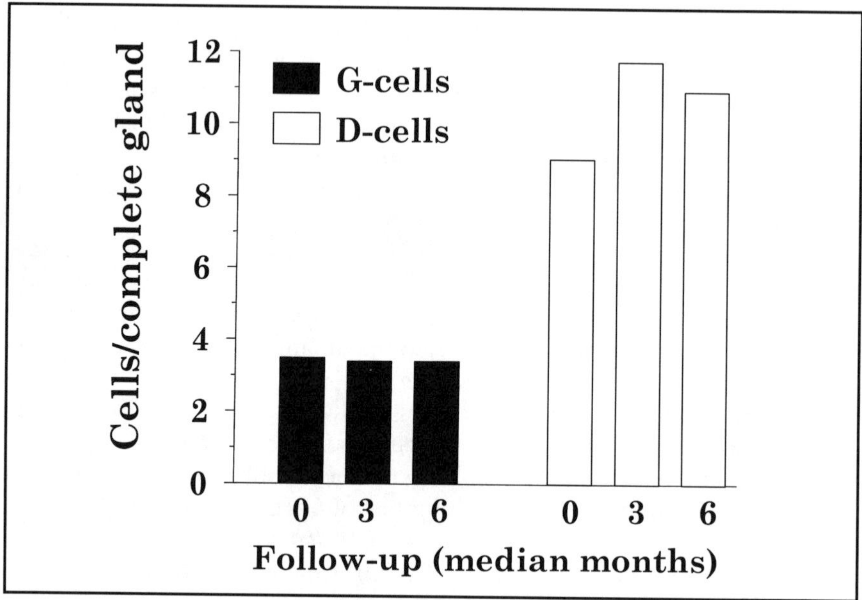

FIGURE 5. *Eradication of* H. pylori *did not result in a significant change in the number of G or D cells per gastric gland during a follow-up of 6 months. Data are shown for before therapy and for the follow-up periods of a median of 2.75 months and 6 months (45).*

Sugamata, et al. reported that in uninfected controls all antral G cells contain abundant gastrin and were easily detected with immunostaining using light microscopy (46). On the contrary, they found that in duodenal ulcer patients with *H. pylori* infection many G-cell granules were electron lucent and that only a few cells stained vividly by immunocytochemistry. They concluded that the number of G-cells might therefore appear to be falsely reduced. We did not find that the number of G cells increased after gastrin release returned to normal levels following *H. pylori* eradication, suggesting that degranulation does not explain the reduced G cell numbers in infected individuals. Another possibility is that low G-cell numbers preceded the infection in a population susceptible to development of duodenal ulcer disease. Current data favor the suggestion that severe inflammation produced by *H. pylori* infection results in irreversible loss of antral G cells. In support of that proposal Crivelli, et al. reported an inverse relationship between the number of antral G cells and the presence and severity of atrophic gastritis (47). The greatest number of G cells was found in those with "normal" histology (defined as no atrophic gastritis), followed by those with histologically atrophic gastritis, with the fewest G cells in those with duodenal ulcer. Other studies have also described reduced antral G-cell numbers with increasingly severe atrophic gastritis (48–50).

Subsequent studies have proposed that reductions in G-cell density were associated with mucosal atrophy, because G cells are rare or absent in antral mucosa with intestinal metaplasia (51, 52). Antral G cell numbers are less in patients with gastric ulcer compared with duodenal ulcer, probably related to the greater frequency of antral mucosal atrophy in gastric ulcer compared with duodenal ulcer. Difference in G-cell numbers between the two *H. pylori* infected groups (duodenal ulcer and asymptomatic gastritis) are probably explained by the fact that antral gastritis is more severe in patients with duodenal ulcer than in *H. pylori*-infected asymptomatic individuals.

Although it has been shown that there is a correlation between maximal acid output and parietal cell density, there is no correlation between parietal cell density and antral G-cell density (51, 53). Current evidence suggests that *H. pylori*-associated increases in gastrin secretion are most likely related, directly or indirectly, to stimulation of G cells (51). Overall, the data support the conclusion that exaggerated gastrin release responses to different stimuli are not the consequence of an increased G-cell mass, but rather reflect greater functional G-cell activity (48, 54). It is not known whether this is through direct stimulation or reduction of inhibition, or both.

Kaneko, et al. reported that *H. pylori* infection was associated with a decrease in imunoreactive somatostatin in human gastric antrum. The degree of decrease correlated with the grade of chronic inflammation (37). Those findings were consistent with an earlier report by Domschke, et al. that the ratio of antral gastrin to somatostatin was greater in patients with duodenal ulcer (and presumably *H. pylori* infection) than in controls (38). Similarly, experiments with organ culture of antral mucosa from duodenal ulcer patients released a greater proportion of antral gastrin into the media and substantially less somatostatin than did non-duodenal ulcer controls (55). In contrast, we found that ratio of G cells to D cells was similar in patients with *H. pylori* infected patients with duodenal ulcer and in uninfected normal individuals (45). Our results support the conclusion that the increased gastrin release response in *H. pylori* infection is not a reflection of increased G-cell or reduced D-cell mass, but rather reflects changes in functional G cell and D cell activities. Reversible decreases in antral somatostatin have been reported in patients with *H. pylori* infection. In addition, somatostatin mRNA/rRNA has been reported to increase after *H. pylori* eradication (56). One must conclude that the details surrounding the changes in gastrin and somatostatin release in relation to *H. pylori* infection remain unsolved. Studies of single events such as synthesis, storage, or release of somatostatin or gastrin provide snap shots that by themselves are difficult to interpret. For example, in animals G-cells can be made to appear or disappear histochemically, by simply fasting or feeding the animal (57). The fact that the gastrin and somatostatin genes appear to be regulated in opposite directions in a coordinated manner (36) does not tell us how, nor does it address differences in post-translational processing or other interactions that may occur (58). To paraphrase Einstein, "God is in the details." The details remain to be elucidated.

H. pylori-*related Perturbation in Acid Secretion*

A logical extension of the evolving concepts of relationships between *H. pylori* and ulcer disease has been that if *H. pylori* were the cause of duodenal ulcer that infection with *H. pylori* may also be responsible for some, if not all, of previously described abnormalities in acid or gastrin secretion. Pentagastrin-stimulated maximum acid output serves as an indirect measure of the parietal cell mass. Study of duodenal ulcer patients has shown that there was either no change or at most a small decrease in maximum acid output after cure of *H. pylori* infection. Any trophic effects of gastrin would not be anticipated to persist for more than 6 months. The failure of the higher than normal parietal cell mass to decrease following cure of the infection did not support the hypothesis that the trophic effect of gastrin was exclusively responsible for producing the high acid output frequently associated with duodenal ulcer disease (21, 29, 59–64).

There was a brief flurry of excitement when it was suggested that acid secretion stimulated by gastrin releasing peptide was exaggerated in patients with duodenal ulcer compared to uninfected or *H. pylori* infected without duodenal ulcer disease (21, 65–67). However, further studies showed that abnormalities in gastric acid secretory responses to gastrin releasing peptide in patients with *H. pylori* infection were not confined to those with duodenal ulcer disease (68) and that the original suggestion was in part related to failure to perform full dose responses. It now appears that the explanation that *H. pylori* infection causes an upward shift in the gastrin-releasing peptide (bombesin) dose response curve for acid secretion independent of clinical presentation is correct. For example, after a maximum dose of gastrin releasing peptide (~40 pmol/k/h), uninfected individuals increased acid secretion to approximately 30% of the maximum pentagastrin-stimulated acid output, whereas patients with *H. pylori* infection, with or without duodenal ulcer, increased to approximately 85% of maximum acid output. Thus, the initial confusion resulted from use of submaximum doses of gastrin releasing peptide and expression of results as the amount of acid secreted rather than the percent of maximum acid output. Because patients with duodenal ulcer tend to have large parietal cell masses, their responses to gastrin releasing peptide appeared excessive when compared to those with *H. pylori* infection and a normal parietal cell mass without ulcer disease. Although cure of infection reverses the upward shift in gastrin releasing peptide-stimulated acid secretion, on average, it does not change the maximum pentagastrin stimulated gastric acid output.

It is now known that the phenomena previously associated with duodenal ulcer disease such as elevated serum pepsinogen levels, reduced inhibition of acid secretion with antral acidification or distention, exaggerated gastrin response to meals, or infusion of bombesin or gastric releasing peptide, exaggerated acid output in response to gastric releasing peptide, and abnormalities in duodenal bicarbonate secretion in response to instillation of acid are all reversible phenomena related to the *H. pylori* infection and are present in patients with and without duodenal ulcer disease (9, 69). The experience learned from the study of previous candidates for genetic factors related to duodenal ulcer disease has suggested minimal criteria for *H. pylori*-related abnormalities in gastric physiology (9, 69). The findings must specifically address whether the event is (i) disease-specific (i.e., to duodenal ulcer disease), (ii) reversible upon cure of the infection and the time course of reversibility, (iii) is it related to the bacteria or a bacterial product (e.g., urease), (iv) to the *H. pylori*-associated inflammation, (v) to a genetics of the host, or (vi) to some combination. In addition, the abnormality must be fully defined (e.g., the full dose response must be examined) and put into perspective with respect to different presentation of *H. pylori* infection (e.g., compare normal patients, those with simple *H. pylori* gastritis, and those with duodenal ulcer disease). Such criteria will largely prevent misidentifying additional reversible epiphenomena with major new disease associated factors. The fact that the greater than normal parietal cell mass remains, following cure of the infection suggests that it the one phenomenon that predates the infection and may in fact predispose development of *H. pylori*-associated duodenal ulcer disease.

H. pylori *and Duodenal Ulcer*

H. pylori organisms are trophic for gastric epithelium but as gastric epithelium is not restricted to the stomach and the organisms can be found whereever ectopic gastric mucosa is present such as inlet patches in the esophagus, ectopic patches in the rectum, and most importantly on ectopic gastric epithelium in the duodenal bulb. The natural mucosal restitution response to duodenal mucosal injury includes production of gastric metaplasia (5). The extent of gastric metaplasia in the duodenum has also been shown to be proportional to gastric acid output. A high duodenal acid load therefore increases the area of gastric metaplasia in the duodenal bulb and provides abundant niches for colonization by *H. pylori. H. pylori* colonization of gastric metaplasia in the duodenal bulb produces inflammation which in turn promotes more gastric metaplasia, resulting in more *H. pylori* colonization and a vicious cycle that culminates in an area of mucosa that becomes increasingly susceptible to ulceration (69, 70). The duodenal ulcer is thought to form at the site of the *H. pylori* infected and inflamed gastric metaplasia and may begin at the junction between inflamed gastric metaplasia and inflamed duodenal mucosa (5).

The actual scenario responsible for producing a duodenal ulcer is unknown. A high duodenal acid load requires relatively unimpeded acid secretion from the gastric corpus. It is thought that the ability to secrete high levels of acid limits the ability of *H. pylori* to interact with corpus mucosa. However, reducing acid secretion by any method such as surgery, anti-secretory therapy, poor diet, etc. may reduce or eliminate this restriction and promote corpus gastritis among those with *H. pylori* infection (5, 6, 69, 71–76). The lack of significant inflammation in the gastric corpus coupled with *H. pylori* associated dysregulations of acid secretion, (e.g., impaired down regulation of acid secretion when the antral pH falls to 3 or less) results in a markedly increased duodenal acid load which is likely the key element responsible for duodenal ulcer disease (69). *H. pylori*-induced inflammation in the duodenal bulb and the damage caused by the duodenal acid load both decrease the duodenal mucosa's ability to secrete bicarbonate and thus further augments the functional duodenal acid load. *H. pylori* growth is inhibited by glycine conjugated bile acids making the normal duodenal bulb a hostile environment for *H. pylori* growth (69, 70). A high duodenal acid load lowers the average duodenal pH and precipitates glycine conjugated bile acids encouraging *H. pylori* colonization in, but rarely beyond, the duodenal bulb. Many factors can promote *H. pylori* colonization of the duodenal bulb via increased duodenal acid load. For example, stress increases basal acid secretion and may also increase the amount of smoking. Smoking is a potent stimulus for an increased duodenal acid load as it increases acid secretion and it inhibits duodenal bulb and pancreatic bicarbonate secretion (69, 70). NSAIDs increase acid secretion and may damage the duodenal mucosa and promote gastric metaplasia, thus providing new niches for *H. pylori* colonization. Similarly, antisecretory therapy by reducing the duodenal acid load may reconstitute the *H. pylori* inhibiting effect of bile and act as a biologic anti-*H. pylori* therapy.

H. pylori is most commonly acquired in childhood, yet duodenal ulcer is typically a disease of adults. Why? According to the physiology outlined above, the development of a duodenal ulcer requires an increased duodenal acid load for long enough to cause sufficient alterations of the duodenum to occur such that *H. pylori* can thrive and cause the disease. Seemingly subtle changes in behavior such as starting or stopping smoking could have major effects on this balance and tip the scale one way or the other. Similarly, as mentioned above use of an antisecretory drug such as an H2-receptor antagonist or antacids would reduce the duodenal acid load and allow the glycine conjugated bile acids to remain in solution and inhibit *H. pylori* growth (69, 70). It is easy to envision many different scenarios where the balance would tip, resulting in exacerbations and remissions in duodenal ulcer disease activity and explaining how and why agents and actions might have influenced ulcer disease in the past. It should be evident that there can be a fine balance that dictates whether an ulcer is present or absent.

SUMMARY

The study of gastric secretion has long focused on the components of gastric acid secretion and comparisons of acid secretion in those with and without duodenal ulcer. Overtime the studies evolved into the detailed examination of factors which regulate gastric acid secretion. The advent of methods to accurately measure gastrointestinal hormones, their receptors, their genes, and as well as beginning to understand the regulation of gene expression and post-translational processing of the gene products has resulted in increasingly detailed descriptions of the factors involved in the regulation of acid secretion. The relationship between ECL cells, G-cells, D-cells, and parietal cells have begun to be explored in detail and these studies have resulted in the generation of a large amount of data relating to neurohumoral interactions between nerves, endocrine cells, secretory targets and the various peptide messengers (3). Each advance seems to only uncover another deeper and richer layer of interactions such that overall science seems to advance with remarkably small steps. In most instances an immense amount of data must be accumulated before synthesis occurs allowing the useful to be separated from the less useful and for the interconnections to be recognized and the nuances explored. The stomach has been the site of many important diseases such that the centuries old interest in the details of how it functions in health and disease has been well placed. The rediscovery of *H. pylori* and realization that a bacteria, bacterial products, inflammation and inflammatory mediators are all potentially critically involved in the disease-associated disregulations of gastric physiology resulted in one of those periods requiring rethinking and reintegration as well as the development of new understandings as old disparate observations and apparent inconsistencies began to make sense. The importance of *H. pylori* also came at the time where it became practical to begin to truly explore what was happening at the level of the cell and of the gene. The number of factors that must now be considered has advanced exponentially, or has it? John H. Walsh was one of the key workers responsible for moving this field forward and his ability to explore, to lead, and to communicate will be sorely missed.

REFERENCES

1. Davenport HW. A history of gastric secretion and digestion Experimental studies to 1975. New York: Oxford University Press, 1992.
2. Hirschowitz BI. Controls of gastric secretion. A roadmap to the choice of treatment for duodenal ulcer. *Am J Gastroenterol* 1982;77:281–293.
3. Sachs G, Prinz CK, Hersey SJ. Acid-related disorders Mystery to mechanism: mechanism to management. Palm Beach, FL: Sushu Publishing, Inc., 1995.
4. Soll AH. Gastric, duodenal, and stress ulcer. In: Sleisenger M and Fordtran J, Eds. *Gastrointestinal Disease.* 5 Ed. Philadelphia: WB Saunders, 1993:580–679.
5. Graham DY. *Campylobacter pylori* and peptic ulcer disease. *Gastroenterology* 1989;96:615–625.
6. Kekki M, Villako K, Tamm A, Siurala M. Dynamics of antral and fundal gastritis in an Estonian rural population sample. *Scand J Gastroenterol* 1977;12:321–324.
7. Rohrer GV, Welsh JD. Correlative study: gastric secretion and histology. *Gastroenterology* 1967;52: 185–191.
8. Funder FF, Weiden S. The correlation between test meal findings and histology of the stomach as shown by gastric biopsy. *Med J Aust* 1952;1:600–602.
9. Graham DY. *Helicobacter pylori* and perturbations in acid secretion: the end of the beginning. *Gastroenterology* 1996;110:1647–1650.
10. Steer HW. The gastro-duodenal epithelium in peptic ulceration. *J Pathol* 1985;146:355–362.
11. Steer HW. Surface morphology of the gastroduodenal mucosa in duodenal ulceration. *Gut* 1984;25: 1203–1210.
12. Steer HW, Colin-Jones DG. Mucosal changes in gastric ulceration and their response to carbenoxolone sodium. *Gut* 1975;16:590–597.
13. Steer HW. Ultrastructure of cell migration through the gastric epithelium and its relationship to bacteria. *J Clin Pathol* 1975;28:639–646.
14. Marshall B. Unidentified curved bacilli on gastric epithelium in active chronic gastritis. *Lancet* 1983; 1:1273–1275.
15. Marshall BJ, Armstrong JA, McGechie DB, Glancy RJ. Attempt to fulfil Koch's postulates for pyloric *Campylobacter. Med J Aust* 1985;142:436–439.
16. Morris A, Nicholson G. Ingestion of *Campylobacter pyloridis* causes gastritis and raised fasting gastric pH. *Am J Gastroenterol* 1987;82:192–199.
17. Morris AJ, Ali MR, Nicholson GI, Perez-Perez GI, Blaser MJ. Long-term follow-up of voluntary ingestion of *Helicobacter pylori. Ann Intern Med* 1991;114:662–663.
18. McNulty CA, Gearty JC, Crump B, Davis M, Donovan IA, Melikian V, Lister DM, Wise R. *Campylobacter pyloridis* and associated gastritis: investigator blind, placebo controlled trial of bismuth salicylate and erythromycin ethylsuccinate. *Br Med J* 1986;293:645–649.
19. Graham DY. Benefits from elimination of *Helicobacter pylori* infection include major reduction in the incidence of peptic ulcer disease, gastric cancer, and primary gastric lymphoma. *Prev Med* 1994;23: 712–716.
20. Graham DY. Present status of research and outlook for the future: what did we accomplish? In: Halter F, Garner A, and Tytgat GNJ, Eds. *Mechanisms of Peptic Ulcer Healing.* Dordrecht: Kluwer Academic Publishers, 1991:303–309.
21. El-Omar EM, Penman ID, Ardill JE, Chittajallu RS, Howie C, McColl KE. *Helicobacter pylori* infection and abnormalities of acid secretion in patients with duodenal ulcer disease. *Gastroenterology* 1995;109:681–691.
22. Graham DY, Opekun A, Lew GM, Evans DJ, Jr., Klein PD, Evans DG. Ablation of exaggerated meal-stimulated gastrin release in duodenal ulcer patients after clearance of *Helicobacter (Campylobacter) pylori* infection. *Am J Gastroenterol* 1990;85:394–398.
23. Levi S, Beardshall K, Haddad G, Playford R, Ghosh P, Calam J. *Campylobacter pylori* and duodenal ulcers: the gastrin link. *Lancet* 1989;1:1167–1168.
24. Levi S, Beardshall K, Swift I, Foulkes W, Playford R, Ghosh P, Calam J. Antral *Helicobacter pylori,* hypergastrinaemia, and duodenal ulcers: effect of eradicating the organism. *Br Med J* 1989;299:1504–1505.

25. McColl KE, Fullarton GM, el Nujumi AM, MacDonald AM, Brown IL, Hilditch TE. Lowered gastrin and gastric acidity after eradication of *Campylobacter pylori* in duodenal ulcer. *Lancet* 1989;2:499–500.

26. Oderda G, Vaira D, Holton J, Ainley C, Altare F, Ansaldi N. Amoxycillin plus tinidazole for *Campylobacter pylori* gastritis in children: assessment by serum IgG antibody, pepsinogen I, and gastrin levels. *Lancet* 1989;1:690–692.

27. Smith JT, Pounder RE, Nwokolo CU, Lanzon Miller S, Evans DG, Graham DY, Evans DJ, Jr. Inappropriate hypergastrinaemia in asymptomatic healthy subjects infected with *Helicobacter pylori*. *Gut* 1990;31:522–525.

28. Graham DY, Dore MP. Perturbations in gastric physiology in *Helicobacter pylori* duodenal ulcer: are they all epiphenomena? *Helicobacter* 1997;2 Suppl 1:S44–9.

29. Peterson WL, Barnett CC, Evans DJ, Jr., Feldman M, Carmody T, Richardson C, Walsh J, Graham DY. Acid secretion and serum gastrin in normal subjects and patients with duodenal ulcer: the role of *Helicobacter pylori*. *Am J Gastroenterol* 1993;88:2038–2043.

30. Graham DY, Opekun A, Lew GM, Klein PD, Walsh JH. *Helicobacter pylori*-associated exaggerated gastrin release in duodenal ulcer patients. The effect of bombesin infusion and urea ingestion. *Gastroenterology* 1991;100:1571–1575.

31. Graham DY, Go MF, Lew GM, Genta RM, Rehfeld JF. *Helicobacter pylori* infection and exaggerated gastrin release: effects of inflammation and progastrin processing. *Scand J Gastroenterol* 1993;28: 690–694.

32. Graham DY, Go MF, Evans DJ, Jr. Urease, gastric ammonium/ammonia, and *Helicobacter pylori*—the past, the present, and recommendations for future research. *Aliment Pharmacol Ther* 1992;6:659–669.

33. Lehmann FS, Golodner EH, Wang J, Chen MC, Avedian D, Calam J, Walsh JH, Dubinett S, Soll AH. Mononuclear cells and cytokines stimulate gastrin release from canine antral cells in primary culture. *Am J Physiol* 1996;270:G783–8.

34. Kramling HJ, Enders G, Teichmann RK, Demmel T, Merkle R, Brendel W. Antigen-induced gastrin release: an immunologic mechanism of gastric antral mucosa. *Adv Exp Med Biol* 1987;216A:427–429.

35. Teichmann RK, Kramling HJ, Merkle T, Merkle R. Opposite effect of interleukin-1 on gastrin and bombesin release in cell suspensions of antral mucosa (Abstract). *Digestion* 1990;46 (Suppl 1):114.

36. Wu V, Sumii K, Tari A, Sumii M, Walsh JH. Regulation of rat antral gastrin and somatostatin gene expression during starvation and after refeeding. *Gastroenterology* 1991;101:1552–1558.

37. Kaneko H, Nakada K, Mitsuma T, Uchida K, Furusawa A, Maeda Y, Morise K. *Helicobacter pylori* infection induces a decrease in immunoreactive-somatostatin concentrations of human stomach. *Dig Dis Sci* 1992;37:409–416.

38. Domschke S, Bloom SR, Adrian TE, Lux G, Bryant MG, Domschke W. Gastroduodenal mucosal hormone content in duodenal ulcer disease. *Hepato-Gastroenterology* 1985;32:198–201.

39. Lichtenberger LM, Nelson AA, Graziani LA. Amine trapping: physical explanation for the inhibitory effect of gastric acidity on the postprandial release of gastrin. Studies on rats and dogs. *Gastroenterology* 1986;90:1223–1231.

40. Chittajallu RS, Neithercut WD, MacDonald AM, McColl KE. Effect of increasing *Helicobacter pylori* ammonia production by urea infusion on plasma gastrin concentrations. *Gut* 1991;32:21–24.

41. Bromberg PA, Robin ED, Forkner CE. The existence of ammonia in blood *in vivo* with observations on the significance of the $NH_4{}^+$-NH_3 system. *J Clin Invest* 1960;39:332–341.

42. Kornberg HL, Davies RE, Wood DR. The activity and function of gastric urease in the cat. *Biochem J* 1954;56:363–372.

43. Kornberg HL, Davies RE. Gastric urease. *Physiol Rev* 1955;35:169–177.

44. Von Korff RW, Ferguson DJ, Glick D. Role of urease in the gastric mucosa II *in vitro* studies with isotopic urea on frog mucosa. *Am J Physiol* 1951;165:688–694.

45. Graham DY, Lew GM, Lechago J. Antral G-cell and D-cell numbers in *Helicobacter pylori* infection: effect of *H. pylori* eradication. *Gastroenterology* 1993;104:1655–1660.

46. Sugamata M, Ihara T, Todate A, Hirakawa R, Yoshida Y, Yamanaka T, Miyata M, Miura M. Ultrastructural study of antral G cells in patients with duodenal ulcer: effect of *Helicobacter pylori* eradication. *Helicobacter* 1997;2:118–122.

47. Crivelli O, Pera A, Ferrari A, Rizzetto M, Lombardo L, Babando G, Verme G. G-cell counts in antral endoscopic biopsies by immunofluorescence. *Scand J Gastroenterol* 1977;12:721–726.

48. Creutzfeldt W, Arnold R, Creutzfeldt C, Track NS. Mucosal gastrin concentration, molecular forms of gastrin, number and ultrastructure of G-cells in patients with duodenal ulcer. *Gut* 1976;17:745–754.

49. Marotta F, Chui DH, Zhong GG, Safran P. Effect of graded intravenous doses of urogastrone on duodenal bicarbonate secretion in conscious rats: evidence of a dose-response pattern. *Digestion* 1990;47:88–94.

50. Keuppens F, Willems G, Vansteenkiste Y, Woussen-Colle MC. Estimation of the antral and duodenal gastrin cell population removed by gastrectomy from patients with peptic ulcer. *Surg Gynecol Obstet* 1978;146:400–406.

51. Stave R, Myren J, Brandtzaeg P, Gjone E. Quantitative studies of gastrin cells (G cells) and parietal cells in relation to gastric acid secretion in patients with peptic ulcer disease. *Scand J Gastroenterol* 1978;13:293–298.

52. Takahashi T, Shimazu H, Yamagishi T, Tani M. G-cell populations in resected stomachs from gastric and duodenal ulcer patients. *Gastroenterology* 1980;78:498–504.

53. Card WI, Marks IN. The relationship between the acid output of the stomach following "maximal" histamine stimulation and the parietal cell mass. *Clin Sci* 1960;19:147–163.

54. Barbara L, Biasco G, Salera M, Baldi F, di Febo G, Miglioli M. Antral G cells and mucosal gastrin concentration in normal subjects and in patients with duodenal ulcer. *Adv Exp Med Biol* 1978;106: 97–104.

55. Harty RF, Aico DG, McGuigan JE. Antral release of gastrin and somatostatin in duodenal ulcer and control subjects. *Gut* 1986;27:652–658.

56. Moss SF, Egon S, Bishop AE, Polak JM, Calam J. Effect of *Helicobacter pylori* on gastric somatostatin in duodenal ulcer disease. *Lancet* 1992;340:930–932.

57. Lichtenberger LM, Lechago J, Johnson LR. Depression of antral and serum gastrin concentration by food deprivation in the rat. *Gastroenterology* 1975;68:1473–1479.

58. Calam J. *Helicobacter pylori* and somatostatin cells. *Eur J Gastroenterol Hepatol* 1998;10:281–283.

59. Moss SF, Calam J. Acid secretion and sensitivity to gastrin in patients with duodenal ulcer: effect of eradication of *Helicobacter pylori*. *Gut* 1993;34:888–892.

60. Calam J. *Helicobacter pylori,* acid and gastrin. *Eur J Gastroenterol Hepatol* 1995;7:310–317.

61. Graham DY. *Helicobacter pylori:* its epidemiology and its role in duodenal ulcer disease. *J Gastroenterol Hepatol* 1991;6:105–113.

62. McColl KE, Fullarton GM, Chittajalu R, el Nujumi AM, MacDonald AM, Dahill SW, Hilditch TE. Plasma gastrin, daytime intragastric pH, and nocturnal acid output before and at 1 and 7 months after eradication of *Helicobacter pylori* in duodenal ulcer subjects. *Scand J Gastroenterol* 1991;26:339–346.

63. Harris AW, Gummett PA, Misiewicz JJ, Baron JH. The effect of eradication of *Helicobacter pylori* on gastric acid output in patients with duodenal ulcer. *Gastroenterology* 108, A109. 1995.

64. Parente F, Maconi G, Sangaletti O, Minguzzi M, Vago L, Bianchi Porro G. Behaviour of acid secretion, gastrin release, serum pepsinogen I, and gastric emptying of liquids over six months from eradication of *Helicobacter pylori* in duodenal ulcer patients. A controlled study. *Gut* 1995;37:210–215.

65. El-Omar E, Penman I, Dorrian CA, Ardill JES, McColl KEL. Eradicating *Helicobacter pylori* infection lowers gastrin mediated acid secretion by two thirds in patients with duodenal ulcer. *Gut* 1993;34:1060–1065.

66. El-Omar E, Penman I, Ardill JE, McColl KE. A substantial proportion of non-ulcer dyspepsia patients have the same abnormality of acid secretion as duodenal ulcer patients. *Gut* 1995;36:534–538.

67. McColl KE, El-Omar E. Review article: gastrin releasing peptide and its value in assessing gastric secretory function. *Aliment Pharmacol Ther* 1995;9:341–347.

68. Olbe L, Hamlet A, Dalenback J, Fandriks L. A mechanism by which *Helicobacter pylori* infection of the antrum contributes to the development of duodenal ulcer. *Gastroenterology* 1996;110:1386–1394.

69. Dore MP, Graham DY. Pathogenesis of duodenal ulcer disease: the rest of the story. *Baillieres Best Pract Res Clin Gastroenterol* 2000;14:97–107.

70. Graham DY, Osato MS. *H. pylori* in the pathogenesis of duodenal ulcer: interaction between duodenal acid load, bile, and *H. pylori*. *Am J Gastroenterol* 2000;95:87–91.

71. Kekki M, Hakkiluoto A, Siurala M. Dynamics of atrophic gastritis in male and female subjects after partial gastric resection—an evaluation by stochastic analysis. *Scand J Gastroenterol* 1976;11:597–601.

72. Tarpila S, Kekki M, Samloff IM, Sipponen P, Siurala M. Morphology and dynamics of the gastric mucosa in duodenal ulcer patients and their first-degree relatives. *Hepato-Gastroenterology* 1983;30:198–201.
73. Kuipers EJ, Lee A, Klinkenberg-Knol EC, Meuwissen SG. Review article: the development of atrophic gastritis—*Helicobacter pylori* and the effects of acid suppressive therapy. *Aliment Pharmacol Ther* 1995;9:331–340.
74. Meining A, Bosseckert H, Caspary WF, Nauert C, Stolte M. H2-receptor antagonists and antacids have an aggravating effect on *Helicobacter pylori* gastritis in duodenal ulcer patients. *Aliment Pharmacol Ther* 1997;11:729–734.
75. Meining A, Kiel G, Stolte M. Changes in *Helicobacter pylori*-induced gastritis in the antrum and corpus during and after 12 months of treatment with ranitidine and lansoprazole in patients with duodenal ulcer disease. *Aliment Pharmacol Ther* 1998;12:735–740.
76. Graham DY. *Helicobacter pylori* infection in the pathogenesis of duodenal ulcer and gastric cancer: a model. *Gastroenterology* 1997;113:1983–1991.

II.

Gut Peptides and their Receptors

Gut-Brain Peptides in the New Millennium, edited by Y. Taché
CURE Foundation, Los Angeles, CA. © 2002

9

Glutathione: Ubiquitous Peptide with Many Functions

Neil Kaplowitz
*University of Southern California Research Center for Liver Diseases,
Department of Medicine, Keck School of Medicine of the
University of Southern California, Los Angeles, CA*

INTRODUCTION

I would like to take this opportunity to pay tribute to the memory and career of John Walsh. I first met John in 1974 when I was being recruited to UCLA and then was a colleague at UCLA-CURE from 1975 to 1990, which spans a period of my career when my research flourished, largely due to the intellectual environment contributed to by many, but most consistently and importantly by John Walsh. Since my interest was glutathione, a tripeptide, and John was an authority on the biology and chemistry of peptide hormones, we shared much in common and had many, nearly daily interactions in the halls of CURE. These were stimulating for both of us. What particularly stands out was John's great curiosity, encyclopedic knowledge and delight in me sharing my latest hypothesis or new finding.

In this chapter I will focus on the current understanding of the functions of glutathione (GSH) as it has been my longitudinal focus. Much of the current understanding of this field has germinated from the seeds laid and nurtured at CURE in the 70's and 80's and has spread to many of my students and postdocs from that era, including Shelly Lu, Laurie DeLeve, Andrew Stolz, Yuichi Sugiyama, Tak Yee Aw, Jose Fernandez-Checa, Murad Ookhtens, Ram Kannan, and others.

Glutathione is a tripeptide which consists of glutamate, cysteine, and glycine. It has several unique properties, most notably a thiol which is far more stable under aerobic conditions than the thiol of cysteine and a unique peptide bond between the gamma carboxyl of glutamate and the amino group of cysteine. This bond resists all proteases in nature except for one enzyme, γ-glutamyl transpeptidase (GGT) which releases glutamate, leaving cysteinylglycine for hydrolysis by dipeptidases. To understand the importance and functions of glutathione, we will consider its transport-interorgan homeostasis and role in detoxification. Since this chapter is a personal view, I will mainly cite my own work and largely reference review articles.

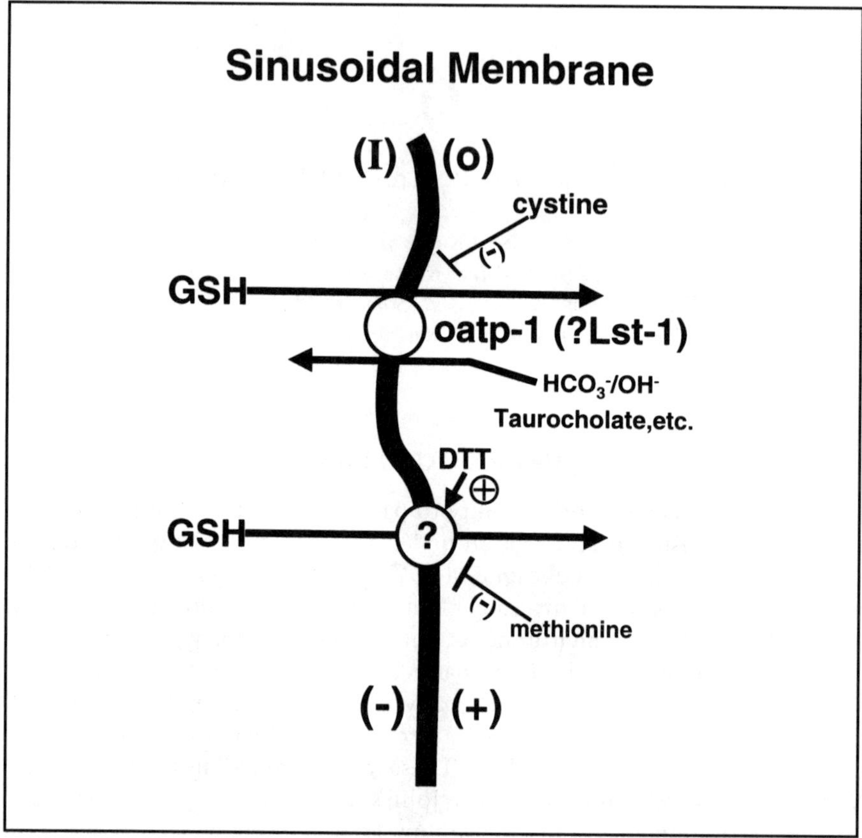

FIGURE 1. *Sinusoidal transport of GSH. At least two transporters exist—(1) oatp-1 which mediates electroneutral exchange of GSH for inorganic and organic anions and is inhibited by cystine, and (2) an unidentified carrier which mediates electrogenic efflux of GSH and is inhibited by methionine and stimulated by DTT. (I) = inside, (O) = outside.*

Transport and Interorgan in Homeostasis

Glutathione is synthesized in the cytosol of all mammalian cells by the sequential activity of two enzymes, γ-glutamylcysteine synthetase and GSH synthetase in reactions which require energy in the form of ATP. Under normal physiological conditions GSH is present in mM concentrations in cells and its turnover is mainly governed by efflux from cells (1, 2). This process appears to be ubiquitous although quantitatively most important in the liver and kidney. At present we do not have a full understanding of all the transporters for GSH. However, in liver, GSH is released at both poles of the cell. Sinusoidal release accounts for nearly all the GSH found in plasma and canalicular release is a major contributor to total liver GSH turnover (3).

On the sinusoidal or basolateral side of hepatocytes, rat oatp-1 has been shown to transport GSH (4). This is an electroneutral exchanger which transports intracellular GSH in exchange for extracellular substrates, such as taurocholate or OH^-/HCO_3^-. The human ortholog is not expressed in liver and it is currently not known if the major family member in human liver, OATP2 (LST-1), transports GSH. Rat oatp2 exhibits little, if any, GSH transport activity. Physiological characterization of GSH transport at the sinusoidal pole suggests that another transporter, not yet identified, accounts for the bulk of this activity. GSH transport appears to be electrogenic, trans-inhibited by methionine, and greatly stimulated by the direct membrane effect of uncharged thiol compounds, such as dithiothreitol (DTT) (3, 5). These properties are not features of oatp-1. In contrast, the transport activity of oatp1 is inhibited by cystine which interferes with GSH transport (Figure 1). Of note, the outwardly directed GSH gradient serves as a driving force for uptake of organic anions by oatp-1 (4, 6).

At the canalicular pole, vesicle studies suggest a low affinity, facilitative transporter (7, 8). However, the absence of GSH secretion in rats with a genetic defect in Mrp2 and increased secretion of GSH in cells overexpressing Mrp2 indicate a close link between Mrp2 and GSH secretion (4). Mrp2 is an ABC transporter which governs the ATP-dependent transport of GSH-conjugates, bilirubin glucuronides, drugs, oxidized glutathione (GSSG) and probably GSH (Figure 2). However, GSH is an extremely low affinity substrate and the direct demonstration of an ATP dependence of GSH transport has been difficult to confirm, although a yeast ABC transporter, YCF-1, appears to do so (4). This leaves open the possibility of a distinct transporter of GSH which is regulated by Mrp2 in an ATP dependent fashion, analogous to the regulation of ATP transport by cystic fibrosis transmembrane regulator (CFTR). A puzzling feature of canalicular GSH secretion is the high concentration of GSH in bile which approaches the cell concentration. Although low affinity, ATP dependent transport of GSH is possible, it seems implausible that this can account for the large secretion capacity for GSH. We and others have demonstrated that GSH may appear in bile by two other mechanisms involving Mrp2. One is transport of labile GSH conjugates and the other is co-transport of GSH and another compound (9) (Figure 2). In either case the transport is of high affinity and results in the appearance of GSH outside the cell. Thus, it is conceivable, and perhaps likely, that the bulk of GSH secretion into bile under physiological conditions in the intact liver is due to one of these mechanisms, such as the formation of labile adducts of GSH with aldehydes which are high affinity substrates for Mrp2.

What purpose does GSH efflux serve? Canalicular secretion may be an important driving force for bile salt independent bile flow but the absence of this phenomenon in Mrp2 mutants or Dubin-Johnson syndrome has no apparent consequences. To understand the importance of GSH efflux, it is

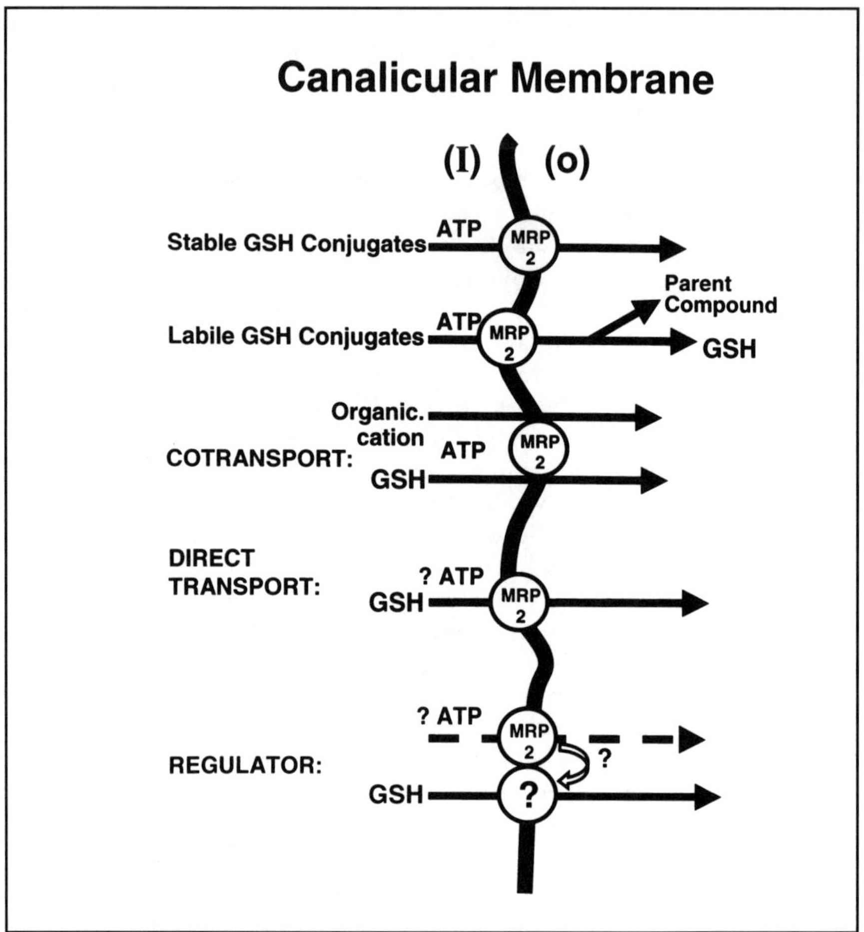

FIGURE 2. *Role of Mrp2 in GSH transport. Various ways in which Mrp2 may mediate GSH secretion are depicted. From top to bottom, Mrp2 transports stable GSH conjugates, labile conjugates which release GSH in the bile, co-transports organic cations (e.g. Vinca Alkaloids) and GSH, may directly transport GSH in an ATP driven process or Mrp2 may regulate the activity of a separate GSH transporter or channel (which may require the interaction of ATP with Mrp2).*

important to recognize that many cell types require plasma cysteine to synthesize GSH and proteins. Some cells do not transport cystine and in general the competition for X_C system transport of cystine by glutamate limits the availability of cystine. Although the hepatocyte can transsulfurate methionine to generate cysteine, this pathway is largely absent elsewhere. Cysteine is very important but has a very short half-life due to auto-oxidation.

The stable thiol of GSH provides a continuous source of cysteine. This requires the hydrolysis of GSH by GGT and dipeptidases which are plasma membrane enzymes whose active sites are oriented externally. Therefore, to release cysteine from its stable storage as GSH requires the release of GSH from cells. This cycle of storage of cysteine as GSH synthesized in cells and recovery of cysteine from GSH outside cells involves two important components—the efflux transport of GSH and the action of GGT (2, 3). Recent studies using GGT null mice have confirmed the critical importance of this cycle as the animals become profoundly cysteine and GSH deficient and their normal development can be restored by treatment with N-acetylcysteine (10).

The cysteine/GSH cycle described above can occur in an autocrine/paracrine fashion within a tissue or can involve interorgan homeostasis. Thus, GSH released from the liver into plasma can supply substrate for GGT in the liver (human hepatocytes express GGT on the sinusoidal pole) or in extrahepatic sites such as the bile ducts, intestine, and kidneys (3).

Another possible fate of hepatic GSH released into plasma is its direct uptake by other tissues. A sodium GSH co-transport process has been described in enterocytes, renal epithelium, alveolar type II cells, lens epithelium and brain capillary endothelium. The existence of such a transporter is strongly supported by physiological data in cells and membrane vesicles (11, 12). However, neither the molecular identity nor the relative contribution of this transport system to GSH homeostasis is known.

GSH and Detoxification

GSH is a substrate for various enzymes of detoxification including GSH S-transferases and selenium-dependent GSH peroxidases (2). The former is illustrated by the detoxification of electrophilic exogenous and endogenous metabolites. In this process the enzyme catalysis preferentially sacrifices the thiol of GSH over chemical reaction with protein thiols. The peroxidases are critical in reducing H_2O_2 and organic peroxides and therefore in defense against oxidative stress.

The subcellular compartmentation of GSH is of critical importance (Figure 3). GSH is synthesized in cytosol and then transported into other compartments. Transport out of the cell has been discussed above in terms of the cysteine/GSH cycle. Extracellular GSH also may be of importance in maintaining the thiols of membrane transporters and receptors, scavenging radicals including NO, and as a substrate for extracellular peroxidase. Within the cell, GSH probably freely enters the nucleus, although some evidence has suggested a nuclear membrane transport. Within the nucleus GSH may be very important in maintaining the reduced thiol status of transcription factors. GSH and GSSG transport in the endoplasmic reticulum are not well characterized but are of obvious importance in protein disulfide formation and protein folding. Of particular importance is GSH transport into mitochondria (13, 14). Evidence supports the role of di- and tri-carboxylate

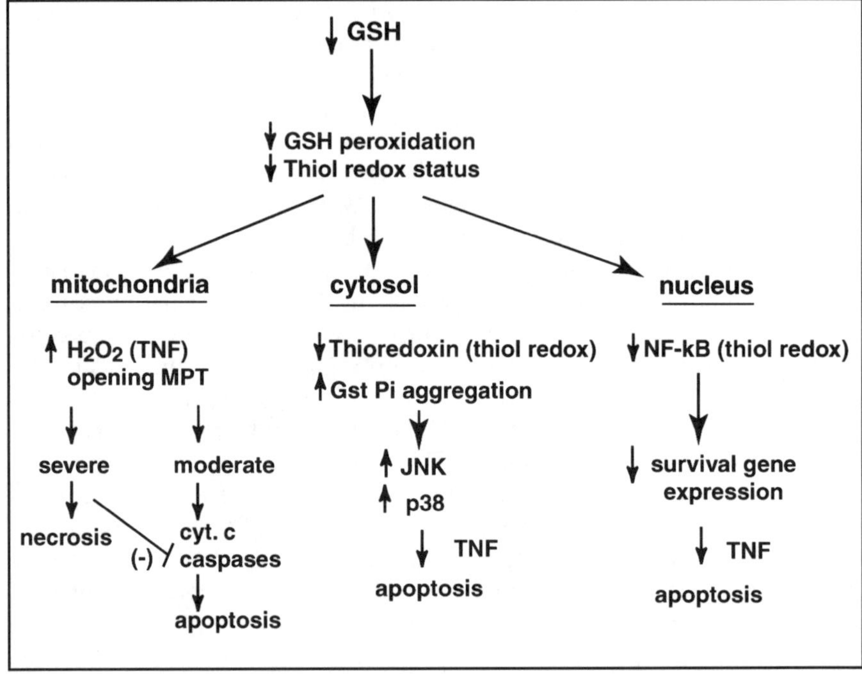

FIGURE 3. *Influence of GSH depletion on cell death. Profound GSH depletion leaves oxidative stress unopposed and alters the redox balance of thiol-disulfides. In mitochondria, these effects, which are amplified by TNF induced oxidative stress, alter mitochondrial permeability which can result in necrotic cell death or promote cytochrome c release and apoptosis. In cytosol, stress kinases (JNK and p38), which are inhibited by thioredoxin and GST Pi, are activated by oxidative stress and redox changes. In the nucleus, redox changes in GSH inhibit DNA binding and transactivation of survival genes by NF-kB. These cytosol and nuclear effects also may sensitize to TNF-induced apopotosis.*

transporters into GSH uptake in renal mitochondria although this has not been fully defined in liver mitochondria. GSH depletion below a critical threshold in mitochondria is lethal to aerobic cells and underscores the fact that mitochondria normally produce H_2O_2 through leak of electrons to O_2^- (physiologic oxidative stress). This process is amplified by uncouplers, GD3 sphingolipids, and bile acids. Tumor necrosis factor (TNFα) signaling leads to interruption of electron transport at complex III leading to increased mitochondrial oxidative stress. Thus, the transport and availability of GSH in mitochondria is of great importance in maintaining defense against oxidative stress. Impairment of this transport due to alcohol feeding renders hepatocytes susceptible to the lethal effects of TNF (15, 16).

Another aspect of the role of GSH is the maintenance of the redox status of protein thiols. When protein thiols are in close proximity (vicinal) it has been empirically demonstrated that the maintenance of the reduced status is defined by $(GSH)^2/(GSSG)$. Thus, aside from the impact of GSSG excess (which is minimized by NADPH GSSG reductase and ABC transporter driven efflux of GSSG), changes in (GSH) in the absence of a change in (GSH)/(GSSG) will influence vicinal dithiols of proteins such as transporters, enzymes and transcription factors. Profound GSH depletion (Figure 3) which includes mitochondria GSH will lead to necrotic cell death which is inhibited by antioxidants. GSH depletion also sensitizes to the lethal action of TNFα due to a dual effect: 1) mitochondrial GSH depletion sensitizes to TNFα induced oxidative stress which tends to cause collapse of mitochondria, loss of ATP, cell swelling and lysis or could cause release of cytochrome C and apoptosis if the oxidative stress is moderate; 2) in contrast, depletion of cytosol/nuclear GSH leads to a redox perturbation which is independent of oxidative stress (antioxidant resistant) and sensitizes to the lethal effects of TNFα. Possible redox sensitive targets include stress kinases (JNK and p38), the mitochondrial permeability pore (MPT) and nuclear factor (NF)-kB binding to DNA and transactivation of survival genes (17) (Figure 3).

In conclusion, I have attempted to provide a concise but broad overview of glutathione, the fascinating peptide which is made in all mammalian cells and performs a variety of critical functions in amino acid homeostasis, detoxification and regulation of redox status. The career of John Walsh, which paralleled much of my career, has served as an inspiration to my work and that of countless others.

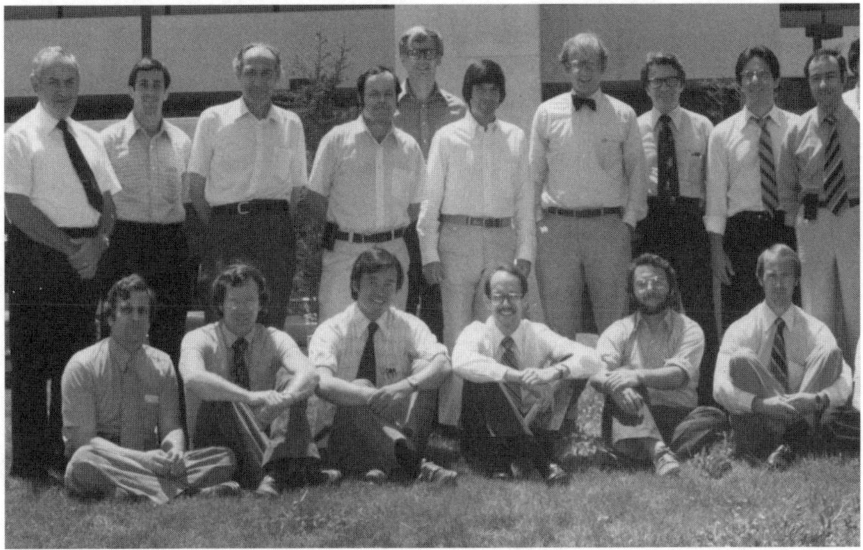

The 1978 CURE group. Upper row, left to right: the late Arthur Schwabe, Al Varner, the late Mort Grossman, a pediatric GI fellow, the late John Walsh (tallest, wearing glasses), Andy Ippoliti, Jon Isenberg, Paul Guth, Steve Weinstock, and Parvis Afshani. Lower row, left to right: Steve Pandol, a GI fellow, Tachi Yamada, Michael Cooper, Neil Kaplowitz, and Dean Jensen.

REFERENCES

1. Kaplowitz N, Ookhtens M, and Aw TY. The regulation of hepatic glutathione. In: *Ann Rev Pharm Tox* 1985;5:715–744.
2. DeLeve L, Kaplowitz N. Glutathione metabolism and its role in hepatotoxicity. *Pharmacology Therapeutics* 1991;52:287–305.
3. Ookhtens M, Kaplowitz N. Role of the liver in interorgan homeostasis of GSH and cysteine. *Seminars in Liver Disease* 1998;18:313–329.
4. Ballatori N, Rebbeor J. Roles of MRP2 and oatp1 in hepatocellular export of reduced glutathione. *Seminars in Liver Disease* 1998;18:377–388.
5. Colell A, Coll O, Garcia-Ruiz C, Paris R, Tiribelli C, Kaplowitz N, Fernandez-Checa J. Tauroursodeoxycholic acid protects hepatocytes from ethanol-fed rats against TNF-induced cell death by replenishing mitochondrial GSH. *Hepatology* 2001;34:964–971.
6. Garcia-Ruiz C, Fernandez-Checa J, Kaplowitz N. Bidirectional mechanism of plasma membrane transport of reduced GSH in hepatocytes and membrane vesicles. *J Biol Chem* 1992;267:22256–22264.
7. Fernandez-Checa J, Takikawa H, Ookhtens M, Kaplowitz N. Canalicular transport of GSH reduced in normal and mutant EHBR rats. *J Biol Chem* 1992;267:1667–1673.
8. Mittur A, Kaplowitz N, Kempner E, Ookhtens M. Structural and functional properties of hepatic canalicular reduced glutathione transport revealed by radiation inactivation. *Am J Physiol* 1998;274: G923–G930.
9. Lou H, Ookhtens M, Stolz A, Kaplowitz N. Chelerythrine stimulates reduced glutathione transport by Mrp2 in MDCK cells. *J Biol Chem* 2002, in press.
10. Lieberman MW, Wiseman A, Shi Z, et al. Growth retardation and cysteine deficiency in γ-glutamyl transpeptidase-deficient mice. *Proc Natl. Acad Sci USA* 1996;93:7923–7926.
11. Kannan R, Mittur A, Bao Y, Tsuruo T, Kaplowitz N. GSH transport in immortalized mouse brain endothelial cells: evidence for apical localization of a sodium-dependent GSH transporter. *J Neurochem* 1999;73:390–399.
12. Kannan R, Chakrabarti R, Tang D, Kim KJ, Kaplowitz N. GSH transport in human cerebrovascular endothelial cells (HCEC) and human astrocytes: evidence for luminal localization of Na^+-dependent GSH transport in HCEC. *Brain Research* 2000;852:374–382.
13. Fernandez-Checa J, Kaplowitz N, Garcia-Ruiz C, et al. GSH transport in mitochondria: defense against TNF-induced oxidative stress and alcohol-induced defect. *Am J Physiol* 1997;273:G7–17.
14. Fernandez-Checa J, Kaplowitz N, Garcia-Ruiz C, Colell A. Mitochondrial GSH: importance and transport. *Seminars in Liver Disease* 1998;18:389–401.
15. Colell A, García-Ruiz C, Miranda M, Ardite E, Marì M, Morales A, Corrales F, Kaplowitz N, Fernández-Checa JC. Selective glutathione depletion of mitochondrial GSH by ethanol sensitizes hepatocytes to tumor necrosis factor. *Gastroenterology* 1998;115:1541–1551.
16. Mittur A, Wolkoff AW, Kaplowitz N. The thiol sensitivity of glutathione transport in sidedness-sorted basolateral liver plasma membrane and in oatp-1 expressing Hela cell membrane. *Mol Pharm*, accepted 2002 (provisional).
17. Kaplowitz N. Hepatotoxicity: The road to death and the role of glutathione. In: *Therapy in Hepatology* (Ed. Arroyo, et al.) Ars Medica 2001;407–410.

Gut-Brain Peptides in the New Millennium, edited by Y. Taché
CURE Foundation, Los Angeles, CA. © 2002

10

Why Do Multiple Molecular Forms of Peptide Hormones Exist? Diverse Biological Activities Can Result from Distinct Peptide Processing

Joseph R. Reeve, Jr., Travis E. Solomon, and David A. Keire
*CURE/Digestive Diseases Research Center, UCLA Division of Digestive Diseases
Department of Medicine and VA Greater Los Angeles Healthcare System
Los Angeles, CA*

Viktor E. Eysselein
Division of Gastroenterology, Harbor/UCLA Medical Center, Torrance, CA

INTRODUCTION

John Walsh came to CURE in 1972 following a fellowship in the laboratory of Dr. Rosalyn Yalow (future Nobel Laureate), where he had learned how to develop radioimmunoassays for peptide hormones. By the late 1970's investigators from around the world were flocking to CURE to work with Dr. Walsh and to use many of the radioimmunoassays he had developed for gastrointestinal peptide hormones. As a testament to the significance of these collaborations, many of these investigators are now leaders in the field of gastrointestinal research.

In the 1970's and 1980's most of the known structures for gastrointestinal peptide hormones were determined. Early on, a number of investigators throughout the world realized that many bioactive peptides exist in multiple molecular forms due to distinct processing of their prohormones. Investigators speculated that these distinct processing products may have physiological relevance. Initially, studies on these different molecular forms of various peptides seemed to show little difference in patterns of physiological response. This suggested that prohormone processing was not a mechanism for regulating physiological events. More recent studies have brought these ideas full circle; differential processing of a propeptide produces multiple molecular forms that have differences in patterns of expression at a single receptor (now known as biased–agonism) (1) or forms with unique receptor subtype selectivity.

Dr. Walsh was on the cutting edge of determining new molecular forms of peptide hormones. He and Dr. Grossman funded one of the first high pressure liquid chromatographs (HPLC, dubbed high priced liquid chromatography) at UCLA and one of the most sensitive amino acid analyzers available at the time. In addition, Dr. Walsh initiated the collaborations with Dr. John E. Shively who was one of the initial developers of peptide microsequencers. This collaboration resulted in the characterization of dozens of new molecular forms of gastrointestinal peptides resulting from differential processing of their prohormone, including the procholecystokinin and the proPYY products that will be discussed here.

On a personal note, we are grateful for having had the privilege of knowing and working with one of the leaders of gastrointestinal research. He always had a stimulating idea for a new experiment: many investigators had to focus on last week's or last month's wonderful experiment because there was not enough time to pursue the many tantalizing ideas emanating from this great scientist. Dr. Walsh had the ability to help young investigators get started and enabled them to develop their own research interests. John was always generous with his money, time and ideas.

When Dr. Keire came to CURE in 1999 to work with Drs. Reeve and Solomon funding for his position was tenuous at best. John did not hesitate to help out financially and also went out of his way to introduce Dr. Keire to other researchers at CURE whose work could be enhanced by 3D conformational studies. This led to a fruitful collaboration with Dr. Rozengurt's laboratory that continues today. Dr. Keire fondly remembers John bursting into Dr. Reeve's office with new ideas and his habit of rearranging papers and pens on the desk in front of him as if he was organizing his thoughts and your office at the same time.

We have said many good things about our mentor, collaborator, and friend, but we would like to supplement these with a few anecdotes. One that immediately comes to mind is the time Dr. Reeve was given the assignment to pick up Professor and Mrs. Gregory at the airport and drive them to their lodgings near CURE. Professor Gregory, held in highest esteem by investigators on both sides of the Atlantic, was the discoverer of gastrin. Unknown to Dr. Walsh, Dr. Reeve's only vehicle at the time was an old dilapidated Volkswagon Bug that had no seat covers (a towel protected one's pants from the seat springs). The legendary scientist and his wife were very gracious about the humble means of transportation, but Dr. Reeve never forgot the experience.

Humble means of transportation was also a common theme for Dr. Walsh. On another occasion, he crowded five scientists into his own diesel Volkswagon (purchased from Grace Rosenquist) to take a visiting scientist (Dr. Frank Cuttitta) to dinner at Spago's. He pulled into a parking lot full of very elegant cars and was met by an unhappy and disapproving parking attendant. During dinner, John ordered "two of everything on the menu". Upon exiting the restaurant, the parking attendant looked even more unhappy. He took John's parking token and started running toward the back of the lot. Soon he was out of sight and ten minutes later an obviously sweating attendant pulled up in the VW with the characteristic clunk-clunk of a diesel engine—the management had not allowed the car to be parked in sight of other customers. Was that the way to treat the car owned by someone who ordered "two of everything"?

The last memory we will describe relates to a gastrointestinal moment taken by Dr. Reeve in a CURE men's room with no stalls. Suddenly the door flew open and in rushed Dr. Walsh followed sheepishly by Dr. Grossman (another revered scientist). John had just had an idea about the chromatography of rat gastrin and could not wait to hear the local biochemist's opinion. To this day, Dr. Reeve wonders what Emily Post would have recommended. Should he have let the moment proceed or should he have waited for his distinguished visitors to leave?

We sincerely miss those lighter moments and we desperately miss the leadership and friendship of a truly great scientist. Thanks for the memories John. This chapter is dedicated to a man who touched many lives and launched numerous careers. The authors of this chapter represent a small percentage of scientists who were enriched professionally and personally by Dr. Walsh.

In this chapter we will review examples where differential processing of proPYY leads to peptides with receptor subtype specificity and how different products of procholecystokinin elicit varied physiological responses mediated by the CCK-A receptor. Furthermore, the role of tertiary structure in the expression of biological activity will be discussed.

Differential Processing of ProPYY Produces Peptides with Y Receptor Selectivity

Many peptides exist in multiple forms that arise from differential processing of their propeptides. Furthermore, these peptide hormones have multiple receptor subtypes at which they can act to illicit a biological response. For a few propeptides, differential processing produces agonists that are selective for certain receptor subtypes. For example, somatostatin-28 binds the SSTR-5 receptor 13-fold more potently than the smaller form, somatostatin-14 (2, 3).

Another example of prohormone processing that leads to altered pharmacology is peptide YY (PYY). PYY was first purified in Viktor Mutt's laboratory as a 36 amino acid peptide. After a post doctoral fellowship with Dr. Walsh, Dr. Eysselein returned to Essen Germany where he and Dr. Grandt set-up a radioimmunoassay for PYY. At that time two Y receptor subtypes were known, the Y_1 receptor that requires full length PYY for

Canine Gastrin Releasing Peptide	
GRP-27	APVPGGQGTVLDKMYPRGNHWAVGHLM*
	↓ DPAP
GRP-25	VPGGQGTVLDKMYPRGNHWAVGHLM*
	↓ DPAP
GRP-23	GGQGTVLDKMYPRGNHWAVGHLM*

Canine PYY	
[1–36]-PYY	YPAKPEAPGEDASPEELSRYYASLRHYLNLVTRQRY*
	↓ DPAP
[3-36]-PYY	AKPEAPGEDASPEELSRYYASLRHYLNLVTRQRY*

Canine Gastrin	
Gastrin 17	pQGPWMEEEEAAYGWMDF*
	↓ PCA Peptidase
Gastrin-16	GPWMEEEEAAYGWMDF*
	↓ DPAP
Gastrin-14	WMEEEEAAYGWMDF*

Rat Gastrin	
Gastrin-17	pQRPPM EEEEEAYGWMDF*
	↓ PCA Peptidase
Gastrin-16	RPPM EEEEEAYGWMDF*
	⚡ DPAP

FIGURE 1. *Role of dipeptidyl aminopeptidase (DPAP) in processing of mammalian bioactive peptides. The ★ denotes the presence of a C-terminal amide group. GRP-23 can be produced from GRP-27 by two steps of DPAP, upper panel. Simarily, [3-36]-PYY can be formed from PYY by one step of DPAP, second panel. Mammalian mini-gastrins (gastrin-14) can be formed via cleavage with pyrrolidinecarboxylic acid peptidase (PCA peptidase) followed by one step of DPAP cleavage, third panel. This is truce for all known mammalian gastrins except for rat gastrin which is not suitable for DPAP cleavage due to a proline in the third position after cleavage by PCA peptidase, lower panel.*

binding, and the Y_2 receptor that binds PYY(22–36) and other synthetic C-terminal fragments not found in nature (4). Drs. Eysselein and Grandt noticed that human colon extracts contained two PYY-like immunoreactive peaks. Microsequence analysis of the two purified peaks demonstrated that one was the expected 36 amino acid peptide, but the other was missing the amino terminal Tyr-Pro- (5). Figure 1 shows the actions of post-proline dipeptidyl amino peptidase (DPAP IV) that removes this dipeptide from PYY/NPY (6). PYY(1–36) and PYY(3–36) forms are also present in colon of dogs (7) and rabbits (8). Furthermore, a post-proline dipeptidyl amino peptidase enzyme may be also important in the processing of gastrin-releasing peptide, and most mammalian gastrins (Figure 1). Until recently DPAP IV was assumed to be the dipeptidyl aminopeptidase that cleaved these peptides after second position prolines. However, a new peptidase has been localized in cell organelles associated with processing of bioactive peptides (9). This peptidase has been named quiescent cell proline dipeptidase (QPP).

The processing of PYY(1–36) into PYY(3–36) changes a peptide that can bind Y_1, Y_2, Y_4 and Y_5 receptors into a peptide that can no longer express its activity at the Y_1 receptor (10, 11). Whether the processing is under physiological regulation, or if there is tissue specific processing has not been determined. However, it has been demonstrated that similar processing occurs for NPY because NPY(3–36) has been isolated from porcine brain (10). This processing results in forms of PYY and NPY that do not act at the Y_1 receptor (a known modulator of satiety in rat models) (12).

We have determined the tertiary structure of porcine, rat PYY by nuclear magnetic resonance (NMR), and have shown that its tertiary solution structure is similar the solution structure of PP (Figure 2) (13). We have proposed a model where PYY(3–36) not only is missing part of its primary structure, but it also has an altered tertiary structure (14). If correct, the model suggests that tertiary structure can also influence receptor subtype selectivity.

Procholecystokinin Processing Produces Biased-agonists

Biased-agonists are molecules that bind to the same receptor, but cause distinct physiological responses. The peptide biased-agonists previously described result from changes in primary structure. For example, pituitary-adenylate cyclase-activating polypeptide (PACAP) has two molecular forms that result from peptide processing of proPACAP: PACAP-27 and PACAP-38 (15). PACAP-27 and PACAP-38 bind the PACAP-1 receptor. The EC_{50} for activation of adenylate cyclase by these two molecular forms shows that PACAP-38 is only two-fold more potent than PACAP-27 at the PACAP-1 receptor. By contrast, the EC_{50}'s for phospholipase C activation show that PACAP-38 is ten-fold more potent than PACAP-27. Therefore, the additional nine

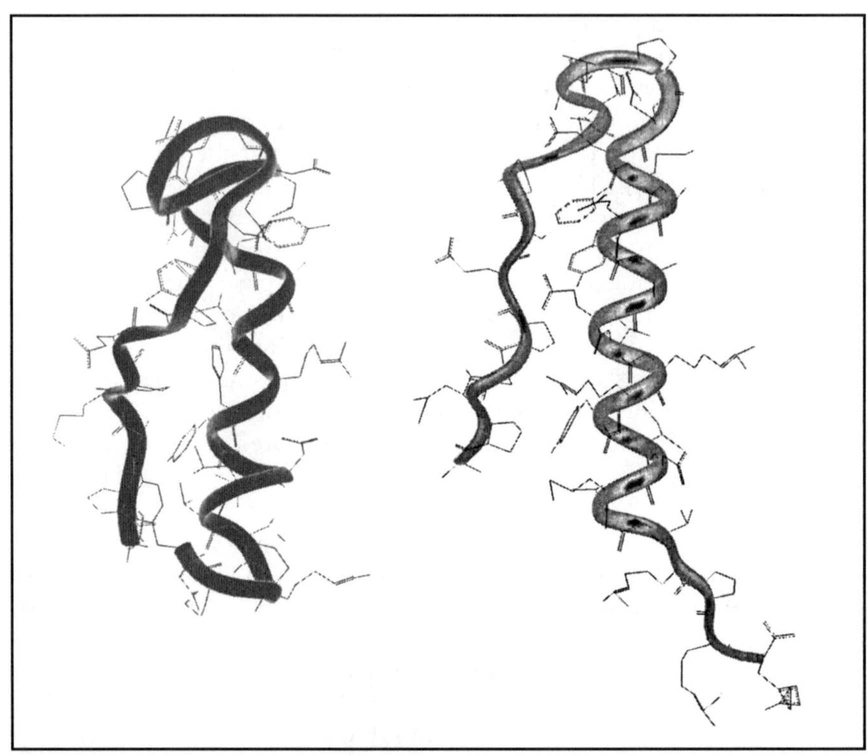

FIGURE 2. *The NMR derived solution structures of porcine PYY (left) (13) and bovine pancreatic polypeptide (33) (right). The backbone residues are visualized with a ribbon representation for each structure. PYY and PP demonstrate a stable juxtaposition of the N- and C-terminal residues. For both peptides, the three C-terminal residues are flexible. In addition, the turn region of PYY (residues 9 to 23) is flexible although the residues 15 to 23 prefer a helical conformation.*

amino acids of PACAP-38 changes the pattern of biological activity enabled via the PACAP-1 receptor. This has been suggested as an initial example of how biased agonists can be produced by peptide processing.

The processing of procholecystokinin also produces biased-agonists. The processing of procholecystokinin produces several molecular forms including: CCK-83, CCK-58, CCK-39, CCK-33, CCK-22, CCK-8, and CCK-5 (Figure 3). As described CCK-5, CCK-8, and CCK-58 have very different patterns of CCK-A mediated physiological response. First, we will describe how CCK-58 was discovered, then we will discuss data that demonstrates that these forms are biased agonists.

One of the international fellows attracted by Dr. Walsh was Dr. Viktor Eysselein from Essen, Germany. He asked Dr. Reeve to help him identify the large form of cholecystokinin immunoreactivity that had been reported by Kothary, et al. (16). At the time, Dr. Reeve was collecting canine intestinal

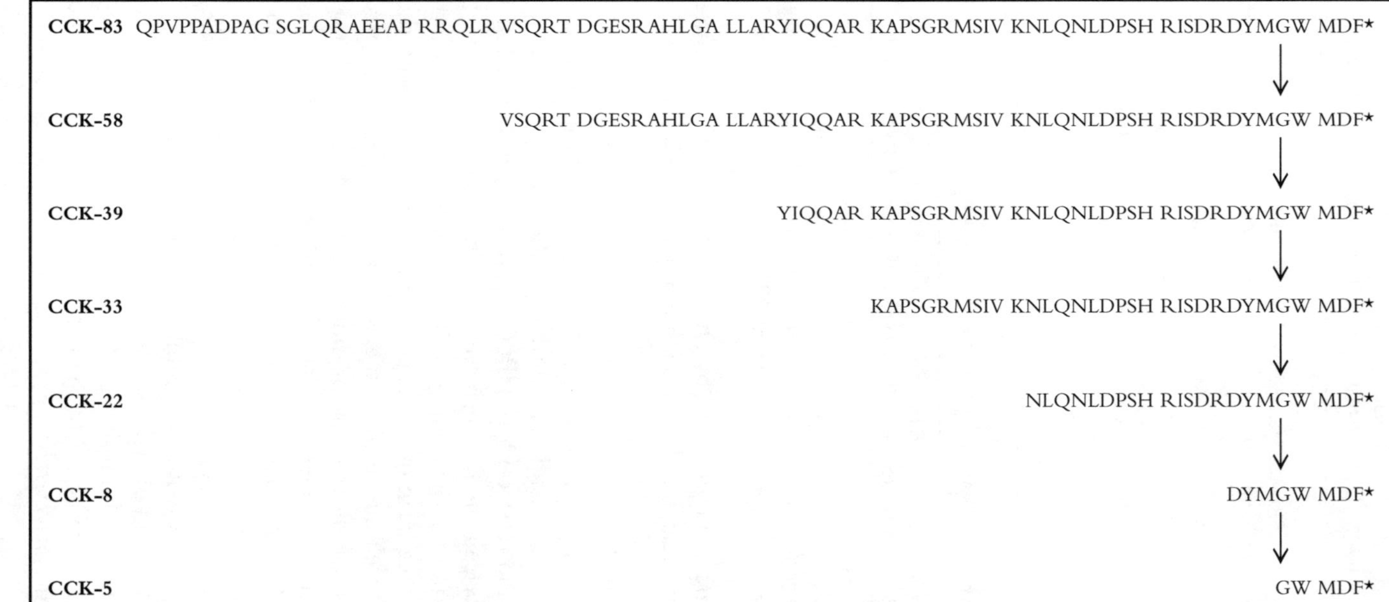

FIGURE 3. *The molecular forms of cholecystokinin. The ★ denotes a C-terminal phenylalanine-amide. The tyrosine at the seventh position from the C-terminus is sulfated in most reported sequences. However, one group has reported the presence of sulfated and non-sulfated tyrosine in a CCK-58 purified from porcine intestines (34). All the peptides shown have been isolated and characterized from more than one species, except CCK-83 which was only purified from human intestines. The presence of a C-terminal amide on CCK-83 shows that amidation can occur before endopeptidase cleavages produce the smaller molecular forms of cholecystokinin.*

Human

VSQRTDGESR AHLGALLARY IQQARKAPSG RMSIVKNLQN LDPSHRISDR DYMGWMDF*

Monkey

AVQRTDGESR AHLGALLARY IQQARKAPSG RMSIIKNLQN LDPSHRISDR DYMGWMDF*

Pig

AVQKVDGESR AHLGALLARY IQQARKAPSG RVSMIKNLQS LDPSHRISDR DYMGWMDF*

Dog

AVQKVDGEPR AHLGALLARY IQQARKAPSG RMSVIKNLQN LDPSHRISDR DYMGWMDF*

Cow

AVPRVDDEPR AQLGALLARY IQQARKAPSG RMSVIKNLQS LDPSHRISDR DYMGWMDF*

Mouse

AVLRPDREPR ARLGALLARY IQQVRKAPSG RMSVLKNLQS LDPSHRISDR DYMGWMDF*

Rat

AVLRPDSEPR ARLGALLARY IQQVRKAPSG RMSVLKNLQG LDPSHRISDR DYMGWMDF*

FIGURE 4. *Species differences in CCK-58. The primary sequence of human, monkey, pig, dog, cow, mouse, and rat CCK-58 are shown. The ★ denotes the presence of a C-terminal amide. The fifty-eight amino acid peptide is conserved in all regions indicating that regions other than the carboxyl terminal region are important for the full expression of cholecystokinin bioactivity.*

muscle (the dog intestines were provided by Dr. Andrew Soll of CURE) for the purification of mammalian bombesin-like immunoreactivity. The mucosa was, therefore, available for Dr. Eysselein for the purification of this intriguing molecular form of cholecystokinin. Dr. Walsh had enough antiserum for affinity chromatography, a step that was used as the initial purification of various molecular forms of cholecystokinin. Further purification by gel-permeation chromatography, and reverse-phase HPLC separation steps resulted in a peak that appeared to be suitable for microsequence analysis.

Of course, this does not tell the entire story of the purification and isolation of this apparently large form of cholecystokinin. Dr. Reeve took on the project to show how to eliminate the artifactual early elution position of what must have been CCK-8 or CCK-33 non-specific binding to a protein. However, after several chromatography steps and treatment of the immunoreactive peak with urea, the CCK immunoreactivity remained in the same early position during gel-permeation chromatography.

The purified peptide was taken out to the City of Hope for microsequence analysis and a peptide with no resemblance to cholecystokinin was sequenced for 16 positions and the fellow running the analyzer was ready to turn off the machine, but fortuitously decided to let it run overnight because it was nearly time to go home. In the morning when he came in and stopped the analysis, the analyzer had proceeded for another 22 residues:

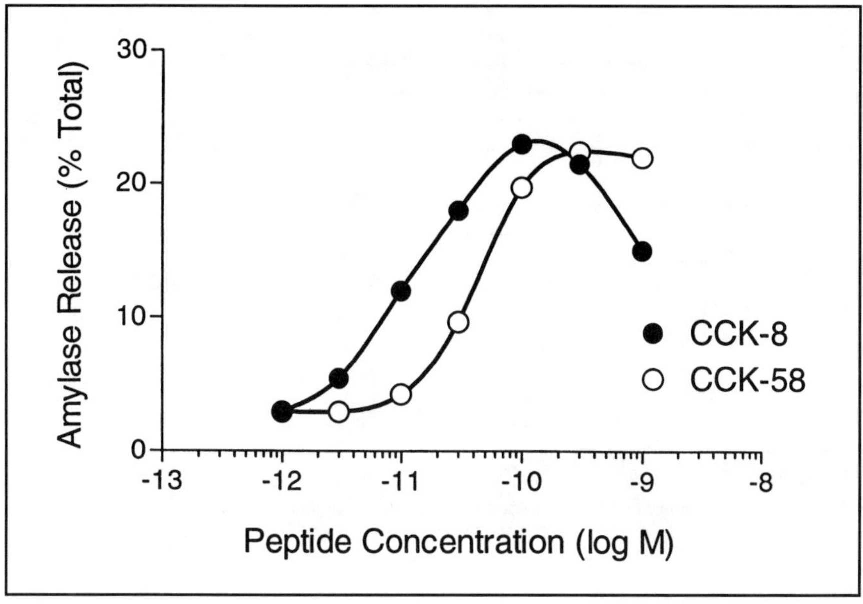

FIGURE 5. *A plot of the percentage of total amylase release from isolated acinar cells stimulated with varying concentrations of CCK-58 (open circles) and CCK-8 (filled circles). CCK-58 is 3-fold less potent than CCK-8 for amylase release. In contrast to CCK-8, CCK-58 does not cause supramaximal inhibition of amylase release.*

three of an unknown sequence and the next 19 surprisingly homologous to porcine CCK-39.

We told John the news from the City of Hope team. That evening John called us to his office and Viktor, John, and Joe started working on a manuscript. By 3 AM we had a completed manuscript that was sent for review. We tentatively named the peptide CCK-58 (17). In the following months we also purified CCK-58 from canine brain (18). After Dr. Eysselein returned to Germany we collaborated on the characterization of CCK-58 from human intestines (19). CCK-58 has also been purified and characterized from the intestines of pig (20), dog (17, 21), cow (22), and rat (23). Monkey (24) and mouse (25) procholecystokinin mRNA sequences have been elucidated. A comparison of the primary sequences of CCK-58 for these species is shown in Figure 4.

In Essen Germany, Dr. Eysselein started characterizing the molecular forms of cholecystokinin in canine blood after stimulation by a fatty meal. He quickly recognized that exogenous CCK-58 was degraded into smaller forms if plasma was collected in the classical manner. He further determined that acidification of the plasma prevented this degradation. If canine blood was acidified, CCK-58 was the major circulating form. Dr. Eysselein next turned his attention to

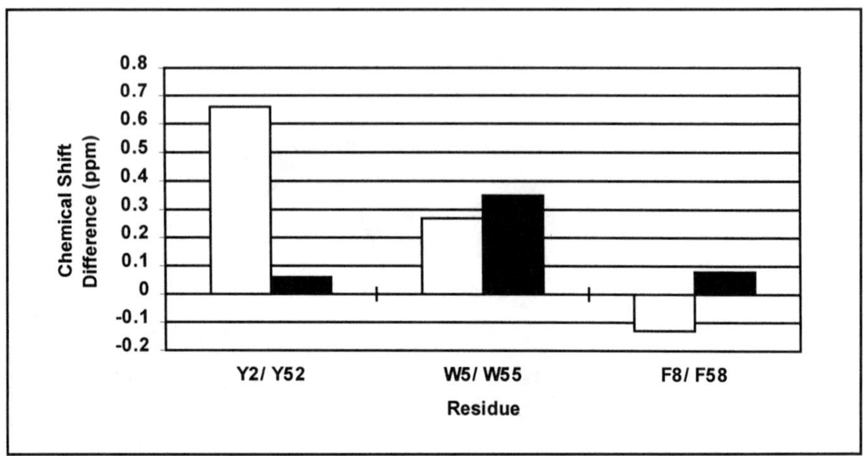

FIGURE 6. *Chemical shift differences for three of the identical amino acids in CCK-8 and canine CCK-58. The open and filled boxes represent NH and $C_\alpha H$ proton differences respectively. ^{1}H-NMR data could only be assigned for the C-terminal Y, W, and F residues, but the differences observed clearly show that CCK-8 and CCK-58 have significantly different solution conformations.*

the molecular forms of cholecystokinin in man. Dr. Reeve watched in disbelief as Dr. Eysselein ate a fatty meal and later drew his own blood. This time the anticipated results were observed, the major form of cholecystokinin in Viktor's blood as well as in five other volunteers was CCK-58.

During Dr. Eysselein's initial studies at CURE the small molecular form of CCK/gastrin was purified from canine intestinal and brain extracts. It was shown that the peptide was the C-terminal pentapeptide of cholecystokinin that is identical with the C-terminal pentapeptide of gastrin. Because gastrin is present in the upper small intestine, it cannot be determined which propeptide (progastrin or procholecystokinin) produces this intestinal form. However, in the brain the cholecystokinin pentapeptide identified came from procholecystokinin because progastrin mRNA is found only in a few specialized regions of the brain while cholecystokinin mRNA is one of the most abundant mRNA's in the brain.

The processing that forms CCK-5 has a profound influence on the biological activity of cholecystokinin. Owyang's group reported that CCK-5 had a different pattern from CCK-8 for stimulating intracellular calcium and amylase release from isolated pancreatic acini (26). CCK-5 causes the spiked pattern of intracellular calcium observed with CCK-8, but does not induce the sustained high levels of intracellular calcium observed at high concentrations of CCK-8. In addition, CCK-5 does not induce supramaximal inhibition of amylase release from isolated pancreatic acini that is seen with CCK-8. This indicates that CCK-5 and CCK-8 are biased-agonists at the CCK-A receptor and this difference is enabled by primary sequence differences (particularly the lack of a sulfated tyrosine in CCK-5). CCK-5 is probably not an endocrine peptide because of its rapid clearance from the circulation. However, CCK-5 could act as a neurocrine agent at the CCK-A or CCK-B receptor in brain or other neural tissue. A more detailed analysis of tissue forms will be necessary to determine if CCK-5 expresses unique actions at one of these receptors.

The common assumption that all the molecular forms of cholecystokinin containing the seven C-terminal amino acids have similar biological activity stems from comparisons of the activity of CCK-8 and CCK-33. These two molecular forms have similar patterns of expression of activity on pancreas (27, 28) and gall bladder (27). In contrast another molecular form of cholecystokinin, CCK-58, purified from canine or procine intestine have different patterns of biological activity from CCK-8. CCK-58 and CCK-8 have different patterns of afferent nerve discharge (29), distinct central catecholaminergic and TSH release, and discrete patterns of gallbladder contraction (20). Data obtained with *in vitro* acini demonstrate that CCK-58 is less potent that CCK-8, but it does not cause the supra-maximal inhibition of amylase release observed with CCK-8 (Figure 5). Preliminary data in collaboration with Dr. Green has shown that CCK-58 has a different pattern for stimulation of pancreatic exocrine secretion from CCK-8 in conscious rats (30). Only CCK-58 stimulated fluid secretion. Furthermore, with continuous infusion of CCK-8 protein output returned to basal by 180 minutes for all doses, while with CCK-58 protein output remained significantly above basal values for the same doses. The CCK-A receptor antagonist, MK-329, abolished both fluid, and protein stimulated by CCK-58 demonstrating that fluid and protein secretion are mediated by the CCK-A receptor. Therefore, CCK-8 and CCK-58 are biased-agonists at the CCK-A receptor.

Further work in our laboratory with Dr. Keire has shown that CCK-58 has a different C-terminal tertiary structure from CCK-8 (Figure 6) (31). We have postulated that this tertiary structure influences biological activity (32). We propose that the differential processing of procholecystokinin that forms CCK-8 and CCK-58 results in peptides with varied C-terminal tertiary structures that enable them to distinctly activate the CCK-A receptor.

SUMMARY

Some of the molecular forms of bioactive peptides may arise during their extraction and purification. For example, our preparative HPLC column used for the purification of cholecystokinin immunoreactivities. This C-18 reverse phase column (2.2 × 25 cm) had immunoreactivity eluting only in the position of CCK-58 the first time the column was used to purify canine intestinal extracts. In subsequent purifications, the relative abundance of

CCK-58 diminished and a new peak that eluted between CCK-8 and CCK-33 (possibly CCK-22?) became the major molecular form of cholecystokinin detected with a CCK radioimmunoassay. New methods that are better controlled than past studies need to be developed before investigations on physiological influence on peptide processing can be determined.

We are still lacking sufficient knowledge of how propeptide processing influences expression of biological activity. A growing body of evidence shows that multiple molecular forms of a peptide can have varied physiogical responses. This mandates careful studies on *in vivo* molecular forms with proper controls.

We have discussed four instances where distinct processing results in varied patterns of physiological response: proPYY, prosomatostatin, proPACAP and procholecystokinin. However, multiple molecular forms are found after processing of proGRP, prosecretin, progastrin, proVIP, promotilin, proneurotensin, and others. Therefore, detailed studies on the patterns of biological expression of their molecular forms may show similar differences to those described in this chapter.

Again, we gratefully acknowledge Dr. Walsh for the role he played in creating the environment that produced so many important discoveries. The description of PYY and CCK are examples where we are just beginning to understand the ramifications of propeptide processing. The legacy of Dr. Walsh will be the development of new methods to answer new and old questions.

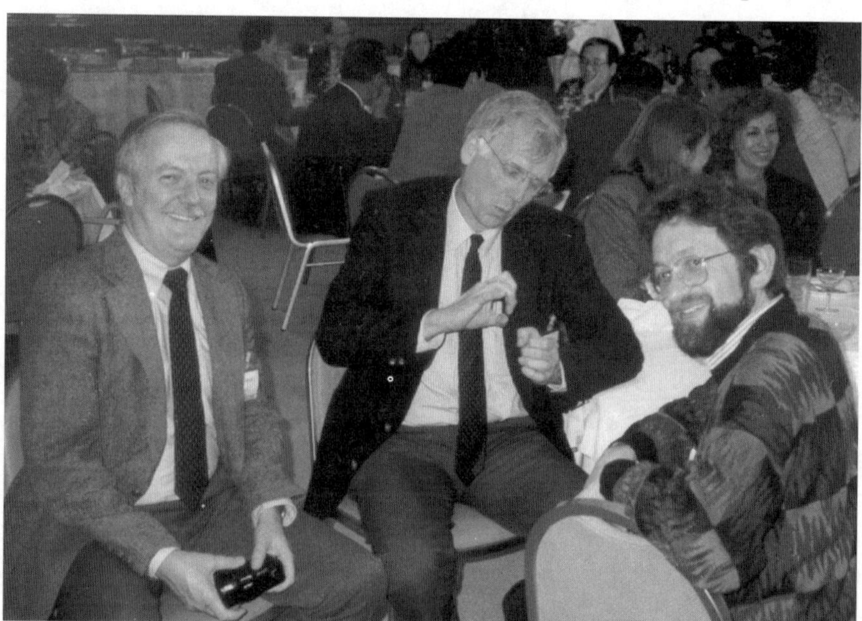

Left to right: J. Reeve, J. Walsh and A. Shulkes at Seventh International Symposium on Gastrointestinal Hormones, Shizuoka, Japan, 1988.

REFERENCES

1. Kenakin T. Inverse, protean, and ligand-selective agonism: matters of receptor conformation. *FASEB J* 2001;5(3):598–611.

2. Panetta R, Greenwood MT, Warszynska A, Demchyshyn LL, Day R, Niznik HB, Srikant CB, Patel YC. Molecular cloning, functional characterization, and chromosomal localization of a human somatostatin receptor (somatostatin receptor type 5) with preferential affinity for somatostatin-28. *Mol Pharmacol* 1994;45:417–427.

3. Yamada Y, Kagimoto S, Kubota A, Yasuda K, Masuda K, Someya Y, Ihara Y, Li Q, Imura H, Seino S. Cloning, functional expression and pharmacological characterization of a fourth (hSSTR4) and a fifth (hSSTR5) human somatostatin receptor subtype. *Biochem Biophys Res Commun* 1993;195:844–852.

4. Wieland HA, Willim K, Doods HN. Receptor binding profiles of NPY analogues and fragments in different tissues and cell lines. *Peptides* 1995;16:1389–1394.

5. Eberlein GA, Eysselein VE, Schaeffer M, Layer P, Grandt D, Goebell H, Niebel W, Davis M, Lee TD, Shively JE, Reeve JR, Jr. A new molecular form of PYY: structural characterization of human PYY(3-36) and PYY(1-36). *Peptides* 1989;10:797–803.

6. Grandt D, Dahms P, Schimiczek M, Eysselein VE, Reeve JR, Jr., Mentlein R. [Proteolytic processing by dipeptidyl aminopeptidase IV generates receptor selectivity for peptide YY (PYY)] Proteolytisches Processing durch Dipeptidyl-Aminopeptidase IV generiert Rezeptorselektivitat fur PeptidYY (PYY). *Med Klin* 1993;88:143–145.

7. Eysselein VE, Eberlein GA, Grandt D, Schaeffer M, Zehres B, Behn U, Schaefer D, Goebell H, Davis M, Lee TD. Structural characterization of canine PYY. *Peptides* 1990;11:111–116.

8. Grandt D, Schimiczek M, Struk K, Shively J, Eysselein VE, Goebell H, Reeve JR, Jr. Characterization of two forms of peptide YY, PYY(1-36) and PYY(3-36), in the rabbit. *Peptides* 1994;15:815–820.

9. Chiravuri M, Agarraberes F, Mathieu SL, Lee H, Huber BT. Vesicular localization and characterization of a novel post-proline-cleaving aminodipeptidase, quiescent cell proline dipeptidase. *J Immun* 2000;165:5695–5702.

10. Grandt D, Schimiczek M, Rascher W, Feth F, Shively J, Lee TD, Davis MT, Reeve JR, Jr., Michel MC. Neuropeptide Y 3-36 is an endogenous ligand selective for Y2 receptors. *Regul Pept* 1996;67:33–37.

11. Grandt D, Teyssen S, Schimiczek M, Reeve JR, Jr., Feth F, Rascher W, Hirche H, Singer MV, Layer P, Goebell H. Novel generation of hormone receptor specificity by amino terminal processing of peptide YY. *Biochem Biophys Res Commun* 1992;186:1299–1306.

12. Kanatani A, Mashiko S, Murai N, Sugimoto N, Ito J, Fukuroda T, Fukami T, Morin N, MacNeil DJ, Van der Ploeg LH, Saga Y, Nishimura S, Ihara M. Role of the Y_1 receptor in the regulation of neuropeptide Y-mediated feeding: comparison of wild-type, Y_1 receptor-deficient, and Y_5 receptor-deficient mice. *Endocrinology* 2000;141:1011–1016.

13. Keire DA, Kobayashi M, Solomon TE, Reeve JR, Jr. Solution structure of monomeric peptide YY supports the functional significance of the PP-fold. *Biochemistry* 2000;15;39:9935–9942.

14. Keire DA, Mannon P, Kobayashi M, Walsh JH, Solomon TE, Reeve JR, Jr. Primary structures of PYY, [Pro(34)]PYY, and PYY-(3-36) confer different conformations and receptor selectivity. *Am J Physiol* 2000;279:G126–G131.

15. Pantaloni C, Brabet P, Bilanges B, Dumuis A, Houssami S, Spengler D, Bockaert J and Journot L. Alternative splicing in the N-terminal extracellular domain of the pituitary adenylate cyclase-activating polypeptide (PACAP) receptor modulates receptor selectivity and relative potencies of PACAP-27 and PACAP-38 in phospholipase C activation. *J Biol Chem* 1996;271:22146–22151.

16. Kothary PC, Vinik AI, Owyang C and Fiddian-Green RG. Immunochemical studies of molecular heterogeneity of cholecystokinin in duodenal perfusates and plasma in humans. *J Biol Chem* 1983;258:2856–2863.

17. Eysselein VE, Reeve JR, Jr., Shively JE, Hawke D and Walsh JH. Partial structure of a large canine cholecystokinin (CCK58): amino acid sequence. *Peptides* 1982:3:687–691.

18. Eysselein VE, Reeve JR, Jr., Shively JE, Miller C and Walsh JH. Isolation of a large cholecystokinin precursor from canine brain. *Proc Natl Acad Sci USA* 1984:81:6565–6568.

19. Eysselein VE, Eberlein GA, Schaeffer M, Grandt D, Goebell H, Niebel W, Rosenquist GL, Meyer HE and Reeve JR, Jr. Characterization of the major form of cholecystokinin in human intestine: CCK-58. *Am J Physiol* 1990;258:G253–G260.

20. Tatemoto K, Jornvall H, Siimesmaa S, Hallden G and Mutt V. Isolation and characterization of cholecystokinin-58 (CCK-58) from porcine brain. *FEBS Lett* 1984;174:289–293.

21. Reeve JR, Jr., Eysselein V, Walsh JH, Ben-Avram CM and Shively JE. New molecular forms of cholecystokinin. Microsequence analysis of forms previously characterized by chromatographic methods. *J Biol Chem* 1986;261:16392–16397.

22. Eng J, Li HR and Yalow RS. Purification of bovine cholecystokinin-58 and sequencing of its N-terminus. *Regul Pept* 1990;30:15–19.

23. Turkelson CM, Solomon TE, Bussjaeger L, Turkelson J, Ronk M, Shively JE, Ho FJ and Reeve JR, Jr. Chemical characterization of rat cholecystokinin-58. *Peptides* 1988;9:1255–1260.

24. Bernal J, Godbout M, Hasel KW, Travis GH and Sutcliffe JG. Patterns of cerebral cortex mRNA expression. *J Neurosci Res* 1990;27:153–158.

25. Vitale M, Vashishtha A, Linzer E, Powell DJ and Friedman JM. Molecular cloning of the mouse CCK gene: expression in different brain regions and during cortical development. *Nucleic Acids Res* 1991;19:169–177.

26. Tsunoda Y, Yoshida H and Owyang C. Structural requirements of CCK analogues to differentiate second messengers and pancreatic secretion. *Am J Physiol* 1996;271:G8–19.

27. Solomon TE, Yamada T, Elashoff J, Wood J and Beglinger C. Bioactivity of cholecystokinin analogues: CCK-8 is not more potent than CCK-33. *Am J Physiol* 1984;247:G105–G111.

28. Liddle RA, Elashoff J and Reeve JR, Jr. Relative bioactivities of cholecystokinins-8 and -33 on rat pancreatic acini. *Peptides* 1986;7:723–727.

29. Kreis ME, Zittel TT, Raybould HE, Reeve JR, Jr., and Grundy D. Prolonged intestinal afferent nerve discharge in response to cholecystokinin-58 compared to cholecystokinin-8 in rats. *Neurosci Lett* 1997;230:89–92.

30. Yamaoto, M, Reeve, JR, Jr., and Green, GM CCK extended structure markedly influences pancreatic secretion in conscious rats. *Digestion* 1999;60: 409.

31. Keire DA, Solomon TE and Reeve JR, Jr. Identical primary sequence but different conformations of the bioactive regions of canine CCK-8 and CCK-58. *Biochem Biophys Res Commun* 1999:266: 400–404.

32. Reeve JR, Jr., Eysselein VE, Rosenquist G, Zeeh J, Regner U, Ho FJ, Chew P, Davis MT, Lee TD, Shively JE, Brazer SR and Liddle RA. Evidence that CCK-58 has structure that influences its biological activity. *Am J Physiol* 1996;270:G860–G868.

33. Li XA, Sutcliffe MJ, Schwartz TW and Dobson CM. Sequence-specific 1H NMR assignments and solution structure of bovine pancreatic polypeptide. *Biochemistry* 1992;31:1245–1253.

34. Bonetto V, Jornvall H, Andersson M, Renlund S, Mutt V and Sillard R. Isolation and characterization of sulphated and nonsulphated forms of cholecystokinin-58 and their action on gallbladder contraction. *Eur J Biochem* 1999;264:336–340.

Gut-Brain Peptides in the New Millennium, edited by Y. Taché
CURE Foundation, Los Angeles, CA. © 2002

11

Motilin

Pierre Poitras
Department of Medicine and Physiology,
Université de Montréal, Montréal, Canada

MOTILIN

March 1978, John Walsh put his cigar away, leaves his office, walks to the lab and opens the door of the refrigerator. Looking at the shelf where stand the vials of peptide antisera, he will choose my future: gastrin RIA is done by Peter Chew and Helen Wong for years; pancreatic polypeptide was mastered by Ian Taylor, somatostatin by Tachi Yamada, bombesin by Joe Reeve and Steve Vigna; Cor Lamers and Arthur Shulkes who recently joined the lab respectively choose CCK, VIP, and GIP. A bottle of motilin antisera 1/100 was left alone at the end of the shelf: "Pierre, this is a Canadian hormone, you will try that."

In this chapter we will review evidence that motilin, a 22 amino acid peptide, is synthesized in endocrine cells of the duodenal mucosa, and is released cyclically into the blood circulation during the interdigestive fasting period to regulate the phase III contraction of the migrating motor complex. Motilin is so far one of the most potent gastrokinetic agents we know.

Motilin Sequence

The sequence of pig motilin was published in 1972 by Brown, et al. (1) working in Vancouver. After observing that instillation of an alkaline buffer in the duodenum increased motor activity in the transplanted gastric pouch of dogs, Brown purified a new peptide of 22 amino acids (molecular weight 2700) through successive chromatographies of a side fraction material obtained during the purification of porcine intestinal secretin by Victor Mutt. He called this peptide motilin because of its effect on gastric motility.

Motilin is subject to an important structural heterogeneity among animal species. Its characterization in dogs (2) and man (3) was important to allow

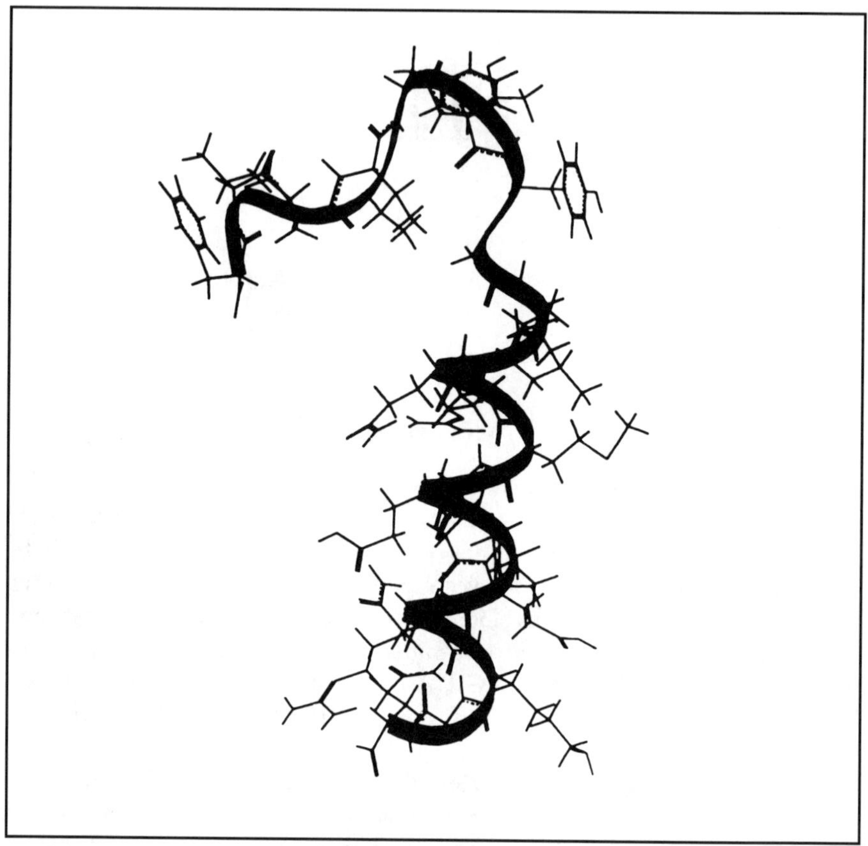

FIGURE 1. *Structure of the 22-amino acid motilin peptide revealed by nuclear magnetic resonance. The N-terminal curved sequence binds to the receptor, while the alpha-helix C-terminal structure protects the molecule* in vivo *bioactivity.*

physiological or pharmacological studies in these species since changes in the peptides structure were shown to impact on the bioactivity of the molecule or on its recognition by the antisera used for RIA. Its structure has now been identified in many other species including chicken, cow, rabbit, etc. Unfortunately, motilin has remained unidentified in mouse and rat; these animals, usually important laboratory tools in biomedical research, could not be of major help in motilin research.

The three dimensional structure of the molecule was identified by nuclear magnetic resonance (4) (Figure 1). Its curved N-terminal sequence was found to interact with the motilin receptor. Structure-activity studies showed that the first 12 amino acids of the molecule were essential for its full binding to its receptor (5, 6); amino acids 1, 4 and 7 appeared most determinant in this respect. The C-terminal sequence, shaped in an alpha-helix structure, seems to play a role in motilin's *in vivo* bioactivity (7), possibly by protecting it from degradation enzymes.

Motilin Receptor

The motilin receptor was sequenced recently by researchers from Merck Laboratories (8). It was cloned from an orphan receptor of the thyroid. The significance of this unexpected localization has still to be clarified. According to motilin's actions documented *in vivo* as *in vitro,* motilin receptors are found in most animal species except mouse and rat and are located on smooth muscle cells of the gastrointestinal tract as well as on intrinsic nerves connecting to these muscle structures (9, 10). Receptor binding studies with motilin analogs have confirmed its structural heterogeneity among species (for example rabbit and man) and clearly supported the concept that muscle and neural receptors correspond to different subtypes that we identified as M and N receptor subtypes (11, 12).

Motilin Action

The most characteristic effect of motilin is to induce motor contraction of the GI tract. Its administration provokes contraction of the lower esophageal sphincter, gastric fundus (tonic contraction) and antrum (phasic contraction), small intestine, colon (sigmoid) and gallbladder. Many of these effects are pharmacological and can be used in therapeutics as described later on. Motilin physiological activity resides in the regulation of interdigestive motility. Indeed, motilin fulfilled all the criteria proposed by the late Morton Grossman. To show that it is a hormone acting as a physiological inducer of the phase III contraction of the migrating motor complex (MMC) in dogs: a) physiological doses of exogenous motilin evoke premature phase III contraction in the stomach and proximal gut; b) plasma motilin is released cyclically during the fasting period, and these cyclical peak increases are synchronized with phase III contractions initiated in the stomach or proximal duodenum (Figure 2); and c) the infusion of motilin antiserum blocks the phase III contraction in the proximal gut (13).

Mechanisms regulating this fascinating interdigestive release of motilin have been studied *in vitro* (14, 15), *ex vivo* (16) and *in vivo* (17–19). They are summarized in Figure 3.

Motilin is also circulating in humans in whom its intermittent peak increases are synchronized with antral phase III contractions. Its mode of action is summarized on Figure 4. Unlike the situation in dogs where motilin cyclical release is completely abolished following a meal, food ingestion in humans induces a very early increase in plasma motilin before interruption of its cyclical secretion (20). This very early release can be mimicked by

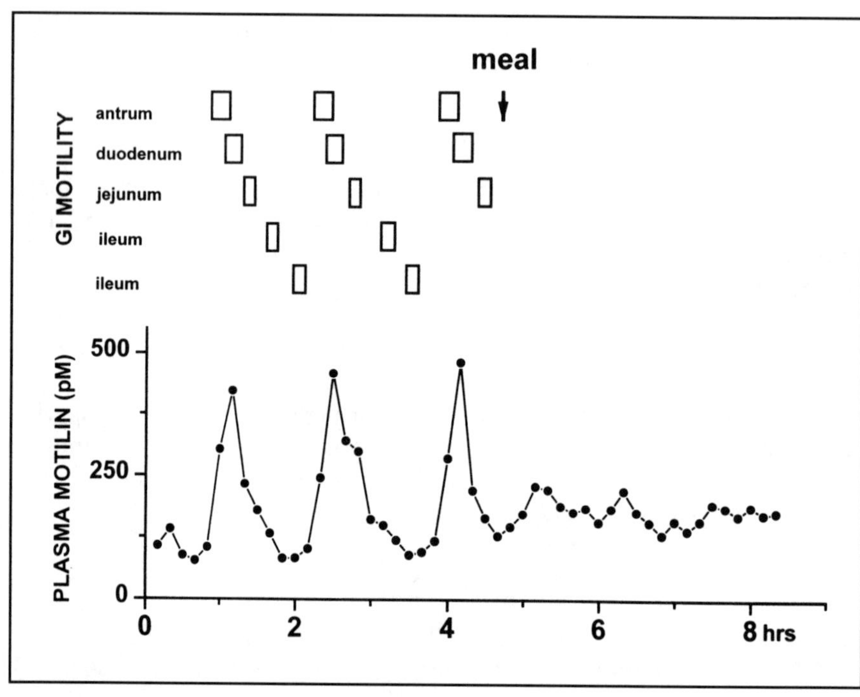

FIGURE 2. *Schematic representation of plasma motilin variations in dog. During the fasting interdigestive period, motilin is released cyclically each 80–120 min (lower panel) to induce phase III contraction of the migrating motor complex from the stomach to the ileum (indicated by clear boxes in the upper panel). After a meal, the motilin cyclical peak increases are abolished for 2 to 8 hours (depending upon the content and nature of the meal) while the fed pattern motility profile is taking place.*

sham feeding or gastric distension (21), but its contribution to the physiological equilibrium remains unknown.

Clinical Application

No clinical disorder has yet been clearly identified as being caused by abnormal motilin release. Motilin hypersecretion has been reported in patients with endocrine tumors, such as pancreatic gastrinoma or intestinal carcinoid tumors, but its pathological contribution to the disease manifestation is uncertain. Motilin hyposecretion was proposed to be an etiological factor in some patients with idiopathic dyspepsia (22) or with gastroparesis following Whipple's duodenal resection for pancreatic tumors (23).

The clinical importance of motilin was mainly recognized by the documentation of erythromycin analogs acting as motilin receptor agonists. Almost by chance, and certainly by perseverance, Zen Itoh discovered that erythromycin could mimic the motor effect of motilin in the canine

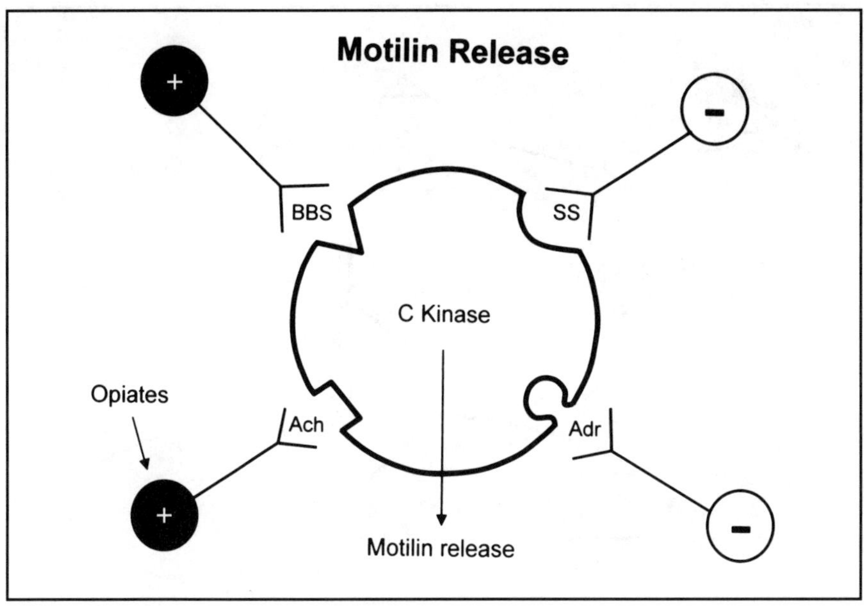

FIGURE 3. *Schematic representation of the mechanisms regulating motilin release from its producing cell in the duodenal mucosa. Acetylcholine (Ach) and bomberin (BBS) act directly on the motilin cell to activate the kinase C intracellular pathway facilitating motilin secretion. The stimulatory action of opiates is exerted via cholinergic nerves. Somatostatin (SST) and adrenaline (adr) receptors are present in the M cell to suppress motilin release.*

stomach (24). Binding experiments later confirmed that erythromycin could displace the I^{125} motilin ligand from its receptor and synthetic motilin receptor antagonists blocked erythromycin action *in vitro* (25). In Leuven, Belgium researchers made the capital observation that erythromycin was a potent stimulant of gastric emptying in patients with severe diabetic gastroparesis (26). Erythromycin derivatives, called motilides (macrolides with motilin behavior but devoid of antibiotic properties), were developed to facilitate the management of hypokinetic gastrointestinal (GI) disorders. Up to now, to our knowledge, three compounds have been tested on humans, but, for various reasons (rapid tachyphylaxis, absence of clinical benefit, presence of serious side effects) none proved to be beneficial. Erythromycin administered intravenously or orally is still used by clinicians for the management of selected and responsive patients with gastroparesis or intestinal pseudo-obstruction, but the full therapeutic potential of motilides have not yet been fully exploited.

Motilin receptor antagonists were desperately needed to, among other things, explore the peptide physiological and pharmacological properties. But up to now, no valid compound has been developed, either from synthetic

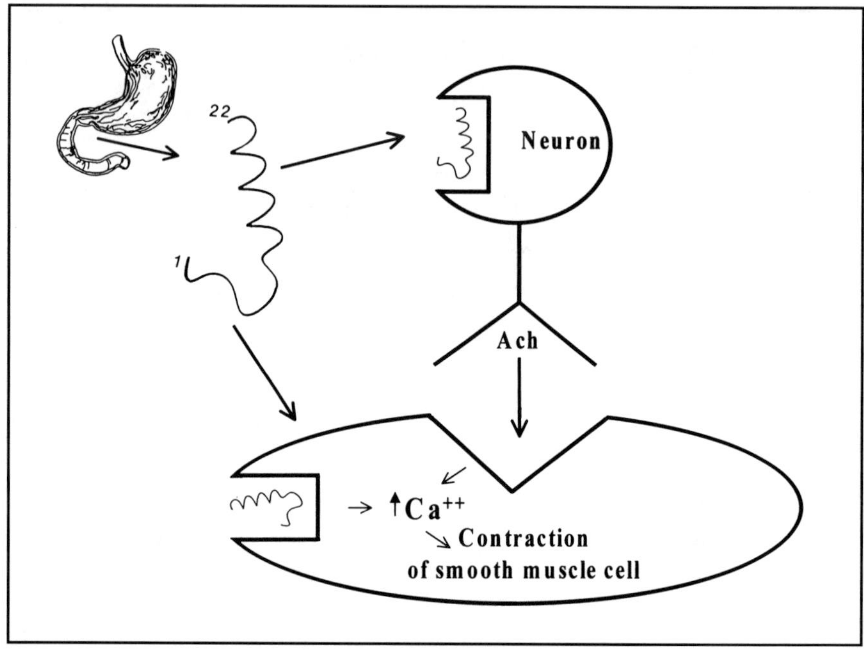

FIGURE 4. *Schematic representation of motilin action on digestive motility. Motilin is released from an endocrine cell of the duodenal mucosa circulates in the blood and acts on motilin receptors located on muscles or on intrinsic (cholinergic) nerves innervating GI muscle cells. Muscular and neural receptors correspond to different specific receptor subtypes (M and N).*

peptide analogs (27) or erythromycin derivatives. Based on the contractile effect of motilin receptor agonists, it could be expected that motilin receptor antagonists could induce an opposite effect, i.e., relaxation of GI muscles. Whether this characteristic could lead to the development of a new family of antispasmodics, with potential use, in patients with irritable bowel syndrome for example remains an hypothesis.

Motilin in the Brain

Most GI peptides are also present in the brain. However, the presence of motilin in the central nervous system remains uncertain (28). The presence of motilin receptors in the brain was clearly suspected, but it certainly needs clarification. Injection of motilin into the lateral brain ventricle stimulated appetite (29), induced the release of growth hormone (30) and reduced anxiety in rats or mice (31). These results were quite unexpected and remain enigmatic since the intracerebroventricular administration of motilin appears effective in species (mice and rat) where the intravenous injection of motilin seem unable to stimulate peripheral motilin receptors that should normally generate motor or secretory actions in the GI tract. In the rabbit, brain examined by autoradiography with I^{125} motilin, motilin binding is intense, mainly in the cerebellum (32, 33). The significance of this observation is unknown and could possibly be put into perspective with the surprising cloning of the motilin receptor from thyroid cells (described earlier) and with the ghrelin story narrated below. As discussed earlier, motilin receptors are present on intrinsic nerves of the intestinal wall, but we have failed to document their localization on extrinsic vagal fibers (33).

Motilin/Ghrelin: A New Family of Peptides?

Tomasetto, et al. (34) from Strasbourg cloned from a murine stomach library a new peptide they called motilin-related-peptide (MTL-RP) because of its structural homogeneity with motilin. At the same time, Japanese researchers purified from rat stomach a new peptide of 28 amino acids they have named ghrelin because of its capacity to bind to growth hormone secretagogue (GHS) receptors of the pituitary and then release growth hormone (35). Ghrelin is produced in endocrine cells of the gastric mucosa in dog and humans. In rodents, its administration promotes food intake, and the peptide appears to represent a major breakthrough in understanding appetite regulation, counter-balancing the satiety effect of leptin through an action on NPY (36). The central impact of ghrelin, i.e., appetite regulation and GH release, therefore completely mimics the unexpected effects previously ascribed to motilin in the rodent brain (29, 30). Furthermore, in the GI tract, we have observed that ghrelin accelerates gastric emptying and small intestinal transit (37). Ghrelin is potent enough to fully restore the gastric emptying function in a model of post-operative ileus. Similarities in the structure and actions of motilin and ghrelin therefore raise, for the first time, the possibility of a motilin peptide family.

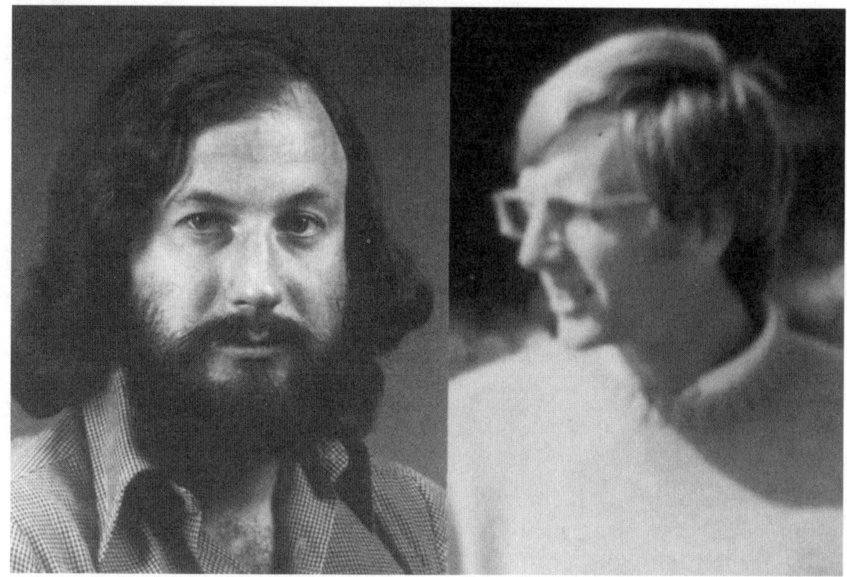

Pierre Poitras (left) and John Walsh (right) in the late 1970's at CURE.

ACKNOWLEDGMENTS

This retrospective preview of our research on motilin is dedicated to John Walsh. Thanks John for the patience you showed for 2 ½ years to this clinical fellow who came to Los Angeles ignorant about laboratory research. I am deeply indebted to you for giving me the tools and spirit that have guided my professional life during the last 20 years (Figure 5).

REFERENCES

1. Brown JC, Cook MA, Dryburgh JR. Motilin, a gastric motor activity stimulating polypeptide: the complete amino acid sequence. *Can J Biochem* 1973;51(5):533–537.

2. Poitras P, Reeve JR, Hunkapiller MW, Walsh JH. Characterization and purification of canine motilin. *Regul Pept* 1983;5:197–208.

3. Dea D, Boileau G, Poitras P, Lahaie RG. Molecular heterogeneity of human motilin like immunoreactivity explained by the processing of prepromotilin. *Gastroenterology* 1989;96:695–703.

4. Boulanger Y, Khiat A, Chen Y, Gagnon D, Poitras P, St-Pierre S. Structural effects of the selective reduction of amide carbonyl groups in motilin 1-12 as determined by NMR. *Int J Peptides Prot Research* 1995;46(6):527–534.

5. Poitras P, Gagnon M, St-Pierre S. N-terminal portion of motilin molecule determines its biological activity. *BBRC* 1992;183:36–40.

6. Miller P, Gagnon D, Dickner M, St-Pierre S, Poitras P. Studies on the structure activity of motilin. *Peptides* 1995;16:11–18.

7. Raymond MC, Boivin M, St-Pierre S, Gagnon D, Poitras P. Studies on the structure-activity of motilin *in vivo*. *Regul Pept* 1994;50:121–126.

8. Feighner SD, Tan CP, McKee KK, Palyha OC, Hreniuk DL, Pong SS, Austin CP, Figueroa D, MacNeil D, Cascieri MA, Nargund R, Bakshi R, Abramovitz M, Stocco R, Kargman S, O'Neill G, Van Der Ploeg LH, Evans J, Patchett AA, Smith RG, Howard AD. Receptor for motilin identified in the human gastrointestinal system. *Science* 1999;284(5423):2184–2188.

9. Poitras P, Lahaie RG, St-Pierre S, Trudel L. Comparative stimulation of motilin duodenal receptor by porcine or canine motilin. *Gastroenterology* 1987;92:658–662.

10. Boivin M, Pinelo LR, St-Pierre S, Poitras P. Neural mediation of the motilin motor effect on the human antrum. *Am J Physiol* 1997;272(1 Pt 1):G71-G76.

11. Poitras P, Miller P, Dickner M, Mao YK, Daniel EE, St-Pierre S, Trudel L. Heterogeneity of motilin receptors in the G.I. tract of the rabbit. *Peptides* 1996;17:701–707.

12. Miller P, Roy A, St-Pierre S, Dagenais M, Lapointe R, Poitras P. Motilin receptors in the human antrum. *Am J Physiol* 2000;278:G18–G23.

13. Poitras P. Motilin is a digestive hormone in the dog. *Gastroenterology* 1984;87:909–913.

14. Poitras P, Dumont A, Cuber JC, Trudel L Cholinergic regulation of motilin release from isolated canine intestinal cells *in vitro*. *Peptides* 1993;14:207–213.

15. Poitras P, Coimbra C, Trudel L. Role of second messengers on motilin release in a preparation of isolated intestinal mucosal cells. *Peptides* 1993;14:767–770.

16. Poitras P, Trudel L, Miller P, Gu CM. Regulation of motilin release: studies with ex vivo perfused canine jejunum. *Am J Physiol* 1997;272(1 Pt 1):G4-G9.

17. Poitras P, Tassé D, Laprise P. Stimulation of motilin release by bombesin in dogs. *Am J Physiol* 1983;8(2):G249–G256.

18. Poitras P, Steinbach JH, VanDeventer G, Walsh JH, Code CF. Motilin independent ectopic front of the interdigestive myoelectric complex in dogs. *Am J Physiol* 1980;239:G215–G220.

19. Poitras P, Boivin M, Lahaie RG, Trudel L. Regulation of plasma motilin by opioids in the dog. *Am J Physiol* 1989;257 (1 Pt 1):G41-G45.

20. Boivin M, Raymond MC, Riberdy M, St-Pierre S, Poitras P. Plasma motilin variation during the interdigestive and the digestive states in man. *J GI Motility* 1990;2:240–246.

21. Boivin M, Bradette M, Riberdy M, Raymond MC, Poitras P. Mechanisms of post prandial motilin release in humans. *Dig Dis Sci* 1992;37:1562–1568.

22. Labo G, Bortolotti M, Vezzadini P, Bonora G, Bersani G. Interdigestive gastroduodenal motility and serum motilin levels in patients with idiopathic delay in gastric emptying. *Gastroenterology* 1986;90(1):20–26.

23. Naritomi G, Tanaka M, Matsunaga H, Yokohata K, Ogawa Y, Chijiiwa K, Yamaguchi K. Pancreatic head resection with and without preservation of the duodenum: different postoperative gastric motility. *Surgery* 1996;120(5):831–837.

24. Itoh Z, Nakaya M, Suzuki T, Arai H, Wakabayashi K. Erythromycin mimics exogenous motilin in gastrointestinal contractile activity in the dog. *Am J Physiol* 1984;247(6 Pt 1):G688–G694.

25. Peeters TL. Erythromycin and other macrolides as prokinetic agents. *Gastroenterology* 1993;105(6):1886–1899.

26. Janssens J, Peeters TL, Vantrappen G, Tack J, Urbain JL, De Roo M, Muls E, Bouillon R. Improvement of gastric emptying in diabetic gastroparesis by erythromycin. Preliminary studies. *N Engl J Med* 1990;322(15):1028–1031.

27. Poitras P, Miller P, Gagnon D, St-Pierre S. Motilin synthetic analogues and motilin receptor antagonists. *BBRC* 1994;205:449–454.

28. Poitras P, Trudel L, Lahaie RG, Pomier-Layrargue G. Motilin-like-immuno-reactivity in intestine and brain of dog. *Life Sciences* 1987;40:1391–1395.

29. Rosenfeld DJ, Garthwaite TL. Central administration of motilin stimulates feeding in rats. *Physiol Behav* 1987;39(6):753–756.

30. Samson WK, Lumpkin MD, Nilaver G, McCann SM. Motilin: a novel growth hormone releasing agent. *Brain Res Bull* 1984;12(1):57–62.

31. Momose K, Inui A, Asakawa A, Ueno N, Nakajima M, Kasuga M. Anxiolytic effect of motilin and reversal with GM-109, a motilin antagonist, in mice. *Peptides* 1998;19(10):1739–1742.

32. Depoortere I, Peeters TL. Demonstration and characterization of motilin-binding sites in the rabbit cerebellum. *Am J Physiol* 1997;272(5 Pt 1):G994-G999.

33. Miller P, Trudel L, Butterworth R, Huet PM, Sharkey K, Rocheleau B, Ho W, Poitras P. Search for motilin receptors on vagus nerves. *Gastroenterology* 1999;116(4):G2740.
34. Tomasetto C, Karam SM, Ribieras S, Masson R, Lefebvre O, Staub, A, Alexander G, Chenard MP, Rio MC. Identification and characterization of a novel gastric peptide hormone: the motilin-related peptide. *Gastroenterology* 2000;119(2):395–405.
35. Kojima M, Hosoda H, Date Y, Nakazato M, Matsuo H, Kangawa K. Ghrelin is a growth-hormone-releasing acylated peptide from stomach. *Nature* 1999;402(6762):656–660.
36. Asakawa A, Inui A, Kaga T, Yuzuriha H, Nagata T, Ueno N, Makino S, Fujimiya M, Niijima A, Fujino MA, Kasuga M. Ghrelin is an appetite-stimulatory signal from stomach with structural resemblance to motilin. *Gastroenterology* 2001;120(2):337–345.
37. Trudel L, Tomasetto C, Rio MC, Plourde V, Eberling P, Poitras P. Motilin related peptide/Ghrelin is a potent gastrokinetic to reverse postoperative ileus in rats. *Am J Physiol.* (Submitted, 2002)

Gut-Brain Peptides in the New Millennium, edited by Y. Taché
CURE Foundation, Los Angeles, CA. © 2002

12

Trefoil Peptides: Regulators of Gastrointestinal Repair and Cancer Progression

Andrew S. Giraud
*Department of Medicine, University of Melbourne, Western Hospital
Footscray, Australia*

JOHN WALSH, GASTRIN, AND TREFOIL PEPTIDES

I was recruited to CURE from Graham Dockray's lab in Liverpool where I was doing a postdoc in mid 1984. The brief was to work up the isolated G (gastrin) cell preparation from the dog, using the elegant elutriation/cell culture technique developed by Marty Sanders and Drew Soll, and then characterize regulatory pathways mediating gastrin expression, especially by bombesin-like peptides (1). The lab was very cosmopolitan, with English falling a distant fifth in frequency of use behind Cantonese, Swedish, Japanese and Italian. At one stage I could say "Beers for everyone please, my friends are paying" in each of these languages, a talent that was to become exceptionally useful at future international meetings.

John proved to be an extremely enthusiastic and scientifically shrewd, as well as rigorous boss. His broad depth of knowledge and enthusiasm for new data often led to long hallway discussions about which experiment should be done next and what it might show, or who in town could provide further insight into solving a particular problem. Highlights were the regular journal and data clubs at John's home in Brentwood (attenuated when the Lakers were playing), CURE research days when new findings were bared for all to scrutinize, and Friday afternoon baseball followed by pizza, beer and camaraderie at Regular Johns (no relation and now sadly defunct).

The 1980's saw the first applications of molecular biology to gastrin research, the rapid understanding of how the gastrin gene and its products are regulated at a molecular level, as well as the realization that non-amidated products of progastrin processing were present in tissue and plasma, and that they might have a significant biological role; an idea which subsequently proved to be correct. In this latter regard I well remember that in the mid '80s John had the entire lab testing C-terminally extended gastrin peptides for biological activity in every bioassay system we could think of, but without result!

In mid 1986, not long after the birth of our twins, my wife Marg (who ran John's office at CURE for several years) and I returned to Australia. My research interests turned to peptides that promote gastrointestinal repair, in part derived from an ongoing interest in regulation of tissue homeostasis by growth factors like bombesin (GRP), as well as the realization, no doubt encouraged by discussions with John Walsh and others, that in order to maintain gut function, efficient tissue repair programs needed to be in place and be functioning optimally. It was about this time that I read papers by Lars Thim and colleagues describing the isolation and characterization of the prototypic trefoil peptide spasmolytic polypeptide from porcine pancreatic extracts (2). The excitement of new peptide discovery, especially evoking the strong parallels with the pioneering work of Rod Gregory on gastrin, with whom I had worked briefly while in Liverpool, and the likely role of trefoils in epithelial repair, encouraged me to begin work on these fascinating regulatory peptides.

In an ironic twist that John would have appreciated, the regulation of gastrin on which I had toiled at CURE in 1985, and the most prevalent trefoil peptide pS2 on which my lab now focuses, may have a functional link which was recently uncovered by a fellow journeyman (and now distinguished Professor) from Liverpool days. At the AGA meeting in Atlanta in 2001, Zara Khan from Rod Dimaline's lab reported that gastrin potently regulates pS2 expression by transfected gastric epithelial cells (3). In addition mutant mice overexpressing gastrin had elevated stomach pS2 mRNA and conversely gastrin knockouts expressed about 60% less pS2. These observations suggest that the physiological repertoire of gastrin may be extended from hormone and mitogen to that of indirect regulator of tissue repair and tumor suppression, an outcome that would have pleased but probably not surprised John Walsh.

WHAT ARE THE TREFOIL PEPTIDES?

The trefoil peptides constitute a small family of regulatory polypeptides synthesized mainly by mucus cells, and which are distinguished by having one or two characteristic 3-looped "trefoil" motifs secured by disulfide bonds between three pairs of cysteine residues in a 1–5, 2–4, 3–6 configuration (31) (Figure 1). Peptides with one trefoil motif form homodimers, and one member has 2 naturally occurring motifs in which the N- and C-terminal regions are coupled by virtue of a fourth disulfide bond forming a looped, loop structure. All trefoils are extremely stable structurally, being particularly resistant to acid proteolysis and are therefore likely to retain biological activity even after secretion into the gut lumen.

There are three known mammalian trefoil peptides and several others expressed by lower vertebrates. Mammalian members are trefoil peptide 1

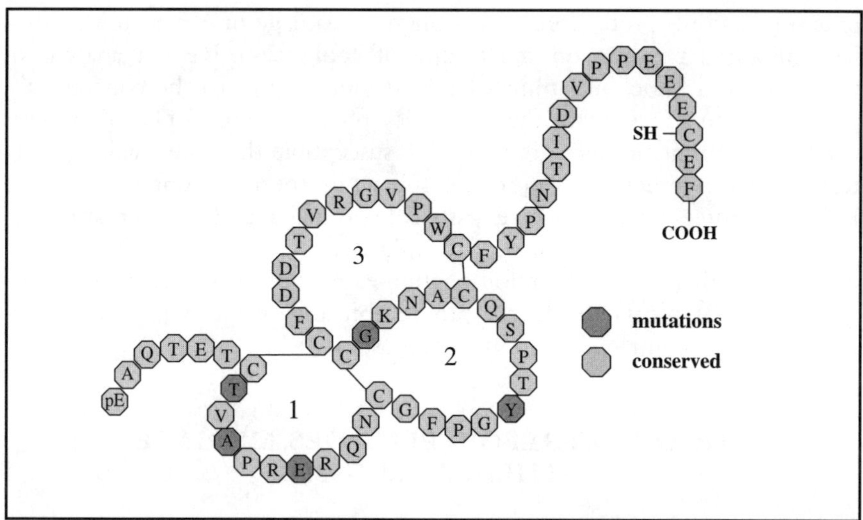

FIGURE 1. *Motif structure of pS2/TFF1. Residues which show somatic mutations are darkly shaded, while conserved residues are lightly shaded. Cysteines which form disulfide bridges are listed as C.*

(TFF1 or pS2; pS2/TFF1) found in surface epithelial cells of the stomach, trefoil peptide 2 (TFF2 or spasmolytic polypeptide; SP/TFF2) expressed by glandular mucus cells of the stomach and Brunner's glands of the duodenum, and trefoil peptide 3 (TFF3 or intestinal trefoil factor; ITF/TFF3) a product of goblet cells of the intestine and colon. The trefoil genes are located together on the long arm of chromosome 21 (21q22.3) in humans, a region characterized by both tumor enhancer and suppressor genes, as well as the prevalence of numerous genes associated with severe CNS pathology including motoneurone disease, Alzheimers disease and bipolar affective disorder. Whether the chromosomal location of the trefoils as a whole is biologically significant is unknown, however pS2/TFF1 has many of the characteristics expected of a gastric-specific tumor suppressor gene, and individuals with Down's syndrome or trisomy of chromosome 21 have a reduced incidence of gastrointestinal cancer if they reach adulthood.

WHAT DO THE TREFOIL PEPTIDES REGULATE AND HOW DO THEY DO SO?

It is now clear that trefoil peptides play a central role in mediating epithelial repair after mucosal injury. They are strongly induced following cryoprobe, chemical or mechanical injury (4, 5, 6), and increased synthesis is maintained in affected regions for many weeks until glandular renewal is complete (7). In addition, application of recombinant trefoil peptides either *in vitro* (5) or

in vivo (8) affords protection against ongoing damage or accelerates epithelial renewal depending on the timing of application. Recent analysis of
transgenic and knockout animals lends further support to the concept of a
primary repair function for these peptides; pS2/TFF1 and ITF/TFF3 overexpressing transgenic mice are much less susceptible than their wildtype lit-
termates to indomethacin injury (9, 10), while the corresponding peptide
knockout mice develop severe gastric hyperplasia and inflammation, or
show increased colonic sensitivity to mild irritants (11, 12). Together these
data suggest that defects in trefoil peptide expression may contribute to inflammatory or ulcerative disease progression and that this peptide family
makes a major contribution to gut homeostasis.

HOW DO TREFOIL PEPTIDES MEDIATE THEIR ACTIONS?

Mucin Interactions

There is substantial indirect evidence that trefoil peptides mediate at least
part of their healing and cytoprotective effects through interactions with secreted mucins (13). Thus trefoils are co-expressed with mucins in the same
cells, and are co-secreted as part of the mucus gel overlying the luminal epithelium. Trefoil cytoprotection is augmented by purified mucin preparations
as is trefoil-induced barrier function of the gastric epithelium to proton permeation (30), and the addition of recombinant trefoils to mucin results in increased light scattering suggesting a specific interaction. Recently elegant
2-hybrid studies have demonstrated such an interaction between trefoils and
the von Willebrand domains (vWD-C) of the secreted (but not membrane-
bound) mucins Muc 5AC and Muc 2 (14). These observations lend weight
to preliminary data by surface plasmon resonance (Giraud, et al. unpublished)
suggesting high affinity binding of TFF2 with Muc 5AC. The full physiological significance of these observations requires elucidation, however ongoing
site-directed mutagenesis of trefoil and vWD-C peptides, as well as further
analysis of the peptide-protein interaction should clarify the issue.

Motogenic Actions/β-catenin

It is now well established that all 3 trefoils are low potency motogens for a
wide variety of epithelial (15, 16) and other cell types, including immuno-
cytes (17). Motogenic thresholds are in the mid to high micromolar range
which is several orders of magnitude less potent than other gut motogens
such as EGF or HGF. Nonetheless, it has been well established that trefoils
are present in high concentrations at sites of epithelial injury and so it is rea-

sonable to surmise that they might regulate local cell migration (restitution) to replace damaged or lost epithelial cells in order to maintain mucosal integrity. This appears to be accomplished by SP/TFF2 and ITF/TFF3 in part by down-regulating E-cadherin -β-catenin complexes, thereby reducing cell-cell adhesion and promoting cell migration (18, 19). One caveat to these data is that they have been derived from colonic or gastric cancer cell lines exclusively, and whether the same holds true for non-transformed gut epithelial cells is yet to be tested.

Apoptosis

Analysis of the phenotype of the ITF/TFF3 null mouse has shown that there is increased proliferation in colonic crypts, yet colonocyte numbers remain unchanged suggesting increased cell death (11). Subsequently an increase in apoptotic cell profiles extending throughout the crypt bases and more apical regions has been demonstrated for both the colon and small intestine of ITF/TFF3 null mice. In addition, *in vitro* studies using both colon carcinoma and non-transformed intestinal epithelial cell lines have confirmed the protective activity of ITF/TFF3 against apoptosis induced by ceramide or serum starvation, and which appears to be accomplished in a bcl-2 and Fas/Fas ligand independent manner (20). It has also been shown that ITF/TFF3 -mediated inhibition of apoptosis induced by loss of substrate adhesion in non-transformed intestinal epithelial cells, is accomplished by signalling through NF-κB (21). Together these observations suggest that ITF/TFF3 (and probably other trefoil peptides as well) not only augment epithelial repair by stimulating restitution, thereby affording protection to the underlying epithelium after damage, but also prevent ongoing apoptotic cell death of cells in the newly reconstituted epithelium.

WHAT ROLE DO TREFOILS PLAY IN CANCER DEVELOPMENT AND PROGRESSION?

In general trefoil peptides show either basal or increased expression in epithelial cancers, particularly of the gut but also the urogenital tract, breast and lung. For example, pS2/TFF1 the most highly expressed trefoil peptide, is a major estrogen-inducible product in breast cancer being expressed by about 70% tumors (22). It is also well represented in tumors of the gut and female reproductive tract as well as the bladder and prostate (23).

The recent application of cDNA array and SAGE technologies to discovering new tumor markers through gene expression analysis has confirmed that particular trefoil peptide genes are specifically up-regulated in certain cancers. Thus SAGE analysis of pancreatic carcinoma has shown that SP/TFF2 is expressed in ~85% pancreatic cell lines and is more highly expressed in SAGE libraries derived from pancreatic adenocarcinomas than normal pancreas (24), while oligonucleotide microarrays of ovarian cancers (25) shows selective up-regulation of ITF/TFF3 (G.M. Hampton, personal communication).

Apart from one exception (described below) it is not clear at this stage whether or not the expression of trefoil peptides in epithelial cancers is an accident of tissue expression or whether these peptides play a role in regulating cancer progression. The motogenic and anti-apoptotic effects of trefoil peptides are clearly advantageous in promoting normal gastrointestinal integrity in the face of a corrosive luminal environment, however these same functions expressed in a cancer setting would both prevent apoptotic targetting of neoplastic cells and promote metastasis. Clearly there must be regulatory mechanisms in place to prevent this occurring, and it is possible that subversion of these may promote malignancy. To date however, there is no evidence for either angiogenic or mitogenic actions of the trefoil peptides. In fact, targeted overexpression of pS2 (10) or ITF (11) in the small intestine of transgenic mice promotes improved mucosal healing rather than augmenting dysplasia or hyperplasia. In addition, ITF over-expression in colonic cancer cell lines and tumors results in inhibition of cell proliferation (26) as does exogenous application of pS2 to the gastric cancer cell line AGS (27).

Although the pS2 gene is upregulated in most gastrointestinal cancers, its expression appears to be selectively inhibited in about 50% of distal cancers of the stomach, and this observation coupled with the discrete phenotype of pS2 null mice, which develop antral adenomas, and in a minority adenocarcinoma, suggests that it functions at this site as a tumor suppressor gene (12). Recent support for this hypothesis comes from studies on a large series of human gastric tumors which show reduced pS2 expression, loss of heterozygosity of the pS2 gene (17%), and numerous somatic mutations confined to the region encoding the trefoil motif and which is essential for biological activity (28).

TREFOILS, RECEPTORS, AND THE WALSH LEGACY

A number of years ago I re-visited CURE after being away for about 10 years. The place was much the same albeit with a new coat of paint and better appointed labs. John was just as enthusiastic as ever and he asked me to present some of my lab's work at a lunchtime seminar. At the end of my talk he asked me whether the effects of trefoil peptides that I had described were receptor mediated, and if so, had the receptors been cloned. We have come a long way since then in understanding trefoil biology, however, if asked the same question now I would answer the same way: no receptors have yet been cloned, despite the fact that binding sites have been demonstrated, second messenger pathways appear to be activated in response to trefoils and at least some effects are mediated through coated pits in membranes (29). A major difficulty has been the fact that trefoils bind a number of different mucins which are components of many systems that might be good sources for receptor identification, as well as the fact that they clearly interact with surface adhesion molecules and are able to transactivate the EGF receptor (29) thereby satisfactorily accounting for many of their biological effects. The existence or not of a trefoil receptor(s) remains the major unresolved question in trefoil biology at present, and an understanding of the full repertoire of trefoil functions will require its resolution. Perhaps we need additional investigators in the field imbued with a sense of the Walsh legacy of insightful problem solving and a passion for gastrointestinal biology to help us.

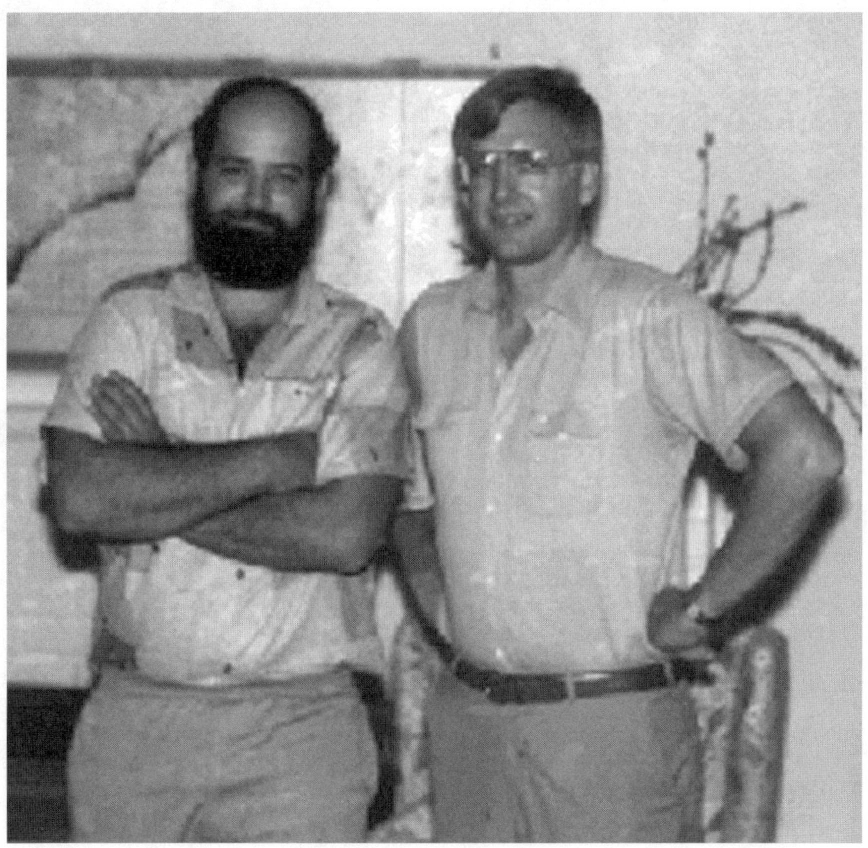

Andy and John, Brentwood 1985.

REFERENCES

1. Giraud AS, Cutitta F, Walsh JH, Soll AH. Bombesin stimulation of gastrin release from canine gastrin cells in primary culture. *Am J Physiol* 1987;252:G413–420.
2. Jorgensen KH, Thim L, Jacobsen HE. Pancreatic spasmolytic polypeptide (PSP): I. Preparation and initial chemical characterization of a new polypeptide from porcine pancreas. *Regul Pept* 1982;3:207–219.
3. Khan ZE, Wang TC, Varro A, Dimaline R. Transcriptional regulation of the TFF1 gene by gastrin. *Gastroenterology* 2001;120:A101.
4. Alison MR, Chinery R, Poulsom R, Ashwood P, Longcroft J, Wright NA. Experimental ulceration leads to sequential expression of spasmolytic polypeptide, intestinal trefoil factor, epidermal growth factor and transforming growth factor a mRNAs in rat stomach. *J Pathology* 1995;175:405–414.
5. Babyatsky MW, de Beaumont M, Thim L, Podolsky DK. Oral trefoil peptides protect against ethanol and indomethacin-induced gastric injury in rats. *Gastroenterology* 1996;110:489–497.
6. Cook GA, Yeomans ND, Giraud AS. Temporal expression of trefoil peptides in the TGFα knockout mouse after gastric ulceration. *Am J Physiol* 1997;272:G1540–1549.
7. Taupin DR, Pedersen J, Familari M, Cook G, Yeomans ND, Giraud AS. Augmented intestinal trefoil factor (TFF3) and loss of pS2 (TFF1) expression precedes metaplastic differentiation of gastric epithelium. *Lab Invest* 2001;81:397–408.
8. Tran C, Whitehead R., Familari MF, Giraud AS. Short chain fatty acids inhibit intestinal trefoil factor (TFF3) gene expression in a colon cancer cells. *Am J Physiol* 1998;275: G85–G94.
9. Playford RJ, Marchbank T, Goodlad RA, Chinery RA, Poulsom R, Hanby AM, et al. Transgenic mice that overexpress the human trefoil peptide pS2 have an increased resistance to intestinal damage. *PNAS* 1996;93:2137–2142.
10. Marchbank T, Cox HM, Goodlad RA, Giraud AS, Moss S, Wright NA, Jankowski RJ, Playford RJ. Effect of ectopic expression of rat intestinal trefoil factor family 3 (TFF3, intestinal trefoil factor) in the jejunum of transgenic mice. *J Biol Chem* 2001;276:24088–24096.
11. Mashimo H, Wu DC, Podolsky DK, Fishman MC. Impaired defense of intestinal mucosa of pS2 expression in mice lacking intestinal trefoil factor. *Science* 1996;274:262–265.
12. Lefebvre O, Chenard MC, Masson R, Linares J, Dierich A, LeMeur M, et al. Gastric mucosal abnormalities and tumorigenesis in mice lacking the pS2 trefoil protein. *Science* 1996;274:259–262.
13. Sands BE, Podolsky DK. The trefoil peptide family. *Ann Rev Physiol* 1996;58:253–273.
14. Tomasetto C, Masson R, Linares JL, Wendling C, Lefebvre O, Chenard MP, Rio MC. PS2/TFF1 interacts directly with the vWFC cysteine-rich domains of mucins. *Gastroenterology* 2000;118:70–80.
15. Dignass A, Lynch-Devaney K, Kindon H, Thim L, Podolsky DK. Trefoil peptides promote epithelial migration through a transforming growth factor β-independent pathway. *J Clin Invest* 1994;94:376–383.
16. Playford RJ, Marchbank T, Chinery R, Evison R, Pignatelli M., et al. Human spasmolytic polypeptide is a cytoprotective agent that stimulates cell migration. *Gastroenterology* 1995;108:108–116.
17. Cook GA, Familari M., Yeomans ND, Thim L, Giraud AS. The trefoil peptides TFF2 and TFF3 are expressed in rat lymphoid tissues and participate in the immune response. *FEBS Letters* 1999;456: 155–159.
18. Liu D, El-Hariry I, Karayiannakis J, Wilding J, Chinery R, Kmiot W, McCrea PD, Gullick WJ, Pignatelli M. Phosphorylation of β-catenin and epidermal growth factor receptor by intestinal trefoil factor. *Lab Investigation* 1997;77:557–563.
19. Moncur PH, Askham J, Markham AF, Morrison EE. Trefoil family factor 2 (TFF2) results in disruption of intercellular junctions facilitating cell migration and restitution. *Gastroenterology* 2000;118:2898.
20. Taupin DR, Kinoshita K, Podolsky DK. Intestinal trefoil factor confers colonic epithelial resistance to apoptosis. *PNAS* 2000;97:799–804.
21. Chen YH, Lu Y, De Plaen IG, Wang LY, Tan XD. Transcription factor NF-κB signals antianoikic function of trefoil factor 3 on intestinal epithelial cells. *Biochem Biophys Res Comm* 2000;11:576–582.
22. Henry JA, Bennet MK, Piggott NH, Levett DL, May FEB, Westley BR. Expression of the pNR-2/pS2 protein in diverse human epithelial tumors. *Br J Cancer* 1991;64:677–682.
23. May FEB, Westley BR. Trefoil proteins: their role in normal and malignant cells. *J Pathol* 1997;183: 4–7.

24. Argani P, Rosty C, Reiter RE, Wilentz RE, Murugesan SR, Leach SD, Ryu B, et al. Discovery of new markers of cancer through serial analysis of gene expression: prostate stem cell antigen is over-expressed in pancreatic carcinoma. *Cancer Res* 2001;61:4320–4324.

25. Welsh JB, Zarrinkar PP, Sapinoso LM, Kern SG, Behling CA, Monk BJ, Lockhart DJ, Burger RA, Hampton GM. Analysis of gene expression profiles in normal and neoplastic ovarian tissue samples identifies candidate molecular markers of epithelial ovarian cancer. *PNAS* 2001;98:1176–1181.

26. Uchino H, Kataoka H, Itoh H, Hamasuna R, Koono M. Overexpression of intestinal trefoil factor in human colon carcinoma cells reduces cellular growth *in vitro* and *in vivo*. *Gastroenterology* 2000;118: 60–69.

27. Calnan DP, Westley BR, May FEB, Floyd DN, Marchbank T, Playford RJ. The trefoil peptide TFF1 inhibits the growth of the human gastric adenocarcinoma cell line *AGS*. *J Pathol* 1999;188:312–317.

28. Park WS, Oh RR, Park JY, Lee JH, Shin MS, Kim HS, Lee HK, et al. Somatic mutations of the trefoil factor family 1 gene in gastric cancer. *Gastroenterology* 2000;119:691–698.

29. Taupin DR, Wu DC, Jeon WK, Devaney K, Wang TC, Podolsky DK. The trefoil gene family are co-ordinately expressed immediate-early genes: EGF receptor-and MAP kinase-dependent interregulation. *J Clin Invest* 1999;103:R31–38.

30. Tanaka S, Podolsky DK, Engel E, Guth PH, Kaunitz JD. Human spasmolytic polypeptide decreases proton permeation through gastric mucus *in vivo* and *in vitro*. *Am J Physiol* 1997;272:G1473–1480.

31. Thim L. Trefoil peptides: from structure to function. *Cell Mol Life Sci* 1997;53:888–903.

Gut-Brain Peptides in the New Millennium, edited by Y. Taché
CURE Foundation, Los Angeles, CA. © 2002

13

The Regulation of Gastric Acid Secretion by Pituitary Adenylate Cyclase Activating Polypeptide (PACAP)

Joseph R. Pisegna
*Division of Gastroenterology and Hepatology, VA Greater Los Angeles Healthcare System,
CURE/Digestive Diseases Research Center, UCLA Division of Digestive Diseases
Department of Medicine, Los Angeles, CA*

INTRODUCTION

The regulation of gastric acid secretion has been a subject of intense interest at the Center for Ulcer Research and Education (CURE). Dr. Morton Grossman was the first to establish this center as a world-renowned gastrointestinal research center. John Walsh who was center director during some of its most active years in the areas of molecular pharmacology has shown the potent effects of gastrin in the regulation of gastric acid secretion. Previously, John was perhaps best known for developing monoclonal and polyclonal antibodies which led to elucidation of the physiology for the majority of peptides and their receptors in the gastrointestinal tract.

A relative latecomer to this center, I wanted to provide a bit of background to reflect as to how this center has expanded my research and that of the PACAP hormone and receptor, which will be discussed later in this chapter. While working in the laboratory of Dr. Stephen Wank, we were able to clone and pharmacologically characterize the receptor for cholecystokinin and gastrin, which was called, CCK-A and CCK-B receptors, respectively. The knowledge gained from cloning these receptors was shared with the Walsh group and led to some of their most prominent applications. Walsh and coworkers developed specific antibodies to these receptors that permitted the mapping of the CCK-A and CCK-B receptors in the gastrointestinal tract. At about this time, I first came to know John Walsh through interactions at scientific meetings.

At the Regulatory Peptides meeting in Santa Barbara in 1995, John and I had a lengthy discussion regarding my research. At the time, my work was focused on the signal transduction for the recently cloned PACAP receptor, now referred to as PAC1. John and I wanted to explore whether this receptor was expressed in the GI tract and what function, if any, could be ascribed to this newly cloned receptor. John initially proposed the development of an anti-PAC1 polyclonal antibody that would allow me to determine where in the GI tract the receptors were localized. John and I sat in his CURE office with the deduced amino acid sequences, which I brought with me from the NIH and John chose the amino acids, which could be used to synthesize a specific polyclonal antibody. In collaboration with George Poy and Steve Wank at NIH, peptides were developed accordingly. These peptides underwent mass spectroscopy with the help of Joe Reeve at the CURE Peptide Core and were conjugated and injected into rabbits to develop sera by Helen Wong at the CURE Antibody Core laboratory. Helen's role was prominent, as she was the person that carefully characterized this antibody. Later, these antibodies were tested both by Western Blot and by immunocytochemistry and shown to be specific.

Now, with the PAC1 specific antibody in hand, we set out to determine whether there were receptors in the GI tract for PACAP. Immunohistochemistry was initially performed with one of my collaborators back at the NIH but the interpretation of the immunostained tissue sections was accomplished with the assistance of Dr. Catia Sternini of the CURE Imaging Core. In these sections, ECL cells appeared to be stained by the anti-PAC1 antibody suggesting the possibility that PACAP could modulate gastric acid secretion. In meetings with John Walsh and Dr. George Sachs, CURE Co-Director, it appeared to be a viable project. In the Sachs laboratory, by Dr. Ning Zeng, a postdoctoral researcher, ECL cells were isolated and the physiology of PACAP on these cells was first characterized. Using molecular tools, we were also able to show the expression of PAC1 splice variants on these cells. Later, in whole animals, and with the assistance of Dr. Gordon Ohning, we were able to demonstrate that PACAP was a potent stimulant of gastric acid secretion. The description of the neural circuitry was done in collaboration with Dr. Marcel Miapambu in the laboratory of Dr. Yvette Taché using the CURE Animal Core facility, results which will be described in more detail in a separate chapter.

What I have described here is what John Walsh saw in the CURE center. Namely, he saw CURE as an outstanding center dedicated to the understanding of the gastrointestinal tract and through his efforts, he developed a group of world-class researchers who working in a collaborative manner could dissect and further our understanding of regulatory systems in the GI tract. I, therefore, am very grateful to his efforts at recruiting me and to furthering the science of this relatively obscure hormone and receptor.

PACAP IS A NEWLY DISCOVERED NEUROENTERIC PEPTIDE

Pituitary Adenylate Cyclase Activating Polypeptide (PACAP) is the most recently discovered neuropeptide in the vasoactive intestinal polypeptide

(VIP), secretin, and glucagon family of peptide hormones. This peptide was first isolated in 1989 by Arimura and coworkers from ovine hypothalamus using assays for adenylyl cyclase. They subsequently discovered that there were actually two peptides that occur biologically, PACAP-38 (P-38) and PACAP-27 (P-27) that are processed from the same gene and share identical 27 N-terminal amino acids (1, 2). Since its discovery, this hormone has been identified in numerous tissues including the brain, gastrointestinal tract, adrenal gland, and testis by radioimmunoassays and immunohisto-chemistry PACAP (3, 4).

In the gastrointestinal tract, PACAP has activity in the esophagus, stomach, duodenum as well as the small and large intestines (5, 6). On smooth muscle cells of the GI tract, PACAP acts as a potent non-adrenergic, non-cholinergic inhibitory neurotransmitter via apamin-sensitive potassium channels (7). PACAP is also able to stimulate cellular growth and differentiation as demonstrated in the AR-42J cells, where PACAP stimulates an increase in ornithine decarboxylase activity and cell proliferation (8) and in the PC-12, pheochromocytoma cell line where PACAP stimulates neurite outgrowth (9). PACAP has been specifically linked to some human motility disorders such as Hirschsprung's disease, where a reduction in PACAP- immunoreactive nerve fibers has been described (10).

CLONING OF THE RAT PACAP RECEPTOR GENE

Prior to the cloning of the PAC1, radioligand-binding data from AR-42J cells as well as hypothalamic and brain membranes suggested the existence of at least three types of PACAP receptors (11, 12). These PACAP receptor subtypes differed in their relative affinities for the ligands P-38, P-27, VIP and helodermin (2, 11). However, cloning of the rat PACAP receptor (rPACAP-R) in 1993 showed that a single high affinity receptor exists for the ligands P-38 and P-27 (12). Although the deduced amino acid sequence of the cloned rPACAP-R shows high homology with VIP and secretin receptors, PACAP-Rs have virtually no affinity for VIP or secretin (12). On the contrary, PACAP has high affinity for VIP_1 and VIP_2 receptors. Cloning of the rat PAC1 cDNA identified it to belong to the VIP and secretin family of peptide receptors (12). The receptor cDNA encoded a putative protein with a molecular weight of 50 kDa containing 495 amino acids (12). Cloning of the rat PAC1 gene identified that the receptor could exist as four major splice variants (13). As shown in Figure 1, the four potential splice variants differed in the length of the third intracellular domain (13). Two exons ("hip" and "hop") can be alternatively spliced and expressed as four major distinct splice variants (13). Each of the splice variants show not only differential tissue expression, but also variable abilities

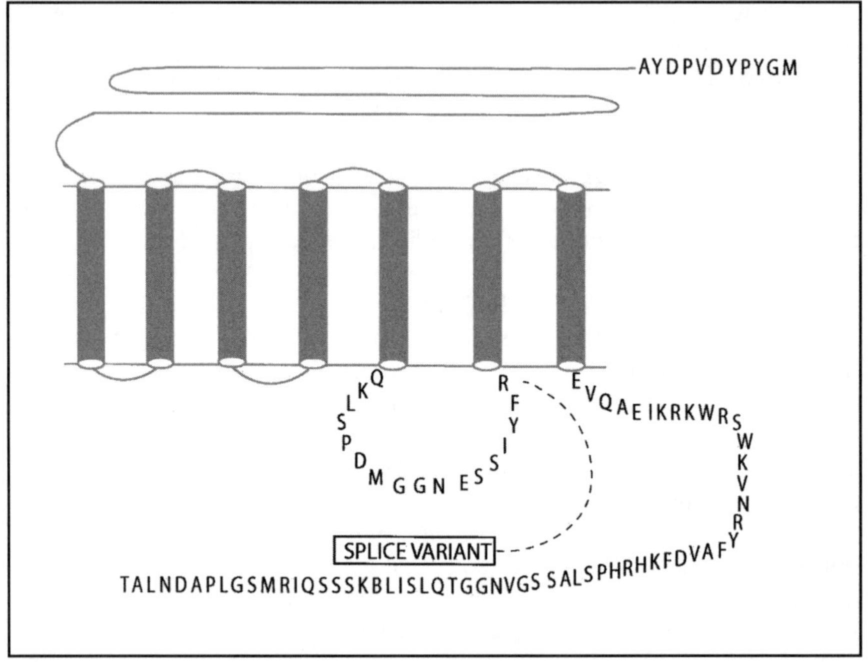

FIGURE 1. *Structure of the PACAP receptor (PAC1). Note the amino acids in block represent splice variant amino acid sequences which can be differentially spliced into the receptor.*

to activate adenylate cyclase (AC) and phospholipase C (PLC). The splice variants ("hip"), demonstrate coupling to only AC, whereas, the remaining three splice variants couple with varying potencies to both AC and PLC. These splice variants were also shown to be variably expressed in different tissues (13).

Subsequent cloning of the human PAC1 revealed a high homology with the rat and mouse receptor and a similar gene organization with two exons, termed SV-1 and SV-2 (14). However, unlike the rat splice variants, the differences in signal transduction coupling were not observed (14). Similar to the rat, the human PAC1 receptor gene has been shown to be large (~50kb). Some species differences do exist in that the gene for PAC1 is localized to chromosome 7 whereas the rat gene is localized on chromosome 4 (15).

Three receptors have been identified and cloned which have high affinity for PACAP hormone. The first of these receptors that was cloned is the classical VIP receptor (VPAC1). Subsequently the PAC1 receptor was cloned and originally called the Type I PACAP Receptor (Table 1). The last receptor in this family to be cloned was the VIP2 receptor (VPAC2) (16). These receptors can be differentiated pharmacologically based on

TABLE 1. *Relative affinities of the three PACAP and VIP receptors for the ligands*

IUPHAR nomenclature	*Relative Affinities*
PAC1	PACAP27 = PACAP38 > >VIP > Helodermin
VPAC1	PACAP27 = PACAP38 = VIP > > Helodermin
VPAC2	Helodermin > PACAP27 = PACAP38 = VIP

their relative affinities for the ligands shown in Table 2 (17). The PAC1 has affinity for only PACAP-38 and PACAP-27 whereas VPAC1 and VPAC2 have nearly identical affinities for the ligands PACAP and VIP (17).

PAC1 SIGNAL TRANSDUCTION

The mammalian heterotrimeric guanine nucleotide-binding proteins (G-proteins) are interposed between the ligand-activated receptor and intracellular second messengers such as cAMP and inositol phosphates (IP). PACAP has been shown in both native cells and in cells transfected with PAC1 cDNAs to have variable degrees of coupling to both adenylate cyclase and phospholipase C. Therefore, PAC1 receptor is coupled to a dual signal transduction pathway (9, 13, 14). This was first demonstrated in PC12 cells (9), however the best characterized native cell systems for evaluating PACAP-Rs are the anterior pituitary-derived somatotrophs and gonadotrophs and adrenal chromaffin cells. In the growth hormone-secreting somatotrophs, PACAP stimulates Ca^{++} influx via a cAMP-dependent mechanism, whereas, in LH-secreting gonadotrophs, PACAP stimulates Ca^{++} release from IP_3-sensitive intracellular stores (18, 19). A fourth transmembrane splice variant was shown not to couple to either adenylyl cyclase or phospholipase C, yet couples to an L-type Ca^{++} channel (15). The region of PAC1 responsible for signal transduction coupling is the COOH- terminus (20). Two critical amino acids Ser and Arg in this region of the receptor coupled to signal transduction intermediates as shown by receptor mutagenesis studies. In addition to stimulating AC and PLC, type 1 PACAP receptors modulate other signal transduction pathways. For example, in colonic smooth muscle, the type 1 PACAP receptor activates apamin-sensitive K^+ channels to induce relaxation. The regions of the PAC1 responsible for ligand recognition have not yet been determined.

The ability of PACAP to stimulate a dual cascade of intracellular effectors may influence cell growth and differentiation by activating immediate early genes such as c-fos, and c-myc that ultimately influence transcriptional activity of a gene. PACAP-induces growth and differentiation in several cell systems such as in the rat pheochromocytoma cell line, PC-12, and in cultured neuroblasts (9). PAC1 is also expressed on several human tumoral cell

TABLE 2. *Nomenclature for PACAP and related VIP receptors*

Receptor Type		Selective Agonists	Selective Antagonists	Fluorescent Agonists	Selective Antagonist
IUPHAR nomenclature	Previous nomenclature				
PAC_1	PACAP Type I PVR1	PACAP-38 PACAP-27 Maxadilan?	PACAP 6-38 PACAP 6-27	Fluor-PACAP	PACAP(6-38)[†]
$VPAC_1$ PACAP Type II	VIP VIP_1 PVR_2 $VIP/PACAP_1$	$[Arg^{16}]$chicken secretin★ $[K^{15}R^{16}L^{27}]VIP(1-7)GRF(8-27)-NH_2$		Fluo-VIP	$[Ac-His^1, D-Phe^2,$ $Lys^{15}, Arg^{16}]$ $VIP(3-7)GRF(8-27)-NH_2$
$VPAC_2$	VIP_2 PACAP-3 PVR3 $VIP/PACAP_2$	Helodermin Ro 25-1553 Ro 25-1392			

lines, such as the neuroblastoma (NB-OK-1), and lung cancer (NCI-N417, NCI-H345) cell lines where PACAP influences growth (21, 22).

LOCALIZATION OF PAC1

The greatest density of PAC1 receptors occurs in the hypothalamus, olfactory bulb, the thalamus and the cerebellum where the null splice variant is the predominant form (15). Similarly, PAC1 is expressed in the retina (23). In peripheral tissues, the greatest density occurs in the adrenals with the "hop" splice variant being predominant (13, 15). The anterior pituitary gland contains abundant expression of PAC1 where again the predominant splice variant is the hop type (24). The human prostate gland and testis also contain PAC1 receptor (15).

With the recent development of the specific anti-PAC1 polyclonal antibodies, we have been able to characterize the localization of both PACAP and PAC1 in the myenteric neurons of the rat stomach and colon (25). PAC1 and VPAC 1 receptors have been identified in the gastrointestinal tract with the PAC1 receptor expressed on the gastric enterochromaffin like (ECL) cells whereas VPAC1 (classical VIP receptor) are expressed on the somatostatin-containing D cells and chief cells of the stomach (26). The smooth muscles of the GI tract contain both VPAC1 and PAC1 (27). We have also recently shown that PAC1 is expressed on the gastrointestinal lymphocytes and appears to regulate their activation and release of cytokines (work in progress by Dr. Patrizia Germano). The colocalization of PACAP and PAC1 will be described in more detail in a subsequent chapter.

PHYSIOLOGY OF PAC 1 IN THE GASTROINTESTINAL TRACT

PACAP and PACAP receptors are localized in the stomach and colon. However, their exact function is unknown. In the stomach, PACAP-containing enteric nerve fibers co-localized with PAC1 receptors in the gastric mucosa (25). PACAP appears to have diverse functions in the stomach that depend on the cell target expressing either PAC1 or VPAC1 because as discussed earlier, PACAP has high affinity to both receptor types. In the rat stomach, PACAP released by enteric neurons innervating the mucosa appear to be involved in gastric acid secretion and may account for the nocturnal increase observed in gastric acid secretion in rats (26). We have also demonstrated that PAC1 activation on ECL cells results in intracellular $Ca++$ release, cAMP stimulation and histamine release. On the contrary, through its activity on the VPAC1 receptor expressed on the surface of the D cell, PACAP inhibits acid secretion by stimulating the release of somatostatin from the gastric D cell (Figure 2).

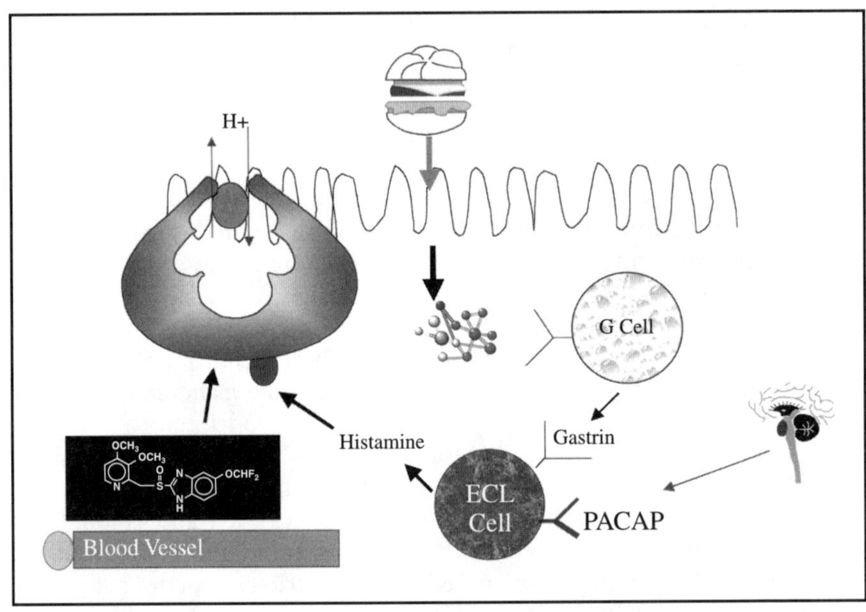

FIGURE 2. *Mechanism for gastric acid secretion. Food stimulates gastric G cell release of gastrin which in turn stimulates the ECL cell via the CCK-2 receptor expressed on the ECL cell. PACAP, released in response to neural stimulation acts at the PAC1 receptor expressed on the ECL cell. Stimulation of either CCK-2 or PAC1 receptors leads to histamine release by the ECL cell. Histamine in turn is the major regulator of parietal cell H^+, K^+ ATPase activity.*

In isolated rabbit glands PACAP induces intracellular Ca^{++} stimulation with consequent stimulation of parietal cell release of acid as detected with acridine orange (26).

Another important effect of PACAP is in the regulation of gastrointestinal motility. As mentioned earlier, PACAP-containing nerve fibers have been localized in the small and large intestine (25). These actions are mainly that of relaxation, being mediated through the VPAC1 receptor. In the rat colon, PACAP stimulates apamin sensitive K^+ channels (27). VIP and PACAP also appear to influence nitric oxide synthase (NOS) (28–31). In the rat pancreas, PACAP has been previously demonstrated to be a potent stimulant of amylase release and to be located in nerve fibers innervating the pancreas supporting a possible role of PACAP in exocrine pancreatic regulation (31).

CONCLUSIONS

PACAP represents one of the newest members of biologically active neuropeptides in the GI tract. Since its discovery in 1989, we are now aware of its importance in the regulation of gastric secretory and gastrointestinal motor function. Despite its early recognition as an important endocrine and neural regulator, much work still needs to be accomplished to further define its role in the GI tract. This will be facilitated by studies to genetically modify mice to better characterize the function of PACAP and its receptor in the GI tract. This chapter has demonstrated that important contributions to the development of a physiological understanding of a specific hormone and receptor can be made by an interdisciplinary approach involving techniques in molecular biology, biochemistry, immunology and classical physiology. We hope to expand these efforts to include that of genetics in the near future. Within the context of this book that defines the role of John Walsh, it is clear that to understand the physiology of gastrointestinal peptides requires a collaborative effort which in the end leads to discoveries.

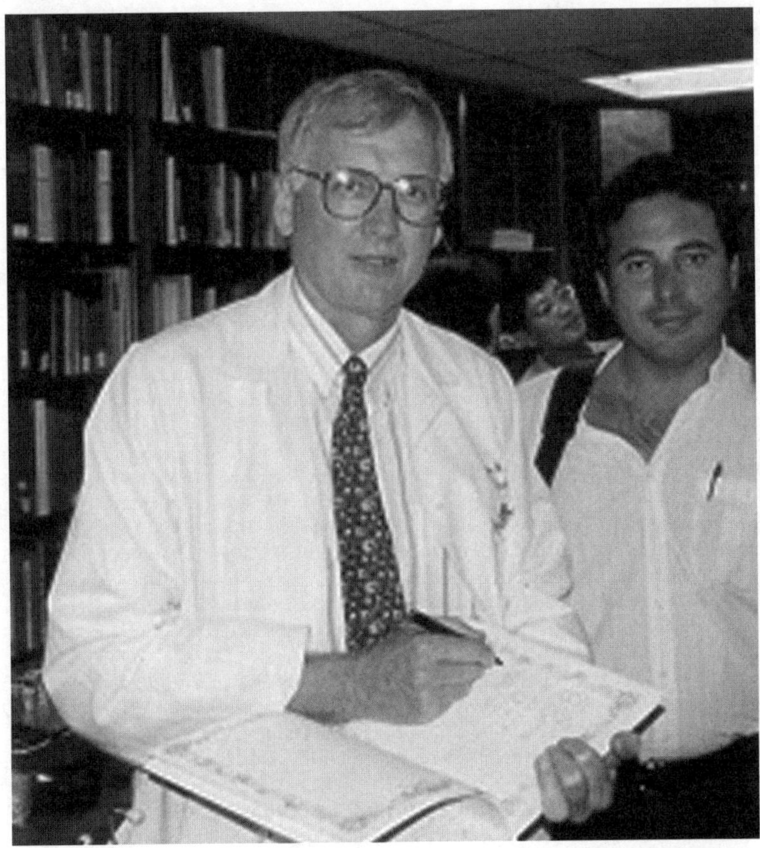

*Drs. Walsh and Pisegna share some humorous moments at one of the
CURE noontime functions held in the Lyon Library in 1999.*

ACKNOWLEDGMENTS

Supported by US VA Merit Review, AGA IRSA, and VA Career Development Award.

REFERENCES

1. Miyata A, Arimura A, Dahl RR, Minamino N, Uheara A, Jiang L, Culler MD, Coy DH. Isolation of a novel 38 residue-hypothalamic polypeptide which stimulates adenylate cyclase in pituitary cells. *Biochem Biophys Res Commun* 1989;164(1):567–74

2. Lam HC, Takahashi K, Ghatei MA, Kanse SM, Polak JM, Bloom SR. Binding sites of a novel neuropeptide pituitary-adenylate-cyclase-activating polypeptide in the rat brain and lung. *Eur J Biochem* 1990;193:725–9.

3. Arimura A, Somogyvari-Vigh A, Miyata A, Mizuno K, Coy DH, Kitada C. Tissue distribution of PACAP as determined by RIA: highly abundant in the rat brain and testes. *Endocrinology* 1991;129(5): 2787–9.

4. Tatsuno I, Somogyvari-Vigh A, Arimura A. Developmental changes of pituitary adenylate cyclase activating polypeptide (PACAP) and its receptor in the rat brain. *Peptides* 1994;15(1):55–60.

5. Mungan Z, Arimura A, Ertan A, Rossowski WJ, Coy DH. Pituitary adenylate cyclase-activating polypeptide relaxes rat gastrointestinal smooth muscle. *Scand J Gastroenterol* 1992;27(5):375–80.

6. Cox HM. Pituitary adenylate cyclase activating polypeptides, PACAP-27 and PACAP-38: stimulators of electrogenic ion secretion in the rat small intestine. *Br J Pharmacol* 1992;106(2):498–502.

7. Schworer H, Katsoulis S, Creutzfeldt W, Schmidt WE. Pituitary adenylate cyclase activating peptide, a novel VIP-like gut-brain peptide, relaxes the guinea-pig taenia caeci via apamin-sensitive potassium channels. *Naunyn Schmiedebergs Arch Pharmacol* 1992;346(5):511–4.

8. Buscail L, Cambillau C, Seva C, Scemama JL, De Neef P, Robberecht P, Christophe J, Susini C, Vaysse N. Stimulation of rat pancreatic tumoral AR4-2J cell proliferation by pituitary adenylate cyclase-activating peptide. *Gastroenterology* 1992;103(3):1002–8.

9. Deutsch PJ, Sun Y. The 38-amino acid form of pituitary adenylate cyclase-activating polypeptide stimulates dual signaling cascades in PC12 cells and promotes neurite outgrowth. *J Biol Chem* 1992; 267(8):5108–13.

10. Shen Z, Larsson LT, Malmfors G, Absood A, Hakanson R, Sundler F. A novel neuropeptide, pituitary adenylate cyclase-activating polypeptide (PACAP), in human intestine: evidence for reduced content in Hirschsprung's disease. *Cell Tissue Res* 1992;269(2):369–74.

11. Shivers BD, Gorcs TJ, Gottschall PE, Arimura A. Two high affinity binding sites for pituitary adenylate cyclase-activating polypeptide have different tissue distributions. *Endocrinology* 1991;128(6):3055–65.

12. Pisegna JR, Wank SA. Molecular cloning and functional expression of the pituitary adenylate cyclase-activating polypeptide type I receptor. *Proc Natl Acad Sci USA* 1993;90(13):6345–9.

13. Spengler D, Waeber C, Pantaloni C, Holsboer F, Bockaert J, Seeburg PH, Journot L. Differential signal transduction by five splice variants of the PACAP receptor. *Nature* 1993;365(6442):170–5.

14. Pisegna JR, Wank SA. Cloning and characterization of the signal transduction of four splice variants of the human pituitary adenylate cyclase activating polypeptide receptor. Evidence for dual coupling to adenylate cyclase and phospholipase C. *J Biol Chem* 1996; 271(29):17267–74.

15. Vaudry D, Gonzalez BJ, Basille M, Yon L, Fournier A, Vaudry H. Pituitary adenylate cyclase-activating polypeptide and its receptors: from structure to functions. *Pharmacol Rev* 2000;52(2):269–324.

16. Lutz EM, Sheward WJ, West KM, Morrow JA, Fink G, Harmar AJ. The VIP2 receptor: molecular characterization of a cDNA encoding a novel receptor for vasoactive intestinal peptide. *FEBS Lett* 1993;334(1):3–8.

17. Harmar AJ, Arimura A, Gozes I, Journot L, Laburthe M, Pisegna JR, Rawlings SR, Robberecht P, Said SI, Sreedharan SP, Wank SA, Waschek JA. International Union of Pharmacology, XVIII. Nomenclature of receptors for vasoactive intestinal peptide and pituitary adenylate cyclase-activating polypeptide. *Pharmacol Rev* 1998;50(2):265–70.

18. Canny BJ, Rawlings SR, Leong DA. Pituitary adenylate cyclase-activating polypeptide specifically increases cytosolic calcium ion concentration in rat gonadotropes and somatotropes. *Endocrinology* 1992;130(1):211–5.

19. Miyata A, Arimura A, Dahl RR, Minamino N, Uehara A, Jiang L, Culler MD, Coy DH. Isolation of a novel 38 residue-hypothalamic polypeptide which stimulates adenylate cyclase in pituitary cells. *Biochem Biophys Res Commun* 1989;164(1):567–74.

20. Lyu RM, Germano PM, Choi JK, Le S, Pisegna J. Identification of an essential amino acid motif within the C terminus of the pituitary adenylate cyclase-activating polypeptide type I receptor that is critical for signal transduction but not for receptor internalization. *J Biol Chem* 2000;275(46):36134–42.

21. Cauvin A, Buscail L, Gourlet P, DeNeef P, Gossen D, Arimura A, Miyata A, Coy DH, Robberecht P, Christophe J. The novel VIP-like hypothalamic polypeptide PACAP interacts with high affinity receptors in the human neuroblastoma cell line NB-OK. *Peptides* 1990;11(4):773–7.

22. Moody TW, Zia F, Makheja L. Pituitary adenylate cyclase activating polypeptide receptors are present on small cell lung cancer cells. *Peptides* 1993;14(2):241–6.

23. Seki T, Shioda S, Izumi S, Arimura A, Koide R. Electron microscopic observation of pituitary adenylate cyclase-activating polypeptide (PACAP)-containing neurons in the rat retina. *Peptides* 2000;21(1):109–13.

24. Rawlings SR, Hezareh M. Pituitary adenylate cyclase-activating polypeptide (PACAP) and PACAP/vasoactive intestinal polypeptide receptors: actions on the anterior pituitary gland. *Endocr Rev* 1996;17(1):4–29.

25. Miampamba M, Germano PM, Arli S, Wong H, Taché Y, Pisegna, J. Expression of pituitary adenylate cyclase activating polypeptide (PACAP) and PACAP Type I receptor (PAC1) in the rat gastric and colonic myenteric neurons. *Regul Pept* 2002, in press.

26. Zeng N, Athmann C, Kang T, Lyu RM, Walsh JH, Ohning GV, Sachs G, Pisegna JR. PACAP type I receptor activation regulates ECL cells and gastric acid secretion. *J Clin Invest* 1999;104(10):1383–91.

27. Schworer H, Katsoulis S, Creutzfeldt W, Schmidt WE. Pituitary adenylate cyclase activating peptide, a novel VIP-like gut-brain peptide, relaxes the guinea-pig taenia caeci via apamin-sensitive potassium channels. *Naunyn Schmiedebergs Arch Pharmacol* 1992;346(5):511–4.

28. Grider JR, Makhlouf GM. Colonic peristaltic reflex: identification of VIP as a mediator of descending relaxation. *Am J Physiol* 1986;251:G40–G45.

29. Grider JR, Katsoulis S, Schmidt WE, Jin JG. Regulation of the descending relaxation phase of intestinal peristalsis by PACAP. *J Auton Nerv Syst* 1994;50:151–159.

30. Grider JR. Interplay of VIP and nitric oxide in the regulation of the descending relaxation phase of peristalsis. *Am J Physiol* 1993;264:G334–G340.

31. Raufman JP, Malhotra R, Singh L. PACAP-38, a novel peptide from ovine hypothalamus, is a potent modulator of amylase release from dispersed acini from rat pancreas. *Regul Pept* 1991;Oct 1:36(1):121–9.

Gut-Brain Peptides in the New Millennium, edited by Y. Taché
CURE Foundation, Los Angeles, CA. © 2002

14

VIP-Specific and PACAP-Specific Receptors in *Tenia Coli*: New Insights into Peptide Signaling and Inhibitory Neurotransmission

Karnam S. Murthy, Baiqin Teng, Ji-Guang Jin,
John R. Grider and Gabriel M. Makhlouf
*Medical College of Virginia, Virginia Commonwealth University
Richmond, VA*

Three PACAP/VIP receptors have been identified: a PACAP-specific receptor (PAC1), which exhibits high affinity for pituitary adenylate cyclase activating peptide (PACAP) and much lower affinity for vasoactive intestinal peptide (VIP) and consists of several splice variants that are coupled with variable efficiency to adenylyl cyclase and phospholipase C-β; and two VIP/PACAP receptors (VPAC1 and VPAC2), which exhibit equally high affinity for VIP and PACAP and are coupled to adenylyl cyclase. Studies in guinea pig (GP) tenia coli have identified two additional receptors: a VIP-specific receptor that does not recognize PACAP but is coupled to adenylyl cyclase, and an apamin-sensitive, PACAP-specific receptor that does not recognize VIP and is not coupled to adenylyl cyclase, which mediates activation of K^+ channels and membrane hyperpolarization. Evidence for the existence of these receptors and characterization of their role in inhibitory neurotransmission is summarized below.

ROLE OF VPAC RECEPTORS IN INHIBITORY NEUROTRANSMISSION TO SMOOTH MUSCLE

In all mammalian species examined so far, inhibitory neurotransmission to smooth muscle of the gut reflects the interplay of nitric oxide (NO) and the neuropeptides, VIP, and its homologues, mainly PACAP. In these tissues, NO is generated in both nerve terminals and smooth muscle cells: NO formed in nerve terminals by the activity of neuronal NO synthase (nNOS) regulates VIP and PACAP release; in turn, these neuropeptides stimulate the formation of NO in smooth muscle cells by activating an endothelial-type NOS (eNOS) (1–3). NO formation in muscle cells is initiated by interaction of VIP or PACAP with a single-transmembrane receptor, the natriuretic peptide clearance receptor, NPR-C, which is coupled via the α subunits of G_{i1} and

G_{i2} to stimulation of Ca^{2+} influx and Ca^{2+}/calmodulin-dependent activation of eNOS (4, 5). Nitric oxide formation leads to the activation of soluble guanylyl cyclase, formation of cGMP, and activation of GMP-dependent protein kinase (PKG). In addition, VIP and PACAP interact with a cognate VPAC2 receptor coupled via $G\alpha_s$ to sequential activation of adenylyl cyclase and cAMP-dependent protein kinase (PKA). PKA and PKG act on various targets to inhibit Ca^{2+} mobilization, stimulate myosin light chain phosphatase activity, and induce membrane hyperpolarization and relaxation of smooth muscle tone. The hyperpolarization (also known as inhibitory junction potential) suppresses rhythmic electrical and contractile activity in smooth muscle.

The GP tenia coli stands as a unique exception to the model of inhibitory neurotransmission described above, which makes it all the more ironic because this tissue had featured prominently in the development of concepts on inhibitory neurotransmission. The singularity of GP tenia coli, however, has been a useful control in constructing a pervasive model of inhibitory signaling in smooth muscle of the gut.

INHIBITORY NEUROTRANSMISSION IN GP TENIA COLI

Inhibitory neurotransmission in GP tenia coli does not involve NO and reflects exclusively the combined effects of VIP and PACAP (6, 7). There is virtually no release of NO during nerve stimulation, and the muscle cells do not express a constitutive nitric oxide synthase (NOS). Smooth muscle cells of the gut in other species and in other regions of the GP gut express VPAC2 receptors that exhibit equal affinity for VIP and PACAP (2, 5, 8). In smooth muscle cells of GP tenia coli, on the other hand, VIP interacts with a VIP-specific receptor coupled via G_s to adenylyl cyclase, whereas PACAP interacts with a PACAP-specific receptor, that may be a molecular variant of the PAC1 receptor coupled to activation of apamin-sensitive K^+ channels (7–9).

Nerve stimulation of tenia muscle strips induces frequency-dependent relaxation and release of both VIP and PACAP, but not NO (7). Peptide release and relaxation are abolished by tetrodotoxin. Relaxation is partially inhibited by pre-incubating the tissue with (i) VIP or PACAP antibodies, (ii) the VIP antagonist, VIP10-28, or the PACAP antagonist, PACAP6-38, and (iii) VIP or PACAP to induce specific receptor desensitization. The effects of combinations of VIP and PACAP antibodies, or VIP and PACAP antagonists, or of pre-treatment of the tissue with both VIP and PACAP, are additive, causing complete inhibition of relaxation at low frequencies of nerve stimulation and strong inhibition (80%) at maximal frequencies. Apamin causes partial inhibition that mimics the effects of PACAP antibody, PACAP antagonist, or desensitization by PACAP; the effect of apamin is additive to that of VIP antibody, VIP antagonist, or desensitization by VIP. Relaxation induced by

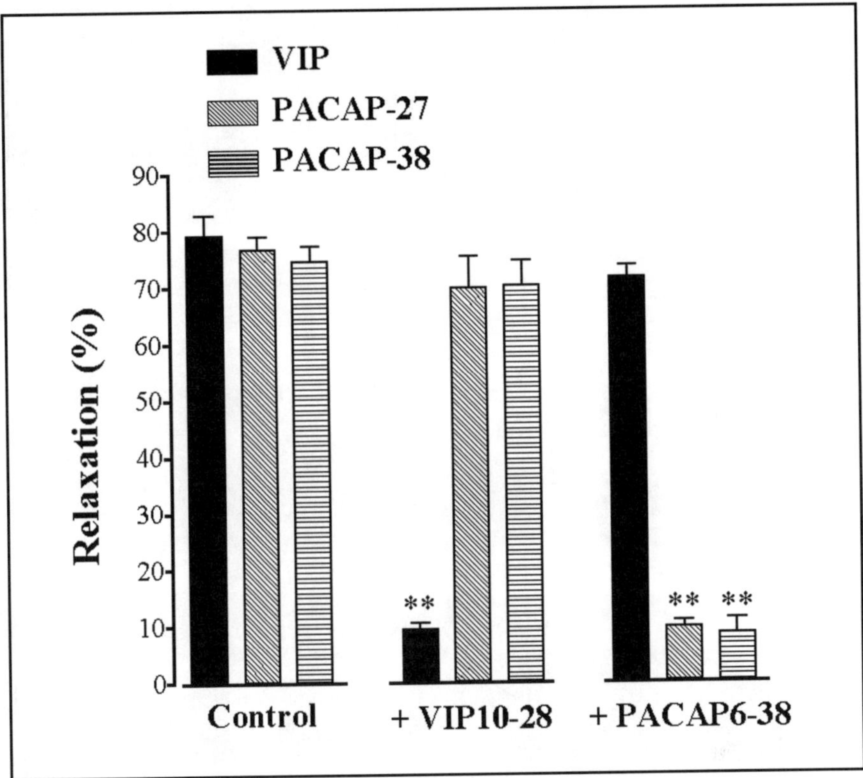

FIGURE 1. *Distinct VIP and PACAP receptors in tenia coli smooth muscle. Relaxation of dispersed tenia coli muscle cells by PACAP-27 or PACAP-38 is inhibited by PACAP6-38, whereas relaxation by VIP is inhibited by VIP10-28. (from ref. 7).*

exogenous PACAP in tenia muscle strips or dispersed muscle cells is selectively inhibited by apamin and PACAP6-38, whereas relaxation induced by VIP is selectively inhibited by VIP10-28 (Figure 1). VIP stimulates cAMP formation in dispersed tenia coli muscle cells, whereas PACAP, despite its name, has no effect. As expected, relaxation induced by VIP but not by PACAP is inhibited by the selective PKA inhibitor, H-89. The pharmacological profile implies that VIP and PACAP interact with distinct receptors, and that only VIP receptors are coupled to activation of adenylyl cyclase.

MOLECULAR CHARACTERIZATION OF VIP RECEPTORS IN GP TENIA COLI

VIP receptors were characterized in freshly dispersed and cultured smooth muscle cells derived from GP stomach or tenia coli by RT-PCR, Northern

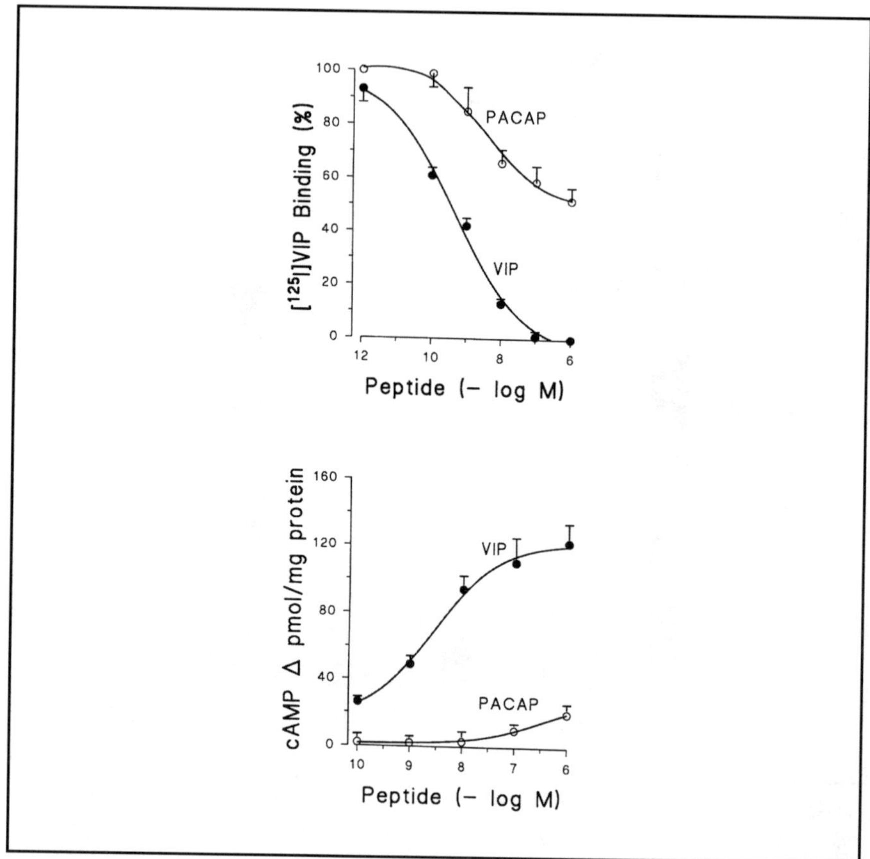

FIGURE 2. *VIP-specific receptor in tenia coli smooth muscle cells. Chimeric receptor consisting of rat VPAC2 receptor with its extracellular domain replaced by the corresponding domain from guinea pig tenia coli receptor was expressed in COS1 cells. The receptor bound VIP but not PACAP and stimulated cAMP in response to VIP but not PACAP. (from ref. 13).*

analysis and cloning of the N–terminal extracellular domain, which is the main determinant of binding (8). All amino acid residues required for VIP binding including all six N–terminal cysteine residues were conserved. The N–terminal sequence was identical in GP stomach and tenia coli except for two adjacent residues (Phe[40] and Phe[41] in GP tenia coli versus Leu[40] and Leu[41] in GP stomach). Leu[40] and Leu[41] are present in all VPAC2 receptors in other species (10–12).

The possibility that the two adjacent residues determined the ability of VIP receptors in GP coli to bind VIP but not PACAP was examined using chimeric receptor constructs in which the N–terminal extracellular domain of rat VPAC2 receptor was replaced by the corresponding domain of GP tenia coli or gastric receptor (13). Wild-type and chimeric receptors were expressed in COS-1 cells and the receptors characterized by VIP and PACAP binding, using [^{125}I]-VIP as radioligand, and by cAMP formation. In both wild-type rat VPAC2 receptor and chimeric rat VPAC2/GP gastric receptor, VIP and PACAP-27 bound with equal affinity (IC$_{50}$ for VIP and PACAP-27 for wild-type VPAC2 receptor: 0.7 ± 0.1 nM and 0.6 ± 0.2 nM; for chimeric GP gastric receptor: 0.3 ± 0.1 nM and 0.4 ± 0.1 nM) and stimulated cAMP with equal potency. In the chimeric rat VPAC2/GP tenia coli receptor, VIP bound with the same high affinity as in wild-type receptor (IC$_{50}$ 0.5 ± 0.1 nM) and stimulated cAMP with the same potency, whereas PACAP-27 exhibited no affinity for the receptor and did not stimulate cAMP (Figure 2). Thus, two adjacent amino acid residues in the N-terminal extracellular domain endow the GP tenia receptor with selectivity for VIP. This is the first and only known example of a VIP-specific receptor. Whether the apamin-sensitive PACAP receptor is a variant of the PACAP-specific receptor, PAC1 (14), or a distinct receptor has not been determined.

SIGNALING VIA NPR-C IN TENIA COLI

The natriuretic peptide clearance receptor, NPR-C, is abundantly expressed in smooth muscle, including tenia coli. Unlike its homologues, NPR-A and NPR-B, which are single-transmembrane receptor-guanylyl cyclases, NPR-C is devoid of kinase or guanylyl cyclase activity. It possesses a truncated 37-amino acid intracellular domain; a 17-amino acid segment in this domain is capable of selectively activating G$_{i1}$ and G$_{i2}$ (4, 15, 16). The receptor exhibits high affinity for natriuretic peptides (e.g., atrial natriuretic peptide, ANP) as well as for VIP and PACAP. Activation of this receptor in smooth muscle of the gut by ANP, VIP or PACAP results in Gα_{i1}- and Gα_{i2}-dependent activation of eNOS, generation of NO, and relaxation (4). In tenia coli smooth muscle, which is eNOS-deficient, activation of NPR-C by ANP or the selective NPR-C ligand, cANP4-23, results in G$\beta\gamma_{i1/2}$-dependent activation of phospholipase C-β3 (PLC-β3), phosphoinositide hydrolysis, and muscle contraction (16). VIP activates both NPR-C initiating this signaling cascade as well as the VIP-specific receptor coupled to cAMP formation, activation of PKA, and muscle relaxation. The predominant effect of VIP in tenia coli is relaxation, which can be reversed to contraction (mediated via NPR-C) upon inhibition of PKA activity.

The G protein-activating domain of NPR-C was identified using synthetic peptide sequences corresponding to the N-terminal, C-terminal, and mid-region of the intracellular domain, and the results confirmed by site-directed mutagenesis of the cloned receptor (15, 17). A 17-amino acid sequence in the middle region of the intracellular domain

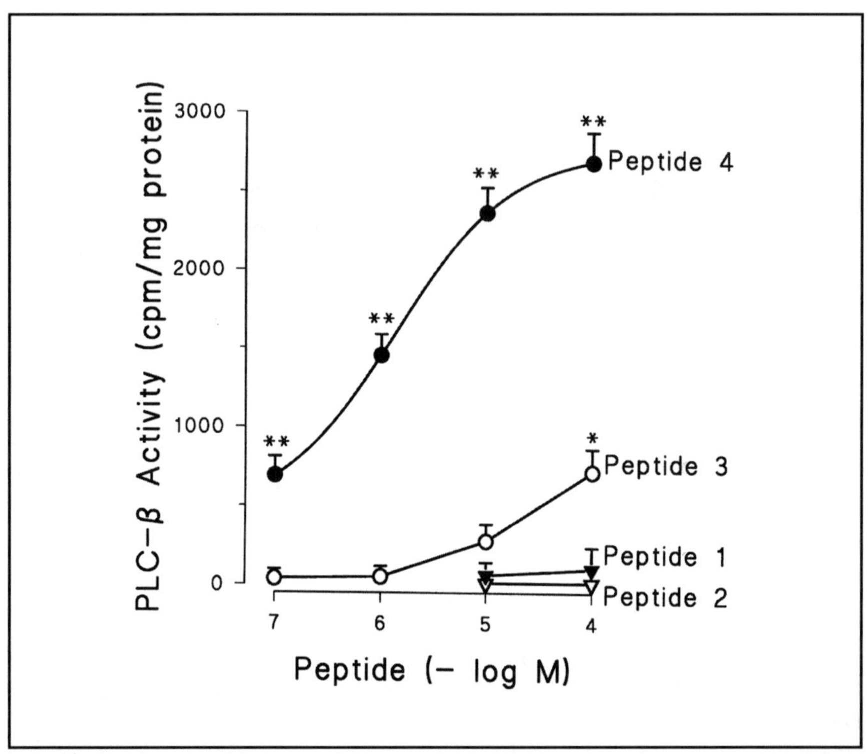

FIGURE 3. *Identification of the G protein-activating sequence in the intracellular domain of NPR-C. (See text for the sequence) Peptide 4 includes the full 17-amino acid sequence, peptide 3 lacks the N-terminal arginine residue, peptide 1 lacks the C-terminal arginine residues, and peptide 1 lacks the entire C-terminal motif. PLC-β activity was fully stimulated by Peptide 4, minimally by Peptide 3, and not at all by Peptides 1 and 2. (from ref. 15).*

(^{508}**RRTQQEESNLGKHREL**^{524}**R**), which possessed two N-terminal basic residues (^{508}**R** ^{509}**R**) and the C-terminal motif **HREL**^{524}**R** (or BBXXB, where B = basic residue in bold and X = non-basic residue) was identified as a specific G_{i1}- and G_{i2}-activating sequence. Treatment of permeabilized tenia coli muscle cells with a synthetic peptide corresponding to this sequence selectively activated both G_{i1} and G_{i2} and stimulated Gβγ-dependent PLC-β3 activity and muscle contraction (Figure 3). Site-directed mutagenesis of NPR-C expressed in COS-1 cells confirmed the essential requirement for a pair of N-terminal arginine residues and the C-terminal motif. Deletion of the entire sequence or substitution of both N-terminal arginine residues blocked the PLC-β response to cANP4-23. Substitution of either arginine residue (^{521}**R** or ^{524}**R**) in the motif virtually abolished the response to cANP4-23; substitution of the histidine residue had a lesser effect shifting the concentration-response curve to the right.

SUMMARY

The unique properties of guinea pig tenia coli smooth muscle have provided new insights into neurotransmission and cell signaling by gut peptides. In mammalian species, including human, smooth muscle cells of the gut express a G protein-coupled constitutive NOS (eNOS) that is activated by VIP and PACAP via the natriuretic peptide clearance receptor, NPR-C, and that mediates muscle relaxation. Smooth muscle cells of tenia coli are devoid of eNOS, and they express a VIP-specific receptor that is not recognized by PACAP and that is coupled via G_s to adenylyl cyclase, and an apamin-sensitive, PACAP-specific receptor that is not recognized by VIP and that is coupled to activation of K^+ channels. VIP and PACAP acting via these receptors mediate inhibitory neurotransmission in tenia coli causing muscle relaxation and membrane hyperpolarization. In the absence of e-NOS, NPR-C in tenia coli is coupled via G_{i1} and G_{i2} to PLC-β3-dependent phosphoinositide hydrolysis and muscle contraction.

ACKNOWLEDGMENTS

Supported by National Institute of Diabetes and Digestive and Kidney Diseases grants DK-28300, DK-15564, and DK-34153.

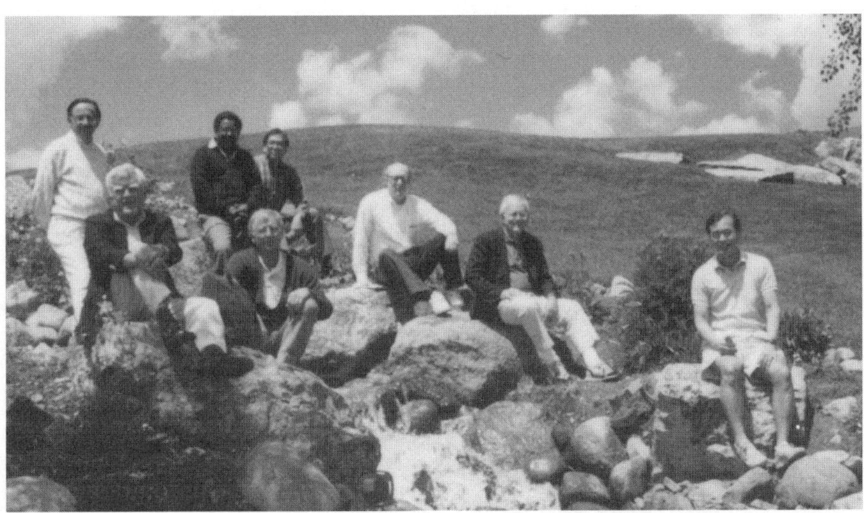

Editorial Board of the Regulatory Peptide Letter *hard at work in Aspen, Colorado, 1991. From top row, left to right: Gabriel Makhlouf, Haile Debas, and Chung Owyang; next row left to right: Jim Thompson, John Walsh, Bob Jensen, and Don Powell, bottom row: Tachi Yamada.*

REFERENCES

1. Jin J-G, Murthy KS, Grider JR, Makhlouf GM. Stoichiometry of neurally induced VIP release, NO formation, and relaxation in rabbit gastric muscle. *Am J Physiol* (Gastrointest Liver Physiol) 1996; 271:G357–369.

2. Murthy KS, Zhang K-M, Jin J-G, Grider JR, Makhlouf GM. VIP-mediated G protein-coupled Ca2+ influx activates a constitutive NOS in dispersed gastric muscle cells. *Am J Physiol* (Gastrointest Liver Physiol) 1993;265:G660–G671.

3. Teng B-Q, Murthy KS, Kuemmerle JK, Grider JR, Makhlouf GM. Expression of endothelial nitric oxide synthase (eNOS) in rabbit and human gastrointestinal smooth muscle cells. *Am J Physiol* (Gastrointest Liver Physiol) 1998;275:G342-G351.

4. Murthy KS, Teng B-Q, Jin J-G, Makhlouf GM. G protein-dependent activation of smooth muscle eNOS via natriuretic peptide clearance receptor. *Am J Physiol* (Cell Physiol.) 1998;275:C1409–C1416.

5. Murthy KS, Jin J-G, Grider JR, Makhlouf GM. Characterization of PACAP receptors and signaling pathways in rabbit gastric muscle cells. *Am J Physiol* (Gastrointest Liver Physiol) 1997;272:G1391-G1399.

6. Gustafsson LE, Wiklund NP, Wiklund CU, Cederqvist B, Persson MG, Moncada S. Modulation of autonomic neuroeffector transmission by nitric oxide-like activity in guinea-pig smooth muscle. In: *Nitric oxide from L-arginine: a bioregulatory system.* Ed, S. Moncada and E.A. Higgs, Ch. 20:177–181, Elsevier Science Publishers, 1990.

7. Jin J-G, Katsoulis S, Schmidt WE, Grider JR. Inhibitory transmission in tenia coli mediated by distinct vasoactive intestinal peptide and apamin-sensitive pituitary adenylate cyclase-activating peptide receptors. *J Pharmacol Exp Ther* 1994;270:433–439.

8. Teng BQ, Murthy KS, Kuemmerle JF, Grider JR, Makhlouf GM. Selective expression of vasoactive intestinal peptide (VIP)$_2$/pituitary adenylate cyclase-activating polypepide (PACAP)$_3$ receptors in rabbit and guinea pig gastric and tenia coli smooth muscle cells. *Regul Pept* 1998;77:127–134.

9. Schworer H, Katsoulis S, Creutzfeldt, Schmidt WE. Pituitary adenylate cyclase activating peptide, a novel VIP-like gut-brain peptide, relaxes the guinea-pig taenia caeci via apamin-sensitive potassium channels. *Nuayn-Schmiedeberg's Arch Pharmacol* 1992;346: 511–514.

10. Couvineau A, Gaudin P, Maoret J-J, Rouyer-Fessard C, Nicole P, Laburthe M. Highly conserved aspartate 68, tryptophan 73 and glycine 109 in the N-terminal extracellular domain of the human VIP receptor are essential for its ability to bind VIP. *Biochem Biophys Res Commun* 1995;206:246–253.

11. Nicole P, Du K, Couvineau A, Laburthe M. Site-directed mutagenesis of human vasoactive intestinal peptide receptor subtypes VIP1 and VIP2: evidence for difference in the structure-function relationship. *J Pharmacol Exp Ther* 1998;284:744–50.

12. Nicole P, Maoret J-J, Couvineau A, Momany FA, Laburthe M. Tryptophan 67 in the human VPAC receptor crucial role for VIP binding. *Biochem Biophys Res Commun* 2000;276:654–659.

13. Teng B-Q, Grider JR, Murthy KS. Identification of a VIP-specific receptor in guinea pig tenia coli. *Am J Physiol* (Gastrointest Liver Physiol) 2001;281: G718–G725.

14. Pisegna JR and Wank SA. Molecular cloning and functional expression of the pituitary adenylate cyclase-activating polypeptide type I receptor. *Proc Natl Acad Sci* 1993;90:6345–6349.

15. Murthy KS and Makhlouf GM. Identification of the G protein-activating domain of the natriuretic peptide clearance receptor (NPR-C). *J Biol Chem* 1999;274:17587–17592.

16. Murthy KS, Teng B-Q, Zhou H, Jin J-G, Grider JR, Makhlouf GM. G_{i-1}/G_{i-2}-dependent signaling by single-transmembrane natriuretic peptide clearance receptor. *Am J Physiol* (Gastrointest Liver Physiol) 2000;278:G974–G980.

17. Zhou H and Murthy KS. Identification of amino acid residues in the C-terminal domain of the natriuretic peptide clearance receptor (NPR-C) that determine G protein coupling by site-directed mutagenesis. *Gastroenterology* 2001;120:A510.

Gut-Brain Peptides in the New Millennium, edited by Y. Taché
CURE Foundation, Los Angeles, CA. © 2002

15

Somatostatin Receptors and the Control of Gastric Acid Secretion

Vicente Martínez
Nervous System Research, Novartis Pharma AG
Basel, Switzerland

INTRODUCTION

From its discovery in the early seventies, somatostatin has been recognized as a peptide that exerts an inhibitory action on a variety of physiological functions, acting as a classical endocrine hormone, as a local (paracrine) regulatory factor or as a neurotransmitter. In the gastrointestinal tract somatostatin displays an extensive variety of inhibitory actions of which the inhibition of gastric acid secretion is regarded as a highly important one (see 1 for review). In canine and human *in vivo* studies, somatostatin has been shown to inhibit gastric acid secretion at doses producing plasma increments of the peptide similar to those observed during postprandial states, therefore suggesting that this is a physiological, rather than a pharmacological, action of somatostatin (1, 2). However, numerous evidence suggests that the influence of somatostatin in acid secretion is a paracrine, rather than endocrine, effect. The physiological effect of somatostatin results from a direct inhibition of parietal cell secretion and indirectly from inhibition of gastrin and histamine release (3). In the stomach, somatostatin is produced in D-cells of the gastric mucosa, which have a close relationship with gastrin-producing cells (G-cells), enterochromaffin-like (ECL) cells, and parietal cells (4, 5). Therefore, the local inhibitory control of gastric acid secretion seems to depend largely on the interplay between gastric D-cells, G-cells, ECL cells and parietal cells (3).

In recent years, the study of the mechanisms through which somatostatin exerts its physiological and pharmacological actions have benefited from the cloning of at least five different types of somatostatin receptors, as well as from the development of somatostatin analogs with receptor-selective agonistic and antagonistic activities. Taking into consideration these advances, this chapter will review our current knowledge of the role of somatostatin in the control of gastric acid secretion with special emphasis on the somatostatin receptors involved. It will summarize how the knowledge of the receptors' structure, the synthesis of receptor-selective agonists and antagonists as well as the genetic manipulation of experimental animals have been used to characterize the gastric somatostatin receptors involved in the control of acid secretion.

Throughout his career John H. Walsh was very much interested in the control of gastric acid secretion and, therefore, in somatostatin. An important part of our knowledge of how somatostatin acts as a physiological inhibitor of gastric acid secretion is derived from his and his collaborators work. For over 20 years, John Walsh provided ideas, tools and the supportive environment that made possible to ascertain the intrincate mechanisms of control of gastric secretion.

GASTRIC SOMATOSTATIN
AND GASTRIC ACID SECRETION

Somatostatin is a potent inhibitor of gastric acid secretion and probably the main inhibitory regulator during the cephalic, gastric and intestinal phases of secretion (3). In the stomach, somatostatin is produced in endocrine D-cells, located both in the fundic and antral mucosa, and released from cytoplasmic processes in the vicinity of its target cells (4, 5). Therefore, although in the gastrointestinal tract somatostatin can also be found in the intestine and pancreas (6), the somatostatin-dependent regulation of gastric acid secretion involves gastric somatostatin acting locally through paracrine, rather than endocrine, mechanisms.

Morphological studies of the gastric mucosa support the hypothesis that somatostatin controls gastric acid secretion in a paracrine fashion (4, 5). Both antral and fundic D-cells have similar morphology, as revealed in immunohistochemical studies, but respond to different stimuli and have different targets of action. Antral D-cells are "open" cells that respond to changes in gastric luminal acidity and are closely associated, by way of cytoplasmic extensions, with their target cells, i.e., G-cells. Stimulation of antral D-cells results in the local release of somatostatin, that in turn inhibits gastrin synthesis and release from G-cells. In contrast, fundic D-cells are of the "closed" type and are stimulated by gastrin and by acetylcholine, as well as by other neuropeptides (7); they are closely associated to parietal cells, also through cytoplasmic extensions, and to ECL cells. Stimulation of antral D-cells results in the release of somatostatin that directly inhibits parietal cell function and histamine release from ECL cells. This organization strongly supports the view that somatostatin exerts its inhibitory effects in a paracrine fashion by reaching its target cells by local diffusion into the intercellular space.

Before (cephalic), during and after the ingestion of a meal, gastric acid secretion is stimulated mainly through the release of gastrin (3). Attenuation of excessive acid secretion can be attributed to the local release of somatostatin that, in turn, regulates the activity of G-cells, ECL cells and parietal cells. Although the interplay between gastrin and somatostatin is a key component of the control of gastric acid secretion, somatostatin secretion depends also on extrinsic (vagal) gastric innervation and the action of other gut regulatory peptides. Physiological effects of somatostatin result from a direct inhibition of parietal cell secretion and indirectly by inhibition of histamine release from ECL cells and gastrin release from G-cells (8, 9, 10). The role of somatostatin in the control of basal (interdigestive) gastric acid secretion is less clear. *In vitro* (luminally perfused stomach preparations) immunoneutralization studies using specific somatostatin antisera suggest that somatostatin tonically inhibits acid secretion (11, 12). In urethane-anesthetized rats, immunoneutralization of somatostatin increases basal gastric acid secretion, probably due to the stimulatory effect of urethane anesthesia on somatostatin synthesis and release (13, 14). However, a similar approach in conscious rats failed to demonstrate changes in basal acid secretion after somatostatin immunoneutralization, while preventing the inhibitory effects of exogenous somatostatin (14).

LOCALIZATION OF SOMATOSTATIN RECEPTORS IN THE STOMACH

To date, five different somatostatin receptor subtypes belonging to the superfamily of G protein coupled receptors, termed sst_{1-5}, have been cloned and pharmacologically characterized in different systems (15, 16). In addition, two splice variants of the sst_2 receptor, $sst_{2(a)}$ and $sst_{2(b)}$ which differ in length and composition of their intracellular carboxy termini, have been isolated and cloned in the mouse and the rat (17). In recent years numerous studies have described the expression and anatomical and cellular distribution of somatostatin receptors in rodent and human tissues as well as in different tumors and cell lines by mRNA analysis, reverse transcriptase–polymerase chain reaction (RT-PCR), ribonuclease protection assay, and *in situ* hybridization (15). Lately, the development of receptor subtype-selective antibodies has allowed the direct localization of somatostatin receptors by immunohistochemistry. These studies revealed an intricate pattern of receptor expression throughout the central nervous system and the periphery, with an overlapping but characteristic pattern that is receptor subtype-selective and tissue- and species-specific.

The first receptor distribution studies in the gastrointestinal tract were based on receptor autoradiography using the $sst_{2/3/5}$-non-selective radioligand, octreotide (SMS 201-995), showing a high density of binding sites in the rat gastric mucosa (18). More recently, tissue distribution studies using ribonuclease protection assays and RT-PCR demonstrated the presence of the five receptor subtypes in the stomach, with a predominance of sst_2 receptor mRNA in ECL cells (19, 20, 21). At a cellular level, *in situ* hybridization studies demonstrated the presence of sst_2 mRNA-containing cells in the gastric mucosa and submucosa as well as in the myenteric plexus and the external muscle layer (22). From these studies, it was proposed that sst_2 receptors could be present on parietal cells, ECL cells and gastrin-producing cells. RT-PCR techniques showed also that the mRNA for both $sst_{2(a)}$ and $sst_{2(b)}$ isoforms is present in the stomach (23). Lastly, immunohistochemical studies using anti-peptide antibodies specific for the $sst_{2(a)}$ and $sst_{2(b)}$ receptors described in detail the cellular distribution of these isoforms in the gastrointestinal tract (24, 25). Both isoforms are extensively expressed in the gastrointestinal tract, including the stomach, but with little overlap, suggesting that they subserve different biological functions. The $sst_{2(a)}$ receptor is abundantly present in the enteric nervous system, in particular in neurons of the myenteric and submucosal plexuses and in fibers innervating the muscle, mucosa and vasculature. Immunoreactive staining was also observed in non–neuronal cells, including interstitial cells of Cajal of the intestine and a small population of ECL cells of the stomach. Interestingly, fibers expressing $sst_{2(a)}$ receptor immunoreactivity were often in close proximity to D cells of the gastric mucosa. This distribution strongly suggest that $sst_{2(a)}$ receptors might mediate somatostatin effects in the gastrointestinal tract via neuronal and paracrine pathways (24). On the other hand, the $sst_{2(b)}$ receptor was mainly localized in parietal cells of the gastric mucosa and also, in high concentration, in ECL cells (24, 25). For both isoforms, receptor immunoreactivity appeared not only on the cell surface but also in the cytoplasm, probably representing internalized or recycling receptors. This observation might suggest that $sst_{2(a)/(b)}$ receptors undergo a tonic agonist stimulation and, as a consequence, internalization. However, it might also indicate the existence of functional intracellular receptors in rat gastric mucosal cells (26). In summary, these morphological observations support the view that somatostatin-dependent control of gastric acid secretion depends mainly on sst_2 receptor activation. The different localization of the $sst_{2(a)}$ and $sst_{2(b)}$ splice variants in the gastric mucosa, ECL-cells and parietal cells, may explain how somatostatin inhibits acid secretion by more than one mechanism.

In vitro studies in isolated canine gastric parietal cells suggest the presence of at least two different subtypes of somatostatin receptors. Functional expression studies indicate that $sst_{2(a)/(b)}$ receptors are associated with inhibitory G proteins (15), however, somatostatin inhibits parietal cell activation via both G-protein-dependent and –independent mechanisms (27), thus suggesting that, in addition to $sst_{2(a)/(b)}$ receptors, at least one other subtype, yet to be determined, should also be present on parietal cells. Furthermore, *in vitro* studies in canine isolated fundic D-cells suggest that somatostatin is able to autoregulate its own secretion by acting in an autocrine fashion via specific receptors on D-cells (28). However, this receptor subtype remains to be characterized, as so far the immunohistochemical studies performed have failed to demonstrate the presence of $sst_{2(a)/(b)}$ receptors in gastric or pancreatic D-cells. Lastly, although somatostatin has been shown to regulate gastrin gene expression and gastrin release from G-cells (1, 7) no somatostatin receptors have been found in gastric G-cells.

FUNCTIONAL EVIDENCE THAT SST₂ RECEPTORS MEDIATE SOMATOSTATIN EFFECTS ON GASTRIC ACID SECRETION

The cloning and characterization of the five somatostatin receptor subtypes has allowed the development of selective agonists and antagonists that could be used as tools to dissect the specific biological actions of each receptor subtype. So far three different types of receptor agonists have been developed: i) non-selective peptide analogs of somatostatin, of which the most frequently used is the octapeptide analog SMS 201-995 (octreotide), that displays high affinity for the receptor subtypes 2 and 5 and moderate affinity for the subtype 3 (15, 16, 29); ii) relatively receptor selective peptide analogs of somatostatin (Table 1) (15, 16, 30, 31, 32, 33); and iii) nonpeptide high-affinity subtype-selective agonists (34, 35). In addition, selective receptor-subtype peptide antagonists have been also described: the somatostatin analog [Ac-4-NO₂-Phe-c(D-Cys-Tyr-D-Trp-Lys-Thr-Cys)-D-Tyr-NH₂], that binds to sst_2 and sst_5 receptors and antagonizes normal receptor effector coupling (36); BIM 23056, that blocks sst_5 signaling and appears to be an antagonist for this subtype although it also acts as a relative sst_3 agonist (37); and PRL-2903 (also known as DC-41-33) that displays relative selectivity in antagonizing sst_2 receptors (38). Most of these compounds have been used both *in vivo* and *in vitro* to characterize the relative involvement of the different somatostatin receptor subtypes in the control of gastric acid secretion in rats, mice, dogs and humans (Table 1).

Earlier acid secretion studies *in vivo* with the non-selective short peptide analog of somatostatin, octreotide, revealed a potent and long-lasting inhibitory activity, similar or higher to that of somatostatin (39, 40). Since octreotide binds with high affinity to sst_2 and with moderate affinity to sst_3 and sst_5 receptors, but does not bind to either sst_1 or sst_4 receptors (15, 16, 29), the potential involvement of sst_2, sst_3 and sst_5 receptor subtypes on somatostatin effects can be inferred. Thereafter several *in vivo* and *in vitro* studies in rats, mice, dogs and humans using different relatively receptor selective peptide analogs of somatostatin (Table 1) identified the sst_2 receptor subtype as the main subtype mediating the inhibitory effects of somatostatin on gastric acid

TABLE 1. *Effect of somatostatin and somatostatin analogs with relative receptor subtype selectivity on gastric acid secretion.*

Peptide	Relative receptor affinity[a]	EC_{50}[b]	Species	Acid secretory state	References
Somatostatin	$sst_1 \sim sst_2 \sim sst_3 \sim sst_4 \sim sst_5$	1.65 nM	Rat (conscious)	Pentagastrin stimulation (iv)	32, 33
		27 nM	Rat (isolated gastric mucosa)	Pentagastrin stimulation	46
		0.05 nmol/kg/h	Dog	8% peptone intraduodenal	44
		12 nmol/kg/h[c]	Mouse (urethane-anesthetized)	Pentagastrin stimulation (iv)	49
Octreotide	$sst_2 > sst_3 \sim sst_5$	15 nM	Rat (isolated gastric mucosa)	Pentagastrin stimulation	46
(SMS 201-995)		10 nmol/kg/h[d]	Rat (pentothal-anesthetized)	Pentagastrin stimulation	41, 42
MK 678	$sst_2 > sst_5 > sst_3$	6 nM	Rat (isolated gastric mucosa)	Pentagastrin stimulation	46
(Seglitide)		0.05 nmol/kg/h[e]	Dog	8% peptone intraduodenal	44
DC-32-87	$sst_2 > sst_3$	1.26 nM	Rat (conscious)	Pentagastrin stimulation (iv)	32, 33
(NC 8-12)		3 nmol/kg/h	Rat (pentothal-anesthetized)	Pentagastrin stimulation (iv)	41, 42
		1 nmol/kg/h	Rat (pentothal-anesthetized)	Bethanecol stimulation (iv)	42
		100 nmol/kg/h	Rat (pentothal-anesthetized)	Histamine stimulation (iv)	42
		~0.05 nmol/kg/h	Dog	8% peptone intragastric	43
		16 nmol/kg/h[b]	Mouse (urethane-anesthetized)	Pentagastrin stimulation (iv)	49
BIM 23058	$sst_3 >> sst_5$	52 nM	Rat (conscious)	Pentagastrin stimulation (iv)	32, 33

Table continues next page

TABLE 1. *Continued*

Peptide	Relative receptor affinity[a]	EC_{50}[b]	Species	Acid secretory state	References
(DC 25-12)		1000 nmol/kg/h	Rat (pentothal-anesthetized)	Pentagastrin stimulation (iv)	41, 42
		100 nmol/kg/h	Rat (pentothal anesthetized)	Bethanecol stimulation (iv)	42
		~3 nmol/kg/h	Dog	8% peptone intragastric	43
DC 25-20	sst_3	63 nM	Rat (conscious)	Pentagastrin stimulation (iv)	32, 33
DC 25-100	$sst_2 > sst_5$	1.44 nM	Rat (conscious)	Pentagastrin stimulation (iv)	32, 33
BIM-23052	$sst_5 > sst_2$	500 nmol/kg/h	Rat (pentothal-anesthetized)	Pentagastrin stimulation (iv)	41, 42
(DC 32-92,		100 nmol/kg/h	Rat (pentothal-anesthetized)	Bethanecol stimulation (iv)	42
DC 23-99)		Not active	Rat (conscious)	Pentagastrin stimulation (iv)	32, 33
		~2.5 nmol/kg/h	Dog	8% peptone intragastric	43
BIM-23027	sst_2	11 nM	Rat (isolated gastric mucosa)	Pentagastrin stimulation	46
BIM-23056	$sst_3 > sst_5$	Not active	Rat (isolated gastric mucosa)	Pentagastrin stimulation	46
L362,855	sst_5	428 nM	Rat (isolated gastric mucosa)	Pentagastrin stimulation	46
L362,823	sst_3	1 nmol/kg/h	Dog	8% peptone intraduodenal	44

[a] Based on binding affinity for cloned human receptors (15, 16, 29, 30, 31, 32).

[b] Dose required to inhibit 50% stimulated gastric acid secretion.

[c] Complete inhibition of stimulated gastric acid secretion.

[d] About 80% inhibition of stimulated gastric acid secretion.

[e] About 96% inhibition of stimulated gastric acid secretion.

secretion. Studies showed that the somatostatin analogs DC 32–87 (sst_2 > sst_3) and DC 25-100 (sst_2 > sst_5) inhibited pentagastrin-stimulated acid secretion in conscious rats with similar potency than somatostatin (32, 33). In the same experiments, the compounds DC 25-20 (sst_3) and DC 25-12 (sst_3 >> sst_5) were at least 50 times less potent, while the compound DC 23-99 (sst_5 > sst_2) was devoid of any effect, thus eliminating sst_3 and sst_5 from this process (32, 33). These results were later confirmed in anesthetized rats and in dogs using the same or relatively similar receptor subtype selective somatostatin analogs (41, 42, 43, 44). In addition, these studies showed that DC 32–87 (sst_2 > sst_3) reduced also bethanecol- and histamine-stimulated acid output, although less effectively than pentagastrin stimulated acid secretion responses (Table 1) (42, 44), thus suggesting that activation of sst_2 receptors might be more effective against acid stimulatory pathways that converge on parietal cells than against those acting directly on parietal cells.

A similar approach was also used in *in vivo* studies in rats and dogs and in *in vitro* studies using rat, dog and human antrum to further characterize the mechanisms through which somatostatin inhibits acid secretion. The use of the relatively selective somatostatin analogs DC 32–87 or BIM-23060 (sst_2), BIM-23058 (sst_3), and BIM-23052 (sst_5) indicated that in these species somatostatin inhibits gastrin and histamine secretion by activating sst_2 receptors located respectively in G-cells and ECL cells (42, 43, 45). These findings were corroborated, *in vitro,* using enriched primary cultures of canine antral G cells and rat fundic ECL cells. In canine antral G cells culture, the relatively selective sst_2 agonist DC 32–87 inhibited by 50% bombesin-stimulated gastrin release, whereas BIM-23058 (sst_3) and BIM-23052 (sst_5) were at least 100-fold less effective (43). In rat fundic ECL cultures DC 32–87 (sst_2) inhibited both the calcium signal induced by gastrin and histamine release at concentrations 1000-fold lower than somatostatin or sst_3 and sst_5 agonists (20). In addition, PCR techniques revealed the expression of sst_2 receptors in rat ECL cells at a significantly higher level than the other receptor subtypes (20). These functional and morphological observations suggest that gastric somatostatin regulates acid secretion by inhibiting gastrin and histamine release through the activation of sst_2 receptor located in G-cells and ECL cells.

Using a rat isolated gastric mucosa preparation Wyatt, et al. showed that the secretory response elicited by direct stimulation of parietal cells with dimaprit or isobutil methylxanthine was inhibited by somatostatin and, with higher potency, by the non-selective somatostatin analogs octreotide and seglitide and the relatively selective sst_2 receptor agonist BIM-23027 (46). In the same experiments, relatively selective sst_3 and sst_5 receptor agonists had little or no effect at all (46). These observations provide strong functional support for the presence of sst_2 receptors on parietal cells where they might mediate a direct inhibitory effect of somatostatin on gastric acid secretion.

Further functional evidence for the involvement of sst$_2$ receptors on somatostatin-dependent control of gastric acid secretion comes from the use of the selective sst$_2$ antagonist PRL-2903 (also known as DC-41-33) (38). Infused intravenously, PRL-2903 dose-dependently inhibited somatostatin-induced inhibition of pentagastrin-stimulated gastric acid secretion in conscious rats, (38). In urethane-anesthetized rats, with low basal gastric acid secretion due to the urethane-induced gastric somatostatin synthesis and release (13), a bolus injection of PRL-2903 produced a transient dose-related increase of basal secretion and of plasma gastrin levels (47). Therefore, acid response to PRL-2903 is most likely mediated by the rise in circulating levels of gastrin, suggesting that somatostatin might be directly inhibiting gastrin release from G-cells.

The most conclusive evidence for the involvement of sst$_2$ receptors in the regulation of gastric acid secretion was provided by the use of mice with a targeted disruption of the somatostatin sst$_2$ receptor gene. Sst$_2$-deficient animals are healthy and reproduce normally, therefore excluding an essential role of sst$_2$ receptors in embryogenesis and development. The only neuroendocrine abnormality detected in these animals is an alteration in the feedback mechanisms that control growth hormone (GH) release (48). Despite this, the animals grow normally, suggesting normal GH secretion. Fasted non-anesthetized sst$_2$ knockout animals seem to have a normal rate of gastric acid secretion compared with wild-type controls (49). However under urethane anesthesia sst$_2$ knockout mice show lower intragastric pH and a basal rate of secretion approximately 10 times higher than wild-type controls, with similar serum gastrin levels (49). *In vivo* gastrin immunoneutralization reduces the elevated acid secretion in sst$_2$ knockout animals to similar levels to those observed in wild-type controls. In parallel, *in vivo* somatostatin immunoneutralization in wild type controls increases basal acid secretion to similar values to those observed in sst$_2$ knockout animals. Lastly, confirming the lack of functional sst$_2$ receptors, neither somatostatin nor the relatively selective sst$_2$ agonist DC 32–87 inhibited the high basal gastric acid output observed in sst$_2$ knockout mice (49). These findings clearly established the crucial role of sst$_2$ receptors and demonstrated that the sst$_2$ receptor alone can account for mediating endogenous somatostatin-induced inhibition of gastric acid secretion through gastrin-dependent mechanisms targeted at gastrin action on ECL cells. Sequence analysis of rat cDNA for sst$_2$ receptors suggests that the smaller transcript (corresponding to the sst$_{2(b)}$ variant) is a spliced product of the larger form (corresponding to the sst$_{2(a)}$ variant) (50). The sst$_2$ knockout mice had a gene deletion of the fragment containing the sst$_{2(a)}$ cDNA, and therefore neither isoform of the receptor was expressed (48). Since both sst$_{2(a)}$ and sst$_{2(b)}$ receptors are lacking in these animals, no information regarding the sst$_2$ isoform mediating somatostatin actions on acid secretion can be derived. Further work with this model would be of interest to determine the involvement of somatostatin in the inhibitory responses of acid secretion elicited by other neuroendocrine mediators.

REFERENCES

1. Chiba T, Yamada T. Gut somatostatin. In Walsh JH, Dockray GJ, Eds. *Gut Peptides.* New York: Raven Press, 1994; pp. 123–145.
2. Seal A, Yamada T, Debas H, Hollinshead J, Osadchey B, Aponte G, Walsh J. Somatostatin-14 and -28: clearance and potency on gastric function in dogs. *Am J Physiol* 1982;243:G97–G102.
3. Lloyd KCK, Walsh J. Gastric secretion. In Walsh JH, Dockray GJ, Eds. *Gut Peptides.* New York: Raven Press, 1994; pp. 633–654.
4. Larsson LI, Goltermann N, de Magistris L, Rehfeld JF, Schwartz TW. Somatostatin cell processes as pathways for paracrine secretion. *Science* 1979;205:1393–1395.
5. Kusumoto Y, Iwanaga T, Ito S, Fujita T. Juxtaposition of somatostatin cell and parietal cell in the dog stomach. *Arch Histol Jpn* 1979;42:459–465.
6. Arimura A, Sato H, Dupont A, Nishi N, Schally AV. Somatostatin: abundance of immunoreactive hormone in rat stomach and pancreas. *Science* 1975;189:1007–1009.
7. Zeng N, Walsh JH, Kang T, Helander KG, Helander HF, Sachs G. Selective ligand-induced intracellular calcium changes in a population of rat isolated gastric endocrine cells. *Gastroenterology* 1996; 110:1835–1846.
8. Vuyyuru L, Schubert ML, Harrington L, Arimura A, Makhlouf GM. Dual inhibitory pathways link antral somatostatin and histamine secretion in human, dog, and rat stomach. *Gastroenterology* 1995; 109:1566–1574.
9. Schubert ML, Makhlouf GM. Neural, hormonal, and paracrine regulation of gastrin and acid secretion. *Yale J Biol Med* 1992;65:553–560.
10. Makhlouf GM, Schubert ML. Gastric somatostatin: a paracrine regulator of acid secretion. *Metabolism* 1990;39 (Suppl 2):138–142.
11. Schubert ML, Edwards NF, Arimura A, Makhlouf GM. Paracrine regulation of gastric acid secretion by fundic somatostatin. *Am J Physiol* 1987;252:G485–G490.
12. Short GM, Doyle JW, Wolfe MM. Effect of antibodies to somatostatin on acid secretion and gastrin release by the isolated perfused rat stomach. *Gastroenterology* 1985;88:984–9888.
13. Yang H, Wong H, Wu V, Walsh JH, Taché Y. Somatostatin monoclonal antibody immunoneutralization increases gastrin and gastric acid secretion in urethane-anesthetized rats. *Gastroenterology* 1990; 99:659–665.
14. Martínez V, Yang H, Wong HC, Walsh JH, Taché Y. Somatostatin antibody does not influence bombesin-induced inhibition of gastric acid secretion in rats. *Peptides* 1995;16:1–6.
15. Patel YC. Somatostatin and its receptor family. *Front Neuroendocrinol* 1999;20:157–198.
16. Reisine T, Bell GI. Molecular biology of somatostatin receptors. *Endocr Rev* 1995;16:427–442.
17. Cole SL, Schindler M. Characterization of somatostatin sst$_2$ receptor splice variants. *J Physiol Paris* 2000;94:217–237.
18. Reubi JC. Somatostatin receptors in the gastrointestinal tract in health and disease. *Yale J Biol Med* 1992;65:493–503.
19. Bruno JF, Xu Y, Song J, Berelowitz M. Tissue distribution of somatostatin receptor subtype messenger ribonucleic acid in the rat. *Endocrinology* 1993;133:2561–2567.
20. Prinz C, Sachs G, Walsh JH, Coy DH, Wu SV. The somatostatin receptor subtype on rat enterochromaffinlike cells. *Gastroenterology* 1994;107:1067–1074.
21. Raulf F, Perez J, Hoyer D, Bruns C. Differential expression of five somatostatin receptor subtypes, SSTR1–5, in the CNS and peripheral tissue. *Digestion* 1994;55 (Suppl 3):46–53.
22. Krempels K, Hunyady B, O'Carroll AM, Mezey E. Distribution of somatostatin receptor messenger RNAs in the rat gastrointestinal tract. *Gastroenterology* 1997;112:1948–1960.
23. Schindler M, Kidd EJ, Carruthers AM, Wyatt MA, Jarvie EM, Sellers LA, Feniuk W, Humphrey PP. Molecular cloning and functional characterization of a rat somatostatin sst$_{2(b)}$ receptor splice variant. *Br J Pharmacol* 1998;125:209–217.

24. Sternini C, Wong H, Wu SV, de Giorgio R, Yang M, Reeve J Jr, Brecha NC, Walsh JH. Somatostatin 2A receptor is expressed by enteric neurons, and by interstitial cells of Cajal and enterochromaffin-like cells of the gastrointestinal tract. *J Comp Neurol* 1997;386:396–408.

25. Schindler M, Humphrey PP. Differential distribution of somatostatin sst2 receptor splice variants in rat gastric mucosa. *Cell Tissue Res* 1999;297:163–168.

26. Reyl FJ, Lewin MJ. Intracellular receptor for somatostatin in gastric mucosal cells: decomposition and reconstitution of somatostatin-stimulated phosphoprotein phosphatases. *Proc Natl Acad Sci USA* 1982;79:978–982.

27. Park J, Chiba T, Yamada T. Mechanisms for direct inhibition of canine gastric parietal cells by somatostatin. *J Biol Chem* 1987;262:14190–14196.

28. Park J, Chiba T, Yokotani K, DelValle J, Yamada T. Somatostatin receptors on canine fundic D-cells: evidence for autocrine regulation of gastric somatostatin. *Am J Physiol* 1989;257:G235–G241.

29. Bruns C, Raulf F, Hoyer D, Schloos J, Lubbert H, Weckbecker G. Binding properties of somatostatin receptor subtypes. *Metabolism* 1996;45(Suppl 1):17–20.

30. Raynor K, Murphy WA, Coy DH, Taylor JE, Moreau JP, Yasuda K, Bell GI, Reisine T. Cloned somatostatin receptors: identification of subtype-selective peptides and demonstration of high affinity binding of linear peptides. *Mol Pharmacol* 1993;43:838–844.

31. Patel YC, Srikant CB. Subtype selectivity of peptide analogs for all five cloned human somatostatin receptors (hsstr 1-5). *Endocrinology* 1994;135:2814–2817.

32. Coy DH, Rossowski WJ. Somatostatin analogues and multiple receptors: possible physiological roles. *Ciba Found Symp* 1995;190:240–252

33. Rossowski WJ, Gu ZF, Akarca US, Jensen RT, Coy DH. Characterization of somatostatin receptor subtypes controlling rat gastric acid and pancreatic amylase release. *Peptides* 1994;15:1421–1424.

34. Rohrer SP, Birzin ET, Mosley RT, Berk SC, Hutchins SM, Shen DM, Xiong Y, Hayes EC, Parmar RM, Foor F, Mitra SW, Degrado SJ, Shu M, Klopp JM, Cai SJ, Blake A, Chan WW, Pasternak A, Yang L, Patchett AA, Smith RG, Chapman KT, Schaeffer JM. Rapid identification of subtype-selective agonists of the somatostatin receptor through combinatorial chemistry. *Science* 1998;282:737–740.

35. Yang L, Berk SC, Rohrer SP, Mosley RT, Guo L, Underwood DJ, Arison BH, Birzin ET, Hayes EC, Mitra SW, Parmar RM, Cheng K, Wu TJ, Butler BS, Foor F, Pasternak A, Pan Y, Silva M, Freidinger RM, Smith RG, Chapman K, Schaeffer JM, Patchett AA. Synthesis and biological activities of potent peptidomimetics selective for somatostatin receptor subtype 2. *Proc Natl Acad Sci USA* 1998; 95:10836–41.

36. Bass RT, Buckwalter BL, Patel BP, Pausch MH, Price LA, Strnad J, Hadcock JR. Identification and characterization of novel somatostatin antagonists. *Mol Pharmacol* 1996 ;50:709–715.

37. Wilkinson GF, Thurlow RJ, Sellers LA, Coote JE, Feniuk W, Humphrey PP. Potent antagonism by BIM-23056 at the human recombinant somatostatin sst$_5$ receptor. *Br J Pharmacol* 1996;118:445–447.

38. Rossowski WJ, Cheng BL, Jiang NY, Coy DH. Examination of somatostatin involvement in the inhibitory action of GIP, GLP-1, amylin and adrenomedullin on gastric acid release using a new SRIF antagonist analogue. *Br J Pharmacol* 1998;125:1081–1087.

39. Karnes WE, Maxwell V, Sytnik B, Chew P, Walsh JH. Prolonged inhibition of meal-stimulated acid secretion and gastrin release following single subcutaneous administration of octreotide (SMS 201–995) in man. *Aliment Pharmacol Ther* 1989;3:527–538.

40. Gyr KE, Meier R. Pharmacodynamic effects of Sandostatin in the gastrointestinal tract. *Digestion* 1993;54(Suppl 1):14–19.

41. Lloyd KC, Wang J, Aurang K, Gronhed P, Coy DH, Walsh JH. Activation of somatostatin receptor subtype 2 inhibits acid secretion in rats. *Am J Physiol* 1995;268:G102-G106.

42. Aurang K, Wang J, Lloyd KC. Somatostatin inhibition of acid and histamine release by activation of somatostatin receptor subtype 2 receptors in rats. *J Pharmacol Exp Ther* 1997;281:245–252.

43. Lloyd KC, Amirmoazzami S, Friedik F, Chew P, Walsh JH. Somatostatin inhibits gastrin release and acid secretion by activating sst$_2$ in dogs. *Am J Physiol* 1997;272:G1481-G1488.

44. Fung LC, Greenberg GR. Characterization of somatostatin receptor subtypes mediating inhibition of nutrient-stimulated gastric acid and gastrin in dogs. *Regul Pept* 1997;68:197–203.

45. Zaki M, Harrington L, McCuen R, Coy DH, Arimura A, Schubert ML. Somatostatin receptor subtype 2 mediates inhibition of gastrin and histamine secretion from human, dog, and rat antrum. *Gastroenterology* 1996;111:919–924.

46. Wyatt MA, Jarvie E, Feniuk W, Humphrey PP. Somatostatin sst2 receptor-mediated inhibition of parietal cell function in rat isolated gastric mucosa. Br J Pharmacol 1996;119:905–910.
47. Kawakubo K, Coy DH, Walsh JH, Taché Y. Urethane-induced somatostatin mediated inhibition of gastric acid: reversal by the somatostatin 2 receptor antagonist, PRL-2903. *Life Sci* 1999;65: PL115–PL120.
48. Zheng H, Bailey A, Jiang MH, Honda K, Chen HY, Trumbauer ME, Van der Ploeg LH, Schaeffer JM, Leng G, Smith RG. Somatostatin receptor subtype 2 knockout mice are refractory to growth hormone-negative feedback on arcuate neurons. *Mol Endocrinol* 1997;11:1709–1717.
49. Martínez V, Curi AP, Torkian B, Schaeffer JM, Wilkinson HA, Walsh JH, Taché Y. High basal gastric acid secretion in somatostatin receptor subtype 2 knockout mice. *Gastroenterology* 1998;114:1125–1132.
50. Patel YC, Greenwood M, Kent G, Panetta R, Srikant CB. Multiple gene transcripts of the somatostatin receptor SSTR2: tissue selective distribution and cAMP regulation. *Biochem Biophys Res Commun* 1993;192:288–294.

Gut-Brain Peptides in the New Millennium, edited by Y. Taché
CURE Foundation, Los Angeles, CA. © 2002

16

Signaling Mechanisms of the Somatostatin Receptor Subtype SSTR1

Chin-Yu Lin and Diane L. Barber
Department of Stomatology, University of California, San Francisco, CA

Alison M. J. Buchan
Department of Physiology, University of British Columbia, Vancouver, Canada

INTRODUCTION

The neuroendocrine peptide somatostatin (SST) has potent inhibitory effects on diverse cell functions such as hormone secretion, neurotransmitter release, smooth muscle contractility and cell proliferation. These effects are mediated by a family of five identified somatostatin receptor subtypes (SSTR1-SSTR5) that belong to the superfamily of seven-transmembrane, G protein-coupled (1–5). The cellular effects of somatostatin are mediated by coupling of these five receptors to different signaling networks and effectors. All SSTR couple to the inhibition of adenylyl cyclase (6) and the activation of tyrosine phosphatases (7–13), while SSTR2-5, but not SSTR1, activate the inwardly rectifying K^+ channel GIRK1 (14). Different SSTR subtypes also selectively regulate distinct signaling mechanisms and effectors. SSTR1 and 2 mediate SST inhibition of voltage-activated Ca^{2+} channels (15–17), SSTR2 and SSTR5 stimulate phospholipase C activity (8, 18), and SSTR4 stimulates phospholipase A2 (19). Moreover, MAP kinase activity is decreased by SSTR2, 3 and 5 (20–22), but increased by SSTR1 and 4 (11, 19). Determining signaling mechanisms regulated by distinct SSTR subtypes is central to understanding their selective cellular actions.

This chapter describes actions of the SSTR1 subtype that are not shared by SSTR2. When stably expressed in CCL39 fibroblasts, SSTR1, but not SSTR2, mediates somatostatin inhibition of the ubiquitously expressed Na-H exchanger NHE1 and decrease in intracellular pH. SST inhibition of NHE1 is also observed in cells expressing SSTR3 and 4, but not SSTR5. A Fasta search and alignment of SSTR reveals distinct amino acid motifs in the second and third intracellular loops of SSTR1, 3 and 4 that are not present in SSTR2 and 5. Site-directed mutatgenesis was used to confirm that these motifs confer signaling to NHE1. NHE1 acts downstream of the low molecular weight GTPase RhoA and this chapter also describes previously unrecognized effects of SSTR1 on inhibiting RhoA activity and the ordered assembly of actin filaments and focal adhesions. Hence, SSTR1 has distinct actions on NHE1, intracellular pH, and the actin cytoskeleton that are not shared by SSTR2. These actions may be key determinants in SSTR1 effects on cell proliferation, secretion, and smooth muscle contractility.

SELECTIVE INHIBITION OF NHE1 BY DISTINCT SSTR SUBTYPES

NHE1 is a ubiquitously expressed plasma membrane ion exchanger that catalyzes an electroneutral exchange of extracellular Na^+ and intracellular H^+. NHE1 activity plays a central role in intracellular pH (pH_i) and cell volume homeostasis. Increased NHE1 activity results in a net efflux of intracellular H^+ and an increase in pH_i. Increased pH_i has a permissive effect in promoting cell secretion, cell proliferation, and tumor progression (reviewed in ref. 23). Previous studies have shown that SST inhibits NHE1 activity and lowers pH_i by acting on endogenously expressed SSTR in primary cultures of enteric endocrine cells (24) and hepatocytes (25). Hou, et al., (26) found that SST inhibits NHE1 activity in mouse muscle Ltk$^-$ fibroblasts expressing human SSTR1, but not SSTR2. In agreement with this later finding, we determined that SST inhibits NHE1 activity and lowers pH_i in CCL39 fibroblasts stably expressing SSTR1 (CCL-R1), but not SSTR2 (CCL-R2).[1] Receptor expression was determined by membrane binding to [^{125}I-*tyr*^{11}]SST-14, and receptor function was confirmed by the ability of both receptor subtypes to mediate a PTX-sensitive inhibition of cAMP accumulation by SST (Figure 1a). In quiescent CCL-R1 and CCL-R2 cells, acute addition of 10% serum results in a pH_i-dependent increase in NHE1 activity, as determined by the rate of pH_i recovery from an NH_4Cl-induced acidification (dpH_i/dt) in cells loaded with the fluorescent pH-sensitive dye BCECF (methods described in ref. 27) (Figure 1b). In the presence of SST (100 nM), increased NHE1 activity by serum is inhibited in CCL-R1 cells, but not in CCL-R2 cells (Figure 1b). Consistent with SSTR1-mediated inhibition of NHE1, increases in steady-state pH_i induced by serum are attenuated by SST in CCL-R1, but not CCL-R2 cells (Figure 1c). These findings indicate a selective coupling of SSTR1 to the inhibtion of NHE1 that is not shared by SSTR2.

We extended our investigation of selective coupling of SSTR subtypes to NHE1 to include studies with heterologously expressed SSTR3, 4 and 5.[1] As described above, SSTR expression was determined by membrane binding to [^{125}I-*tyr*^{11}]SST-14, and SSTR function was confirmed by the ability

---

[1] Lin, et al., manuscript submitted.

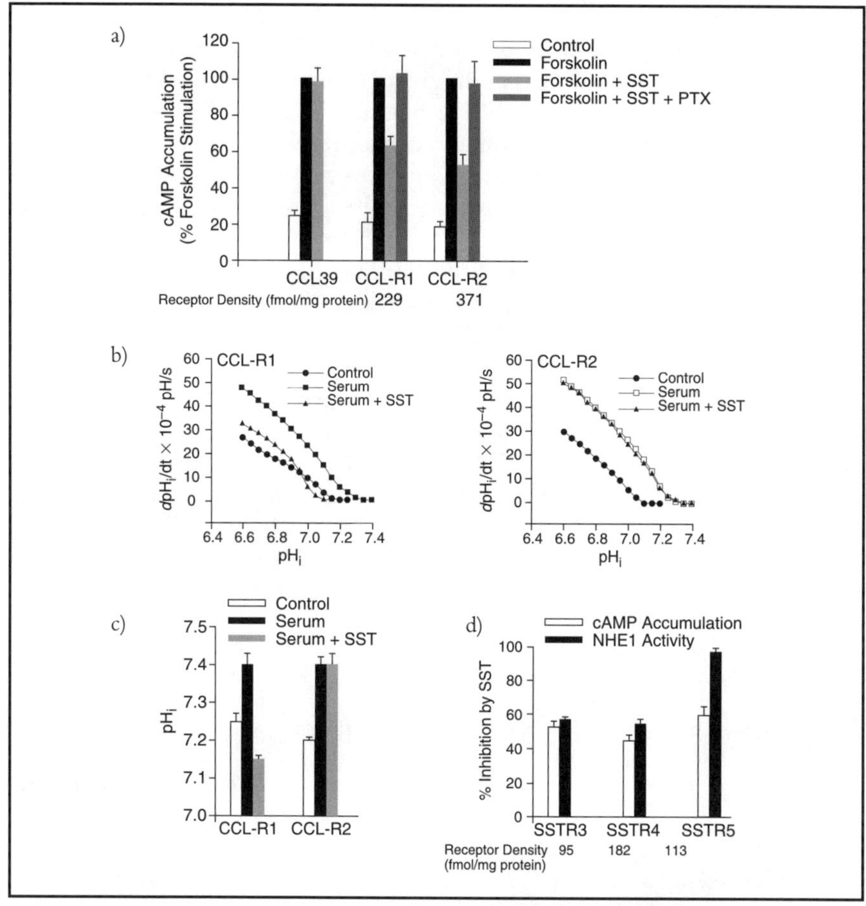

FIGURE 1. *SST inhibits cAMP accumulation and NHE1. (a) cAMP accumulation was determined in wild-type CCL39 cells and in CCL39 cells stably expressing SSTR1 (CCL-R1) and SSTR2 (CCL-R2). Data are expressed as a percentage of forskolin (10 μM) stimulation. Also included are data of cAMP accumulation by forskolin (10 μM) plus SST (100 nM) with and without pretreament with PTX (100 ng/ml for 18 h). Forskolin-induced increases in cAMP accumulation were not significantly different in the absence and presence of PTX (data not shown). Expression of SSTR1 and SSTR2 was determined by radioligand binding of cell membranes with [^{125}I-tyr^{11}]SST-14 and expressed as fmol/mg protein. Data represent the means ± s.e.m. of three separate cell preparations for cAMP accumulation, and the means of four separate membrane preparations for radioligand binding. (b) NHE1 activity was determined as the rate of pH$_i$ recovery (dpH$_i$/dt) from an acid load and expressed as pH$_i$-dependent recoveries in quiescent CCL39 cells expressing SSTR1 (CCL-R1) or SSTR2 (CCL-R2), and in cells treated with serum (10%) in the absence or presence of SST (100 nM). (c) Steady-state pH$_i$ in the absence and presence of SST. Results are expressed as the mean ± s.e.m. four cell passages. (d) The percent inhibition by SST of forskolin-induced cAMP accumulation and serum-induced NHE1 activity at pH$_i$ 6.6 in cells expressing SSTR3-5 is shown as the means (s.e.m. of 4–6 separate cell preparations. Receptor expression was determined by radioligand binding of cell membranes with [^{125}I-tyr^{11}]SST-14 and expressed as fmol/mg protein.*

to mediate SST inhibition of cAMP accumulation (Figure 1d). These data are consistent with previous findings that all five SSTR couple to the inhibition of adenylyl cyclase (6). SST inhibits NHE1 activity, however, only in cells expressing SSTR3 and SSTR4, but not SSTR5 (Figure 1d). These findings, together with those of our previous study (26), indicate that SSTR subtypes 1, 3, and 4, but not 2 and 5, couple to the inhibition of NHE1. On the basis of sequence homology and affinity to conformationally restricted analogs, SSTR are classified into two subgroups (28). SSTR1 and SSTR4, comprising one subgroup, share 70% homology between their transmembrane domains and a 57% overall sequence homology. The second subgroup contains SSTR2, SSTR3, and SSTR5. Within this subgroup, SSTR3 and SSTR5 share the next highest homology, 69% between the transmembrane domains and 52% overall; SSTR2 shares 61% homology with SSTR5 and 62% with SSTR3 between their transmembrane domains. Although all five receptors share similar affinities for the naturally occurring peptide somatostatin-14, the SSTR2, 3, and 5 subgroup is characterized as having higher affinities for the synthetic analogs RC-160, SMS201-995 and BIM 23014. On the basis of signaling mechanisms, however, this subclass distinction may not be applicable. Our findings on the regulation of NHE place SSTR3 in a functional subgroup with SSTR1 and SSTR4.

SSTR MOTIFS CONFER INHIBITION OF NHE1

To determine whether specific SSTR determinants confer coupling to NHE1, we previously studied the action of SSTR2/SSTR1 chimeras (26). Mutant SSTR2 receptors that contain collective, but not individual, replacement of intracellular domains i2 and i3 with those of SSTR1 are capable of mediating SST inhibition of NHE1. These findings indicate that an interaction between the second and third cytoplasmic domains of SSTR1 might be critical for this effect. We, therefore, examined the sequence of all five receptor subtypes by performing a Fasta search of the Swiss-Prot database and aligning i2 and i3 of 16 SSTR retrieved with pile up. Comparing the amino acid sequences of SSTR1, 3, and 4 with those of SSTR2 and 5 revealed a number of potentially important changes, both in i2 and in i3 (Figure 2a). All species of SSTR2 and SSTR5 have an arginine in i2 (R16) that is absent in SSTR1, 3, and 4. This signifies an important difference in charge and may play a role in an i2–i3 interaction of the receptor that may be important for NHE coupling. SSTR1, 3 and 4 have a polar residue, glutamine (Q8), which is not present in SSTR2 or 5. Focusing on these selective residues, we used site-directed mutagenesis of SSTR2 to replace the RT motif in i2 with that of TV found in the cognate position of SSTR1, and the SSK motif in i3 with WQQ found in SSTR1 (Figure 2a, 2b).

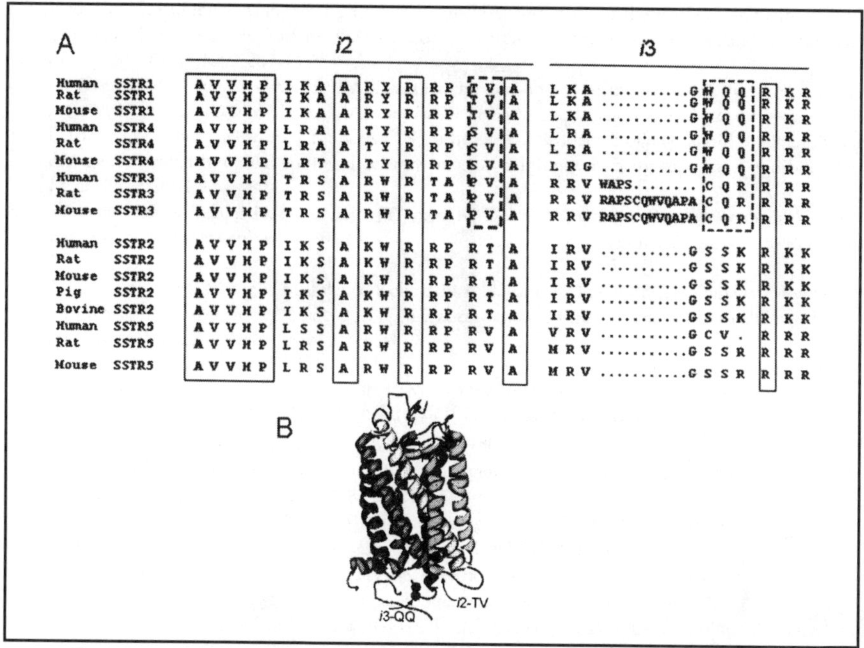

FIGURE 2. *(A) Sequence alignment of segments of intracellular domains i2 and i3 for SSTR. Conserved residues shared by all five subtypes are indicated by boxes with solid lines. Conserved residues found in SSTR1, 3, and 4, but not SSTR2 and 5, are indicated by boxes with dashed lines. (B) Predicted structure of SSTR, with filled circles indicating the i2-TV and i3-QQ substitutions.*

SSTR2 mutant receptors containing either individual or collective i2 and i3 substitutions were stably expressed in CCL39 fibroblasts and their function was confirmed by their ability to mediate SST inhibition of cAMP accumulation (Figure 3a). Consistent with our previous finding that SSTR2/SSTR1 chimeras with collective replacements of i2 and i3 from SSTR1 inhibit NHE1 (26), the collective, but not individual, substitution of a TV motif in i2 and a WQQ motif in i3 is sufficient for mutant SSTR2 to mediate SST inhibition of the exchanger and a decrease in pH$_i$ (Figure 3b). Interestingly, the i2 TV and i3 QQ sequences are found at cognate sites in the the D2-dopamine and (α2β-adrenergic receptors, which both regulate NHE1 (29, 30). These residues, therefore, may represent an evolutionarily conserved signaling motif.

SSTR1, BUT NOT SSTR2, INHIBITS RHOA AND IMPAIRS CYTOSKELETAL ORGANIZATION

NHE1 activity is stimulated by a number of G protein-coupled receptors, including those for thrombin and lysophosphatidic acid, through a signaling cascade mediated by the heterotrimeric GTPase Gα13, the low molecular

Lin, Buchan, and Barber

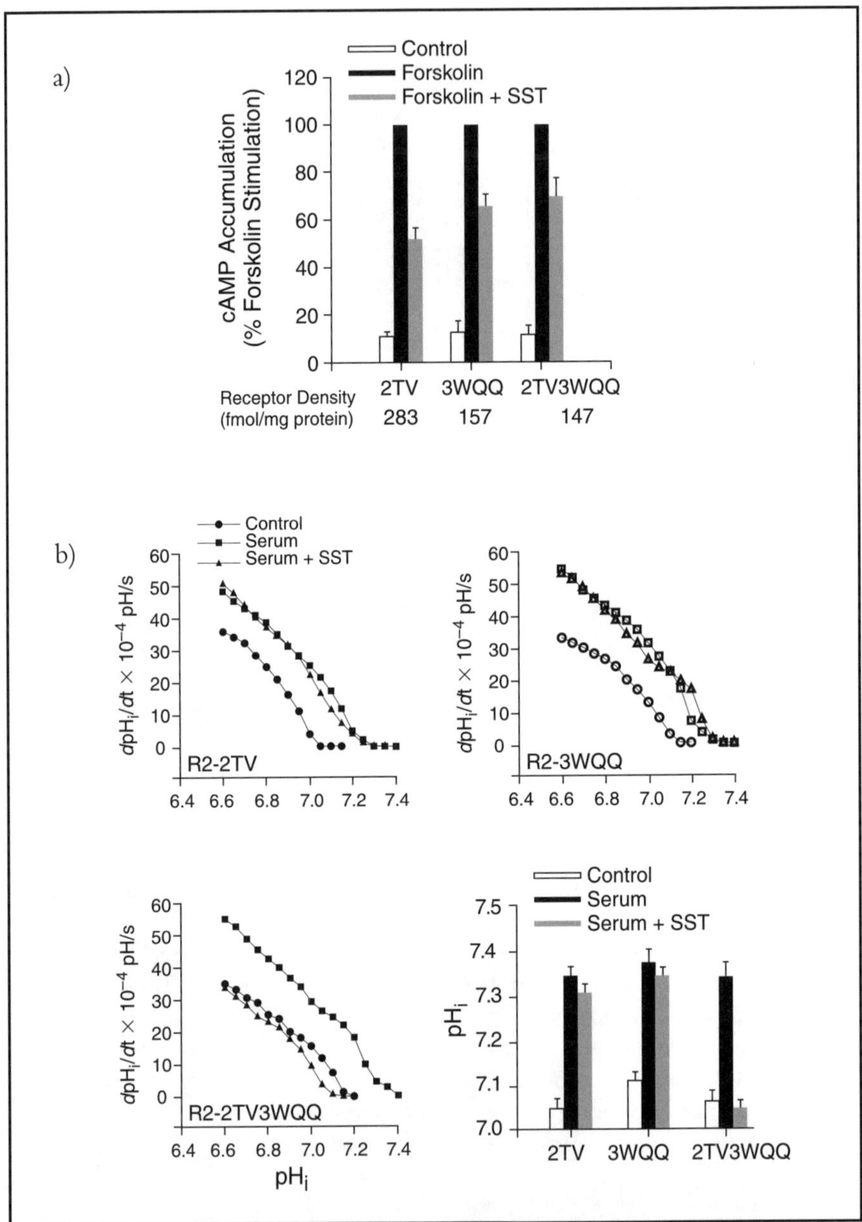

FIGURE 3. *(a) cAMP accumulation and receptor density in CCL39 cells stably expressing SSTR2 containing the indicated i2 and i3 amino acid substitutions, either individually (2TV; 3WQQ) or collectively (2TV3WQQ). (b) NHE1 activity, expressed as the rate of pH_i recovery (dpH_i/dt) from an acid load, and steady-state pH_i in CCL39 cells stably expressing SSTR2 with the indicated i2 and i3 amino acid substitutions.*

weight GTPase RhoA and the RhoA-associated kinase ROCK, which directly phosphorylates NHE1 (27, 31) (Figure 4a). RhoA and ROCK also mediate activation of NHE1 by integrin receptors (32) (Figure 4a). RhoA and ROCK play a central role in regulating dynamic reorganization of the actin-based cytoskeleton (33), and their activation of NHE1 is critical for the ordered assembly of actin filaments and focal adhesions (27, 32, 34, 35).

Because the SSTR1 subtype inhibits NHE1, we reasoned that it might also inhibit the upstream regulator RhoA and impair cytoskeletal organization. RhoA activity was determined by measuring abundance of GTP-bound Rho complexed to a GST-fusion protein of the Rho-binding domain of its effector, ROCK (36). Thrombin (30 nM; 20 min) increases the abundance of RhoA-GTP in CCL39 cells, and in the presence of SST (100 nM), RhoA activation by thrombin is inhibited by 75% in CCL-R1 cells expressing SSTR1, but is unchanged in wild-type CCL39 cells and in CCL-R2 cells expressing SSTR2 (Figure 4b).[2] In the absence of thrombin, SST has no effect on the abundance of RhoA-GTP in all three cell types (data not shown), indicating that SSTR1 inhibits stimulated, but not basal, RhoA activity. Consistent with the inhibition of RhoA, activation of SSTR1 also impairs actin filament assembly. CCL39 cells treated with thrombin (30 nM; 20 min) have long parallel arrays of actin stress fibers that extend throughout the cell (Figure 4c). In the presence of SST (100 nM), thrombin-induced stress fiber formation is unchanged in wild-type CCL39 cells and in CCL-R2, but is strikingly inhibited in CCL-R1 cells (Figure 4c). In CCL-R1 cells treated with thrombin and SST, actin stress fibers are absent in the cell body, and their abundance and size are markedly decreased in the cortex.

SSTR1 also inhibits activation of RhoA by integrins.[2] Compared to control cells plated on poly-L-lysine, plating on fibronectin for 60 min, which activates $\alpha_5\beta_1$ integrins in CCL39 cells (32), increases RhoA activity (Figure 5a). Although preincubating cells with SST for 5 min prior to plating has no effect on cell attachment (data not shown), it inhibits RhoA activation by fibronectin in CCL-R1 cells, but not in CCL-R2 cells (Figure 5a). Moreover, SST treatment has a dramatic effect on the assembly of focal adhesions and stress fibers induced by fibronectin in CCL-R1 cells. In the absence of SST, immunostaining showed that the focal adhesion-associated protein paxillin is localized in densely packed bundles within peripheral focal adhesions, and phalloidin staining reveals densely packed actin filaments predominantly at the cortex (Figure 5b). With SST treatment, however, paxillin immunostaining revealed smaller, punctate focal complexes, indicating impaired assembly of focal adhesions (Figure 5b). Additionally, in the presence of SST, fibronectin-induced stress fiber formation is dramatically inhibited in both the cell body and cortex (Figure 5b). Hence, SSTR1, but not SSTR2, inhibits activation of RhoA and cytoskeletal reorganization in response to signals from both G protein-coupled receptors and integrins.

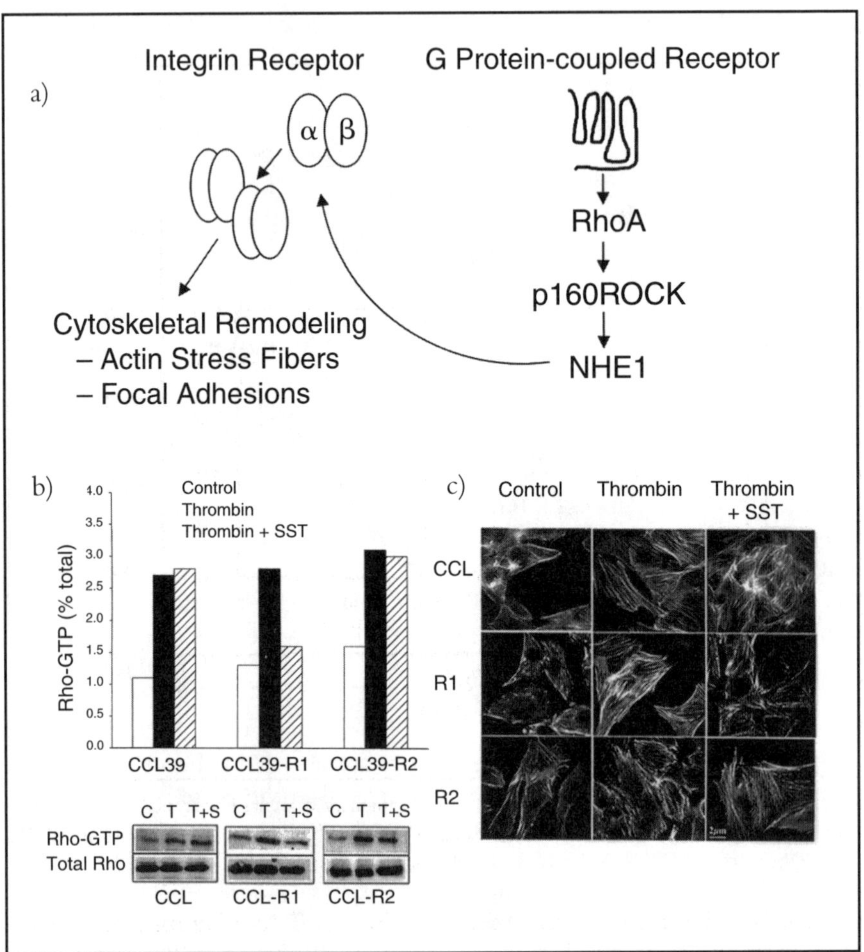

FIGURE 4. *(a) Schematic diagram demonstrating the RhoA-dependent activation of NHE1 by G protein-coupled receptors and by integrins. (b) The regulation of Rho-GTP abundance and immunoblots of Rho-GTP and total Rho acquired from wild-type CCL39 cells and CCL39-R1 and CCL39-R2 cells. Data were obtained from quiescent cells (control) and cells treated with thrombin (30 nM; 20 min) in the absence and presence of SST (100 nM), and are representative of five separate cell preparations. (c) Phalloidin labeling of actin filaments in quiescent cells (control) and cells treated with thrombin in the absence and presence of SST.*

CONCLUSIONS

We have described actions of the SSTR1 subtype that are not shared by SSTR2, including inhibition of NHE1 and RhoA activities, and inhibition of actin filament and focal adhesion assembly. Inhibition of NHE1 is also shared by SSTR3 and 4, but not by SSTR5. Whether SSTR3 and 4 also

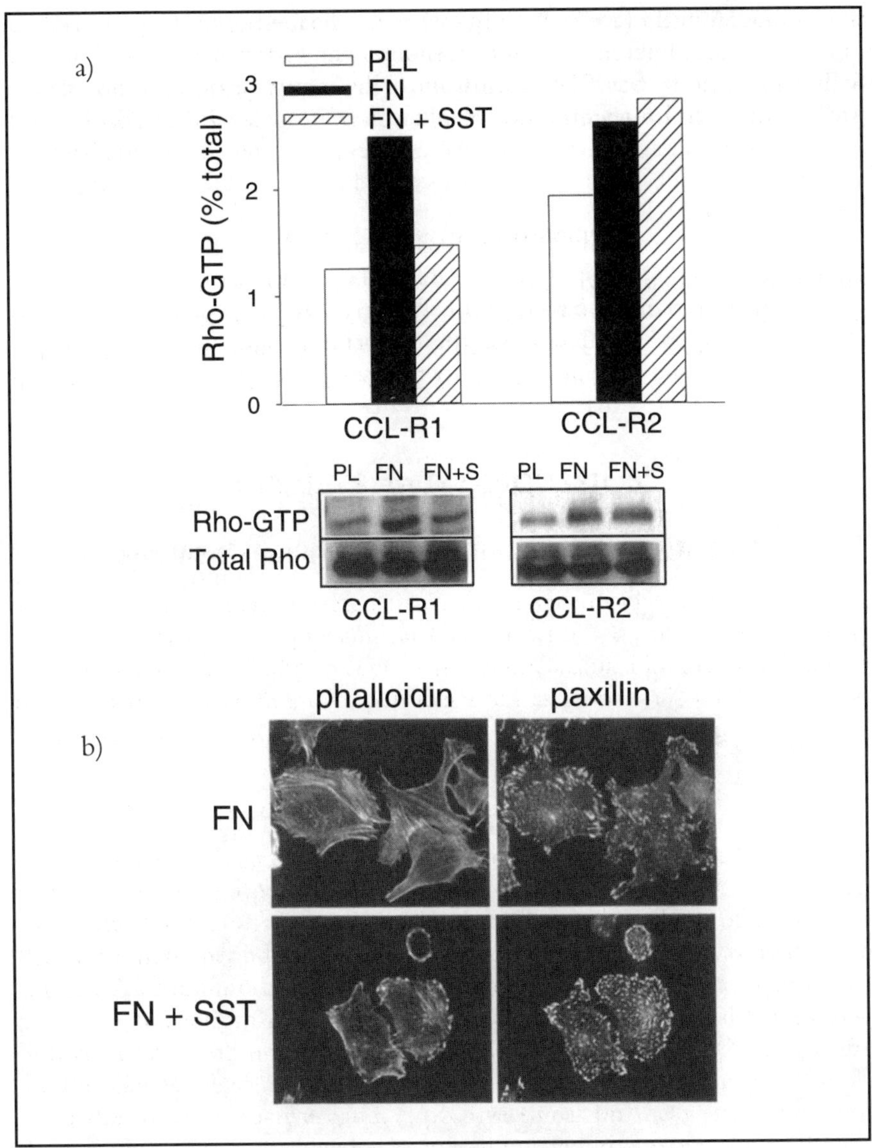

FIGURE 5. *(a) The abundance of GTP-bound Rho complexed with the Rho-binding domain of ROCK and total Rho in CCL-R1 and CCL-R2 cells was determined by immunoblotting, and the abundance of Rho-GTP was expressed as a percentage of total Rho immunoreactivity. Data were obtained from cells plated for 60 min on poly-L-lysine (PL) (control) or fibronectin in the absence (FN) or presence of SST (FN + S), and are representative of three separate cell preparations. (b) The abundance of abundance of actin filaments, determined by phalloidin labeling, and focal adhesions, determined by paxillin staining, are shown for CCL-R1 cells plated for 60 min on fibronectin in the absence (FN) and presence of somatostatin (FN + SST).*

inhibit RhoA and cytoskeletal organization remains to be determined. An important future direction is to establish the functional significance of SSTR inhibition of NHE1, RhoA and cytoskeletal organization with regard to the cellular effects of SST. Because increased NHE1 (35, 37) and RhoA (38, 39) activities promote cell proliferation, their inhibition by SST might be a mechanism contributing to the antiproliferative effects of SSTR. Increased RhoA activity also stimulates secretion (40, 41) and smooth muscle contractility (42, 43), which are cellular effects generally inhibited by SST (44). Moreover increased NHE1 and RhoA activities stimulate neoplastic transformation and cell migration (45–48) suggesting roles in tumor growth and metastasis. The majority of human tumors express SSTRs (49), hence therapeutic agents that selectively target their coupling to NHE1 and RhoA may be a novel means for halting tumor progression.

ACKNOWLEDGMENTS

This work was supported by grants from the National Institutes of Health to DLB (DK40259 and GM58642) and to C-Y.L (T32DE07204) and from the Canadian Institutes of Health Research to A.M.J.B.

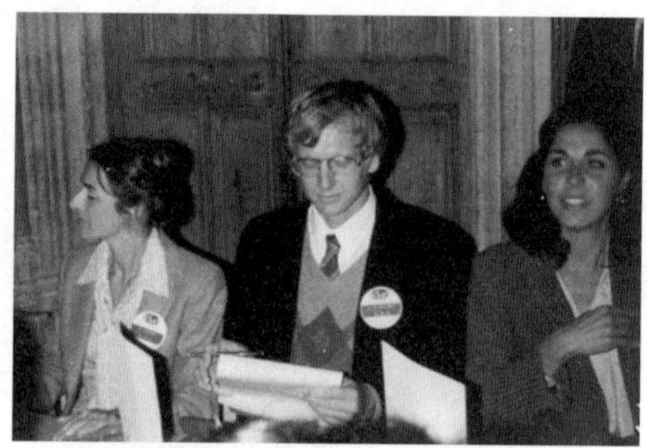

Yvette Taché, John Walsh and Diane Barber, 1980.
Gut Peptide meeting in Cambridge, England.

REFERENCES

1. Yamada Y, Post SR, Wang K, Tager HS, Bell GI, Seino S. Cloning and functional characterization of a family of human and mouse somatostatin receptors expressed in brain, gastrointestinal tract, and kidney. *Proc Natl Acad Sci USA* 1992;89(1):251–5.
2. Yasuda K, Rens-Domiano S, Breder CD, Law SF, Saper CB, Reisine T, Bell GI. Cloning of a novel somatostatin receptor, SSTR3, coupled to adenylylcyclase. *J Biol Chem* 1992;267(28):20422–8.
3. Bruno JF, Xu Y, Song J, Berelowitz M. Molecular cloning and functional expression of a brain-specific somatostatin receptor. *Proc Natl Acad Sci USA* 1992;89(23):11151–5.
4. Meyerhof W, Wulfsen I, Schonrock C, Fehr S, Richter D. Molecular cloning of a somatostatin-28 receptor and comparison of its expression pattern with that of a somatostatin-14 receptor in rat brain. *Proc Natl Acad Sci USA* 1992;89(21):10267–71.
5. O'Carroll AM, Lolait SJ, Konig M, Mahan LC. Molecular cloning and expression of a pituitary somatostatin receptor with preferential affinity for somatostatin-28. *Mol Pharmacol* 1992;42(6):939–46.
6. Patel YC, Greenwood MT, Warszynska A, Panetta R, Srikant CB. All five cloned human somatostatin receptors (hSSTR1–5) are functionally coupled to adenylyl cyclase. *Biochem Biophys Res Commun* 1994;198(2):605–12.
7. Buscail L, Delesque N, Esteve JP, Saint-Laurent N, Prats H, Clerc P, Robberecht P, Bell GI, Liebow C, Schally AV, Vaysse N, Susini C. Stimulation of tyrosine phosphatase and inhibition of cell proliferation by somatostatin analogues: mediation by human somatostatin receptor subtypes SSTR1 and SSTR2. *Proc Natl Acad Sci USA* 1994;91(6):2315–9.
8. Buscail L, Esteve JP, Saint-Laurent N, Bertrand V, Reisine T, O'Carroll AM, Bell GI, Schally AV, Vaysse N, Susini C. Inhibition of cell proliferation by the somatostatin analogue RC-160 is mediated by somatostatin receptor subtypes SSTR2 and SSTR5 through different mechanisms. *Proc Natl Acad Sci USA* 1995;92(5):1580–4.
9. Florio T, Rim C, Hershberger RE, Loda M, Stork PJ. The somatostatin receptor SSTR1 is coupled to phosphotyrosine phosphatase activity in CHO-K1 cells. *Mol Endocrinol* 1994;8(10):1289–97.
10. Florio T, Scorizello A, Fattore M, D'Alto V, Salzano S, Rossi G, Berlingieri MT, Fusco A, Schettini G. Somatostatin inhibits PC Cl3 thyroid cell proliferation through the modulation of phosphotyrosine activity. Impairment of the somatostatinergic effects by stable expression of E1A viral oncogene. *J Biol Chem* 1996;271(11):6129–36.
11. Florio T, Yao H, Carey KD, Dillon TJ, Stork PJ. Somatostatin activation of mitogen-activated protein kinase via somatostatin receptor 1 (SSTR1). *Mol Endocrinol* 1999;13(1):24–37.
12. Reardon DB, Wood SL, Brautigan DL, Bell GI, Dent P, Sturgill TW. Activation of a protein tyrosine phosphatase and inactivation of Raf-1 by somatostatin. *Biochem J* 1996;314 (Pt 2):401–4.
13. Sharma K, Patel YC, Srikant CB. C-terminal region of human somatostatin receptor 5 is required for induction of Rb and G1 cell cycle arrest. *Mol Endocrinol* 1999;13(1):82–90.
14. Kreienkamp HJ, Honck HH, Richter D. Coupling of rat somatostatin receptor subtypes to a G-protein gated inwardly rectifying potassium channel (GIRK1). *FEBS Lett* 1997;419(1):92–4.
15. Fujii Y, Gonoi T, Yamada Y, Chihara K, Inagaki N, Seino S. Somatostatin receptor subtype SSTR2 mediates the inhibition of high-voltage-activated calcium channels by somatostatin and its analogue SMS 201–995. *FEBS Lett* 1994;355(2):117–20.
16. Roosterman D, Glassmeier G, Baumeister H, Scherubl H, Meyerhof W. A somatostatin receptor 1 selective ligand inhibits Ca^{2+} currents in rat insulinoma 1046–38 cells. *FEBS Lett* 1998;425(1):137–40.
17. Viana F, Hille B. Modulation of high voltage-activated calcium channels by somatostatin in acutely isolated rat amygdaloid neurons. *J Neurosci* 1996;16(19):6000–11.
18. Tomura H, Okajima F, Akbar M, Abdul Majid M, Sho K, Kondo Y. Transfected human somatostatin receptor type 2, SSTR2, not only inhibits adenylate cyclase but also stimulates phospholipase C and Ca^{2+} mobilization. *Biochem Biophys Res Commun* 1994;200(2):986–92.
19. Bito H, Mori M, Sakanaka C, Takano T, Honda Z, Gotoh Y, Nishida E, Shimizu T. Functional coupling of SSTR4, a major hippocampal somatostatin receptor, to adenylate cyclase inhibition, arachidonate release and activation of the mitogen-activated protein kinase cascade. *J Biol Chem* 1994;269(17):12722–30.

                    Lin, Buchan, and Barber

20. Cattaneo MG, Amoroso D, Gussoni G, Sanguini AM, Vicentini LM. A somatostatin analogue inhibits MAP kinase activation and cell proliferation in human neuroblastoma and in human small cell lung carcinoma cell lines. *FEBS Lett* 1996;397(2–3):164–8.

21. Cordelier P, Esteve JP, Bousquet C, Delesque N, O'Carroll AM, Schally AV, Vaysse N, Susini C, Buscail L. Characterization of the antiproliferative signal mediated by the somatostatin receptor subtype sst$_5$. *Proc Natl Acad Sci USA* 1997;94(17):9343–8.

22. Yoshitomi H, Fujii Y, Miyazaki M, Nakajima N, Inagaki N, Seino S. Involvement of MAP kinase and c-fos signaling in the inhibition of cell growth by somatostatin. *Am J Physiol* 1997;272(5 Pt 1): E769–74.

23. Putney LK, Denker SP, Barber DL. The changing face of the Na$^+$/H$^+$ Exchanger, NHE1: Structure, regulation, and cellular actions. In: *Annual Review of Pharmacology and Toxicology,* Schekman R, Goldstein LB, McKnight SL, Rossant J, editors. Palo Alto; 2002.

24. Barber DL, McGuire ME, Ganz MB. Beta-adrenergic and somatostatin receptors regulate Na-H exchange independent of cAMP. *J Biol Chem* 1989;264(35):21038–42.

25. Ye WZ, Mathieu S, Marteau C. Somatostatin inhibits the Na$^+$/H$^+$ exchange activity of rat hepatocytes in short term primary culture. *Cell Mol Biol* (Noisy-le-grand) 1999;45(8):1183–9.

26. Hou C, Gilbert RL, Barber DL. Subtype-specific signaling mechanisms of somatostatin receptors SSTR1 and SSTR2. *J Biol Chem* 1994;269(14):10357–62.

27. Tominaga T, Ishizaki T, Narumiya S, Barber DL. p160ROCK mediates RhoA activation of Na-H exchange. *Embo J* 1998;17(16):4712–22.

28. Patel YC, Greenwood MT, Panetta R, Demchyshyn L, Niznik H, Srikant CB. The somatostatin receptor family. *Life Sci* 1995;57(13):1249–65.

29. Ganz MB, Pachter JA, Barber DL. Multiple receptors coupled to adenylate cyclase regulate Na-H exchange independent of cAMP. *J Biol Chem* 1990;265(16):8989–92.

30. Pihlavisto M, Scheinin M. Functional assessment of recombinant human alpha(2)-adrenoceptor subtypes with cytosensor microphysiometry. *Eur J Pharmacol* 1999;385(2–3):247–53.

31. Hooley R, Yu CY, Symons M, Barber DL. G alpha 13 stimulates Na$^+$-H$^+$ exchange through distinct Cdc42-dependent and RhoA-dependent pathways. *J Biol Chem* 1996;271(11):6152–8.

32. Tominaga T, Barber DL. Na-H exchange acts downstream of RhoA to regulate integrin-induced cell adhesion and spreading. *Mol Biol Cell* 1998;9(8):2287–303.

33. Bishop AL, Hall A. Rho GTPases and their effector proteins. Biochem J 2000;348 Pt 2:241–55.

34. Vexler ZS, Symons M, Barber DL. Activation of Na$^+$-H$^+$ exchange is necessary for RhoA-induced stress fiber formation. *J Biol Chem* 1996;271(37):22281–4.

35. Denker SP, Huang DC, Orlowski J, Furthmayr H, Barber DL. Direct binding of the Na—H exchanger NHE1 to ERM proteins regulates the cortical cytoskeleton and cell shape independently of H(+) translocation. *Mol Cell* 2000;6(6):1425–36.

36. Kranenburg O, Poland M, van Horck FP, Drechsel D, Hall A, Moolenaar WH. Activation of RhoA by lysophosphatidic acid and Galpha12/13 subunits in neuronal cells: induction of neurite retraction. *Mol Biol Cell* 1999;10(6):1851–7.

37. Kapus A, Grinstein S, Wasan S, Kandasamy R, Orlowski J. Functional characterization of three isoforms of the Na$^+$/H$^+$ exchanger stably expressed in Chinese hamster ovary cells. ATP dependence, osmotic sensitivity, and role in cell proliferation. *J Biol Chem* 1994;269(38):23544–52.

38. Sahai E, Olson MF, Marshall CJ. Cross-talk between Ras and Rho signalling pathways in transformation favours proliferation and increased motility. *Embo J* 2001;20(4):755–66.

39. Danen EH, Sonneveld P, Sonnenberg A, Yamada KM. Dual stimulation of Ras/mitogen-activated protein kinase and RhoA by cell adhesion to fibronectin supports growth factor-stimulated cell cycle progression. *J Cell Biol* 2000;151(7):1413–22.

40. Holt MR, Koffer A. Rho GTPases: secretion and actin dynamics in permeabilized mast cells. *Methods Enzymol* 2000;325:356–69.

41. Nozu F, Tsunoda Y, Ibitayo AI, Bitar KN, Owyang C. Involvement of RhoA and its interaction with protein kinase C and Src in CCK-stimulated pancreatic acini. *Am J Physiol* 1999;276(4 Pt 1):G915–23.

42. Somlyo AP, Somlyo AV. Signal transduction by G-proteins, rho-kinase and protein phosphatase to smooth muscle and non-muscle myosin II. *J Physiol* 2000;522 Pt 2:177–85.

43. Wang P, Bitar KN. Rho A regulates sustained smooth muscle contraction through cytoskeletal reorganization of HSP27. *Am J Physiol* 1998;275(6 Pt 1):G1454–62.

44. Patel YC. Somatostatin and its receptor family. *Front Neuroendocrinol* 1999;20(3):157–98.

45. Klein M, Seeger P, Schuricht B, Alper SL, Schwab A. Polarization of Na(+)/H(+) and Cl(-)/HCO(3)(-) exchangers in migrating renal epithelial cells. *J Gen Physiol* 2000;115(5):599–608.

46. Reshkin SJ, Bellizzi A, Albarani V, Guerra L, Tommasino M, Paradiso A, Casavole V. Phosphoinositide 3-kinase is involved in the tumor-specific activation of human breast cancer cell Na(+)/H(+) exchange, motility, and invasion induced by serum deprivation. *J Biol Chem* 2000;275(8):5361–9.

47. Evers EE, Zondag GC, Malliri A, Price LS, ten Klooster JP, van der Kammen RA, Collard JG. Rho family proteins in cell adhesion and cell migration. *Eur J Cancer* 2000;36(10):1269–74.

48. Ridley AJ. Rho GTPases and cell migration. *J Cell Sci* 2001;114(Pt 15):2713–22.

49. Patel YC. Molecular pharmacology of somatostatin receptor subtypes. *J Endocrinol Invest* 1997;20(6):348–67.

50. Palczewski K, Kumasaka T, Hori T, Behnke CA, Motoshima H, Fox BA, Trong I, Teller DC, Okada T, Stenkamp RE, Yamamoto M. Crystal structure of rhodopsin: A G protein-coupled receptor. *Science* 2000;289:739–745.

Gut-Brain Peptides in the New Millennium, edited by Y. Taché
CURE Foundation, Los Angeles, CA. © 2002

17

Gastrointestinal Peptide Signaling

Enrique Rozengurt
Department of Medicine, School of Medicine and Molecular Biology Institute, University of California, Los Angeles, CA

INTRODUCTION

Gastrointestinal (GI) peptides, neuropeptides or regulatory peptides are over-lapping terms that design a structurally diverse group of molecular messengers that function in a rich network of intercellular exchange of information throughout the organism. Produced by neural or endocrine cells, these structurally diverse signaling neuropeptides, including mammalian bombesin-like peptides, gastrin, cholecystokinin (CCK) and neurotensin, reach their targets as neurotransmitters, paracrine regulators or systemic hormones. Neuropeptides play a crucial role in the regulation of exocrine and endocrine secretion, smooth-muscle contraction, pain transmission, fluid homeostasis, blood pressure and inflammation. In the CNS, neuropeptides regulate food intake, body temperature, and behavioral responses. The function and regulation of GI hormones in general and of gastrin in particular, was the major scientific interest of John Walsh during his brilliant and productive career. His work has been central for establishing that gastrin, produced by the G cells in the gastric antrum, is the circulating hormone responsible for stimulation of acid secretion from the parietal cell.

In addition to these traditional functions, GI peptides, including bombesin/gastrin-releasing peptide (GRP) and gastrin also act as potent cellular growth factors (1, 2). Several lines of evidence including gene knock-out studies indicate that the mitogenic effects of neuropeptides are relevant for a variety of normal biological processes including development, inflammation and cell proliferation under physiological conditions (3, 4). It is also increasingly recognized that multiple neuropeptides including those of the bombesin family, play an important role as autocrine/paracrine growth factors for human cancer cells including lung, colon, and pancreatic cancer (3, 5).

I was very excited when in 1992, John Walsh decided to come to my laboratory (then at the Imperial Cancer Research Fund, London) for a sabbatical period. Our central interest was to delineate the intracellular signal transduction pathways that mediate the growth-promoting effects induced by bombesin/GRP and other neuropeptides in normal and cancer cells. The sabbatical period that John spent in ICRF not only cemented our friendship but also influenced his scientific outlook. As he put it succinctly in his incomparable style, the time for those interested in understanding the mechanism of action of GI hormones has come to move *from the outside of the cell to the inside*. This chapter which as the rest of this book is dedicated to John Walsh, will summarize some recent developments in the mechanism of action of bombesin/GRP in Swiss 3T3 cells, a model system studied in our laboratory for the last 20 years.

SIGNAL TRANSDUCTION PATHWAYS IN THE ACTION OF GI PEPTIDES

The binding of a neuropeptide to its cognate heptahelical G protein-coupled receptor (GPCR) triggers the activation of a network of signaling events that act in a synergistic and combinatorial fashion to relay the mitogenic signal to the nucleus and promote progression through the cell cycle leading to cell proliferation. The model of signal transduction to be discussed in this chapter is that a single type of GPCR (e.g., the bombesin/GRP) couples to several heterotrimeric G proteins thereby initiating the activation of multiple parallel pathways, as indicated in Figure 1.

SIGNALING THROUGH Gq

Bombesin/GRP and gastrin activate pertussis toxin-insensitive Gq, promoting its dissociation into Gαq and Gβγ and the exchange of GDP bound to the Gαq for GTP. The resulting GTP-Gαq complex activates the β isoforms of phospholipase C (PLC) via interaction with the carboxy-terminal region of the enzyme. As depicted in Figure 1, PLC catalyzes the hydrolysis of phosphatidylinositol 4,5-biphosphate to produce two second messengers: Ins $(1,4,5)P_3$ and diacylglycerol (DAG). Ins $(1,4,5)P_3$ binds to its intracellular receptor, a ligand-gated Ca^{2+} channel located in the endoplasmic reticulum, and triggers the release of Ca^{2+} from internal stores. DAG directly activates protein kinase C (PKC), a multi-gene family that encodes at least eleven distinct isoforms, which are differentially expressed in cells and tissues. This bifurcating signaling pathway has been reviewed recently by us (2, 3) and others (6).

All members of the PKC family, i.e., conventional PKCs (α, βI, βII, γ), novel PKCs (δ, ε, η, θ) and atypical PKCs (ζ, λ, ι), are characterized by a highly conserved catalytic domain. Most of the variation between the PKC isoforms occurs in the regulatory domain. It is thought that individual PKC

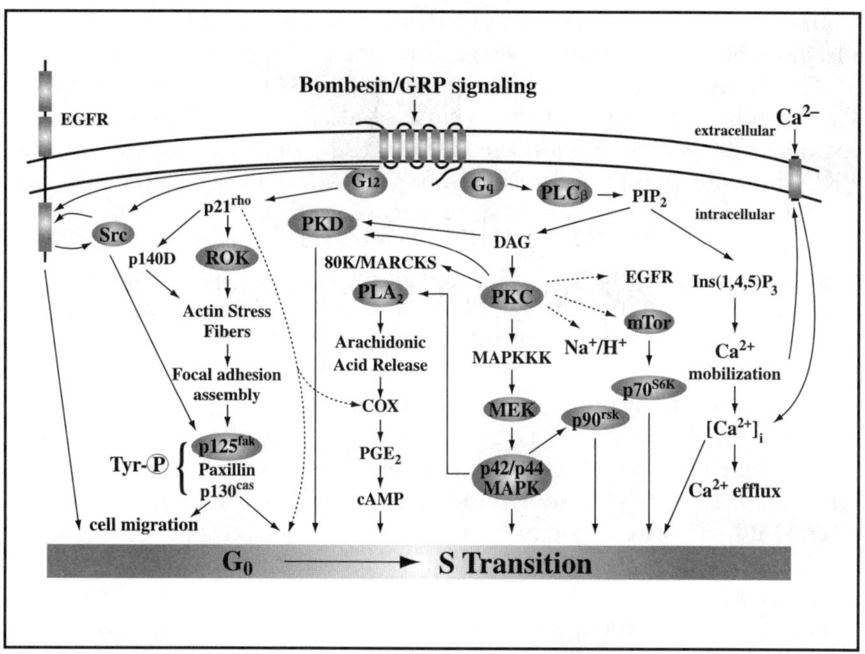

FIGURE 1. *Signal transduction pathways activated by engagement of the bombesin/GRP receptor. See text for details and abbreviations.*

isoforms differ with respect to their roles in growth control and other biologic effects by executing distinct cellular functions at different subcellular locations. A large number of cellular studies using the potent tumor promoters of the phorbol ester family which substitute for DAG in PKC activation, implicated PKC in a wide range of fundamental biological effects, including changes in ion flux, secretion, contraction, adhesion, gene expression, cell differentiation and, in particular, in the regulation of cell proliferation.

The importance of PKC-mediated pathways in bombesin-mediated mitogenesis is underscored by the fact that phorbol ester-mediated down-regulation of conventional and novel PKCs inhibits the stimulation of DNA synthesis induced by bombesin in Swiss 3T3 cells. These studies indicate that PKC occupies a pivotal position in neuropeptide receptor signal transduction (Figure 1). However, the events downstream to individual PKC isoforms have remained poorly understood.

Protein Kinase D (PKD): A Downstream Target of PKC

Protein kinase D (PKD) is a serine/threonine protein kinase with distinct structural features and enzymological properties that has been cloned in our laboratory (7). PKD is a protein of 918 amino acids with a predicted molecular mass of 102 kDa that consists of catalytic and regulatory domains.

The catalytic domain of PKD (residues 557-845) is distantly related to Ca^{2+}-regulated kinases and shows little similarity to the highly conserved regions of the kinase subdomains of the PKC family. Consistent with this, PKD does not phosphorylate a number of known PKC substrates *in vitro,* indicating that PKD has a distinct substrate specificity (7).

In contrast to all known PKCs, the NH_2-terminal region of PKD contains a pleckstrin homology (PH) domain (residues 429-557) that regulates enzyme activity (8). In addition, PKD contains a tandem repeat of cysteine-rich, zinc finger-like motifs (cys-1 and cys-2) that bind phorbol esters and the second messenger DAG (7) and mediate the intracellular translocation of this enzyme, from the cytosol to the membrane, in response to bombesin receptor stimulation (9). PKD, and its homologue PKCµ (10), can be activated *in vitro* by either DAG or biologically active phorbol esters in the presence of phosphatidyl-L-serine indicating that PKD/PKCµ are phorbol ester/DAG-stimulated protein kinases.

The catalytic activity of PKD is rapidly activated by cell stimulation with a variety of neuropeptide agonists including bombesin and gastrin/CCK which signal through Gq-coupled receptors (11). Gαq-mediated signaling is sufficient to promote PKD activation in intact COS-1 cells and endogenous Gαq mediates PKD activation in response to bombesin receptor stimulation (12). Several lines of evidence including the use of selective PKC inhibitors and cotransfection of PKD with constitutively active mutants of PKC ε and η indicate that PKD is activated by phosphorylation in living cells through a novel PKC-dependent signal transduction pathway. More recent studies from our laboratory demonstrated that PKD forms a molecular complex with PKC η. In particular, the residues Ser-744 and Ser-748, located in the activation loop of PKD, have been identified as critical phosphorylation sites in PKD activation (13). These results revealed an unsuspected connection between PKCs and PKD, implied that PKD can function downstream of PKCs and identified a novel phosphorylation cascade activated by neuropeptide agonists.

Our recent results indicate that PKD plays an important role in bombesin-induced mitogenesis. Specifically, PKD overexpression in Swiss 3T3 cells selectively potentiates the stimulation of DNA synthesis and cell proliferation induced by bombesin in these cells (14). Furthermore, cell stimulation with bombesin induces a transient nuclear accumulation of PKD that is prevented by inhibiting PKC activity (15). Thus, PKD is emerging as an important element in bombesin-induced cell proliferation and it is attractive to hypothesize that the nuclear translocation of PKD contributes to the transduction of the mitogenic signal generated by bombesin/GRP receptor stimulation.

SIGNALING VIA G$_{12}$: TYROSINE PHOSPHORYLATION AND ACTIN REMODELING

Our own studies demonstrated that GI peptides could induce cellular mitogenesis not only through PKC-dependent but also via PKC-independent routes (1). These findings stimulated the search for novel signal transduction pathways in the action of GI peptides.

We demonstrated that in addition to eliciting the synthesis of classic second messengers (e.g., Ca^{2+}, DAG, cAMP) and the consequent stimulation of serine/threonine protein kinase cascades, GI peptide receptor activation also induces a rapid increase in the tyrosine phosphorylation of multiple substrates within target cells (2, 3). These initial findings were surprising because they demonstrated that activation of GPCRs, which are characterized by seven putative transmembrane α helices, also induces tyrosine phosphorylation of multiple proteins in their target cells, apparently through stimulation of protein tyrosine kinase activity.

The non-receptor tyrosine kinase p125 focal adhesion kinase (FAK) and the adaptor proteins p130 Crk-associated substrate (CAS) and paxillin have been identified as prominent targets of GI peptide-stimulated tyrosine phosphorylation (16). The importance of FAK-mediated signal transduction is underscored by recent experiments showing that this tyrosine kinase is implicated in embryonic development and in the control of cell migration, proliferation and apoptosis (16, 17). In addition, there is increasing evidence linking overexpression of FAK to the invasive properties of cancer cells. The adaptor protein CAS has recently been identified as a downstream mediator of FAK-mediated cell migration.

We also found that GI peptides induce a rapid and transient activation of the protooncogene Src (18) and recent reports from several laboratories suggest that GPCR agonists lead to epidermal growth factor receptor (EGFR) transactivation (19). All of these findings indicate that tyrosine phosphorylation plays a critical role in GI peptide-induced cellular migration and mitogenesis.

Specific Tyrosine Phosphorylation Sites of FAK in Bombesin-stimulated Cells

Tyr-397, the only apparent site of FAK autophosphorylation, has emerged as a critical residue in FAK-mediated signaling (20). The phosphorylation of FAK at Tyr-397 triggers the formation of molecular complexes with other signaling proteins including Src-family kinases, the p85 regulatory subunit phosphatidylinositol 3-kinase, phospholipase Cγ-1, the adapter proteins Grb-7 and Shc and the tumor suppressor PTEN (see (21) and refs. therein). These findings suggest that FAK autophosphorylation promotes the activation of multiple effector pathways.

The best characterized function of FAK autophosphorylation at Tyr-397 is the creation of a high affinity-binding site for the SH2 domain of Src family members. Given that competition for the SH2 and/or SH3 domains of Src by high affinity allosteric ligands promotes enzymatic activation of this kinase, the association of Src with FAK should lead to the formation of a molecular complex in which Src kinases are activated. A model has recently been proposed that envisages reciprocal catalytic activation of FAK and Src-family kinases (22). In the framework of this model, Src activated by binding to FAK Tyr-397, phosphorylates FAK at Tyr-576 and 577 which are located in the activation loop of the kinase catalytic domain of FAK and thereby promotes maximal FAK catalytic activity.

Our recent results demonstrate that stimulation of intact Swiss 3T3 cells with bombesin induces a rapid increase in FAK phosphorylation at both, Tyr-397 and Tyr-577, as revealed using antibodies that specifically recognized these residues in their phosphorylated form (21, 23). These findings show that activation of GPCRs, like engagement of integrins, induces rapid multi-site tyrosine phosphorylation of FAK, leading to FAK/Src complex formation in intact cells.

Signal Transduction Pathways Leading to FAK Tyrosine Phosphorylation: Cytoskeletal Link

A salient feature of FAK is its subcellular localization to focal adhesions, discrete macromolecular complexes that function in cell attachment and signal transduction and that form at the termini of actin stress fibers (24). We demonstrated that bombesin-induced FAK tyrosine phosphorylation is completely blocked by treatment with cytochalasin D, which disrupts the actin filament network and prevents focal adhesion assembly (25). We proposed that FAK tyrosine phosphorylation induced by bombesin is downstream of focal adhesion assembly and actin reorganization and occurs in parallel with PLC-mediated events, as illustrated in Figure 1.

The small GTP-binding protein Rho, which belongs to the Ras related super family, is implicated in directing the assembly of focal adhesions and in promoting the formation of actin stress fibers in Swiss 3T3 cells. Bombesin/GRP induces a rapid increase in stress fibers and focal adhesions via Rho activation in these cells. Treatment of Swiss 3T3 cells with *Clostridium botulinum* C3 exotransferase, which ADP ribosylates and inactivates Rho, attenuates FAK tyrosine phosphorylation induced by subsequent exposure to bombesin (16).

Our additional experiments with bacterial toxins that selectively activate Rho, including cytotoxic necrotizing factor (CNF) from *E. coli* and dermonecrotic toxin (DNT) from *B. bronchiseptica,* also indicate that Rho activation leads to stress fiber formation, focal adhesion assembly and tyrosine phosphorylation of focal adhesion proteins (26), including FAK phosphorylation at Tyr-397 (27). Moreover, CNF and DNT stimulate DNA synthesis providing additional evidence for a novel Rho-dependent signaling pathway that leads to entry into the S phase of the cell cycle in Swiss 3T3 (26). All these findings strongly suggest the existence of a mitogenic pathway activated by GPCRs in which Rho is upstream of cytoskeletal reorganization and tyrosine phosphorylation of focal adhesion proteins, as indicated in Figure 1.

Rho has multiple effectors, including the serine/threonine protein kinase ROK (Rho-kinase), which transduces Rho activation into cytoskeletal responses. ROK activation increases the phosphorylation of the regulatory MLC, primarily by phosphorylation and inhibition of the myosin-associated MLC phosphatase (see (28) and refs. therein). MLC phosphorylation promotes the formation of stress fibers and the assembly of focal adhesions (Figure 1), thereby leading to clustering and tyrosine phosphorylation of focal adhesion proteins (24). Accordingly, calyculin-A, a potent inhibitor of MLC phosphatase, induces focal adhesion assembly and tyrosine phosphorylation of FAK (28) whereas exposure to ROK inhibitors prevents formation of actin stress fibers, assembly of focal contacts and tyrosine phosphorylation of FAK in response to neuropeptides (29). Thus, FAK tyrosine phosphorylation and activation is downstream of Rho and ROK.

$G\alpha_{12}$ and $G\alpha_{13}$ Stimulate Tyrosine Phosphorylation

How do GPCRs stimulate Rho activation? Recent work has demonstrated that $G\alpha_{12}$ and $G\alpha_{13}$ induce Rho activation via Rho guanine nucleotide exchange factors that contain a domain closely related to that of regulators of G protein signaling (RGS) including p115RhoGEF (30, 31). In fact, expression of constitutively active $G\alpha_{12}$ or of $G\alpha_{13}$ stimulates Rho-dependent biological responses, including tyrosine phosphorylation of FAK, paxillin and CAS (32). Thus, neuropeptide-mediated GPCR activation stimulates PLC-mediated phosphoinositide hydrolysis via Gq and Rho-dependent ROK activation, stress fiber formation, focal adhesion assembly and tyrosine phosphorylation of FAK, CAS and paxillin through $G\alpha_{12}$/ $G\alpha_{13}$ (Figure 1). It is increasingly recognized that there are cross-talks between these pathways, including a role of Rho in promoting PKC-dependent PKD activation (33).

Neuropeptides Activate Additional Tyrosine Kinase Pathways: Src-family Kinases and EGFR Transactivation

GPCR agonists induce a rapid and transient increase in the kinase activity of the Src-family of tyrosine kinases (18, 23). Cytochalasin D, at concentrations that prevent FAK tyrosine phosphorylation, does not impair Src-family kinase activation induced by neuropeptides (18). Thus, the signal transduction pathway leading to Src-family kinase activation can be separated from tyrosine phosphorylation of FAK in GPCR-stimulated cells but the precise mechanism(s) of Src activation in response to bombesin remains unclear. In this context, Src has been shown to associate either with arrestin recruited to phosphorylated GPCRs (34) or directly to GPCRs (35) thereby leading to Src activation. In addition, Src has also been reported to be stimulated *in vitro* by α subunits of heterotrimeric G proteins (Gs and Gi) (36). Whether or not GI peptides promote Src activation through any of these pathways or others, as yet unidentified, remains an important challenge for the future.

The EGFR is a single-pass transmembrane tyrosine kinase that is activated by direct binding of at least six EGF-related ligands that are synthesized as transmembrane precursors (19). GPCR agonists also induce a rapid increase in EGFR tyrosine autophosphorylation, leading to the assembly of signaling complexes in several cell types, a receptor cross-talk mediated, at least in part, by rapid proteolytic generation of EGFR ligands (e.g., heparin binding EGF) at the cell surface, termed transactivation (19). These recent findings demonstrated the existence of multiple signal transduction pathways leading to protein tyrosine phosphorylation in neuropeptide-stimulated cells.

GI PEPTIDE STIMULATION OF MITOGEN-ACTIVATED PROTEIN KINASE (MAPK) PATHWAYS

The MAPKs are a family of highly conserved serine/threonine kinases that are activated by multiple upstream signals, including GPCRs, via protein phosphorylation cascades which relay mitogenic signals to the nucleus. The two best characterized isoforms, p42^{mapk} (ERK-2) and p44^{mapk} (ERK-1), which are clearly implicated in cell proliferation, are directly activated by phosphorylation on specific tyrosine and threonine residues by the dual-specificity ERK kinase (or MEK). Several pathways leading to MEK activation have been identified. Tyrosine kinase receptors induce ERK activation via the complex between the adaptor protein Grb-2 and the guanine nucleotide release factor SOS which binds to tyrosine kinase receptors and promotes Ras-GTP accumulation, which then in turn recruits Raf-1 to the plasma membrane and activates a kinase cascade comprising Raf-1, MEK and ERK (37).

Gq-coupled neuropeptide receptors induce ERK activation via PKC-dependent and PKC-independent pathways (2, 3). The precise mechanism(s) by which the PKCs activate the ERKs remains incompletely understood. In some cells, PKC appears to directly phosphorylate and activate Raf-1 (38), whereas in other cell types PKC induces the ERK cascade via SOS-Grb2-mediated accumulation of Ras-GTP (39). Neuropeptide agonists also stimulate PKC-independent ERK activation via rapid tyrosine phosphorylation of Shc, which recruits the SOS-Grb2 complex leading to Ras activation, thus resembling the pathway utilized by receptor tyrosine kinases. Several neuropeptide-stimulated tyrosine kinases have been implicated as upstream regulators of this pathway, including Src, FAK and the FAK-homologue Pyk2, which promote ERK activation via tyrosine phosphorylation of adaptor proteins including Shc (2). Another potential pathway is transactivation of the EGF receptor which also leads to Ras-dependent ERK activation in a variety of cell types (19, 40). These tyrosine phosphorylation pathways were discussed above.

Studies with GPCRs expressed in different cells revealed that neuropeptides frequently stimulate the ERKs via separate pathways in different cell types (40). In Swiss 3T3 cells, PKC mediates bombesin-induced activation of Raf/MEK/ERK, leading to increased expression of immediate early response genes (e.g., c-fos/c-jun, c-myc) and subsequent regulation of cell cycle events (2, 41–43).

CONCLUSIONS AND IMPLICATIONS

It is now recognized that neuropeptides act as potent cellular growth factors for multiple cell types, including cancer cells. Studies on the signaling pathways activated by mitogenic GPCRs have revealed previously unsuspected connections and complexities. These include the realization that GPCRs interact with several rather than a single G protein, that heterotrimeric G proteins regulate small monomeric G proteins, that these receptors not only stimulate the synthesis of conventional second messengers but also induce multiple pathways leading to tyrosine phosphorylation events. GPCR signaling via G protein-independent pathways (e.g. direct binding of Src to the receptors) has also been proposed. It is also conceivable that these signaling pathways are modulated by other GPCRs that are also expressed in the GI tract (44). A major task for the future will be to identify all the contributing molecules, define their functional importance and elucidate the spatial and temporal relationships of this complicated signaling network. As John Walsh would have said…*these are exciting times in GPCR signaling.*

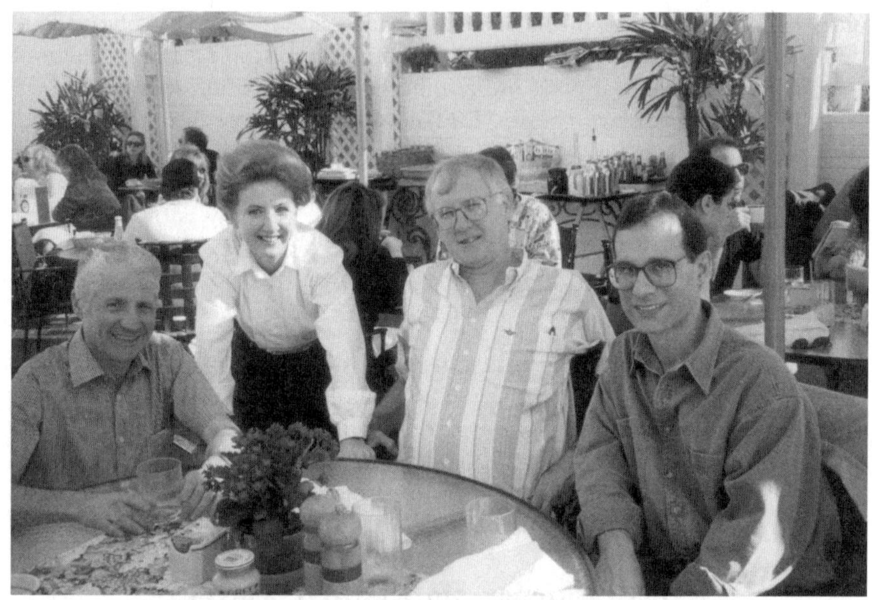

From left to right: Enrique Rozengurt, Nora Rozengurt, John Walsh, and Jim Sinnett-Smith,
January, 1996.

REFERENCES

1. Rozengurt E. Early signals in the mitogenic response. *Science* 1986;234:161–166.
2. Rozengurt E. Signal transduction pathways in the mitogenic response to G protein-coupled neuropeptide receptor agonists. *J Cell Physiol* 1998;177:507–517.
3. Rozengurt E and Walsh JH. Gastrin, CCK, signaling, and cancer. *Ann Rev Physiol* 2001;63:49–76.
4. Rozengurt E. Neuropeptides as growth factors for normal and cancer cells. *Trends Endocrinol Metabol* 2002;13:128–134.
5. Rozengurt E. Autocrine loops, signal transduction, and cell cycle abnormalities in the molecular biology of lung cancer. *Curr Opin Oncol* 1999;11:116–122.
6. Rhee SG. Regulation of phosphoinositide-specific phospholipase C. *Ann Rev Biochem* 2001;70: 281–312.
7. Valverde AM, Sinnett-Smith J, Van Lint J, Rozengurt E. Molecular cloning and characterization of protein kinase D: a target for diacylglycerol and phorbol esters with a distinctive catalytic domain. *Proc Natl Acad Sci USA* 1994;91:8572–8576.
8. Iglesias T and Rozengurt E. Protein kinase D activation by mutations within its pleckstrin homology domain. *J Biol Chem* 1998;273:410–416.
9. Rey O, Young SH, Cantrell D, Rozengurt E. Rapid Protein Kinase D Translocation in Response to G Protein-coupled Receptor Activation. Dependence on Protein Kinase C. *J Biol Chem* 2001;276: 32616–32626.
10. Johannes FJ, Prestle J, Eis S, Oberhagemann P, Pfizenmaier K. PKCu is a novel, atypical member of the protein kinase C family. *J Biol Chem* 1994;269:6140–6148.
11. Zugaza JL, Waldron RT, Sinnett-Smith J, Rozengurt E. Bombesin, vasopressin, endothelin, bradykinin, and platelet-derived growth factor rapidly activate protein kinase D through a protein kinase C-dependent signal transduction pathway. *J Biol Chem* 1997;272:23952–23960.

12. Yuan JZ, Slice L, Walsh JH, Rozengurt E. Activation of protein kinase D by signaling through the alpha subunit of the heterotrimeric G protein G(q). *J Biol Chem* 2000;275:2157–2164.

13. Waldron RT, Rey O, Iglesias T, Tugal T, Cantrell D, Rozengurt E. Activation Loop Ser744 and Ser748 in Protein Kinase D Are Transphosphorylated in Vivo. *J Biol Chem* 2001;276:32606–32615.

14. Zhukova E, Sinnett-Smith J, Rozengurt E. Protein Kinase D Potentiates DNA Synthesis and Cell Proliferation Induced by Bombesin, Vasopressin, or Phorbol Esters in Swiss 3T3 Cells. *J Biol Chem* 2001;276:40298–40305.

15. Rey O, Sinnett-Smith J, Zhukova E, Rozengurt E. Regulated Nucleocytoplasmic Transport of Protein Kinase D in Response to G Protein-coupled Receptor Activation. *J Biol. Chem* 2001;276: 49228–49235.

16. Rozengurt E. Gastrointestinal Peptide Signaling through Tyrosine Phosphorylation of Focal Adhesion Proteins. *Am J Physiol* 1998;275:G177–G182.

17. Ilic D, Damsky CH, Yamamoto T. Focal adhesion kinase: at the crossroads of signal transduction. *J Cell Sci* 1997;110:401–407.

18. Rodríguez-Fernández JL and Rozengurt E. Bombesin, bradykinin, vasopressin, and phorbol esters rapidly and transiently activate Src family tyrosine kinases in Swiss 3T3 cells. Dissociation from tyrosine phosphorylation of p125 focal adhesion kinase. *J Biol Chem* 1996;271:27895–27901.

19. Carpenter G. Employment of the epidermal growth factor receptor in growth factor-independent signaling pathways. *J Cell Biol* 1999;146:697–702.

20. Schlaepfer DD, Hauck CR, Sieg DJ. Signaling through focal adhesion kinase. *Progress in Biophysics and Molecular Biology* 1999;71:435–478.

21. Salazar EP and Rozengurt E. Src Family Kinases Are Required for Integrin-mediated but Not for G Protein-coupled Receptor Stimulation of Focal Adhesion Kinase Autophosphorylation at Tyr-397. *J Biol Chem* 2001;276:17788–17795.

22. Owen JD, Ruest PJ, Fry DW, Hanks SK. Induced focal adhesion kinase (FAK) expression in FAK-null cells enhances cell spreading and migration requiring both auto- and activation loop phosphorylation sites and inhibits adhesion-dependent tyrosine phosphorylation of Pyk2. *Mol Cell Biol* 1999;19:4806–4818.

23. Salazar EP and Rozengurt E. Bombesin and platelet-derived growth factor induce association of endogenous focal adhesion kinase with Src in intact Swiss 3T3 cells. *J Biol Chem* 1999;274:28371–28378.

24. Burridge K and Chrzanowska-Wodnicka M. Focal adhesions, contractility, and signaling. *Ann Rev Cell Dev Biol* 1996;12:463–518.

25. Sinnett-Smith J, Zachary I, Valverde AM, Rozengurt E. Bombesin stimulation of p125 focal adhesion kinase tyrosine phosphorylation. Role of protein kinase C, Ca2+ mobilization, and the actin cytoskeleton. *J Biol Chem* 1993;268:14261–14268.

26. Lacerda HM, Pullinger GD, Lax AJ, Rozengurt E. Cytotoxic necrotizing factor 1 from Escherichia coli and dermonecrotic toxin from Bordetella bronchiseptica induce p21(rho)-dependent tyrosine phosphorylation of focal adhesion kinase and paxillin in Swiss 3T3 cells. *J Biol Chem* 1997;272: 9587–9596.

27. Thomas W, Pullinger GD, Lax AJ, Rozengurt E. Escherichia coli Cytotoxic Necrotizing Factor and Pasteurella multocida Toxin Induce Focal Adhesion Kinase Autophosphorylation and Src Association. *Infect Immun* 2001;69: 5931–5935.

28. Leopoldt D, Yee HF, Rozengurt E. Calyculin-A induces focal adhesion assembly and tyrosine phosphorylation of p125Fak, p130Cas, and paxillin in Swiss 3T3 cells. *J Cell Physiol* 2001;188:106–119.

29. Sinnett-Smith J, Lunn JA, Leopoldt D, Rozengurt E. Y-27632, an inhibitor of Rho-associated kinases, prevents tyrosine phosphorylation of focal adhesion kinase and paxillin induced by bombesin: Dissociation from tyrosine phosphorylation of p130cas. *Exp Cell Res* 2001;266:292–302.

30. Kozasa T, Jiang X, Hart MJ, Sternweis PM, Singer WD, Gilman AG, Bollag G, Sternweis PC. p115 RhoGEF, a GTPase activating protein for Galpha12 and Galpha13. *Science* 1998;280:2109–2111.

31. Hart MJ, Jiang X, Kozasa T, Roscoe W, Singer WD, Gilman AG, Sternweis PC, Bollag G. Direct stimulation of the guanine nucleotide exchange activity of p115RhoGEF by Galpha13. *Science* 1998;280:2112–2114.

32. Needham LK and Rozengurt E. G-alpha-12 and G-alpha-13 stimulate Rho-dependent tyrosine phosphorylation of focal adhesion kinase, paxillin, and p130 Crk-associated substrate. *J Biol Chem* 1998;273:14626–14632.

33. Yuan J, Slice LW, Rozengurt E. Activation of Protein Kinase D by Signaling through Rho and the alpha Subunit of the Heterotrimeric G Protein G13. *J Biol Chem* 2001;276:38619–38627.

34. Luttrell LM, Ferguson SSNG, Daaka Y, Miller WE, Maudsley S, Della Rocca GJ, Lin F-T, Kawakatsu H, Owada K, Luttrell DK, Caron MG, Lefkowitz RJ. Beta-Arrestin-Dependent Formation of 2 Adrenergic Receptor-Src Protein Kinase Complexes. *Science* 1999;283:655–661.

35. Cao W, Luttrell LM, Medvedev AV, Pierce KL, Daniel KW, Dixon TM, Lefkowitz RJ, Collins S. Direct Binding of Activated c-Src to the beta 3-Adrenergic Receptor Is Required for MAP Kinase Activation. *J Biol Chem* 2000;275:38131–38134.

36. Ma Y-C, Huang J, Ali S, Lowry W, Huang X-Y. Src tyrosine kinase is a novel direct effector of G proteins. *Cell* 2000;102:635–646.

37. Widmann C, Gibson S, Jarpe MB, Johnson GL. Mitogen-activated protein kinase: conservation of a three-kinase module from yeast to human. *Physiol Rev* 1999;79:143–180.

38. Cai H, Smola U, Wixler V, Eisenmann-Tappe I, Diaz-Meco MT, Moscat J, Rapp U, Cooper GM. Role of diacylglycerol-regulated protein kinase C isotypes in growth factor activation of the Raf-1 protein kinase. *Mol Cell Biol* 1997;17:732–741.

39. Marais R, Light Y, Mason C, Paterson H, Olson MF, Marshall CJ. Requirement of Ras-GTP-Raf complexes for activation of Raf-1 by protein kinase C. *Science* 1998;280:109–112.

40. Santiskulvong C, Sinnett-Smith J, Rozengurt E. EGF receptor function is required in late G(1) for cell cycle progression induced by bombesin and bradykinin. *Amer J Physiol-Cell Physiol* 2001;281: C886–C898.

41. Seufferlein T, Withers DJ, Rozengurt E. Reduced requirement of mitogen-activated protein kinase (MAPK) activity for entry into the S phase of the cell cycle in Swiss 3T3 fibroblasts stimulated by bombesin and insulin. *J Biol Chem* 1996;271:21471–21477.

42. Withers DJ, Seufferlein T, Mann D, Garcia, B, Jones N, Rozengurt E. Rapamycin dissociates p70(S6K) activation from DNA synthesis stimulated by bombesin and insulin in Swiss 3T3 cells. *J Biol Chem* 1997;272:2509–2514.

43. Mann DJ, Higgins T, Jones NC, Rozengurt E. Differential control of cyclins D1 and D3 and the cdk inhibitor p27Kip1 by diverse signalling pathways in Swiss 3T3 cells. *Oncogene* 1997;14:1759–1766.

44. Wu SV, Rozengurt N, Yang M, Young SH, Sinnett-Smith J, Rozengurt E. Expression of bitter taste receptors of the T2R family in the gastrointestinal tract and enteroendocrine STC-1 cells. *Proc Natl Acad Sci USA* 2002;99:2392–2397.

Gut-Brain Peptides in the New Millennium, edited by Y. Taché
CURE Foundation, Los Angeles, CA. © 2002

18

Gastrin Releasing Peptide-dependent Cyclooxygenase-2 Expression in Fibroblasts

Lee W. Slice
CURE/Digestive Diseases Research Center, UCLA Division of Digestive Diseases
Department of Medicine and VA Greater Los Angeles Healthcare System
Los Angeles, CA

INTRODUCTION

Prostaglandins play a pivotal role in a broad range of physiological and pathological processes including inflammation, pain transmission, maintenance of gastrointestinal integrity, and progression of colorectal cancer (1–4). The rate-limiting enzymes for production of prostaglandins are cyclooxygenases (COX) type 1 and 2 (5–7). COX-1 is constitutively expressed in cells, whereas COX-2 expression is induced as an immediate-early gene in response to pro-inflammatory cytokines, tumor promoters, and growth factors (8–11). COX-2 is over-expressed in cancers of the colon, stomach, and breast (12–15), and chronic inhibition of COX activity has been associated with chemopreventive effects on colon cancer (16–19). Recent studies have shown COX-2 expression in stromal fibroblasts of human and rodent colorectal carcinomas (20), suggesting the possible role of bioactive prostaglandins in promoting tumor growth by a "Landscaping Effect" (21). One study showed the growth of a lung cancer cell line was attenuated if xenographed onto $COX2^{-/-}$ versus wild-type control mice (22) highlighting the important role played by COX-2 expression in fibroblasts within the microenvironment of a tumor.

Previous studies in fibroblasts showed the induction of COX-2 expression by epidermal growth factor (EGF), forskolin, serum, and platlet-derived growth factor (PDGF) (23, 24). Transcriptional activation of the COX-2 promoter can be induced by tyrosine kinase receptors, G-protein coupled receptors and is activated by a large number of distinct signaling pathways mediated by protein kinase A (PKA), protein kinase C (PKC), and mitogen-activated protein kinase MAPK (25). Here, we demonstrate COX-2 expression in fibroblasts induced by the gastrin releasing peptide (GRP) receptor, through a novel, Rho-dependent signaling pathway.

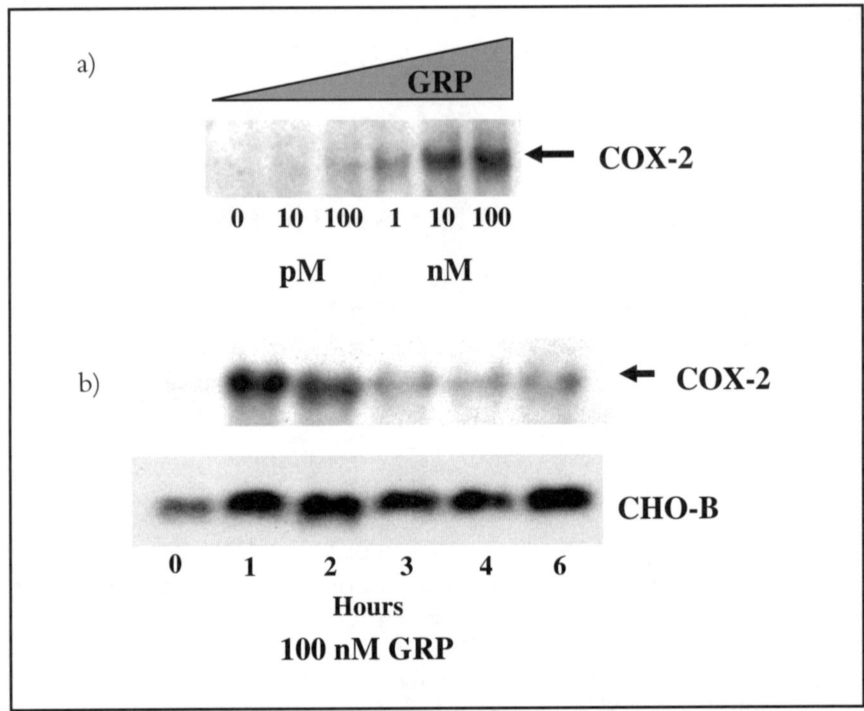

FIGURE 1. *GRP-dependent expression of COX-2 mRNA. (a) Confluent, serum-starved Swiss 3T3 cells were treated with increasing amounts of GRP for 1 h and the RNA analyzed by Northern blot using murine COX-2 cDNA as a probe. (b) Swiss 3T3 cells were treated with GRP (100 nM) for up to 6 h and the RNA analyzed by Northern blot. The Northern blot was re-screened with a probe for CHOB.*

METHODS

Cell Line and Transfection

Swiss 3T3 and NIH 3T3 cells were cultured in Dulbecco's modified Eagles' medium (DMEM) supplemented with 10% fetal bovine serum, 2.92 mg/ml of L-glutamine, 1000 U/ml of penicillin G and streptomycin at 37°C, 5% CO_2. NIH 3T3 cells were transfected using Superfect (Qiagen) as described (26).

Expression and Reporter Plasmids

The COX-2 reporter plasmids, pTIS-10L, pTIS-10s, pTIS-10(-80) and pTIS-10(-40) encodes the luciferase cDNA under the control of the murine COX-2 promoter, −963/+70, −371/+70, −80/+3, and −40/+3, respectively. The pTIS-10sCRE★ and pTIS-10(-80)CRE★ are the CRE/ATF sites mutated (27). The −300, −250, −200, and −150 COX-2 reporter plasmids were produced by PCR such that the luciferase cDNA was under the control of the proximal COX-2 promoter truncated at −300/+3, −250/+3, −200/+3, and −150/+3, respectively. The expression vectors for v-src and C3 toxin were provided by H. Herschman (UCLA) and R. Treisman (ICRF), respectively. The expression plasmid for lbc-no DH was provided by D. Toksoz (Tufts University).

Northern Blot and Western Blot Analysis

Swiss 3T3 cells were treated with GRP and then RNA isolated as described (28). The RNA was size separated by electrophoresis and then transferred to nylon membranes. Murine cDNA's for COX-2, GAPDH, and CHOb were radiolabeled using ^{32}P and used as probes (28).

Protein extracts from treated Swiss 3T3 cells were size separated using SDS polyacrylamide electrophoresis and then electrotransferred onto PVDF membranes. An anti-COX-2 antibody and ECL were used to detect the COX-2 protein (28).

Statistical Analysis

Results are reported as the mean ± standard error from at least 3 independent experiments. Differences were analyzed by one way analysis of variance and the Student-Newman-Kuel's test with $P < 0.05$ considered to be significant.

RESULTS AND DISCUSSION

Induction of COX-2 mRNA by GRP

GRP induced the production of COX-2 mRNA in Swiss 3T3 fibroblasts (Figure 1). COX-2 mRNA induction was dose dependent, with an EC_{50} of 1 nM GRP. The induction of COX-2 mRNA was transient with a maximal induction level after 1 h of GRP exposure followed by reduction of COX-2 mRNA (Figure 1b). Pretreatment with either cycloheximide (70 μM, 30 m) or pertussis toxin (100 ng/ml, 18 h) prior to induction with GRP did not block the COX-2 mRNA induction (data not shown). This indicates that GRP induces COX-2 mRNA as an immediate/early gene without *de novo* protein synthesis. COX-2 mRNA induction in perussis toxin treated cells indicates that induction by the GRP receptor is not through Gi.

Induction of COX-2 Protein by GRP

Untreated Swiss 3T3 cells did not show detectable amounts of COX-2 protein and required GRP concentrations greater than 1 nM for detectable levels

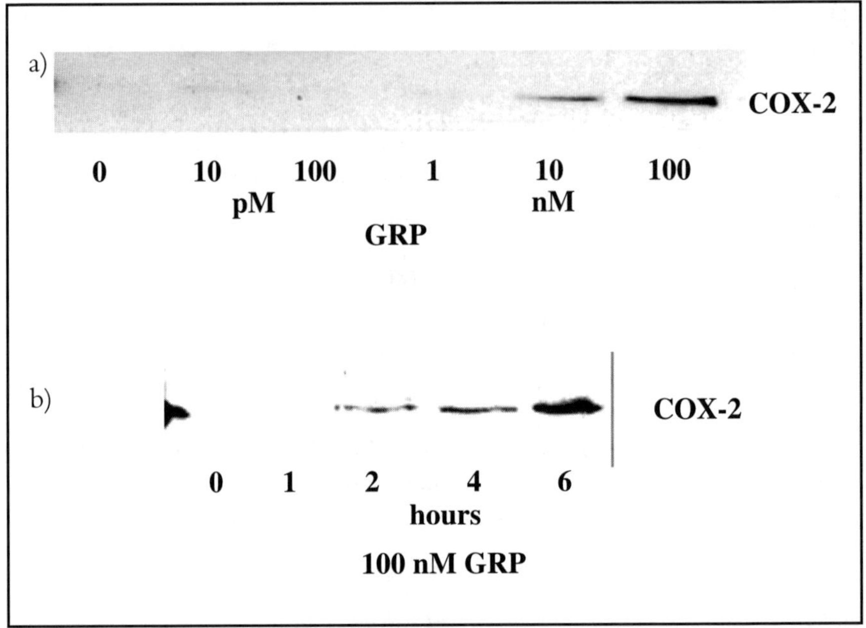

FIGURE 2. *GRP-dependent expression of COX-2 protein. (a) Confluent, serum-starved Swiss 3T3 cells were treated with increasing amounts of GRP for 18 h. The proteins were analyzed by Western blot using anti-COX-2 antibody. (b) Swiss 3T3 cells were treated with GRP (100 nM) for the indicated times and the proteins analyzed by Western blot.*

of proteins to appear (Figure 2a). GRP caused detectable levels of COX-2 protein after 2 h with levels increasing up to 6 h (Figure 2b). This demonstrates that the induction of COX-2 mRNA leads to increased expression of COX-2 protein.

Induction of the COX-2 Promoter by GRP

To determine whether GRP can regulate the COX-2 promoter, NIH 3T3 cells were co-transfected with a reporter plasmid in which the production of luciferase is driven by the murine COX-2 promoter (Figure 3) and an expression vector encoding the rat GRP receptor. GRP (100 nM, 5 h) induced luciferase expression by over 4-fold in transfected cells (Figure 4a). Luciferase induction was dependent on co-transfection of the GRP receptor expression vector indicating that the NIH 3T3 cells did not express indigenous receptors for GRP.

The COX-2 promoter contains several cis-acting promoter elements that respond to multiple signal transduction pathways (29–32). Platelet-derived growth factor, serum, v-src, MEKK, and p38 MAPK promote COX-2 expression through Ras and Rac-mediated increases in extracellular signal-

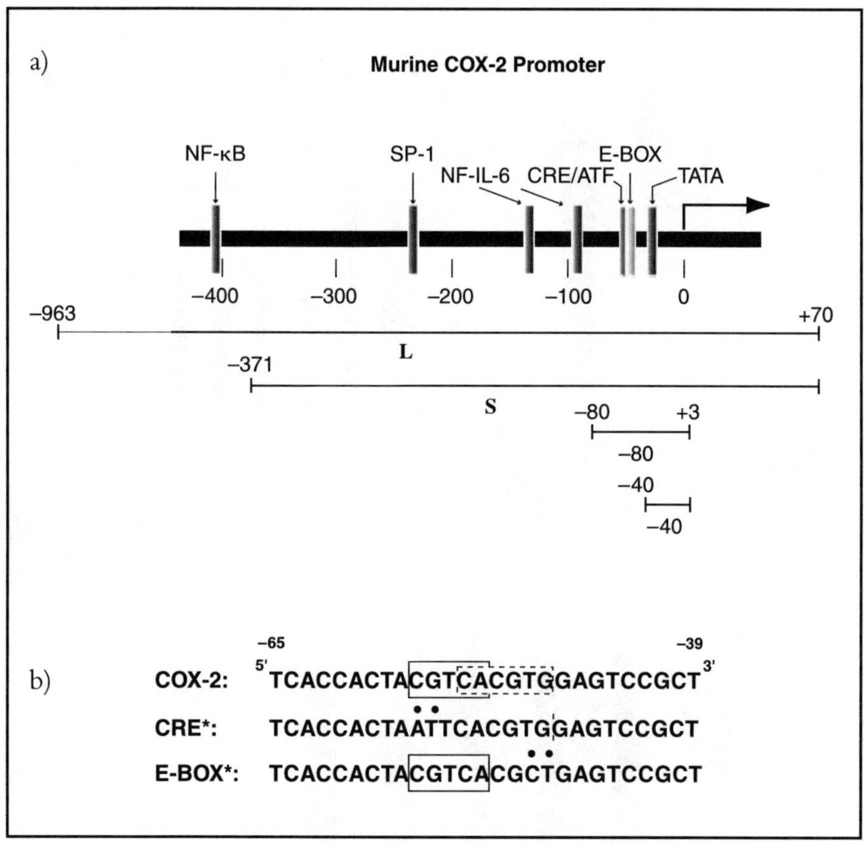

FIGURE 3. *COX-2 promoter and CRE and E-box mutations. (a) The murine COX-2 promoter contains several cis-acting transcriptional elements including NF-κB at −402, CRE/ATF at −56, and E-box at −53. The series of COX-2 promoter plasmids containing progressive 5′ truncation are shown. (b) The CRE consensus site (rec. box, solid lines) was mutated by converting $C^{-56}G^{-55}$ to $A^{-56}T^{-55}$. The E-box consensus site (rec. box, dashed lines) was mutated by converting $T^{-49}G^{-48}$ to $C^{-49}T^{-48}$.*

related kinase and c-Jun NH_2-terminal kinase pathways in NIH 3T3 cells (33–36). Agonists that signal through cAMP induce COX-2 expression through cAMP response element binding transcription factor (37). These pathways converge onto a common regulatory region, the CRE/ATF response element located between −56 to −48 of the murine COX-2 promoter (Figure 3). Progressive 5′ deletion of the COX-2 promoter revealed two regions that are responsive to GRP. The pTIS-10s reporter vector (which corresponds to −371) and the -963 reporter vector showed to highest level of luciferase induction by GRP (Figure 4b). Removal of 5′ nucleotides to −300 of the COX-2 promoter decreased the level of GRP induction to just over 2-fold. GRP induction was lost when the COX-2

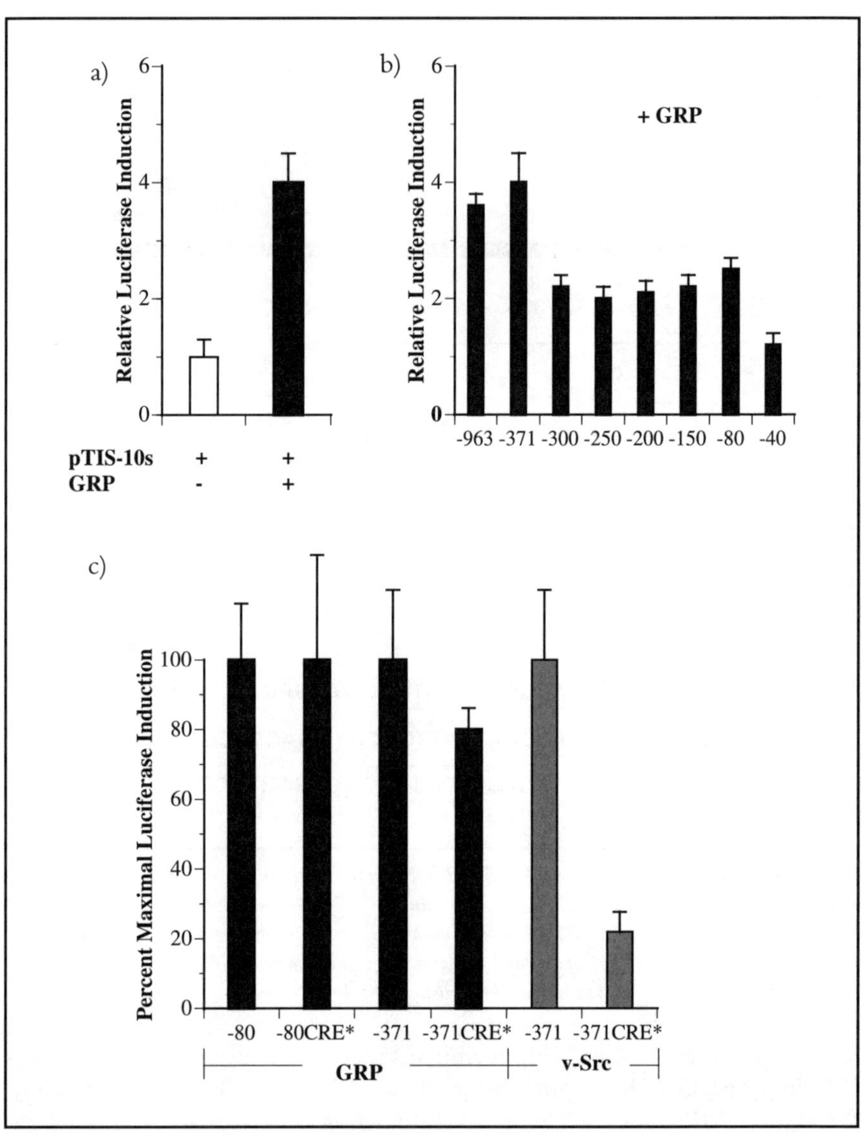

FIGURE 4. *(a) Transcriptional Activation of the COX-2 Promoter by GRP. NIH 3T3 cells were co-transfected with the GRP receptor expression vector and the COX-2 promoter reporter plasmid, pTIS-10s (−371). Cells were treated with GRP (100 nM, 5 h). Luciferase activity was measured. (b) NIH 3T3 cells were co-transfected with the GRP receptor expression vector and COX-2 reporter plasmids containing 5′ deletions from the proximal promoter region. Luciferase was induced by GRP (100 nM, 5 h). (c) NIH 3T3 cells were co-transfected with the GRP receptor expression vector and COX-2 reporter plasmids containing the COX-2 promoter (starting at −371 or −80). A second set of transfections used COX-2 reporter plasmids containing mutations in the CRE site. These cells were induced with GRP (100 nM, 5 h). Control cells were co-transfected with an expression vector encoding v-src.*

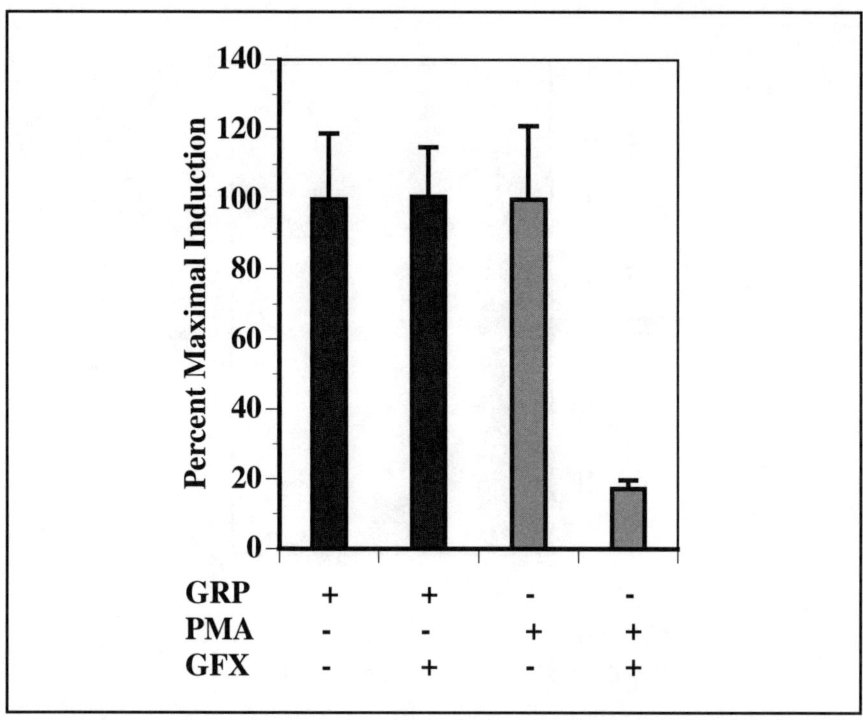

FIGURE 5. *Transcriptional Activation of the COX-2 Promoter by GRP is independent of Protein Kinase C Activity. NIH 3T3 cells were co-transfected with the GRP receptor expression vector and the COX-2 (−371) reporter plasmid. Cells were induced with either GRP (100 nM, 5 h) or PMA (200 nM, 5 h). Protein kinase C activity was inhibited in cells that were pretreated for 30 m with GFX (1 µM).*

promoter was truncated to position −40. This suggests that there are two regions of the proximal COX-2 promoter (−371 to −300, and −80 to −40) contain elements that are responsive to GRP.

To determine whether the GRP receptor signals through the CRE/ATF element on the COX-2 promoter, mutations were made in the CRE/ATF element in the −371 and −80 reporter vectors (Figure 3b). The CRE element was not required for GRP induction (Figure 4c) for either the −371 or −80 COX-2 reporter plasmid. Induction by v-src was inhibited by the CRE mutation. These results suggest a novel signaling pathway used by the GRP receptor to induce the COX-2 promoter.

COX-2 Promoter Induction by GRP Is Independent of PKC Activity

The GRP receptor is coupled to the Gq family of heterotrimeric G-proteins (38). Because protein kinase C activation induces COX-2 expression

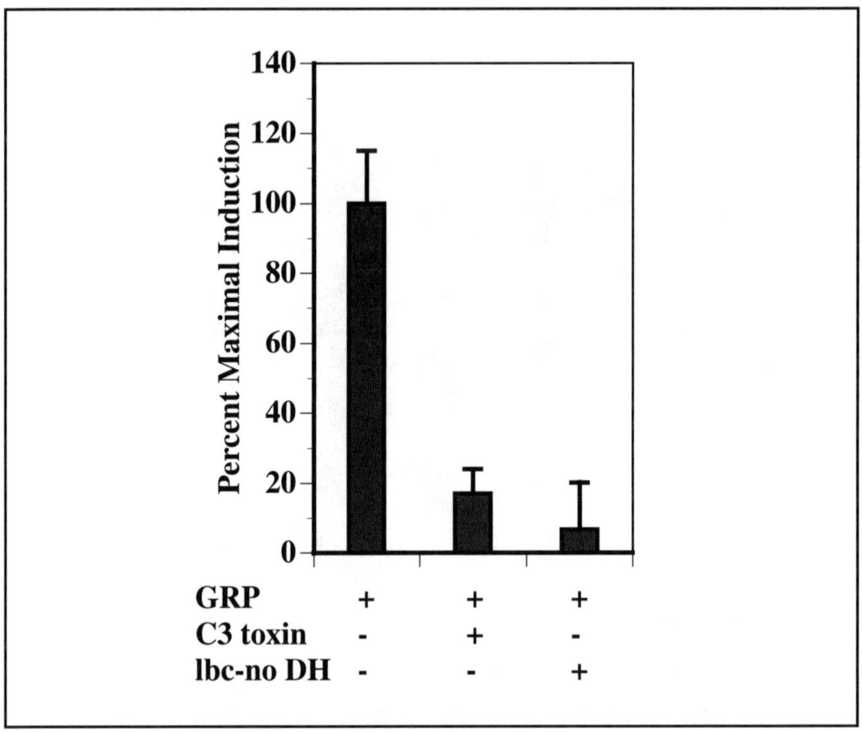

FIGURE 6. *Transcriptional Activation of the COX-2 Promoter by GRP is dependent on Rho. NIH 3T3 cells were co-transfected with the GRP receptor expression vector and the COX-2 (−371) reporter plasmid with and without the expression vectors encoding C3 toxin or lbc-no DH. Cells were induced with GRP (100 nM, 5 h) and then luciferase activity was measured.*

(39), it is expected that $G\alpha q$, which activates phospholipase $C\beta$ and thereby the production of inositol 1,4,5-trisphosphate, which mobilizes Ca^{2+} from internal stores, and diacylglycerol, which activates protein kinase C, contributes to COX-2 transcriptional activation. Surprisingly, inhibition of protein kinase C activity using bisindolylmaleimide (GFX) did not inhibit COX-2 promoter activation by GRP (Figure 5). Activation of the COX-2 promoter by PMA was blocked by GFX. This indicates that the primary signaling pathway used by the GRP receptor to induce transcription of the COX-2 promoter is not through protein kinase C.

Rho-dependent Transcriptional Activation of the COX-2 Promoter by GRP

It has been demonstrated that in fibroblasts, the GRP receptor activates Rho (40) and that Rho induces gene transcription via the serum response element (SRE) by activation of the serum response factor (SRF) that is independent of signaling by Ras and Rac. To determine whether activation of the COX-2 promoter by the GRP receptor is Rho-dependent, NIH 3T3 cells were co-transfected with the expression vector for *Clostridium botulinum* C3 toxin, which specifically ADP-ribosylates Rho at residue 41 and impairs its function (41). C3 toxin inhibited GRP-induction of the COX-2 promoter (Figure 6). C3 toxin did not inhibit cAMP mediated induction of the COX-2 promoter by forksolin in transfected NIH 3T3 cells (26). Next, a dominant negative form of the specific Rho-GEF, lbc (42, 43), lbc-no DH was expressed in transfected NIH 3T3 cells. Lbc-no DH also inhibited GRP induction of the COX-2 promoter. These results delineate a novel, Rho-dependent signaling pathway that is used by the GRP receptor that leads to transcriptional activation of the COX-2 promoter.

CONCLUDING REMARKS

We have identified a novel, Rho-dependent signaling pathway, initiated by the GRP receptor that rapidly induces the COX-2 promoter in fibroblasts. The *cis*-acting elements on the COX-2 promoter have been mapped to two regions (−371 to −300 and −80 to −40). The nucleotide sequence within these regions do not have apparent homology to other known *cis*-acting elements including the Rho responsive SRF element. The CRE/ATF element which is critical for promoter induction by Ras and Rac signaling is not required for GRP receptor mediated induction of the COX-2 promoter.

It is likely that induction of COX-2 occurs by the action of other agonists that active G-protein coupled receptors that induce Rho activity in fibroblasts. Given the increasing evidence that COX-2 expression in the stroma plays a role in the progression of colorectal cancer, it is important to understand the regulation of COX-2 expression in fibroblasts by agonists that active Rho.

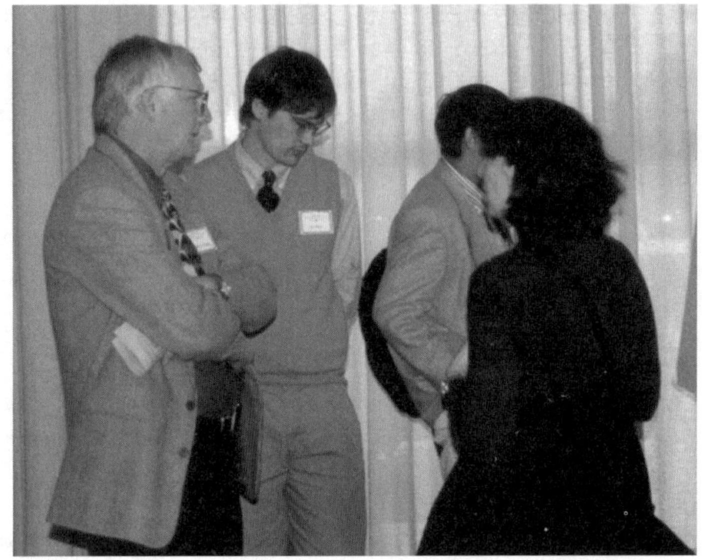

Drs. John Walsh and Lee Slice at the CURE Annual Meeting, 1997.

ACKNOWLEDGMENTS

I thank Dr. John Walsh for his mentorship and his scientific leadership at CURE. I also thank Dr. Enrique Rozengurt (UCLA) for his support and encouragement especially after Dr. Walsh's death.

REFERENCES

1. Anderson GD, Hauser SD, McGarity KL, Bremer ME, Isakson PC, Gregory SA. Selective inhibition of cyclooxygenase (COX)-2 reverses inflammation and expression of COX-2 and interleukin 6 in rat adjuvant arthritis. *J Clin Invest* 1996;97:2672–9.
2. Boolbol SK, Dannenberg AJ, Chadburn A, Martucci C, Guo XJ, Ramonetti JT, Abreu-Goris M, Newmark HL, Lipkin ML, DeCosse JJ, Bertagnolli MM. Cyclooxygenase-2 overexpression and tumor formation are blocked by sulindac in a murine model of familial adenomatous polyposis. *Cancer Res* 1996;56:2556–60.
3. DuBois RN, Eberhart CF, Williams CS. Introduction to eicosanoids and the gastroenteric tract. *Gastroenterol Clin North Am* 1996;25:267–77.
4. DuBois RN, Radhika A, Reddy BS, Entingh AJ. Increased cyclooxygenase-2 levels in carcinogen-induced rat colonic tumors. *Gastroenterology* 1996;110:1259–62.
5. Crofford LJ. COX-1 and COX-2 tissue expression: implications and predictions. *J Rheumatol* 1997;24 Suppl 49:15–9.
6. Herschman HR. Prostaglandin synthase 2. *Biochim Biophys Acta* 1996;1299:125–40.
7. Smith WL, Dewitt DL. Prostaglandin endoperoxide H synthases-1 and -2. *Adv Immunol* 1996;62:167–215.
8. Fletcher BS, Lim RW, Varnum BC, Kujubu DA, Koski RA, Herschman HR. Structure and expression of TIS21, a primary response gene induced by growth factors and tumor promoters. *J Biol Chem* 1991;266:14511–8.

9. Fletcher BS, Kujubu DA, Perrin DM, Herschman HR. Structure of the mitogen-inducible TIS10 gene and demonstration that the TIS10-encoded protein is a functional prostaglandin G/H synthase. *J Biol Chem* 1992;267:4338–44.

10. DeWitt DL, Kraemer SA, Meade EA. Serum induction and superinduction of PGG/H synthase mRNA levels in 3T3 fibroblasts. *Adv Prostaglandin Thromboxane Leukot Res* 1991;21A:65–8.

11. DuBois RN, Awad J, Morrow J, Roberts LJN, Bishop PR. Regulation of eicosanoid production and mitogenesis in rat intestinal epithelial cells by transforming growth factor-alpha and phorbol ester. *J Clin Invest* 1994;93:493–8.

12. Subbaramaiah K, Telang N, Ramonetti JT, Araki R, DeVito B, Weksler BB, Dannenberg AJ. Transcription of cyclooxygenase-2 is enhanced in transformed mammary epithelial cells. *Cancer Res* 1996;56:4424–9.

13. Tsuji S, Kawano S, Sawaoka H, Takei Y, Kobayashi I, Nagano K, Fusamoto H, Kamada T. Evidences for involvement of cyclooxygenase-2 in proliferation of two gastrointestinal cancer cell lines. *Prostaglandins Leukot Essent Fatty Acids* 1996;55:179–83.

14. Tsujii M, Kawano S, DuBois RN. Cyclooxygenase-2 expression in human colon cancer cells increases metastatic potential. *Proc Natl Acad Sci USA* 1997;94:3336–40.

15. Ristimaki A, Honkanen N, Jankala H, Sipponen P, Harkonen M. Expression of cyclooxygenase-2 in human gastric carcinoma. *Cancer Res* 1997;57:1276–80.

16. Ligumsky M, Grossman MI, Kauffman GL, Jr. Endogenous gastric mucosal prostaglandins: their role in mucosal integrity. *Am J Physiol* 1982;242:G337–41.

17. Subbaramaiah K, Zakim D, Weksler BB, Dannenberg AJ. Inhibition of cyclooxygenase: a novel approach to cancer prevention. *Proc Soc Exp Biol Med* 1997;216:201–10.

18. Kawamori T, Rao CV, Seibert K, Reddy BS. Chemopreventive activity of celecoxib, a specific cyclooxygenase-2 inhibitor, against colon carcinogenesis. *Cancer Res* 1998;58:409–12.

19. Masferrer JL, Leahy KM, Koki AT, Zweifel BS, Settle SL, Woerner BM, Edwards DA, Flickinger AG, Moore RJ, Seibert K. Antiangiogenic and antitumor activities of cyclooxygenase-2 inhibitors. *Cancer Res* 2000;60:1306–11.

20. Shattuck-Brandt RL, Varilek GW, Radhika A, Yang F, Washington MK, DuBois RN. Cyclooxygenase 2 expression is increased in the stroma of colon carcinomas from IL-10(–/–) mice. *Gastroenterology* 2000;118:337–45.

21. Kinzler KW, Vogelstein B. Landscaping the cancer terrain. *Science* 1998;280:1036–7.

22. Williams CS, Tsujii M, Reese J, Dey SK, DuBois RN. Host cyclooxygenase-2 modulates carcinoma growth. *J Clin Invest* 2000;105:1589–94.

23. Yamagata K, Andreasson KI, Kaufmann WE, Barnes CA, Worley PF. Expression of a mitogen-inducible cyclooxygenase in brain neurons: regulation by synaptic activity and glucocorticoids. *Neuron* 1993;11:371–86.

24. Ryseck RP, Raynoschek C, Macdonald-Bravo H, Dorfman K, Mattei MG, Bravo R. Identification of an immediate early gene, pghs-B, whose protein product has prostaglandin synthase/cyclooxygenase activity. *Cell Growth Differ* 1992;3:443–50.

25. Herschman HR. Function and regulation of prostaglandin synthase 2. *Adv Exp Med Biol* 1999;469:3–8.

26. Slice LW, Walsh JH, Rozengurt E. Galpha(13) stimulates Rho-dependent activation of the cyclooxygenase-2 promoter. *J Biol Chem* 1999;274:27562–6.

27. Slice LW, Bui L, Mak C, Walsh JH. Differential regulation of COX-2 transcription by Ras- and Rho-family of GTPases. *Biochem Biophys Res Commun* 2000;276:406–10.

28. Hecht JR, Duque J, Reddy ST, Herschman HR, Walsh JH, Slice LW. Gastrin-releasing peptide-induced expression of prostaglandin synthase-2 in Swiss 3T3 cells. *Prostaglandins* 1997;54:757–68.

29. Dean JL, Brook M, Clark AR, Saklatvala J. p38 mitogen-activated protein kinase regulates cyclooxygenase-2 mRNA stability and transcription in lipopolysaccharide-treated human monocytes. *J Biol Chem* 1999;274:264–9.

30. DuBois RN, Tsujii M, Bishop P, Awad JA, Makita K, Lanahan A. Cloning and characterization of a growth factor-inducible cyclooxygenase gene from rat intestinal epithelial cells. *Am J Physiol* 1994;266:G822–7.

31. Kim Y, Fischer SM. Transcriptional regulation of cyclooxygenase-2 in mouse skin carcinoma cells. Regulatory role of CCAAT/enhancer-binding proteins in the differential expression of cyclooxygenase-2 in normal and neoplastic tissues. *J Biol Chem* 1998;273:27686–94.

32. Morris JK, Richards JS. An E-box region within the prostaglandin endoperoxide synthase-2 (PGS-2) promoter is required for transcription in rat ovarian granulosa cells. *J Biol Chem* 1996;271:16633–43.

33. Montaner S, Perona R, Saniger L, Lacal JC. Multiple signalling pathways lead to the activation of the nuclear factor kappaB by the Rho family of GTPases. *J Biol Chem* 1998;273:12779–85.

34. Xie W, Fletcher BS, Andersen RD, Herschman HR. v-src induction of the TIS10/PGS2 prostaglandin synthase gene is mediated by an ATF/CRE transcription response element. *Mol Cell Biol* 1994;14:6531–9.

35. Xie W, Herschman HR. v-src induces prostaglandin synthase 2 gene expression by activation of the c-Jun N-terminal kinase and the c-Jun transcription factor. *J Biol Chem* 1995;270:27622–8.

36. Xie W, Herschman HR. Transcriptional regulation of prostaglandin synthase 2 gene expression by platelet-derived growth factor and serum. *J Biol Chem* 1996;271:31742–8.

37. Miller C, Zhang M, He Y, Zhao J, Pelletier JP, Martel-Pelletier J, Di Battista JA. Transcriptional induction of cyclooxygenase-2 gene by okadaic acid inhibition of phosphatase activity in human chondrocytes: co-stimulation of AP-1 and CRE nuclear binding proteins. *J Cell Biochem* 1998;69: 392–413.

38. Rozengurt E. Signal transduction pathways in the mitogenic response to G protein-coupled neuropeptide receptor agonists. *J Cell Physiol* 1998;177:507–17.

39. Herschman HR, Kujubu DA, Fletcher BS, Ma Q, Varnum BC, Gilbert RS, Reddy ST. The tis genes, primary response genes induced by growth factors and tumor promoters in 3T3 cells. *Prog Nucleic Acid Res Mol Biol* 1994;47:113–48.

40. Nobes CD, Hawkins P, Stephens L, Hall A. Activation of the small GTP-binding proteins rho and rac by growth factor receptors. *J Cell Sci* 1995;108 (Pt 1):225–33.

41. Hill CS, Wynne J, Treisman R. The Rho family GTPases RhoA, Rac1, and CDC42Hs regulate transcriptional activation by SRF. *Cell* 1995;81:1159–70.

42. Olson MF, Sterpetti P, Nagata K, Toksoz D, Hall A. Distinct roles for DH and PH domains in the Lbc oncogene. *Oncogene* 1997;15:2827–31.

43. Sterpetti P, Hack AA, Bashar MP, Park B, Cheng SD, Knoll JH, Urano T, Feig LA, Toksoz D. Activation of the Lbc Rho exchange factor proto-oncogene by truncation of an extended C terminus that regulates transformation and targeting. *Mol Cell Biol* 1999;19:1334–45.

Gut-Brain Peptides in the New Millennium, edited by Y. Taché
CURE Foundation, Los Angeles, CA. © 2002

19

Inhibition of Forskolin and PGE$_2$-dependent Increases in cAMP by Galanin Receptor 1 in Transfected Epithelial Cells

Helen Wong, John H. Walsh, and Lee W. Slice
*CURE/Digestive Diseases Research Center, UCLA Division of Digestive Diseases
Department of Medicine and VA Greater Los Angeles Healthcare System
Los Angeles, CA*

INTRODUCTION

Galanin is a 29 or 30 amino acids long neuroendocrine peptide that was originally isolated from porcine upper intestine (1), but is found throughout the GI tract (2) and the peripheral and central nervous system (3). In the central nervous system, galanin acts to stimulate fat intake (4) and impair cognitive performance (5); whereas in the GI tract, galanin modulates motility (6), pancreatic exocrine and endocrine secretions (7, 8) and inhibits acid secretion (9, 11).

Galanin acts through specific cell surface receptors. Three subtypes of human and rat galanin receptors have been cloned, denoted as Gal R1, Gal R2, and Gal R3 (12–14). All three Gal R's are G-protein coupled receptors (GPCR). Gal R1, the most widely expressed galanin receptor is coupled to G_I (15) and has been shown to inhibit agonist stimulated release of histamine in ECL cells in the stomach (10). In order to facilitate our studies of the inhibition of cell signaling by Gal R1, we expressed rat Gal R1 in transfected KNRK cells and determined the effects of galanin on forskolin and PGE$_2$ stimulated cAMP levels in these cells.

METHODS

Cell Line and Transfection

KNRK cells were cultured in Dulbecco's modified Eagles' medium (DMEM) supplemented with 10% fetal bovine serum, 2.92 mg/ml of L-glutamine, 1000 U/ml of penicillin G and streptomycin at 37°C, 5% CO$_2$. Cells were

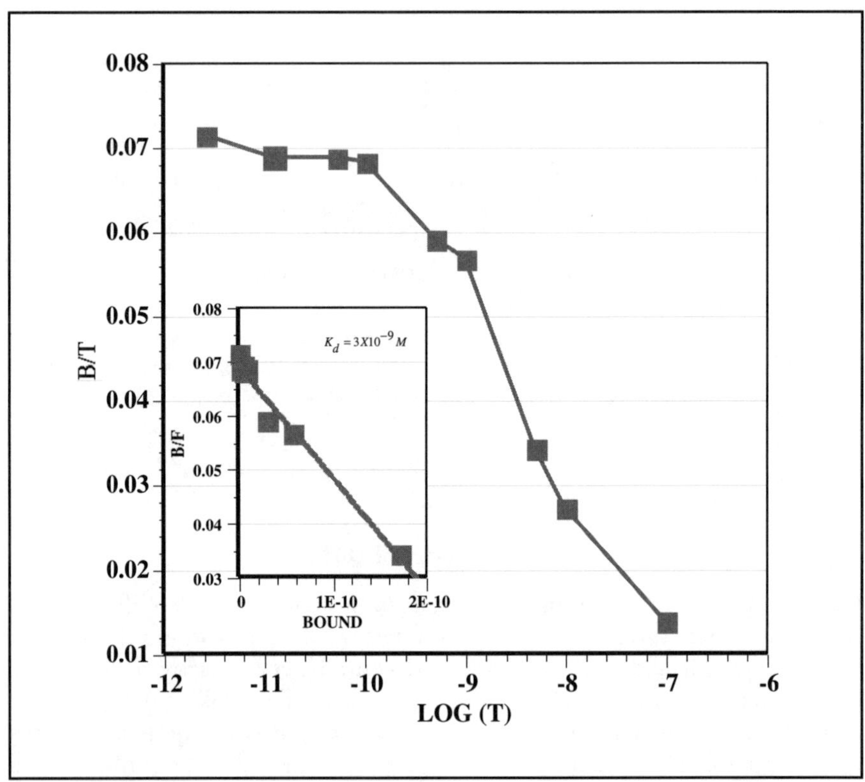

FIGURE 1. *Scatchard Analysis of Galanin Binding. Radiolabeled galanin was bound to transfected KNRK cells expressing the Gal R1. Unlabeled galanin was able to compete for binding indicting a Kd of 3 nM with an average of 500,000 receptors per cell.*

transfected with pcDNA-3 encoding the rat Galanin receptor 1 (provided by Bristol-Myers Squibb Pharmaceutical Research Institute, Wallingford, CT) using Transfectam (Promega Corp.). Cells were grown for two weeks in media containing G418 (400 µg/ml) and then clonally selected.

Binding Assays, Internalization Assays, and cAMP Analysis

Galanin was labeled with ^{125}I by the lactose peroxidase method followed by HPLC. Cells were incubated (4°C, 1 hr) with 1 nM of ^{125}I-galanin in the presence of increasing amounts of cold competitor peptide.

For internalization assays, cells were grown on 12-well plates. Cells were incubated with 200,000 cpm of ^{125}I-galanin in 0.5 ml per well (4°C, 1 hr). The temperature was increased to 37°C for 10–30 minutes prior to washing with PBS, 0.1 % BSA. Surface bound galanin was collected by incubating cells in 0.5 M KSCN (0.5 ml, 4°C, 10 min). The cell associated galanin was collected by lysing the cells in 0.1% SDS (0.5 ml). Each fraction was counted for radioactivity. Each condition was done in triplicate.

Radioimmunoassay was used to measure cAMP according to manufacturers instructions using Biotrak cellular communication assay for cAMP (Amersham Life Science, RPA 509).

Gal R1 Specific Antibody

Polyclonal antibodies were produced in rabbits using standard procedures that were developed at the CURE Antibody Core (9). Ab #96202 was made using a synthetic peptide to the third intracellular loop (225–238) of the Gal R1 (YLHKKLKNMSKKSEA) as the antigen.

RESULTS AND DISCUSSION

Specific Galanin Binding to Transfected KNRK Cells

Scatchard analysis demonstrated that galanin specifically bound to clonally selected KNRK cells expressing rat Gal R1 with a K_d of 3 nM (Figure 1) and an average of 500,000 receptors per cell. Galanin binding could not be displaced by non-competitive peptides such as gastrin-17, CCK-8, SS-14, VIP, GRP, secretin, CGRP or PACAP.

Galanin Receptor Specific Antibody

The presence of the recombinant Gal R1 could also be detected by western blot analysis using a polyclonal antibody specific to the Gal R1 (Figure 2). Antibody #96202 was targeted to the third intracellular loop of the rat Gal R1. A synthetic peptide (residues 225 to 238 of the Gal R1) was used as the antigen. An immunoreactive band corresponding to 70 kD was detected in protein extracts from KNRK cells transfected with the rat Gal R1 expression vector but not in non-transfected KNRK cells. Ab #96202 was specific for the Gal R1 because pre-absorption using the antigenic peptide abolished the immunoreactive band. A positive signal on the western blot and the specific binding of labeled galanin demonstrate the expression of the recombinant Gal R1 in the KNRK cells.

Galanin Internalization in Transfected KNRK Cells

Fluorescent Cy3-galanin binds to the surface of KNRK cells that are expressing the Gal R1 (Figure 3a). Warming the cells to 37°C from 4°C, initiates internalization of bound galanin. By 30 minutes, the internalized

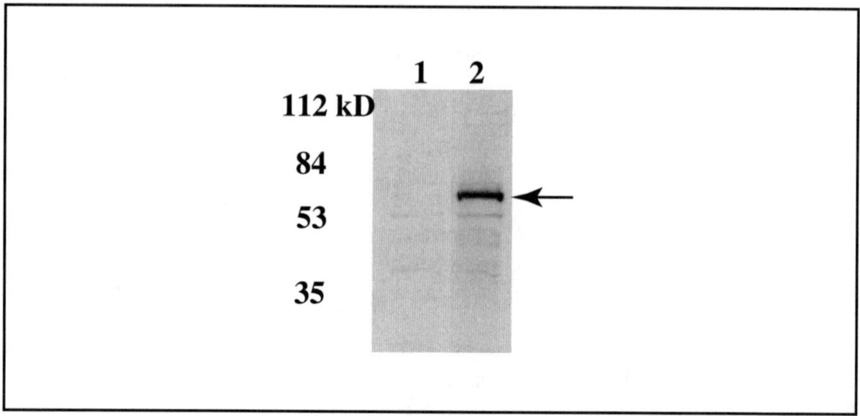

FIGURE 2. *Galanin Receptor Specific Antibodies. Proteins from transfected KNRK cells (25 μg) were size separate using PAGE and then electroblotted onto PVDF paper. Ab #96202 was using (1:3000 dilution) to detect the expressed Gal R1 (lane 2, arrow). The antibody was specific to Gal R1 because pre-incubation with the antigenic peptide eliminated the immunoreactive band (lane 1).*

galanin has accumulated into perinuclear locations. This process requires galanin binding to the Gal R1 because no internalization is present either in non-transfected KNRK cells or in KNRK cells expressing Gal R1 in the presence of saturating amounts of non-fluorescent galanin (data not shown). This is consistent with the current model of initiation of Gal R1 internalization into early endosomes by the binding of galanin at the cell surface. The Gal R1-galanin complex contained in early endosomes continues on to late endosomal compartments. The fluorescent signal accumulates in perinuclear compartments that could correspond to lysosomes. It is unknown whether the Gal R1 is also present in the lysosomes or has been previously sorted away from the internalized galanin.

Clathrin-dependent Internalization of Galanin

Internalization of galanin by the Gal R1 is mediated by clathrin-coat formation but not by Protein Kinase C (PKC). Internalization of ^{125}I-labeled galanin occurs rapidly at 37°C, reaching a plateau after 20 minutes (Figure 3b). Activation of PKC by treatment with phorbol 12-myristate-13-acetate (PMA) did not affect galanin internalization. Inhibition of PKC activity using bisindolylmaleimide also did not affect galanin internalization. Disruption of clathrin-coat formation did inhibit galanin internalization. Pretreatment of cells with hyperosmotic sucrose (16) or phenylarsine oxide (PAO) (17), or potassium depletion (18) of the cells blocks clathrin-coat formation and endocytosis via clathrin-coated pits. Galanin internalization

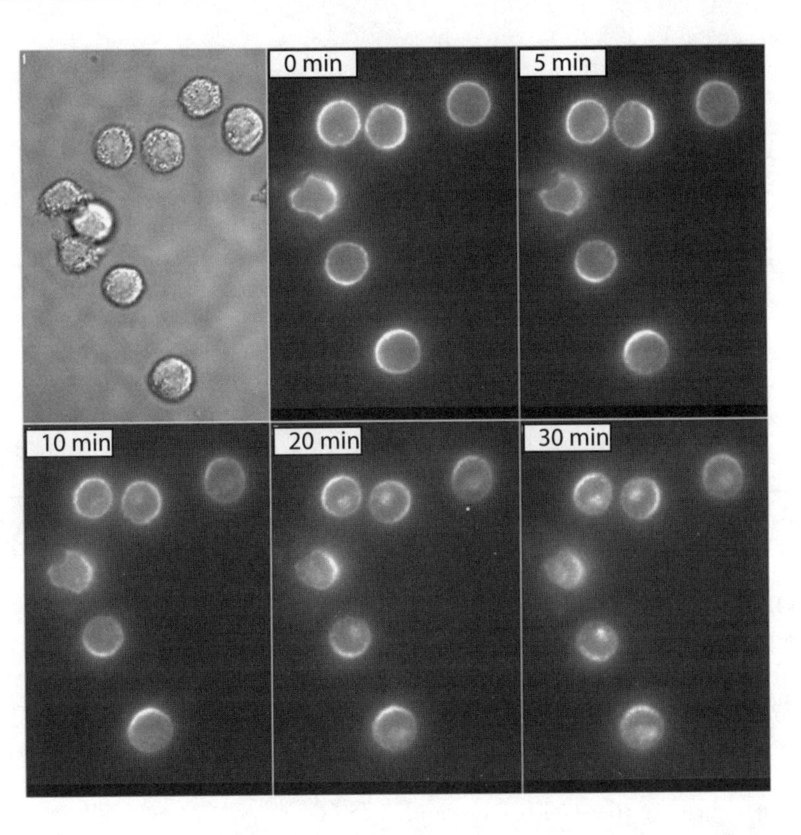

FIGURE 3a. *Internalization of Labeled Galanin. Transfected KNRK cells, grown on glass coverslips, were incubated with fluorescent Cy3 labeled galanin at 4°C for 1 hr. Internalization of surface bound Cy3-galanin was initiated by warming the cells to 37°C. Images were taken using a CCD camera by a fluorescent microscope (Olympus) at 0, 5, 10, 15, and 30 min. Internalized galanin accumulated in a perinuclear location.*

is inhibited when clathrin-coat formation is inhibited which indicates that Gal R1 endocytosis is mediated through early endosomes requiring clathrin-coat formation. This demonstrates that the recombinant Gal R1 is functionally active in transfected KNRK cells.

Galanin Inhibits Basal Levels of cAMP

To determine the effects of Gal R1 activation on cell signaling pathways, cellular cAMP concentrations were measured in the presence of increasing amounts of galanin (Figure 4a). Galanin in the presence of the phosphodiesterase

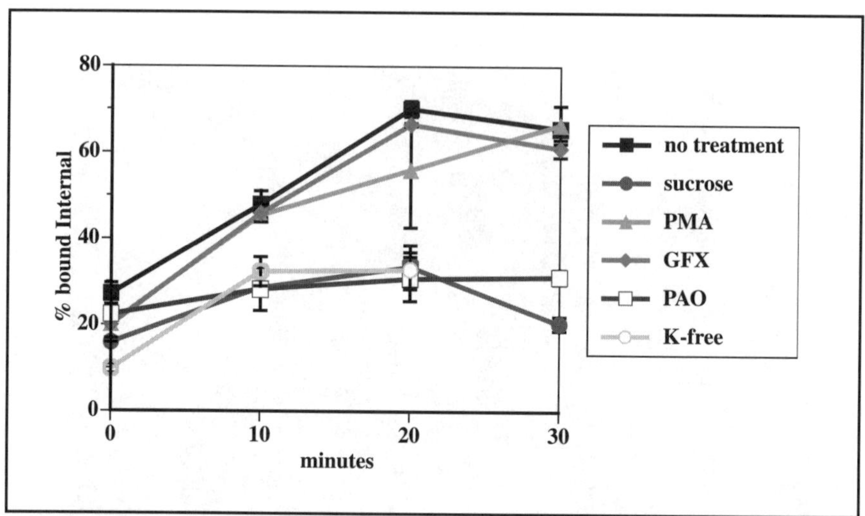

FIGURE 3b. *Surface bound ^{125}I-galanin was rapidly internalized into KNRK cells expressing Gal R1. Neither activation of PKC by pre-treatment with PMA (200 nM) nor inhibition of PKC by bisindolylamide (GFX, 3.5 μM) did not alter galanin internalization. Inhibition of clathrin-mediated endocytosis by pre-treatment with sucrose (0.45 M), phenyl arsine oxide (PAO, 80 μM) or potassium depleted cells (K-free) inhibited galanin internalization.*

inhibitor, isobutyl methylxanthine (IBMX) showed a decrease in the basal levels of cAMP in cells treated with IBMX alone. Inhibition of Gi signaling in cells treated with pertussis toxin (PTX) blocked the inhibitory effects of galanin indicating that Gal R1 is coupled to Gi.

Galanin Inhibits Forskolin-induced Increases in cAMP Levels

Forskolin increases significantly cAMP levels in transfected KNRK cells in a dose dependent manner (Figure 4b). Co-treatment with galanin blocks the effects of forskolin on cAMP in the cell. Inhibition of Gi signaling with PTX inhibits galanin's ability to block the increase in cAMP levels by forskolin. This demonstrates that the Gal R1 is able to inhibit forskolin-induced adenylate cyclase activity via signaling through Gi.

Galanin Inhibits PGE$_2$-induced Increases in cAMP Levels

PGE$_2$, acting through endogenous receptors, dose dependently increases cAMP in transfected KNRK cells (Figure 4c). Galanin is able to block the increase in cAMP levels in response to PGE$_2$. Pretreatment of cells with PTX, blocked the effects of galanin. This demonstrates that the Gal R1 is

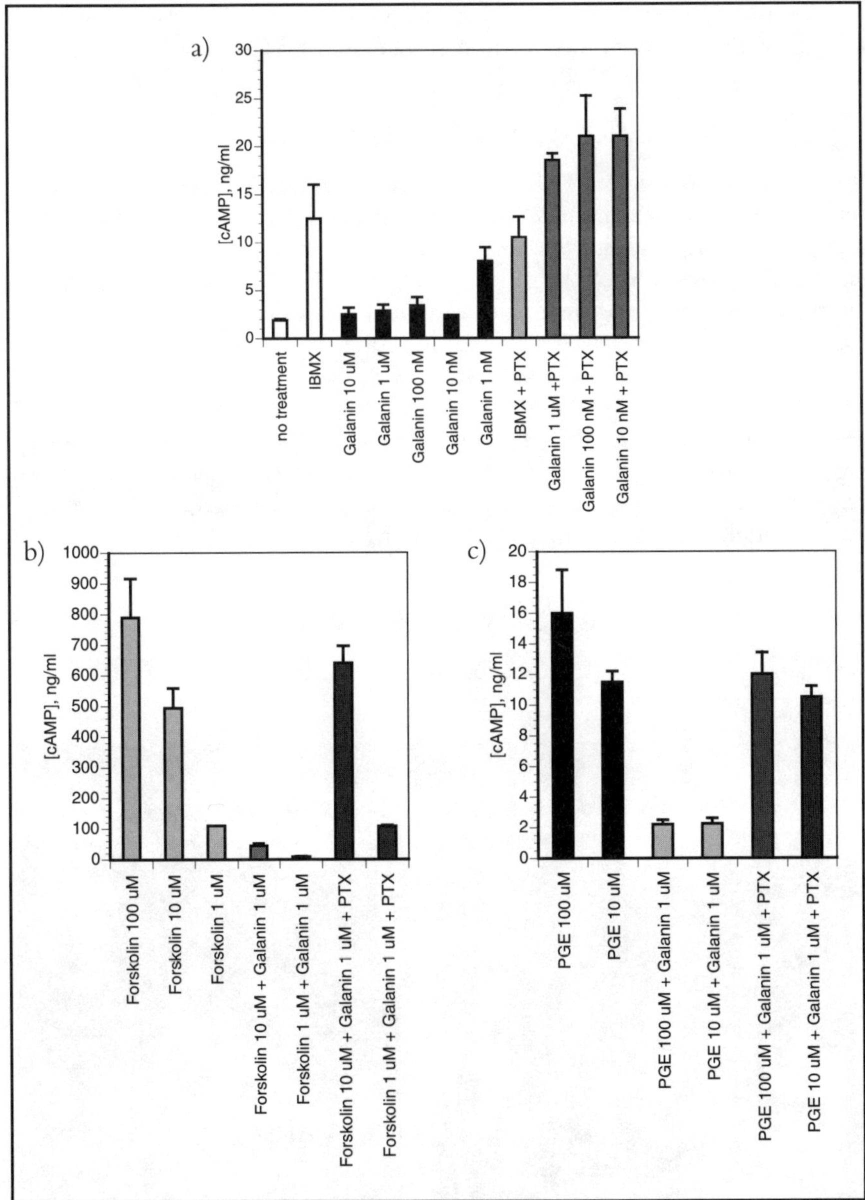

FIGURE 4. *Inhibition of cAMP Levels by Gal R1 in Transfected KNRK cells. (a) Transfected KNRK cells expressing Gal R1 were treated with increasing amounts of galanin for 30 min, 37°C with IBMX. At concentrations over 1 nM, galanin inhibited the basal level of cAMP. Pretreatment with PTX (500 ng/ml, 24 hr), blocked the effects of galanin on basal levels of cAMP. Forskolin (b) and PGE_2 (c) dose dependently increased cAMP. Co-stimulation with galanin inhibited the increase in cAMP levels. Pretreatment with PTX blocked the effects of galanin.*

able to inhibit adenylate cyclase activation by the endogenous receptors to PGE_2 and that this inhibitory action is mediated by Gi.

CONCLUDING REMARKS

We have expressed the rat Gal R1 in KNRK cells and have demonstrated receptor function in three areas. First, the expressed receptor specifically binds galanin with high affinity. Second, galanin binding to the receptor results in rapid endocytosis of the agonist bound receptor via clathrin-coated pits. The internalized galanin progresses from early endosomes to late endosomal compartments near the nucleus. Third, galanin acting through the Gal R1 decreases the basal level of cAMP in transfected cells. Agonist activated Gal R1 inhibits cAMP increases by forskolin and by PGE_2. All of Gal R1 effects on cAMP levels in transfected KNRK cells were blocked by PTX, that indicates signaling by the Gal R1 is through Gi. This cell system mimics galanin's inhibitory actions on cell signaling in acutely isolated primary cells and will serve as a useful model for studying the mechanism of inhibition by the Gal R1.

ACKNOWLEDGMENTS

We thank Dr. Hal Yee (UCLA) for use of his fluorescent microscope and imaging system.

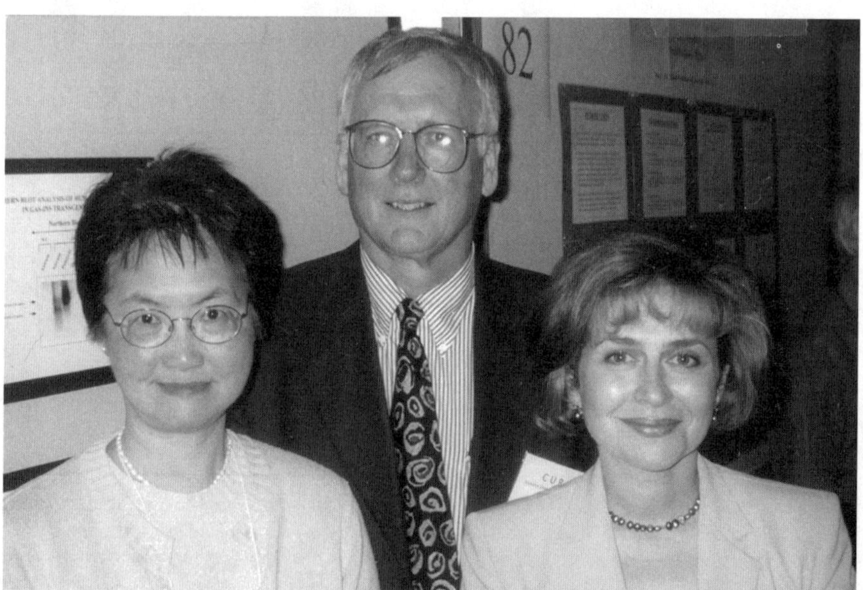

Photo taken at the 1999 CURE Meeting
(left to right: Helen Wong, John Walsh, and Elena Zhukova).

REFERENCES

1. Tatemoto K, Rokaeus A, Jornvall H, McDonald TJ, Mutt V. Galanin—a novel biologically active peptide from porcine intestine. *FEBS Lett* 1983;164:124–8.
2. Melander T, Hokfelt T, Rokaeus A, Fahrenkrug J, Tatemoto K, Mutt V. Distribution of galanin-like immunoreactivity in the gastrointestinal tract of several mammalian species. *Cell Tissue Res* 1985;239: 253–70.
3. Bartfai T, Fisone G, Langel U. Galanin and galanin antagonists: molecular and biochemical perspectives. *Trends Pharmacol Sci* 1992;13:312–7.
4. Jhanwar-Uniyal M, Chua SC, Jr. Critical effects of aging and nutritional state on hypothalamic neuropeptide Y and galanin gene expression in lean and genetically obese Zucker rats. *Brain Res Mol Brain Res* 1993;19:195–202.
5. Crawley JN. Functional interactions of galanin and acetylcholine: relevance to memory and Alzheimer's disease. *Behav Brain Res* 1993;57:133–41.
6. Haring H, Tottrup A. Motility regulating effects of galanin on smooth muscle of porcine ileum. *Regul Pept* 1991;34:251–60.
7. Rossowski WJ, Zacharia S, Jiang NY, Mungan Z, Mills M, Ertan A, Coy DH. Galanin: structure-dependent effect on pancreatic amylase secretion and jejunal strip contraction. *Eur J Pharmacol* 1993; 240:259–67.
8. McDonald TJ, Dupre J, Tatemoto K, Greenberg GR, Radziuk J, Mutt V. Galanin inhibits insulin secretion and induces hyperglycemia in dogs. *Diabetes* 1985;34:192–6.
9. Wong HC, Sternini C, Yang H, Pham T, Walsh JH. Monoclonal antibody to rat galanin: production, characterization, and *in vivo* immunoneutralization activity. *Hybridoma* 2001;20:109–15.
10. Lindstrom E, Lerner UH, Hakanson R. Isolated rat stomach ECL cells generate prostaglandin E(2) in response to interleukin-1 beta, tumor necrosis factor-alpha and bradykinin. *Eur J Pharmacol* 2001; 416:255–63.
11. Rossowski WJ, Coy DH. Inhibitory action of galanin on gastric acid secretion in pentobarbital-anesthetized rats. *Life Sci* 1989;44:1807–13.
12. Lorimer DD, Benya RV. Cloning and quantification of galanin-1 receptor expression by mucosal cells lining the human gastrointestinal tract. *Biochem Biophys Res Commun* 1996;222:379–85.
13. Floren A, Land T, Langel U. Galanin receptor subtypes and ligand binding. *Neuropeptides* 2000;34: 331–7.
14. Habert-Ortoli E, Amiranoff B, Loquet I, Laburthe M, Mayaux JF. Molecular cloning of a functional human galanin receptor. *Proc Natl Acad Sci USA* 1994;91:9780–3.
15. de Mazancourt P, Goldsmith PK, Weinstein LS. Inhibition of adenylate cyclase activity by galanin in rat insulinoma cells is mediated by the G-protein Gi3. *Biochem J* 1994;303 (Pt 2):369–75.
16. Heuser JE, Anderson RG. Hypertonic media inhibit receptor-mediated endocytosis by blocking clathrin-coated pit formation. *J Cell Biol* 1989;108:389–400.
17. Frost SC, Lane MD, Gibbs EM. Effect of phenylarsine oxide on fluid phase endocytosis: further evidence for activation of the glucose transporter. *J Cell Physiol* 1989;141:467–74.
18. Larkin JM, Brown MS, Goldstein JL, Anderson RG. Depletion of intracellular potassium arrests coated pit formation and receptor-mediated endocytosis in fibroblasts. *Cell* 1983;33:273–85.

III.

Pathophysiology of
Nerve-Gut Interactions

Gut-Brain Peptides in the New Millennium, edited by Y. Taché
CURE Foundation, Los Angeles, CA. © 2002

20

Brain Medullary Peptides and the Vagal Regulation of Gastric Secretion

Yvette Taché
CURE: Digestive Diseases Research Center
VA Greater Los Angeles Healthcare System, Department of Medicine and
Brain Research Institute, University of California at Los Angeles
Los Angeles, CA

INTRODUCTION

The study of cellular mechanisms through which gut peptides regulate gastric acid secretion was one of the sustained research interests of John Walsh throughout his productive academic career (1). He was among the first in 1979 to characterize the presence of bombesin-like peptides in both the brain and the gut (2) lending support to the emerging concept of the peptidergic brain-gut axis. Two years later, he reported that peripheral bombesin had high potency to stimulate gastrin release and acid secretion in humans (3). At the same time, we found that bombesin administered into the rat brain induced a potent inhibition of gastric acid secretion in rats (4). These initial observations led us to visit John at CURE in 1980 to talk about assessing the role of gastrin in the gastric acid alterations induced by central injection of peptides using his gastrin antibody (4, 5). This first meeting was the start of a sustained collaboration for two decades. Throughout these years, we appreciated John's relentless intellectual curiosity which he applied to new fields of research. Most of all, we would like to pay tribute to John for his dedication to CURE/Digestive Diseases Research Center (DDRC). He created a very stimulating and supportive milieu which fostered the development of several research programs.

The present chapter will focus on the physiological role of brain medullary thyrotropin releasing hormone (TRH) in the vagal regulation of gastric function. Central and peripheral vagal mechanisms through which TRH stimulates gastric acid secretion and alters the resistance of the gastric mucosa to injury will be also reviewed.

MEDULLARY TRH AS A PHYSIOLOGICAL VAGAL STIMULANT OF GASTRIC FUNCTION

TRH was initially isolated from mammalian hypothalami and named after its property to stimulate the release of pituitary thyroid-stimulating hormone (TSH). Soon after, a number of reports showed that TRH displays several features of a neurotransmitter and exerts behavioral actions unrelated to its endocrine effects. In particular, we found that TRH acts centrally to influence autonomic outflow to the viscera independently from its TSH releasing action in rats (4). This provided the first evidence that central injection of a peptide stimulates gastric acid secretion. However, to ascertain whether a brain neuropeptide plays a physiological role in the vagal regulation of gastric function at the level of preganglionic vagal motoneurons, several other criteria are required in addition to show a biological action upon central injection. First, the neuropeptide should be localized in fibers/terminals innervating preganglionic vagal motoneurons in the dorsal motor nucleus of the vagus (DMN). Secondly, receptors for this peptide should be present within the DMN circuitry and their activation by the ligand should induce changes in vagal activity which impact gastric function. Lastly, blockade of the peptide receptors and/or ligand within the DMN site should prevent vagal alterations of gastric function induced by known stimuli. So far TRH is the only brain stimulatory peptide for which these combined criteria have been fulfilled (6).

Neuroanatomical and Electrophysiological Evidence

Neuroanatomical studies in humans established that TRH immunoreactive (TRH-IR) fibers represent the most prominent network innervating the DMN compared with twelve other neuropeptides investigated (7). Likewise in rodents, the dorsal vagal complex (DVC) that encompasses the DMN and nucleus tractus solitarius (NTS), is densely innervated by TRH containing fibers and nerve terminals which make synaptic contacts on dendrites of DMN neurons projecting to the stomach (8). Retrograde labeling demonstrated that TRH-IR fibers in the DVC originate exclusively from cell-bodies located in the raphe pallidus (Rpa), raphe obscurus (Rob) and parapyramidal region (9). The abundant distribution of TRH-IR fibers and terminals in the DVC is matched with the presence of specific TRH receptors on DMN neurons. Autoradiographic localization of TRH binding sites showed that the highest density is found in the medial DMN column (10) which contains the majority of preganglionic cell bodies contributing vagal efferent innervation to the stomach (11). To date two TRH receptor subtypes 1 (TRH_1) and 2 (TRH_2) have been cloned (12). Mapping TRH receptor distribution by *in situ* hybridization revealed that DMN and NTS neurons expressed only the TRH_1 receptor (13).

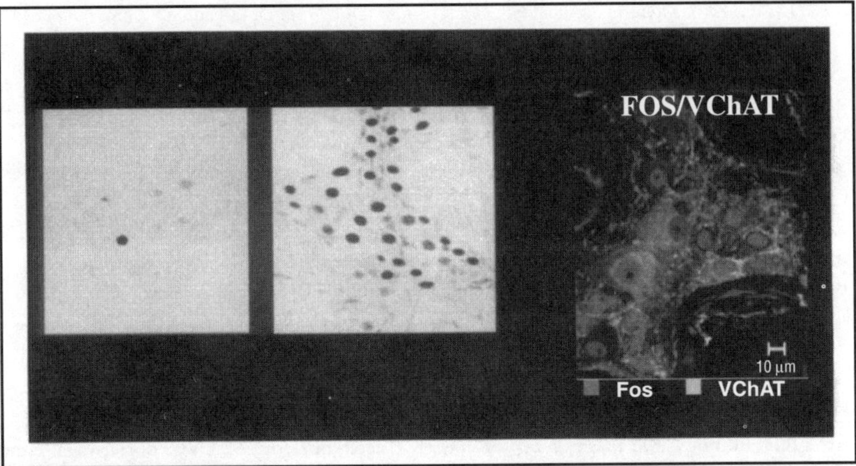

FIGURE 1. *Left panel: photomicrographs of Fos immunoreactivity in the corpus myenteric ganglia of the corpus 90 min after intracisternal (ic) injection of saline or the stable TRH analog, RX-77368 in conscious fasted rats. Fos immunoreactivity nuclei are rare in the myenteric ganglia after intracisternal saline (left). A marked increase in the number of Fos expression is induced by the TRH analog (right). Right pannel: rats injected ic with the stable TRH analog: confocal microscope images of gastric longitudinal muscle myenteric preparations double labeled with the monoclonal mouse anti-Fos (TF161) and polyclonal rabbit anti-vesicular acetylcholine transferase (VAChT). Adapted from reference 15.*

Electrophysiological studies demonstrated that intracisternal (ic) injection of TRH or the stable TRH analog, RX 77368 induces a sustained stimulation of gastric vagal efferent discharges (14). This results in a nicotinic dependent activation of gastric myenteric cells as shown by Fos expression (15) (Figure 1). Further reports established that TRH exerts a direct postsynaptic excitatory effect on DMN motoneurons and characterized the underlying cellular events (16). These observations provided convergent neuroanatomical and electrophysiological evidence that TRH directly excites DMN neurons and gastric vagal efferent discharges which translates in nicotinic activation of gastric myenteric neurons in rats.

Functional Evidence

Relevant strategies to assess the physiological role of endogenous transmitters and peptides involve the selective blockade of receptor or ligand under study by specific antagonists. However, with regard to TRH, no specific receptor antagonists are yet available. Alternative strategies rely on TRH_1 receptor antisense oligodeoxynucleotides to inhibit *in vivo* TRH_1 receptor expressed in the DVC (17). We also used polyclonal TRH antibody developed by G. Ohning, H. Wong and J. Walsh (CURE/DDRC Antibody Core)

TABLE 1. *Vagal cholinergic stimulation of gastric function by stimuli: inhibition by TRH antibody or* TRH_1 *receptor antisense oligodeoxynucleotides injected centrally (ic, DVC) in rats.*

Stimuli	Gastric Responses	Blockade	References
Sham feeding	acid secretion	AS	27
2-Deoxy-D-glucose, iv	emptying, erosion formation	Ab	25, 28
Cold (2–3h)	emptying	AS	29
Cold (2–3 h)	acid secretion, erosion	Ab	30
Intragastric low + high acid	adaptive gastric protection	Ab	26
Rpa cell bodies activation (low)	ethanol injury protection	Ab	22
Rpa cell bodies activation (high)	acid, motility and erosions	Ab	18, 21
Rob cell bodies activation	motility	AS	17

Ab: TRH antibody; AS: TRH_1 receptor antisense deoxynucleotides; DVC: dorsal vagal complex; ic: intercisternal; Rpa: raphe pallidus; Rob: raphe obscurus.

to immunoneutralize endogenous TRH (18). In a series of experiments initiated by Yang et al. (18), cell bodies containing TRH synthesizing neurons located in the Rpa, Rob and parapyramidal region (9) were selectively activated by microinjection of kainic acid (18). This resulted in the vagal dependent, atropine-sensitive stimulation of gastric acid secretion, motility and mucosal blood flow, and alterations of the resistance of the gastric mucosa to injury similar to changes elicited by TRH microinjected into the DMN in rats (18–24). In addition, TRH antibody injected into the cisterna magna or selectively microinjected bilaterally into the DVC, or ic pretreatment with TRH_1 receptor antisense oligodeoxynucleotides prevented the stimulation of gastric function (acid and motility) and changes in the resistance of the gastric mucosa to injury induced by microinjection of kainic acid into the Rob or Rpa (17-19, 21–25) (Table 1). Together these results indicate that the excitation of TRH synthesizing raphe medullary neurons is coupled with TRH release and TRH_1 receptor activation within the DMN which leads to vagal cholinergic stimulation of gastric function.

Additional studies established that medullary TRH pathways contribute to the gastric responses to known gastric vagal stimulants. TRH antibody microinjected into the DVC or the cisterna magna or ic pretreatment with the TRH_1 receptor antisense oligodeoxynucleotides prevented the vagal dependent gastric responses to various stimuli outlined in Table 1 (25–30). In further support of the medullary TRH involvement of cold exposure in rats activates TRH synthesizing neurons in the Rpa, Rob and parapyramidal region as shown by double labeling with Fos and prepro-TRH (23, 31). Cold also induces Fos expression in DMN neurons (31), stimulates vagal efferent discharge (32), which induces a vagal dependent activation of gastric myenteric neurons (33). There is also a time-related increase in proTRH mRNA expression in raphe nuclei (34). By contrast, these TRH blocking pretreatments did not influence the vagal gastric responses to central injection of somatostatin analog or peptide PYY or the basal gastric function showing their specificity (29, 35). Collectively, these data indicate that endogenous brain medullary TRH is involved in the gastric responses to established vagal stimulants such as 2-deoxy-D-glucose, sham feeding, and cold exposure in rats. However, this pathway does not contribute to the basal regulation of gastric function in the experimental models investigated.

MODULATION OF MEDULLARY TRH ACTION BY OTHER BRAIN PEPTIDES

There is growing evidence that TRH excitatory action on DMN neurons does occur in concert with other modulatory influences. These are exerted by neuropeptides or neurotransmitters co-localized with TRH in raphe nuclei and co-released in the DVC. For instance, the proteolytic cleavage of TRH prohormone generates TRH and the connecting peptide, prepro-TRH-(160-169) (Ps4), which are both co-released (36). When co-injected into the DMN Ps4 potentiates the acid secretion stimulated by TRH while having no effect by itself (37). Serotonin (5-HT) is co-localized with TRH synthesizing neurons in medullary raphe nuclei and parapyramidal region (24) and released in the DVC in response to excitation of medullary raphe neurons (38). Functional studies showed that this 5-HT pathway potentiates TRH stimulatory action through 5-HT$_2$ receptors in the DMN while by itself, 5-HT microinjected into the DMN did not alter basal gastric secretion (39).

Several peptides innervating the DVC exert an inhibitory influence on TRH stimulatory action. TRH containing neurons in the Rpa, Rob and parapyramidal region projecting to the DVC also expressed substance P (SP) (24). Retrograde labeling studies identified DMN neurons projecting to the stomach that are in contact with SP terminals as well as the presence of neurokinin-1 receptor (NK$_1$), the preferential receptor for SP, on these DMN neurons (40). The biological consequence of activation of NK$_1$ receptors in the DMN is the reduction of gastric secretory and motor responses to exogenous TRH (DVC microinjection) or endogenous TRH (released by stimulation of Rpa or Rob) (41, 42). Therefore, co-released SP with TRH in the DVC dampens the excitatory action of TRH. Several other brain peptides co-injected with TRH into the DMN also inhibit the vagal dependent stimulation of gastric secretory and motor function. These peptides include those that play a role in the immune (interleukin-1, tumor necrosis factor-α), or stress (corticotrophin releasing factor, CRF, urocortin, opioid peptides) responses, as well as peptides innervating the DVC through their projections from the paraventricular nucleus of the hypothalamic (gastrin releasing peptide/bombesin) or central amygdala (calcitonin gene related peptide, CGRP/adrenomedullin) (24, 43–45). Cellular mechanisms through which these peptides inhibit TRH excitatory effect on DMN neurons need to be further investigated.

PERIPHERAL STIMULATORY MECHANISMS INVOLVED IN THE VAGALLY MEDIATED GASTRIC ACID RESPONSE TO TRH

Central injection of TRH provided a relevant physiological tool to unravel peripheral mechanisms through which vagal activation influences gastric function. Previous results using electrical vagal stimulation may be confounded by concomitant activation of vagal afferents (which constitute 90% of vagal fibers) and related release of transmitters at their terminals in the NTS and the stomach (46).

Gastrin Does Not Play a Primary Role in the Acid Response to Central TRH

Convergent findings indicate that the stimulation of gastric acid secretion induced by ic injection of TRH is largely independent from gastrin release. When TRH was injected ic at a dose that resulted in a 4-fold increase in gastric acid output, there was no associated changes in serum gastrin as monitored in conscious rats with pylorus ligation for 2 h (47). Time course studies in urethane anesthetized rats revealed a non-significant transient gastrin peak at 5–10 min, while acid secretion remained significantly elevated for 90 min (47). In addition, immunoneutralization of endogenous gastrin by intravenous injection of gastrin monoclonal antibody 28-2 developed by H. Wong and J.H. Walsh attenuated the maximal acid response to TRH injected ic or into the DMN by only 33% and 22%, respectively (48). The gastrin antibody injected at a dose blocking the acid response to gastrin-17, did not influence the peak acid secretion elicited by the stable TRH analog injected ic or the cholinergic agonist carbachol infused intravenously (48–50). However in our models, gastrin stimulation may have been dampened by negative feedback under conditions of sustained low intraluminal gastric pH after pylorus-ligation, or somatostatin release induced by urethane anesthesia (51). Further experiments in conscious rats without pylorus ligation demonstrated that ic injection of TRH analog resulted in a significant 3-fold peak increase in plasma gastrin at 30 min followed by a lower, but significant elevation for 240 min (52). The gastrin elevation was not prevented by atropine injected at a dose that had no effect on basal gastrin release but blocked the acid response to ic TRH analog (4, 52). Together these findings indicate that other non-gastrin dependent mechanisms play a primary role in driving acid secretion after ic injection of TRH or TRH analog.

Role of Gastric Myenteric Activation and Muscarinic Receptors

Using Fos as a marker of neuronal activation, and double labeling with the neuronal marker, PGP 9.5, Miampamba et al. (15) showed that ic injection of TRH analog induced Fos expression in the majority of neuronal cell bodies located in the corpus and antral myenteric ganglia. Fos expression was observed in neurons densely surrounded with cholinergic fibers identified by the vesicular acetylcholine transporter (Figure. 1) (15). The Fos response was abolished by hexamethonium while atropine had no effect supporting a mediation through nicotinic receptor activation (15). Double labeling also showed that activated gastric myenteric neurons encompass a population of intrinsic cholinergic neurons (15). Muscarinic antagonists-induced complete blockade of the acid response to ic injection of TRH or medullary raphe activation in rats and cats support the primary role of this cholinergic pathway (4, 6, 50).

Role of Gastric Histamine Release and Histamine-2 Receptors

RX-77368 injected ic increases histamine levels in the hepatic portal plasma, and corpus submucosal interstitial fluid in urethane-anesthetized rats and histamine output in gastric secretion of conscious pylorus-ligated rats (49, 50). The histamine increase in hepatic portal blood was maximal at 30 min and prevented by cervical vagotomy and atropine. By contrast, gastrin antibody had no effect when administered under conditions blocking the acid response to gastrin-17 infused intravenously in urethane anesthetized rats (49). In the isolated vascularly perfused rat stomach, Sandvik et al. (53) showed also that electrical vagal stimulation induced histamine release through atropine sensitive pathways (53). TRH analog stimulates histidine decarboxylase activity (HDC) in the corpus mucosa with a peak response at 4 h which was confirmed by the increased number of HDC immunoreactive cells in conscious rats (52). Such a HDC response is dependent upon gastrin release which occurs through non-muscarinic activation in conscious rats (52). Therefore, ic TRH analog stimulates gastric histamine release and HDC activity through muscarinic and non-muscarinic mechanisms, respectively (49, 52).

Gastric histamine release has functional significance since the H_2 receptor antagonist, cimetidine, reduced the acid response to an ic injection of the TRH stable analog by 62% (50). By contrast, cimetidine completely abolished similar levels of gastric acid secretion induced by intravenous infusion of histamine (50). Therefore, both muscarinic and H_2 receptor activation contribute to the acid response by central vagal efferent activation.

MODULATION OF THE ACID RESPONSE TO CENTRAL TRH BY VAGALLY MEDIATED RELEASE OF ACID INHIBITORS

Vagal stimulation by ic TRH also induces the release of a number of gastric transmitters and the acid response represents the net effect of vagally mediated increase of stimulants (mainly histamine and acetylcholine) and inhibitors (prostranglandins, serotonin, CGRP) (Figure 2).

Role of Gastric Prostaglandins, 5-HT and CGRP

TRH or its analog injected ic, induced a dose-related and vagal dependent increase in prostaglandin E_2 (PGE_2) secretion monitored in the interstitial fluid sampled from corpus submucosa (54). The released gastric PGE_2 exerts antisecretory and gastroprotective effects on the gastric mucosa most notably under conditions of submaximal vagal stimulation (14, 55–57). For instance, TRH injected ic at a subthreshold dose to induce gastric acid secretion, stimulates gastric vagal efferent activity and mucosal blood flow, and confers gastric protection against ethanol injury through vagal pathways (14, 55, 57). The lack of gastric acid secretion in the presence of vagal activation results from the antisecretory effect of gastric prostaglandins (55–57). Similarly, when Rpa neurons are injected with kainic acid at a subthreshold to induce acid secretion, this results in vagal dependent gastric hyperemia (19). The acid response can be unmasked by pretreatment with indomethacin showing an inhibitory influence of gastric prostaglandins released by endogenous TRH (19). Other studies established that the release of gastric prostaglandins also contribute to the gastric protection against intragastric ethanol-induced gastric injury, but do not contribute to the increase in blood flow induced by ic RX 77368 (56, 57). The submaximal or maximal acid responses to ic RX 77368 are, however, not significantly further enhanced by prostaglandin blockade (54, 56).

The release of 5-HT from enterochromaffin cells (EC) is also under vagal control. TRH microinjected into the DMN or intracisternally results in a vagal-atropine sensitive increase in gastric secretion of 5-HT (58). 5-HT exerts an inhibitory effect on the acid response to RX 77368 injected ic at a submaximal secretory dose through mechanisms that are likely neurally mediated (59).

We previously showed the potent inhibitory action of CGRP on gastric acid secretion (60). Ablation of capsaicin sensitive afferents containing CGRP and peripheral administration of CGRP receptor antagonist result in gastric acid secretion when RX 77368 is injected ic at a subthreshold acid secretory dose, which induced a pronounced increase in gastric mucosal blood flow (57). The implication of CGRP in modulating the acid response appears less

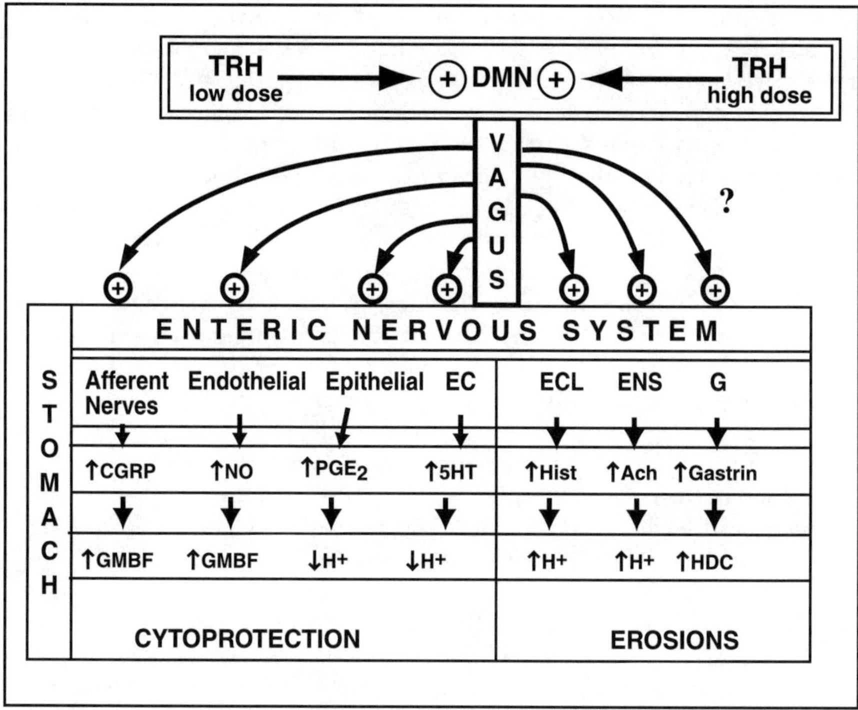

FIGURE 2. *Schematic representation of the vagal cholinergic mechanisms involved in the dual gastric mucosal protective and erosive effects induced by low or high dose of TRH injected into the dorsal motor nucleus of the vagus (DMN) or cisterna magna. Ach: acetylcholine; CGRP: calcitonin gene-related peptide; EC: enterochromaffin cells; ECL: enterochromaffin-like cells; G: gastrin cells; GMBF: gastric mucosal blood flow; HDC: histamine decarboxylase; NO: nitric oxide. Hist: histamine.*

prominent in comparison with its main role in mediating the vagal cholinergic gastric hyperemia induced by ic RX 77368 (57).

DUAL GASTRIC PROTECTIVE AND EROSIVE ACTIONS OF THE VAGUS RELATED TO LEVELS OF ACTIVATION

Central administration of TRH at increasing doses have allowed us to unravel the dual opposite actions of the vagus on the resistance of the gastric mucosa to injury (61) (Figure 2). Under conditions of submaximal stimulation of vagal efferent activity induced by low doses of TRH injected into the cisterna magna, there is a robust gastric hyperemia while acid secretion is inhibited. This results from the vagal cholinergic dependent activation of capsaicin sensitive CGRP/nitric oxide (NO) vasodilatory pathways (54, 56, 57). At these low doses, ic TRH injected into the cisterna magna or DCV confer gastric protection against ethanol-induced mucosal lesions. The gastric protection is brought out by vagal cholinergic dependent release of gastric prostaglandins and NO, as well as the activation of a local effector function of capsaicin-sensitive splanchnic afferents containing CGRP and related gastric hyperemia (55). Likewise, the endogenous release of TRH in the DVC induced by the low activation of TRH cell bodies in the Rpa is gastroprotective (19) (Table 1). Other phenomena, such as the vagal dependent adaptive gastric protection, whereby a mild gastric irritant reduced the damaging effect of a strong irritant are also mediated by TRH in the brain medulla (26). In view of these findings, it may be speculated that the cephalic phase of gastric secretion, which results in a mild vagal stimulation, may have beneficial effects on the gastric mucosa by triggering these mucosal protective mechanisms. Conversely, deficient cephalic phase may facilitate the damaging effect of ulcerogenic stimuli due to the diminished or absence of vagally recruited protective mechanisms.

By contrast, at maximal effective doses of TRH or TRH analogs, the stimulation of acid secretion by histamine and acetylcholine (49, 50) is no longer influenced by the inhibitory effects of prostaglandins, CGRP or 5-HT (54, 56). Under these conditions, the sustained vagal activation induced prolonged stimulation of gastric acid, pepsin, and motility leading to the development of gastric hemorrhagic lesions in 24 h fasted rats (61). These observations support the notion that various transmitters are released in the stomach by central vagal cholinergic stimulation. Their interplay varies with the degree of vagal activation and contributes to the differential patterns of gastric responses elicited by low or high levels of vagal efferent drive (Figure 2).

ACKNOWLEDGMENTS

The research was supported by the NIHDDK grants DK 30110 (YT), DK 33061 (YT) and the Center grant DK 41301 (John Walsh). We are profoundly grateful to John (Figure 3) for his generosity in providing key reagents and for stimulating discussions. He expanded the frontiers of knowledge in the field of peptide gastroenterology.

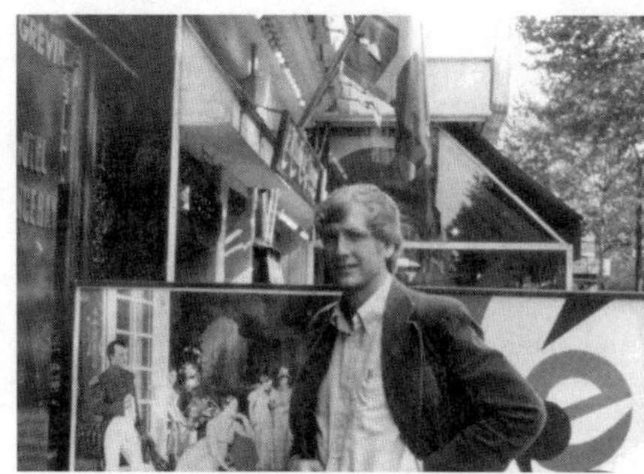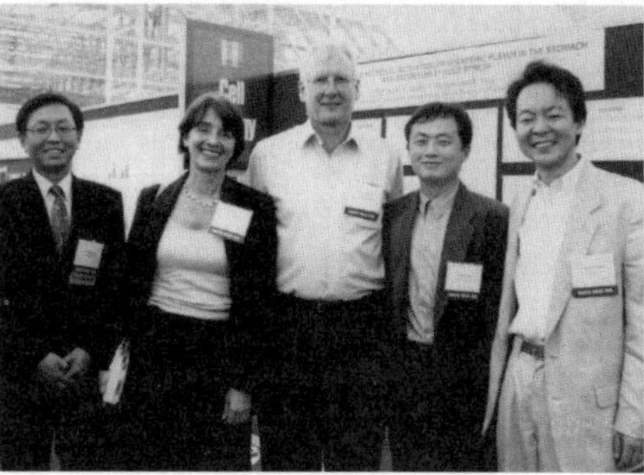

Left panel: John Walsh doing a Napolean imitation at the Grevin Museum in Paris, 1980.
Right panel: John Walsh viewing posters at the AGA in San Diego, 2000: from left to right:
Drs. Pu Qing Yuan, Yvette Taché, John Walsh, Chih-Yen Chen, and Kazuyoshi Kuratani.

REFERENCES

1. Walsh JH. Peptides as regulators of gastric acid secretion. *Annu Rev Physiol* 1988;50:41–63.
2. Walsh JH, Wong HC, Dockray GJ. Bombesin-like peptides in mammals. *Fed Proc* 1979;38:2315–2319.
3. Varner AA, Modlin IM, Walsh JH. High potency of bombesin for stimulation of human gastrin release and gastric acid secretion. *Regul Pept* 1981;1:289–296.
4. Taché Y, Vale W, Rivier J, Brown M. Brain regulation of gastric secretion: influence of neuropeptides. *Proc Natl Acad Sci USA* 1980;77:5515–5519.
5. Taché Y, Vale W, Brown M. Thyrotropin-releasing hormone-CNS action to stimulate gastric acid secretion. *Nature* 1980;287:149–151.
6. Taché Y, Yang H, Yoneda M. Vagal regulation of gastric function involves thyrotropin-releasing hormone in the medullary raphe nuclei and dorsal vagal complex. *Digestion* 1993;54:65–72.
7. Fodor M, Pammer C, Gorcs T, Palkovits M. Neuropeptides in the human dorsal vagal complex: an immunohistochemical study. *J Chem Neuroanat* 1994;7:141–157.
8. Rinaman L and Miselis RR. Thyrotropin-releasing hormone-immunoreactive nerve terminals synapse on the dentrites of gastric vagal motoneurons in the rat. *J Comp Neurol* 1990;294:235–251.
9. Lynn RB, Kreider MS, Miselis RR. Thyrotropin-releasing hormone-immunoreactive projections to the dorsal motor nucleus and the nucleus of the solitary tract of the rat. *J Comp Neurol* 1991;311:271–288.
10. Manaker S and Rizio G. Autoradiographic localization of thyrotropin-releasing hormone and substance P receptors in the rat dorsal vagal complex. *J Comp Neurol* 1989;290:516–526.
11. Powley TL, Berthoud H-R, Prechtl JC, Fox AE. Fibers of the vagus regulating gastrointestinal function. In: *Brain-gut interactions.* Taché Y, Wingate D, eds., Boca Raton. CRC Press 1991:73–82.
12. Cao J, O'Donnell D, Vu H, Payza K, Pou C, Godbout C, Jakob A, Pelletier M, Lembo P, Ahmad S, Walker P. Cloning and characterization of a cDNA encoding a novel subtype of rat thyrotropin-releasing hormone receptor. *J Biol Chem* 1998;273:32281–32287.
13. Heuer H, Schafer MK, O'Donnell D, Walker P, Bauer K. Expression of thyrotropin-releasing hormone receptor 2 (TRH-R2) in the central nervous system of rats. *J Comp Neurol* 2000;428:319–336.
14. O-Lee TJ, Wei JY, Taché Y. Intracisternal TRH and RX 77368 potently activate vagal efferent discharge in rats. *Peptides* 1997;18:213–219.
15. Miampamba M, Yang H, Sharkey KA, Taché Y. Intracisternal TRH analog induces Fos expression in gastric myenteric neurons and glia in conscious rats. *Am J Physiol Gastrointest Liver Physiol* 2001;280:G979–G991.
16. Travagli RA, Gillis RA, Vicini S. Effects of thyrotropin-releasing hormone on neurons in the rat dorsal motor nucleus of the vagus, *in vitro. Am J Physiol* 1992;263:G508–G517.

17. Sivarao DV, Krowicki ZK, Abrahams TP, Hornby PJ. Intracisternal antisense oligonucleotides to TRH receptor abolish TRH- evoked gastric motor excitation. *Am J Physiol* 1997;272:G1372–G1381.
18. Yang H, Ohning G, Taché Y. TRH in dorsal vagal complex mediates acid response to excitation of raphe pallidus neurons in rats. *Am J Physiol* 1993;265:G880–G886.
19. Kaneko H, Kaunitz J, Taché Y. Vagal mechanisms underlying gastric protection induced by chemical activation of the raphe pallidus in rats. *Am J Physiol* 1998;275:G1056–G1062.
20. Yang H, Kawakubo K, Taché Y. Kainic acid into the parapyramidal region protects against gastric injury by ethanol. *Eur J Pharmacol* 1999;372:R1–R3.
21. Kaneko H, Taché Y. TRH in the dorsal motor nucleus of the vagus is involved in gastric erosion induced by excitation of raphe pallidus in rats. *Brain Res* 1995;699:97–102.
22. Kaneko H, Yang H, Ohning G, Taché Y. Medullary TRH is involved in gastric protection induced by low dose of kainic acid into the raphe pallidus. *Am J Physiol* 1995;268:G548–G552.
23. Yang H, Yuan PQ, Wang L, Taché Y. Activation of the parapyramidal region in the ventral medulla stimulates gastric acid secretion through vagal pathways in rats. *Neuroscience* 2000;95:773–779.
24. Taché Y, Yang H, Kaneko H. Caudal raphe-dorsal vagal complex peptidergic projections: role in gastric vagal control. *Peptides* 1995;16:431–435.
25. Okumura T, Grant AP, Taylor IL, Ohning G, Taché Y, Pappas TN. Gastric mucosal damage induced by 2-deoxy-D-glucose involves medullary TRH in the rat. *Regul Pept* 1995;55:311–319.
26. Kaneko H, Kato K, Ohning G, Taché Y. Medullary thyrotropin-releasing hormone mediates vagal-dependent adaptive gastric protection induced by mild acid in rats. *Gastroenterology* 1995;109:861–865.
27. Barrachina MD, Wu V, Taché Y. Central TRH receptors are involved in the gastric secretory response to sham-feeding in rats. *Gastroenterology* 1997;112:A1130.
28. Okumura T, Taylor IL, Ohning G, Taché Y, Pappas TN. Intracisternal injection of TRH antibody blocks gastric emptying stimulated by 2-deoxy-D-glucose in rats. *Brain Res* 1995;674:137–141.
29. Martinez V, Wu SV, Taché Y. Intracisternal antisense oligodeoxynucleotides to the thyrotropin-releasing hormone receptor blocked vagal-dependent stimulation of gastric emptying induced by acute cold in rats. *Endocrinology* 1998;139:3730–3735.
30. Niida H, Takeuchi K, Okabe S. Role of thyrotropin-releasing hormone in acid secretory response induced by lowering of body temperature in the rat. *Eur J Pharmacol* 1991;198:137–142.
31. Bonaz B and Taché Y. Induction of Fos immunoreactivity in the rat brain after cold-restraint induced gastric lesions and fecal excretion. *Brain Res* 1994;652:56–64.
32. Cho CH, Qui BS, Bruce IC. Vagal hyperactivity in stress induced gastric ulceration in rats. *J Gastroenterol Hepatol* 1996;11:125–128.
33. Yuan PQ, Taché Y, Miampamba M, Yang H. Acute cold exposure induces vagally mediated Fos expression in gastric myenteric neurons in conscious rats. *Am J Physiol* 2001;281:G560–G568.
34. Yang H, Wu SV, Ishikawa T, Taché Y. Cold exposure elevates thyrotropin-releasing hormone gene expression in medullary raphe nuclei: relationship with vagally mediated gastric erosions. *Neuroscience* 1994;61:655–663.
35. Yang H, Kawakubo K, Taché Y. Intracisternal PYY increases gastric mucosal resistance: role of cholinergic, CGRP, and NO pathways. *Am J Physiol* 1999;277:G555–G562.
36. Ladram A, Bulant M, Delfour A, Montagne JJ, Vaudry H, Nicolas P. Modulation of the biological activity of thyrotropin-releasing hormone by alternate processing of pro-TRH. *Biochimie* 1994;76:320–328.
37. Yang H and Taché Y. Prepro-TRH-(160-169) potentiates gastric acid secretion stimulated by TRH microinjected into the dorsal motor nucleus of the vagus. *Neurosci Lett* 1994;174:43–46.
38. Stephen RL, Jr. Disparate effects of intracisternal RX 77368 and ODT8-SS on gastric acid and serotonin release: role of adrenal catecholamines. *Regul Pept* 1991;36:21–28.
39. Yoneda M and Taché Y. Serotonin enhances gastric acid response to TRH analog in dorsal vagal complex through 5-HT2 receptors in rats. *Am J Physiol* 1995;269:R1–R6.
40. Ladic LA and Buchan AM. Association of substance P and its receptor with efferent neurons projecting to the greater curvature of the rat stomach. *J Auton Nerv Syst* 1996;58:25–34.
41. Yang H and Taché Y. Substance P in the dorsal vagal complex inhibits medullary TRH-induced gastric acid secretion in rats. *Am J Physiol* 1997;272:G987–G993.

42. Krowicki ZK and Hornby PJ. Substance P in the dorsal motor nucleus of the vagus evokes gastric motor inhibition via neurokinin 1 receptor in rat. *J Pharmacol Exp Ther* 2000;293:214–221.

43. Hermann GE, Tovar CA, Rogers RC. Induction of endogenous tumor necrosis factor-alpha: suppression of centrally stimulated gastric motility. *Am J Physiol* 1999;276:R59–R68.

44. Martinez V and Taché Y. Bombesin and the brain-gut axis. *Peptides* 2000;21:1617–1625.

45. Taché Y and Saperas E. Potent inhibition of gastric acid secretion and ulcer formation by centrally and peripherally administered interleukin-1. *Ann NY Acad Sci* 1992;659:353–368.

46. Wang FB and Powley TL. Topographic inventories of vagal afferents in gastrointestinal muscle. *J Comp Neurol* 2000;421:302–324.

47. Taché Y, Goto Y, Hamel D, Pekary A, Novin D. Mechanisms underlying intracisternal TRH-induced stimulation of gastric acid secretion in rats. *Regul Pept* 1985;13:21–30.

48. Yang H, Wong H, Walsh JH, Taché Y. Effect of gastrin monoclonal antibody 28.2 on acid response to chemical vagal stimulation in rats. *Life Sci* 1989;45:2413–2418.

49. Yanagisawa K and Taché Y. Intracisternal TRH analog RX 77368 stimulates gastric histamine release in rats. *Am J Physiol* 1990;259:G599–G604.

50. Yanagisawa K, Yang H, Walsh JH, Taché Y. Role of acetylcholine, histamine and gastrin in the acid response to intracisternal injection of TRH analog, RX 77368, in the rat. *Regul Pept* 1990;27:161–170.

51. Yang H, Wong H, Wu V, Walsh JH, Taché Y. Somatostatin monoclonal antibody immunoneutralization increases gastrin and gastric acid secretion in urethane-anesthetized rats. *Gastroenterology* 1990;99:659–665.

52. Song M, Yang H, Walsh JH, Ohning G, Wong H, Taché Y. Intracisternal TRH analog increases gastrin release and corpus histidine decarboxylase activity in rats. *Am J Physiol* 1999;276:G901–G908.

53. Sandvik AK, Kleveland PM, Waldum HL. Muscarinic M2 stimulation releases histamine in the totally isolated, vascularly perfused rat stomach. *Scand J Gastroenterol* 1988;23:1049–1056.

54. Yoneda M and Taché Y. Vagal regulation of gastric prostaglandin E2 release by central TRH in rats. *Am J Physiol* 1993;264:G231–G236.

55. Taché Y, Yoneda M, Kato K, Kiràly A, Sütö G, Kaneko H. Intracisternal thyrotropin-releasing hormone-induced vagally mediated gastric protection against ethanol lesions: central and peripheral mechanisms. *J Gastroenterol Hepatol* 1994;9:S29–S35.

56. Cardin S, Soll AH, Taché Y. Different effects of indomethacin and nabumetone on prostaglandin-mediated gastric responses to central vagal activation in rats. *J Pharmacol Exp Ther* 1995;275:667–673.

57. Kiràly A, Sütö G, Guth PH, Taché Y. Mechanisms mediating gastric hyperemic and acid responses to central TRH analog at a cytoprotective dose. *Am J Physiol* 1997;273:G31–G38.

58. Yang H, Stephens RL, Taché Y. TRH analogue microinjected into specific medullary nuclei stimulates gastric serotonin secretion in rats. *Am J Physiol* 1992;262:G216–G222.

59. Stephens RL, Garrick T, Weiner H, Taché Y. Serotonin depletion potentiates gastric secretory and motor responses to vagal but not peripheral gastric stimulants. *J Pharmacol Exp Ther* 1989;251:524–530.

60. Taché Y. Inhibition of gastric acid secretion and ulcers by calcitonin gene-related peptide. *Ann NY Acad Sci* 1992;657:240–247.

61. Taché Y and Yoneda M. Central action of TRH to induce vagally mediated gastric cytoprotection and ulcer formation in rats. *J Clin Gastroenterol* 1993;17(Suppl. 1):S58–S63.

Gut-Brain Peptides in the New Millennium, edited by Y. Taché
CURE Foundation, Los Angeles, CA. © 2002

21

Hypothyroidism and Autonomic Changes: Role of Medullary TRH

Hong Yang
*CURE/Digestive Diseases Research Center, UCLA Division of Digestive Diseases
Departments of Medicine and VA Greater Los Angeles Healthcare System
Los Angeles, CA*

INTRODUCTION

An important component of Dr. Walsh's career was his leadership as the Director of CURE. During his tenure, neuroscience in gastroenterology was one of the key research disciplines in CURE that flourished under his tutelage. Studies on brain regulation of gastrointestinal (GI) functions and the gut-brain signaling have contributed significantly on revealing the neural and endocrine mechanisms regulating the gut functions. Recently, the discovery that particular circulating hormones display central vagal regulatory actions has shed new light on our understanding of the interactions between the two major visceral regulatory systems, the autonomic nervous system and the endocrine system.

It is well known from clinical and experimental observations that hypothyroidism is associated with disorders of autonomic nervous system regulated visceral functions. Symptoms like sinus bradycardia and abdominal pain, disorders like altered gastrointestinal (GI) motility and gastric acid secretion are widely known (37, 38). In animal experiments, gastric acid secretion and ulcer formation are increased in hypothyroid animals (6, 13) while decreased in hyperthyroid animals (16, 32).

Attempts to show a direct relationship between the known calorigenic effects of thyroid hormone and the viscera alterations have been unsuccessful (9). It is also unlikely that the alterations result from an indirect effect on calcium metabolism (9). The exact nature of interactions between thyroid status and autonomic nervous activities in the control of visceral organs, particularly the central mechanisms, are still poorly understood. This chapter will review our recent findings that revealed a possible central mechanism through which thyroid hormone regulates vagal mediated visceral functions.

Medullary Thyrotropin-releasing Hormone (TRH)-containing Caudal Raphe Nuclei/Parapyramidal Regions (PPR)-dorsal Vagal Complex (DVC) Pathways Play Important Roles in the Central Regulation of Vagal Activities

Neuronal terminals arising from specific nuclei located in the ventral regions of the medulla, namely the raphe pallidus (Rpa), raphe obscurus (Rob) and the PPR, directly innervate the dorsal motor nucleus of the vagus (DMN) (27). Thyrotropin-releasing hormone (TRH), substance P (SP) and serotonin (5-HT) are among the neurotransmitters synthesized by neurons in these nuclei and released in the DMN from the neuronal terminals which modulate the function of preganglionic motoneurons of the vagus (27, 42). Dense TRH-containing nerve terminals and TRH receptors are located in the nucleus ambiguus (Amb) and dorsal vagal complex (DVC), composed of the DMN and the nucleus tractus solitarius (NTS) (28, 35). The DMN and Amb are the main medullary sources of vagal innervation of the GI tract and heart, respectively (26). The direct effects of TRH on neurons in the DVC are to excite DMN neurons and inhibit NTS neurons (30).

During the last two decades, studies in Dr. Taché's lab and other labs have well established the gastric regulatory function of medullary TRH (42). TRH exogenousely microinjected into the DMN (15), or endogenously released into the DMN after chemical stimulation of the neurons in the Rpa (8, 18, 45), Rob (41) or PPR (48), activates vagal efferent activity (33), increases gastric acid secretion (45, 48), motility (8, 41) and induces ulcer formation (18). The gastric secretory and motor changes induced by chemical stimulation of the Rpa or Rob could be prevented by pretreatment either with TRH antibody microinjected into the DVC (45) or with antisense oligodeoxynucleotides of TRH receptor injected intracisternally (ic) (29, 41, 44). In addition, we have observed that TRH analog microinjected into the DVC or chemical stimulation of the Rpa neurons induces vagal-mediated bradycardia. The effect of Rpa stimulation could be prevented by pretreatment with TRH antibody microinjected into the Amb (unpublished observations).

The physiological role of medullary TRH in regulating vagal efferent activity has been evidenced in the animal model of cold exposure, which is wildly used to induce vagally mediated gastric ulceration (1, 2, 46). Cold exposure induces Fos expression in the Rpa, Rob, PPR and DVC neurons (4, 48), and enhances medullary TRH gene expression, especially in the Rpa and Rob (46). Cold induced gastric ulceration was prevented by intracerebroventricular injection (icv) of TRH antiserum (3). Both exogenous ic injection of TRH (31) and cold exposure (50) activate gastric myenteric neurons through vagal preganglionic stimulatory input and nicotinic synapse.

Thyroid Hormone Action on Medullary TRH Containing Rpa/Rob/PPR Neurons May Play an Important Role in the Autonomic Disorders Observed in Altered Thyroid Status

The possibility that thyroid hormone acts centrally to regulate the vagal and sympathetic outflow is supported by the facts that all the autonomic disorders observed in altered thyroid status could be ascribed to abnormal parasympathetic or sympathetic activities. However, central regulation of thyroid hormone on autonomic function has received little attention though thyroid hormone has been reported to have profound effects in the central nervous system. Interestingly, alterations in gastric and heart functions observed in hypothyroidism are similar to the vagally mediated gastric and heart responses to activated medullary TRH pathways. Using rat hypothyroid and hyperthyroid models, our studies demonstrate that thyroid hormone induced alterations of TRH gene expression in the Rpa, Rob and PPR neurons might be one of the central pathophysiological mechanisms mediating the autonomic disorders of altered thyroid statues.

Thyroid Hormone Feedback Regulates Medullary TRH Gene Expression in the Rpa, Rob and PPR

The negative feedback regulation of TRH gene expression by thyroid hormone has been well documented in neurons of the medial paraventricular nucleus of the hypothalamus (PVN) (22, 39). The simultaneous occurrence of increased TRH mRNA and the TRH prohormone in PVN cells in hypothyroid animals indicates that hypothyroidism may induce both transcription and translation of the TRH prohormone (22, 39). The medullary caudal raphe nuclei and the PPR contain the most abundant group of TRH synthesizing neurons outside of the hypothalamus (22, 46). Our recent studies revealed that medullary TRH synthesizing neurons are also targets of thyroid hormone regulation (47, 49, 51, 52).

Medullary pro-TRH mRNAs are localized in the Rpa, Rob and PPR (Figure 1). Quantitative analysis of Northern blot signals in the brainstem showed that TRH mRNA levels significantly increased by 73% at one week after thyroidectomy compared with sham operated controls. A plateau (133% increase) is reached at the third week, which was maintained until after the 5 week thyroidectomy. During this period, the serum T_4 levels were reduced by 75% in the first week and kept in this level or slightly lower (−87%) during the next 4 weeks. The increase of TRH mRNA levels in hypothyroid rats was reversed to euthyroid levels by daily T_4 replacement (47). Similar results were obtained by *in situ* hybridization. In addition, hyperthyroidism induced by daily T_4 injection significantly increased the serum T_4 levels and reduced the TRH mRNA signals in the Rpa, Rob and PPR (51) (Figure 1).

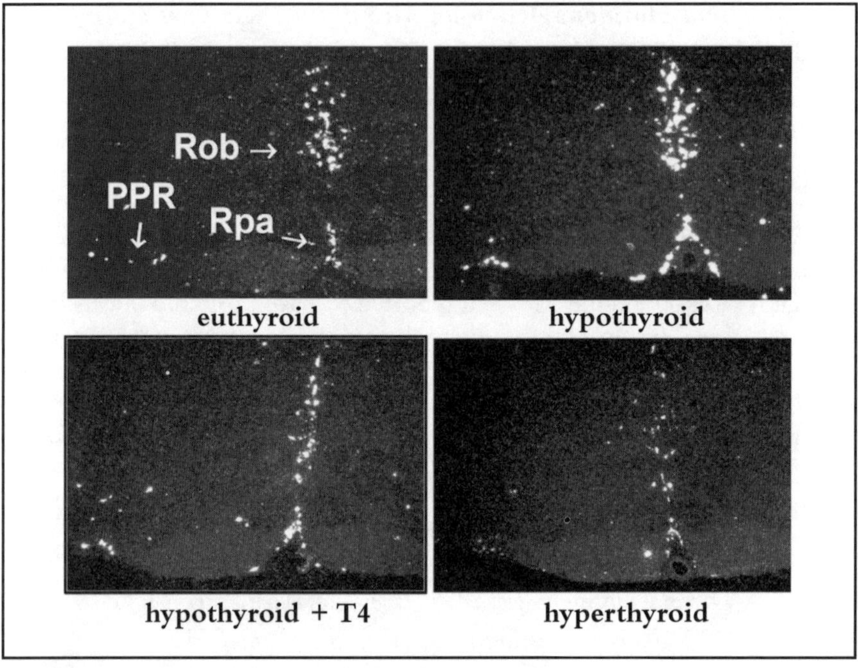

FIGURE 1. *Darkfield view micrographs (interaural −3.72 mm [10]) showing pro-TRH mRNA signals in medullary raphe pallidus (Rpa), raphe obscurus (Rob) and the parapyramidal regions (PPR) in rats with different thyroid statuses (30 days after the surgery). (a) euthyroid: sham operation/vehicle (ip daily for 30 days); (b) hypothyroid: thyroidectomy/vehicle; (c) hypothyroid + T_4: thyroidectomy/T_4 (2 µg/100 g/day); (d) hyperthyroid: sham operation/T_4 (20 µg/100 g/day). Bar = 80 µm. Adapted from Reference 51.*

Recent studies have revealed that nutritional state alters the negative feedback regulation of thyroid hormone on TRH biosynthesis and secretion in hypophysiotropic neurons of the PVN (11, 23). The diminution of the thyroid hormone feedback regulation of TRH gene expression in the PVN induced by fasting could be completely reversed by systemic administration of leptin to fasting animals (23). Likewise, we found that fasting also weakens the feedback regulatory action of thyroid hormone on medullary TRH gene expression. Thyroidectomized (30 days) rats fed normally showed a 2.8-fold higher increase in medullary TRH mRNA levels compared with thyroidectomized/24 h fasted rats (47).

Hypothyroidism Induces Fos Expression in the TRH Synthesizing Neurons in the Rpa, Rob, and PPR

Fos is the product of *c-fos* gene, and is a member of the set of cellular inducible transcription factors (ITFs) (12). These factors are induced by diverse extracellular stimuli and interact with DNA to influence the

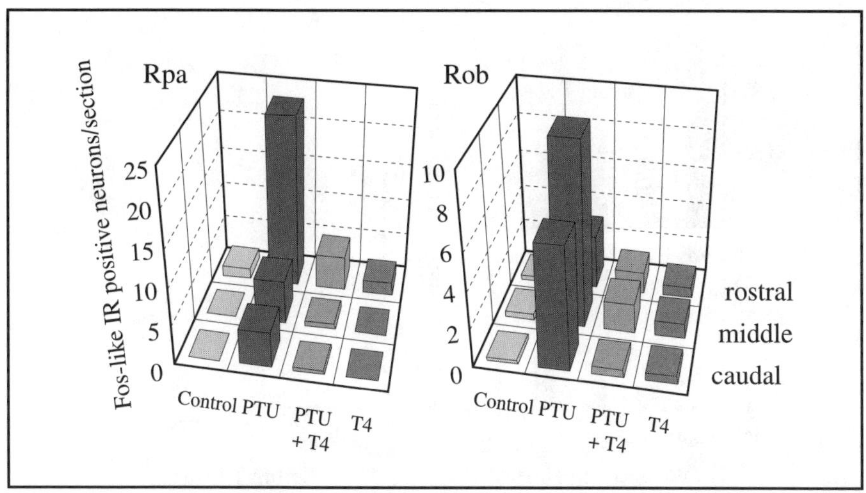

FIGURE 2. *Fos-like IR positive neurons in the Rpa and Rob under different thyroid statuses for 4 weeks. Each column represents mean of 20 sections/region/rat and 4-6 rats/group. Control, euthyroid; PTU, hypothyroid rat induced by 0.1% PTU in drinking water; PTU +T₄, hypothyroid +T₄ replacement (2 μg/100 g/day, ip); T₄, hyperthyroid rat induced by T₄ injection (10 μg/100g/day, ip). Rostral, interaural −1.80 to −2.60 mm; middle, −2.60 to −4.30 mm; caudal, −4.30 to −5.08 mm according to atlas of Paxinos and Watson (34). Adapted from Reference 52.*

transcription of specific genes, including the TRH gene (40). The expressions of Fos and other ITFs in the central nervous system are therefore widely used as markers of neuronal activation by specific stimuli (14). In particular, Fos may be involved in the feedback regulation of TRH gene expression by thyroid hormones (19). Decreased thyroid hormone levels caused by thyroidectomy induce Fos expression in the TRH synthesizing neurons in the PVN (19).

The number of Fos-immunoreactive (IR) neurons in the medullary Rpa, Rob and PPR were low in euthyroid rats (0–2/section). Adding 1% 6-N-propyl-2-thiouracil (PTU) to the rat drinking water gradually decreased thyroid hormone levels in the rat serum and selectively increased the number of Fos-like IR neurons in the Rpa, Rob (Figures 2, 3) and PPR. After 4 weeks, Fos-IR neurons were 10 to 70-fold higher compared with the euthyroid controls (52). The increase of Fos expression in the Rpa, Rob and PPR was prevented by simultaneous T₄ replacement (Figure 2). Hyperthyroidism did not induce Fos expression in these medullary nuclei (Figure 2).

Double immunostaining revealed that most of the Fos-IR cells induced by hypothyroidism in the Rpa, Rob and PPR were located in pro-TRH positive neurons (52; also in the cover page of *American Journal of Physiology, Endocrine and Metabolism, Jan.–June, 2000*). The noticeable pro-TRH

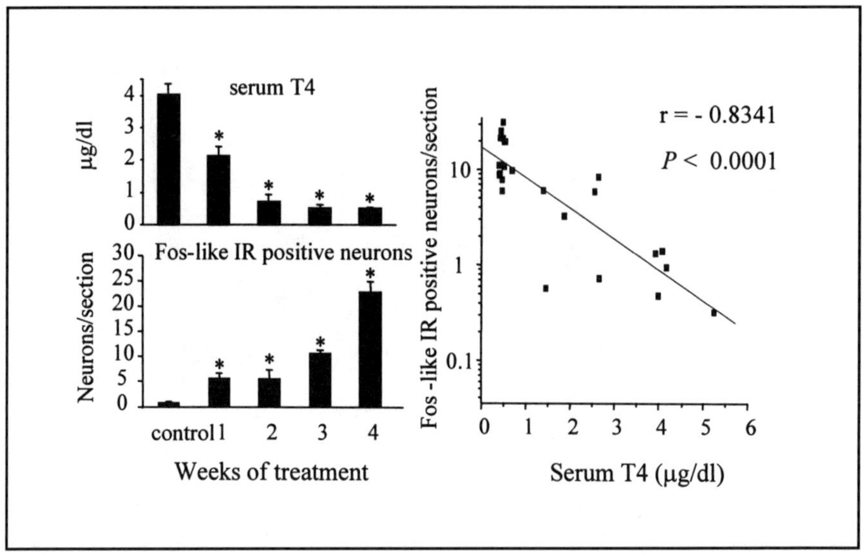

FIGURE 3. *Time courses of serum T_4 levels (a) and number of Fos-like IR positive neurons (b) in rostral Rpa during the progression of hypothyroidism in rats. Columns are means ± SE of 4–6 rats. ★ P < 0.05 compared with control levels. (c) Correlation between serum T_4 levels and number of Fos-like IR positive neurons in the rostral Rpa. r. Correlation coefficient. Adapted from Reference 52.*

staining observed in brainstem sections of hypothyroid rats without colchicine treatment indicates that hypothyroidism increases pro-TRH peptide content in the Rpa, Rob and PPR neurons, since the pro-TRH immunostaining was undetectable in euthyroid rats (52). There were significant negative correlations between serum T_4 levels and the numbers of Fos-like IR positive neurons in the Rpa (Figure 3), Rob and PPR (52). The selective and sustained induction of Fos-like IR in TRH-synthesizing neurons in the Rpa, Rob and PPR in hypothyroid rats is consistent with the enhanced TRH gene expression in these locations (47) and strongly suggest that the activation of these nuclei may attribute to the mechanism responsible for the autonomic disorders observed in hypothyroidism.

Thyroid Hormone Receptors Are Localized in the Medullary TRH Synthesizing Neurons in the Rpa, Rob, and PPR

The TRH gene belongs to a family of triiodothyronine (T_3) responsible genes, whose expression is negatively regulated by T_3 at the level of gene transcription (7). The negative regulation of murine TRH gene expression by thyroid hormone requires thyroid hormone receptors (TRs) (36). The TRs include TRα and TRβ subtypes encoded by separate genes, c-erbAα and c-erbAβ (5). Both TRα and TRβ give rise to several isoforms of which three, $TR\alpha_1$, $TR\beta_1$ and $TR\beta_2$ bind T_3 and mediate the action of thyroid hormone (21). The TRs are nuclear transactivating proteins involved in the regulation of gene expression. Unliganded $TR\alpha_1$, $TR\beta_1$ and $TR\beta_2$ significantly activated basal promoter activity of the TRH gene while TR-T_3 complexes presented the T_3-dependent inhibitory regulation of the TRH promoter (7). There were reports showing the absence of TR isoform specificity on T_3 inhibition of TRH gene (7, 36). However, in cultured embryonic chick hypothalamic cells, only $TR\beta$-dependent TRH transcription was differentially modulated by physiological concentration of T_3 (24). In cultured CV-1 cell line, $TR\beta_2$ achieved significantly greater ligand-independent activation on TRH gene than either $TR\beta_1$ or $TR\alpha_1$ and yielded greater ligand-dependent repression versus the other isoforms (20). Using *in vivo* gene transferred mice model, all forms of $TR\beta$ gave T_3-dependent regulation of TRH transcription, whereas transcription was T_3 insensitive with each $TR\alpha$ tested (10). These studies indicate a unique effect of $TR\beta$, especially $TR\beta_2$ on the negative regulation of TRH gene by T_3.

To support that the feedback regulation of medullary TRH gene expression by thyroid hormone is a direct action of thyroid hormone on the TRH-synthesizing neurons, we localized the immunoreactivities for $TR\alpha_1$, $TR\alpha_2$, $TR\beta_1$ and $TR\beta_2$, as well as the mRNA of $TR\alpha_1$ in the Rpa, Rob and PPR (49).

$TR\beta_2$ IR was widely distributed throughout the gray matter in the medulla. No immunostaining was present in white matter fiber tracts. Within the ventral medulla, many neuronal groups contained some $TR\beta_2$ IR positive cells with different immunostaining density. Dense accumulations of $TR\beta_2$ IR were particularly apparent in the cells of the Rpa, Rob and PPR that extended throughout the entire rostral-caudal extent of the nuclei. The reaction product was primarily confined to the cell nuclei (49).

It was reported that $TR\beta_2$ expression is strongly regulated by thyroid hormone in both *in vitro* (17) and *in vivo* (43) systems. In particular, Li and Boyages (25) found that the number and the staining of the $TR\beta_2$ IR positive cells in the pituitary gland were increased in hypothyroid rats when detected with immunocytochemistry. Therefore we also investigated whether thyroid status influences the number of $TR\beta_2$ IR positive cells in the medulla. However, there was no significant difference in the numbers of $TR\beta_2$ IR positive cells in the Rpa, Rob and PPR between euthyroid and hypothyroid rats (49).

Double staining of $TR\beta_2$ IR using immunohistochemistry and pro-TRH mRNA using *in situ* hybridization with digoxigenin-labeled probe revealed that the $TR\beta_2$ IR was present in all nuclei of pro-TRH mRNA positive neurons in the Rpa, Rob and PPR. These results provide an anatomical substrate for a direct regulatory action of thyroid hormone on TRH gene expression in these nuclei.

SUMMARY

Our recent studies provide evidence that thyroid hormone exerts a negative feedback regulation on medullary TRH gene expression. Hypothyroidism increased, while hyperthyroidism decreased the pro-TRH mRNA signals in the Rpa, Rob and PPR. Hypothyroidism stimulated remarkable Fos expression in the TRH synthesizing neurons in these nuclei. The effects-induced by hypothyroidism were prevented by simultaneous thyroid hormone replacement. The localization of thyroid hormone receptor subtypes, especially the $TR\beta_2$ in the Rpa, Rob and PPR provide anatomical support for a direct action of thyroid hormone on TRH synthesizing neurons in these medullary nuclei. These findings, together with the well established role of brain medullary TRH on the central regulation of autonomic regulation, demonstrate that the thyroid hormone action on TRH gene expression might be an important component of the pathophysiological mechanism through which autonomic disorders are induced by altered thyroid states.

ACKNOWLEDGMENTS

Studies on thyroid hormone regulation of medullary TRH-containing system were supported by grant from the National Institute of Diabetes and Digestive and Kidney Diseases, DK-50255 (Hong Yang).

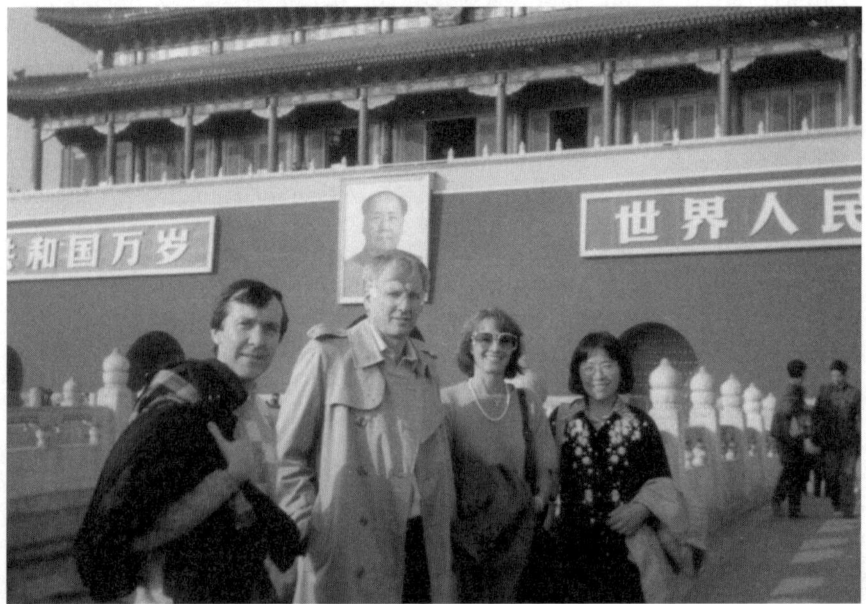

This picture was taken during the Beijing International Conference on Brain-Gut Peptides November, 1988. (From left to right: Graham Dockray, John Walsh, Yvette Taché, Hong Yang.)

REFERENCES

1. Arai I, Muramatsu M, Aihara H. Body temperature dependency of gastric regional blood flow, acid secretion and ulcer formation in restraint and water-immersion stressed rats. *Jpn J Pharmacol* 1986a; 40:501–504.

2. Arai I, Muramatsu M, Aihara H. Body temperature dependent decrease of gastric blood flow in restraint and water-immersion stressed rats. *J Pharmacobiodyn* 1986b;9:678–682.

3. Basso N, Bagarani M, Pekary AE, Genco A, Materia A. Role of thyrotropin-releasing hormone in stress ulcer formation in the rat. *Dig Dis Sci* 1988;33:819–823.

4. Bonaz B, Taché Y. Induction of Fos immunoreactivity in the rat brain after cold-restraint induced gastric lesions and fecal excretion. *Brain Res* 1994;652:56–64.

5. Brent GA, Moore DD, Larsen PR. Thyroid hormone regulation of gene expression. *Annual Rev Physiol* 1991;53:17–35.

6. Chang HC, Sloan JH. Influence of experimental hypothyroidism upon gastric secretion. *Am J Physiol* 1927;80:732–734.

7. Feng P, Li QL, Satoh T, Wilber JF. Ligand (T3) dependent and independent effects of thyroid hormone receptors upon human TRH gene transcription in neuroblastoma cells. *Biochem Biophys Res Commun* 1994;200:171–177.

8. Garrick T, Prince M, Yang H, Ohning G, Taché Y. Raphe pallidus stimulation increases gastric contractility via TRH projections to the dorsal vagal complex in rats. *Brain Res* 1994;636:343–347.

9. Goldsmith DPJ, Nasset ES. Relation of thyroid to gastric acid secretin in the anesthetized rat. *Am J Physiol* 1959;197:1–4.

10. Guissouma H, Ghorbel MT, Seugnet I, Ouatas T, Demeneix BA. Physiological regulation of hypothalamic TRH transcription *in vivo* is T3 receptor isoform specific. *FASEB J* 1998;12:1755–1764.

11. Harris M, Aschkenasi C, Elias CF, Chandrankunnel A, Nillni EA, Bjorbaek C, Elmquist JK, Flier JS, Hollenberg AN. Transcriptional regulation of the thyrotropin-releasing hormone gene by leptin and melanocortin signaling. *J Clin Invest* 2001;107:111–120.

12. Herdegen T, Leah JD. Inducible and constitutive transcription factors in the mammalian nervous system: control of gene expression by Jun, Fos and Krox, and CREB/ATF proteins. *Brain Res Rev* 1998;28:370–490.

13. Hernandez DE, Walker CH, Mason GA. Influence of thyroid states on stress gastric ulcer formation. *Life Sci* 1988;42:1757–1764.

14. Hoffman GE, Lee WS, Smith MS, Abbud R, Roberts MM, Robinson AG, Verbalis JG. c-Fos and Fos-related antigens as markers for neuronal activity: perspectives from neuroendocrine systems. *NIDA Res Monogr* 1993;125:117–133.

15. Ishikawa T, Yang H, Taché Y. Medullary sites of action of the TRH analogue, RX 77368, for stimulation of gastric acid secretion in the rat. *Gastroenterology* 1988;95:1470–1476.

16. Johansson H, Nylander G. Effects of thyroxine and thiouracil treatment on gastric secretion and gastric ulcer incidence in the Shay rat. *Acta Chir Scand* 1964;127:527–535.

17. Jones KE, Yaffe BM, Chin WW. Regulation of thyroid hormone receptor beta-2 mRNA levels by retinoic acid. *Mol Cell Endocrinol* 1993;91:113–118.

18. Kaneko H, Taché Y. TRH in the dorsal motor nucleus of vagus is involved in gastric erosion induced by excitation of raphe pallidus in rats. *Brain Res* 1995;699:97–102.

19. Koibuchi N, Gibbs RB, Suzuki M, Pfaff DW. Thyroidectomy induces Fos-like immunoreactivity within thyrotropin- releasing hormone-expressing neurons located in the paraventricular nucleus of the adult rat hypothalamus. *Endocrinology* 1991;129:3208–3216.

20. Langlois MF, Zanger K, Monden T, Safer JD, Hollenberg AN, Wondisford FE. A unique role of the beta-2 thyroid hormone receptor isoform in negative regulation by thyroid hormone. Mapping of a novel amino- terminal domain important for ligand-independent activation. *J Biol Chem* 1997; 272:24927–24933.

21. Lechan RM, Qi Y, Berrodin TJ, Davis KD, Schwartz HL, Strait KA, Oppenheimer JH, Lazar MA. Immunocytochemical delineation of thyroid hormone receptor beta 2-like immunoreactivity in the rat central nervous system. *Endocrinology* 1993;132:2461–2469.

22. Lechan RM, Segerson TP. Pro-TRH gene expression and precursor peptides in rat brain. Observations by hybridization analysis and immunocytochemistry. *Ann NY Acad Sci* 1989;553:29–59.

23. Legradi G, Emerson CH, Ahima RS, Flier JS, Lechan RM. Leptin prevents fasting-induced suppression of prothyrotropin-releasing hormone messenger ribonucleic acid in neurons of the hypothalamic paraventricular nucleus. *Endocrinology* 1997;138:2569–2576.

24. Lezoualch F, Hassan AH, Giraud P, Loeffler JP, Lee SL, Demeneix BA. Assignment of the beta-thyroid hormone receptor to 3,5,3′- triiodothyronine-dependent inhibition of transcription from the thyrotropin-releasing hormone promoter in chick hypothalamic neurons. *Mol Endocrinol* 1992;6:1797–1804.

25. Li M and Boyages SC. Expression of beta2-thyroid hormone receptor in euthyroid and hypothyroid rat pituitary gland: An *in situ* hybridization and immunocytochemical study. *Brain Res* 1997;773:125–131.

26. Loewy AD, Spyer KM. Vagal preganglionic neurons. In: *Central regulation of autonomic function*, edited by Loewy AD and Spyer KM, London: Oxford University Press, 1990 p. 68–87.

27. Lynn RB, Kreider MS, Miselis RR. Thyrotropin-releasing hormone-immunoreactive projections to the dorsal motor nucleus and the nucleus of the solitary tract of the rat. *J Comp Neurol* 1991;311:271–288.

28. Manaker S, Rizio G. Autoradiographic localization of thyrotropin-releasing hormone and substance P receptors in the rat dorsal vagal complex. *J Comp Neurol* 1989;290:516–526.

29. Martinez V, Wu SV, Taché Y. Intracisternal antisense oligodeoxynucleotides to the TRH receptor blocked vagal dependent stimulation of gastric emptying induced by acute cold in rats. *Endocrinology* 1998;139:3730–3735.

30. McCann MJ, Hermann GE, Rogers RC. Thyrotropin-releasing hormone: effects on identified neurons of the dorsal vagal complex. *J Auton Nerv Syst* 1989;26:107–112.

31. Miampamba M, Yang H, Sharkey KA, Taché Y. Intracisternal TRH analog induces Fos expression in gastric myenteric neurons and glia in conscious rats. *Am J Physiol Gastrointest Liver Physiol* 2001;280: G979-G991.

32. Nasset ES, Logan VW, Kelley ML, Thomas M. Inhibition of gastric secretion by thyroid preparations. *Am J Physiol* 1959;196:1262–1265.

33. O-Lee TJ, Wei JY, Taché Y. Intracisternal TRH and RX 77368 potently activate gastric vagal efferent discharge in rats. *Peptides* 1997;18: 213–219.

34. Paxinos G, Watson C: The Rat Brain in Stereotaxic Coordinates. San Diego: *Academic Press,* 1997 pp. 1–79.

35. Rinaman L, Miselis RR, Kreider MS. Ultrastructural localization of thyrotropin-releasing hormone immunoreactivity in the dorsal vagal complex in rat. *Neurosci Lett* 1989;104:7–12.

36. Satoh T, Yamada M, Iwasaki T, Mori M. Negative regulation of the gene for the preprothyrotropin-releasing hormone from the mouse by thyroid hormone requires additional factors in conjunction with thyroid hormone receptors. *J Biol Chem* 1996;271:27919–27926.

37. Seely EW, Williams GH. Gastrointestinal manifestations of endocrine disease. In: *Principles and Practice of Endocrinology and Metabolism,* edited by Becker KL, Philadelphia: JB Lippincott Company, 1990a, p. 1503–1506.

38. Seely EW, Williams GH. The cardiovascular system and endocrine disease. In: *Principles and Practice of Endocrinology and Metabolism,* edited by Becker KL, Philadelphia: JB Lippincott Company, 1990b, p. 1496–1501.

39. Segerson TP, Kauer J, Wolfe HC, Mobtaker H, Wu P, Jackson IM, Lechan RM. Thyroid hormone regulates TRH biosynthesis in the paraventricular nucleus of the rat hypothalamus. *Science* 1987; 238:78–80.

40. Sheng M, Greenberg ME. The regulation and function of c-fos and other immediate early genes in the nervous system. *Neuron* 1990;4:477–485.

41. Sivarao DV, Krowicki ZK, Abrahams TP, Hornby PJ. Intracisternal antisense oligonucleotides to TRH receptor abolish TRH- evoked gastric motor excitation. *Am J Physiol* 1997;272:G1372–G1381.

42. Taché Y, Yang H. Role of medullary TRH in the vagal regulation of gastric function. In: *Innervation of the Gut: Pathophysiological Implications,* edited by Wingate DL and Butkd TF, Boca Raton: CRC, 1994, p. 67–80.

43. Ulisse S, Esslemont G, Baker BS, Krishna V, Chatterjee K, Tata JR. Dominant-negative mutant thyroid hormone receptors prevent transcription from Xenopus thyroid hormone receptor beta gene promoter in response to thyroid hormone in Xenopus tadpoles *in vivo. Proc Natl Acad Sci USA* 1996;93:1205–1209.

44. Yang H, Kawakubo K, Taché Y. Intracisternal PYY increases gastric mucosal resistance: role of cholinergic, CGRP, and NO pathways. *Am J Physiol* 1999;277:G555-G562.

45. Yang H, Ohning GV, Taché Y. TRH in dorsal vagal complex mediates acid response to excitation of raphe pallidus neurons in rats. *Am J Physiol* 1993;265:G880-G886.

46. Yang H, Wu SV, Ishikawa T, Taché Y. Cold exposure elevates thyrotropin-releasing hormone gene expression in medullary raphe nuclei: relationship with vagally mediated gastric erosions. *Neuroscience* 1994;61:655–663.

47. Yang H, Yuan P, Wu V, Taché Y. Feedback regulation of thyrotropin-releasing hormone gene expression by thyroid hormone in the caudal raphe nuclei in rats. *Endocrinology* 1999;140:43–49.

48. Yang H, Yuan PQ, Wang L, Taché Y. Activation of the parapyramidal region in the ventral medulla stimulates gastric acid secretion through vagal pathways in rats. *Neuroscience* 2000;95:773–779.

49. Yuan P, Yang H. Localization of thyroid hormone receptor beta2 in the ventral medullary neurons that synthesize thyrotropin-releasing hormone. *Brain Res* 2000;868:22–30.

50. Yuan PQ, Taché Y, Miampamba M, Yang H. Acute cold exposure induces vagally mediated Fos expression in gastric myenteric neurons in conscious rats. *Am J Physiol Gastrointest Liver Physiol* 2001; 281:G560-G568.

51. Yuan PQ, Yang H. Hyperthyroidism decreases thyrotropin-releasing hormone gene expression in the caudal raphe nuclei and the parapyramidal regions in rats. *Neurosci Lett* 1999a;276:189–192.

52. Yuan PQ, Yang H. Hypothyroidism induces Fos-like immunoreactivity in ventral medullary neurons that synthesize TRH. *Am J Physiol* 1999b;277:E927-E936.

53. Cover. Endocrinology and Metabolism, *Am J Physiol* 2000;278(1–6).

22

Peptides in the Enteric Nervous System

John B. Furness and Daniel P. Poole
*Department of Anatomy and Cell Biology, The University of Melbourne
Victoria, Australia*

INTRODUCTION

Studies of peptides in neurons of the gastrointestinal tract have played an important part in the demonstration that peptides occur in neurons and in showing that they are neurotransmitters. Studies of enteric innervation have also been a trigger for the development of the concept of neurons being chemically coded.

SUBSTANCE P—THE FIRST NEUROPEPTIDE TO BE DISCOVERED

The first neuropeptide, substance P, was initially isolated from the equine brain and intestine in 1931 by Gaddum and Euler (1) and its biological activity was assayed in terms of contraction of the isolated rabbit jejunum (2). In fact, the first peptide suggested to be a transmitter was substance P, proposed by Lembeck in 1953 to be a transmitter of primary afferent neurons (3). However, possibly the first published pharmacological evidence that substance P (or any peptide) might be a transmitter, comes from work on the intestine published in a slightly obscure abstract in 1966 (4). These authors reported that a crude extract containing substance P reduced the responses of the guinea pig ileum to the stimulation of intramural nerves, in preparations in which responses to acetylcholine had been blocked. The conclusion depended on the idea that substances could cause a specific desensitization of their own receptors (5). Pure substance P became available

---

Abbreviations: ACh, acetylcholine; ATP, adenosine triphosphate; BN, bombesin (the mammalian form also referred to as GRP, below); CCK, cholecystokinin; ChAT, choline acetyltransferase; CGRP, calcitonin gene related peptide; DYN, dynorphin; ENK, enkephalin; GABA, gamma aminobutyric acid; GAL, galanin; GRP, gastrin releasing peptide (mammalian bombesin); 5-HT, 5-hydroxytryptamine; NFP, neurofilament protein; NK, neurokinin; NMU, neuromedin U; NOS, nitric oxide synthase; NPY, neuropeptide Y; PACAP, pituitary adenylyl cyclase activating peptide; PHI, peptide histidine-isoleucine; SOM, somatostatin; TK, tachykinin; VIP, vasoactive intestinal peptide.

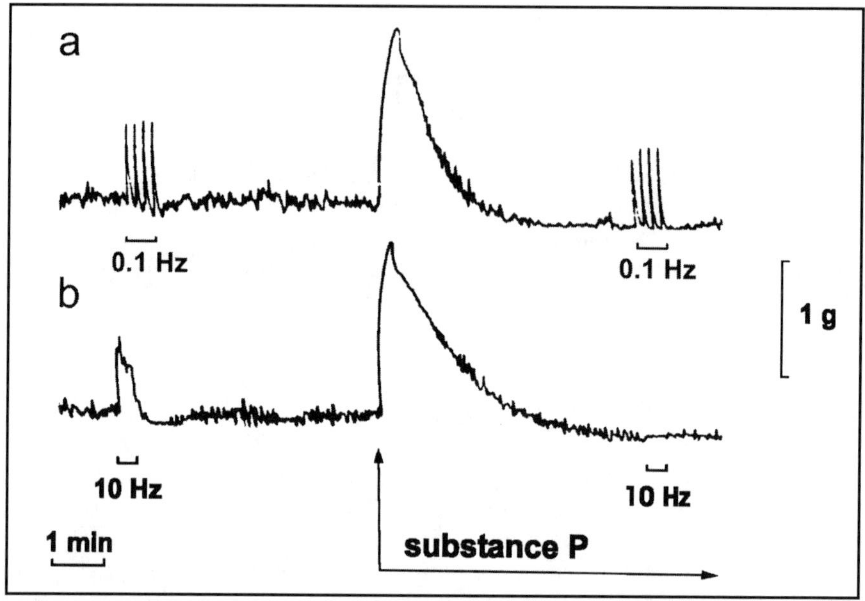

FIGURE 1. *Some of the first pharmacological evidence for a transmitter role of tachykinins in the intestine. In this experiment, the pharmacology of transmission to the longitudinal muscle of the guinea pig ileum was examined. Intramural nerves were stimulated with pulses at 1 Hz, or at 10 Hz after muscarinic receptors were blocked. In both cases, transmission caused contraction of the muscle. Transmission at 1 Hz was blocked by the muscarinic antagonist, hyoscine. Excitatory transmission in response to stimulation of the intramural nerves at 10 Hz was blocked by desensitizing tachykinin receptors with substance P (75 nM). Record from reference 7.*

only after it was sequenced in 1971 (6). Using the newly available pure peptide, in 1979 Franco et al. (7) showed that non-cholinergic transmission to gut muscle was antagonized when the receptors for substance P were desensitized (Figure 1). They also showed that desensitization was specific, in that responses to 5-HT, carbachol, nicotinic agonists and bradykinin were unaffected. In other experiments, release of substance P-like material in response to stimulation of intestinal nerves and blockade of transmission by antagonists that had no agonist activity were demonstrated (8). These findings established the idea that substance P, or closely related peptides, were enteric neurotransmitters (8).

More recent studies indicate that there are three receptor types for substance P, and that substance P belongs to a family of peptides called tachykinins, that in mammals include substance P, neurokinin A and neurokinin B. Tachykinins are in fact co-transmitters of excitatory neurons innervating gut muscle. The primary transmitter of the excitatory neurons is acetylcholine, which acts on the muscle through muscarinic receptors (9). Tachykinins have a lesser role than acetylcholine, except perhaps in the rat small intestine (8, 10, 11). The

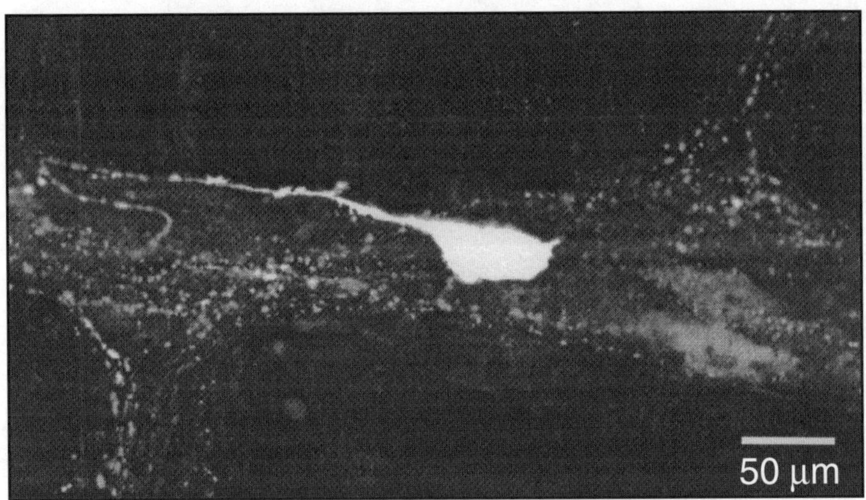

FIGURE 2. *Immunohistochemical localization of a neuropeptide, NPY, in a wholemount of guinea pig myenteric plexus. This illustrates the utility of peptide immunohistochemistry in wholemounts, developed in 1979 and 1980, for investigation of the distribution of enteric neuropeptides. NPY immunoreactivity occurs in the strongly reactive cell bodies of secretomotor neurons, in more weakly reactive Dogiel type I neurons and in nerve fibers in the myenteric ganglia. .*

tachykinins present in enteric neurons are substance P, neurokinin A, neuropeptide K, and neuropeptide γ. There is direct experimental evidence for the involvement of two of these, substance P and neurokinin A, in neuromuscular transmission (12). Immunohistochemical studies and quantitative electron microscopy show that acetylcholine and tachykinins are contained in the same excitatory muscle motor neurons (13, 14).

Tachykinins are also transmitters at neuro-neuronal synapses in the enteric nervous system, where their actions are mediated through slow excitatory post-synaptic potentials (15–18). Studies of the effects of tachykinin receptor antagonists on enteric motility reflexes confirm roles for tachykinins in physiological responses of the intestine (19–21).

The Advent of Peptide Immunohistochemistry

Methods to generate effective antibodies to relatively small molecules such as neuropeptides, and immunohistochemical methods to exploit these antibodies to locate neuropeptides burst on the scene in 1974 and 1975, mainly through the work of Tomas Hökfelt and his collaborators. The intestine was examined in some of the early studies, and neurons in the intestine were soon revealed with antibodies against somatostatin (22), substance P (23), enkephalin (24) and VIP (25). Many more neuropeptides were revealed in subsequent years, and the number of neuropeptides that are localized in enteric neurons now numbers about 30 (some of which are listed in Table 1). The structure of the intestine lends itself to the preparations of wholemounts, in which the enteric plexuses are laid out in two dimensions. Very quickly methods were developed to improve antibody penetration into the tissue and peptide immunhistochemistry in wholemounts became a method of choice for the analysis of the distributions and projections of enteric neurons (Figure 2) (26, 27).

At this time, in the mid to late 1970's, John Walsh saw the great potential of antibodies to peptides as tools to probe their distributions and functions. With Helen Wong, he set up the CURE Antibody Core Facility. Very soon, high quality antibodies were being produced and were used through John's generosity by numerous laboratories throughout the world. This far-sighted approach accelerated the accumulation of data concerning the distribution and roles of neuropeptides in the gastrointestinal tract.

The Chemical Coding Hypothesis

It was quickly realized with the outcome and availability of new tools and antibody probes that peptides were often colocalized in neurons, either with other peptides, or with other chemicals that defined classes of neurons (Table 1). These discoveries were made in several parts of the nervous system, but it was in the enteric nervous system that the major exploration of colocalization was made, leading to the hypothesis that neurons that have particular places in nerve circuits, and hence defined functions, could be identified by the combinations of chemicals that they contain, that is, by a chemical code (28–30). The reasons for the large numbers of peptides in enteric (and other) neurons are unknown. It is clear that some of these peptides contribute to neurotransmission, and examples of peptide neurotransmission are given below. However, some peptides do not appear to have transmitter, or any identified, roles. It has been argued that some peptides might be expressed by neurons, but have no functional role (31).

Plurichemical Transmission

The evidence that individual neurons contain several substances with potential to be neurotransmitters led to studies to evaluate their relative roles. It was soon discovered that transmission from individual enteric neurons generally involved two or more transmitters. This was against the commonly held view that each neuron has a unique transmitter, but was consistent with data that was being obtained in other regions, for example, the innervation of blood vessels and sympathetic ganglia (32). In the intestine and elsewhere, there often appears to be one substance with a dominant role in neurotransmission (the

TABLE 1. *Chemical coding of enteric neurons of the guinea pig small intestine (references: 30, 55). Neuropeptides in enteric neurons are indicated in bold.*

Myenteric Neurons	*Chemical Coding*	*Function/Comments*
Excitatory circular muscle motor neurons	*Short:* ChAT/**TK/ENK/**GABA *Long:* ChAT/**TK/ENK/**NFP	Primary transmitter ACh, cotransmitter **TK**
Inhibitory circular muscle motor neurons	*Short:* NOS/**VIP/PACAP/****ENK/NPY**/GABA *Long:* NOS/ **VIP/PACAP/****DYN/BN**/NFP	Several cotransmitters with varying prominence: NO, ATP, **VIP, PACAP**
Excitatory longitudinal muscle motor neurons	ChAT/Calretinin/**TK**	primary transmitter ACh, cotransmitter **TK**
Inhibitory longitudinal muscle motor neurons	NOS/**VIP/PACAP**/GABA	Several cotransmitters with varying prominence: NO, ATP, **VIP, PACAP**
Ascending interneurons	ChAT/Calretinin/**ENK/****TK**	primary transmitter ACh
Descending interneurons (local reflex)	ChAT/NOS/**VIP/PACAP**± **BN** ± **NPY**	primary transmitter ACh, ATP may be a cotransmitter
Descending interneurons (secretomotor reflex)	ChAT/5-HT	primary transmitters ACh, 5-HT (at 5-HT$_3$ receptors)
Descending interneurons (migrating myoelectric complex)	ChAT/**SOM**	primary transmitter ACh
Myenteric intrinsic primary afferent (primary sensory) neurons	ChAT/Calbindin/**TK/****NMU** ± **SOM**	primary transmitter **TK**
Intestinofugal neurons	ChAT/**BN/VIP/CCK/****CGRP/ENK/DYN**	primary transmitter ACh
Submucosal Neurons	*Chemical Coding*	*Function/Comments*
Non-cholinergic secreto-motor/vasodilator neurons	**VIP/GAL/DYN/NMU**	primary transmitter **VIP**
Cholinergic secretomotor/ vasodilator neurons	ChAT/Calretinin/**DYN**	primary transmitter ACh
Cholinergic secretomotor (non-vasodilator) neurons	ChAT/**NPY/CCK/GAL/****SOM/CGRP/DYN/****NMU**	primary transmitter ACh
Submucosal intrinsic primary afferent (primary sensory) neurons	ChAT/**TK**/calbindin/**NMU**	Calbindin-IR, seen with some antisera only. Primary transmitter ACh, TK may also have transmitter role

primary transmitter), and other substances with subsidiary roles. For example, acetylcholine is the primary transmitter of excitatory muscle motor neurons and tachykinins have lesser roles. For the enteric inhibitory neurons, which have been extensively investigated, there appear to be three or four transmitters: nitric oxide, ATP, VIP and PACAP. Interestingly, the relative importances of the transmitters appear to differ between regions and species (33).

Other Peptides with Transmitter Roles in the Intestine

In addition to tachykinins, which are discussed previously, there is good evidence that gastrin releasing peptide is a neurotransmitter to gastrin cells in the antrum, that VIP is a transmitter of inhibitory motor neurons and enteric secretomotor neurons, and that PACAP is also a transmitter of enteric inhibitory neurons. Some of the data is reviewed below. There is also evidence that somatostatin is a transmitter of inhibitory synaptic inputs to secretomotor neurons (34) and that opioid peptides are enteric neurotransmitters (35).

VIP as a Transmitter of Enteric Inhibitory Neurons

Enteric inhibitory neurons innervate the muscle of all parts of the gastrointestinal tract; in all regions and all mammalian species they are immunoreactive for VIP (36). Evidence that VIP is one of the neurotransmitters of these neurons was amongst the earliest evidence for peptide neurotransmitters (9, 37). VIP relaxes intestinal muscle throughout the gastrointestinal tract. An important part of the evidence for a transmitter role was the discovery by Farhenkrug and colleagues that VIP was released into the venous effluent of the stomach when the enteric inhibitory neurons were activated reflexly (38). Further evidence for VIP release was obtained when reflexes in intestinal segments were elicited (39, 40).

VIP in Secretomotor and Vasodilator Neurons

There are two types of intestinal secretomotor neurons: cholinergic and noncholinergic. The noncholinergic neurons appear to mediate most of the local reflex response, and utilize VIP, or a related peptide (e.g., PHI or PACAP), as their primary transmitter (41, 42). VIP is a stimulant of secretion that occurs in the non-cholinergic secretomotor neurons (see Table 1), and when these neurons are electrically stimulated, their effects are diminished by antagonists of VIP receptors (42). Furthermore, VIP is released when enteric secretomotor reflexes are evoked (43) and secretomotor reflex responses are antagonized by VIP receptor antagonists, by immunoneutralization or by desensitization of VIP receptors (44, 45).

The same VIP neurons that innervate the mucosa have collaterals to arterioles in the submucosa and it has been deduced that VIP could be a vasodilator transmitter released from these neurons (46).

PACAP

PACAP is closely related to VIP, both structurally and in its effects at receptors. It is, therefore, reasonable to assume that pharmacological data that has implicated VIP as a neurotransmitter could equally well implicate PACAP, which seems to be colocalized with VIP in many enteric neurons. Direct evidence for PACAP mediated transmission has been reported (47, 48).

Gastrin Releasing Peptide

GRP (mammalian bombesin) is a powerful stimulant of gastrin secretion that is found in nerve fibres innervating the antral mucosa, where gastrin secreting endocrine cells occur. Evidence for a transmitter role includes the observation that GRP immunoneutralization decreases nerve mediated gastric acid secretion by about 60% (49).

Differences Between Species and Regions

There are systematic differences in the peptide content and chemical coding of homologous neurons between regions of the gastrointestinal tract (50) and between the same regions in different species (51–54). These differences may reflect differences in the roles of peptides between regions and species, although this hypothesis needs more thorough investigation. Nevertheless, peptides that have demonstrated functional roles appear to be conserved. For example, in all species and regions, excitatory neurons to the external muscle contain tachykinins and inhibitory neurons contain VIP. Another example, is that in all cases, the mucosa of the small and large intestine is innervated by VIP immunoreactive secretomotor neurons. This leads us to suggest that peptides that have roles that are significant for the function of enteric neurons tend to be conserved between species, while those that have little functional relevance (the superfluous peptides of Bowers, ref 31) may be less often conserved.

CONCLUSIONS

The discovery of peptides in enteric neurons in the mid 1970s laid the foundation for studies that defined the circuitry of the enteric nervous system through peptide immunohistochemistry, and defined roles of peptides as neurotransmitters. Work on the enteric nervous system was instrumental in the development of the chemical coding hypothesis and was important in the discovery that many neurons have multiple transmitters. In only some cases (e.g., neurokinin and opioid receptors), adequately potent, systemically effective and specific receptor antagonists have been discovered. It is anticipated that further development of neuropeptide antagonists will better define their roles, and may lead to therapeutically useful compounds.

REFERENCES

1. Von Euler US, Gaddum JH. An unidentified depressor substance in certain tissue extracts. *J Physiol* (Lond) 1931;72:74–87.
2. Von Euler US. Herstellung und Eigenschaften von Substanz P. *Acta Physiol Scand* 1942;4:373–375.
3. Lembeck F. Zur Fragen der zentralen Übertragung afferenter Impulse. III Mitteilung: Das Vorkommen und die Bedeutung der Substanz P in den dorsalen Wirzeln des Rückenmarks. *Naunyn Schmiedeberg's Arch Pharmacol* 1953;219:197–213.
4. Paton WDM, Zar MA. Evidence for transmission of nerve effects by substance P in guinea-pig longitudinal muscle strip. *Abstracts of III Int Pharmacol Cong,* Sao Paulo, Brazil, 1966;9.
5. Gaddum JH. Tryptamine receptors. *J Physiol* (Lond) 1953;119:363–368.
6. Chang MM, Leeman SE, Niall HD. Amino-acid sequence of substance P. *Nature New Biol* 1971; 232:86–87.
7. Franco R, Costa M, Furness JB. Evidence for the release of endogenous substance P from intestinal nerves. *Naunyn Schmiedeberg's Arch Pharmacol* 1979;306:195–201.
8. Barthó L and Holzer P. Search for a physiological role of substance P in gastrointestinal motility. *Neuroscience* 1985;16:1–32.
9. Furness JB, Costa M. *The Enteric Nervous System.* Churchill Livingstone, Edinburgh, 1987.
10. Ruwart MJ, Klepper MS, Rush BD. Evidence for noncholinergic mediation of small intestinal transit in the rat. *J Pharm Exp Ther* 1979;209:462–465.
11. Zagorodnyuk V, Santicioli P, Maggi CA. Tachykinin NK1 but not NK2 receptors mediate noncholinergic excitatory junction potentials in the circular muscle of guinea-pig colon. *Br J Pharmacol* 1993;110:795–803.
12. Lippi A, Santicioli P, Criscuoli M, Maggi CA. Depolarization evoked co-release of tachykinins from enteric nerves in the guinea-pig proximal colon. *Naunyn Schmiedeberg's Arch Pharmacol* 1998;357: 245–251.
13. Llewellyn Smith IJ, Furness JB, Gibbins IL, Costa M. Quantitative ultrastructural analysis of enkephalin-, substance P-, and VIP-immunoreactive nerve fibers in the circular muscle of the guinea-pig small intestine. *J Comp Neurol* 1988;272:139–148.
14. Brookes SJH, Steele PA, Costa M. Identification and immunohistochemistry of cholinergic and noncholinergic circular muscle motor neurons in the guinea-pig small intestine. *Neuroscience* 1991;42: 863–878.
15. Mawe GM. Tachykinins as mediators of slow EPSPs in guinea-pig gall-bladder ganglia: involvement of neurokinin-3-receptors. *J Physiol* (Lond) 1995;485:513–524.
16. Neunlist M and Schemann M. Projections and neurochemical coding of myenteric neurons innervating the mucosa of the guinea pig proximal colon. *Cell Tissue Res* 1997;287:119-125.
17. Alex G, Kunze WAA, Furness JB, Clerc N. Comparison of the effects of neurokinin-3 receptor blockade on two forms of slow synaptic transmission in myenteric AH neurons. *Neuroscience* 2001; 104:263–269.
18. Alex G, Clerc N, Kunze WAA, Furness JB. Responses of myenteric S neurons to low frequency stimulation of their synaptic inputs. *Neuroscience* 2002;110:361–373.
19. Grider JR. Tachykinins as transmitters of ascending contractile component of the peristaltic reflex. *Am J Physiol* 1989;257:709–714.
20. Johnson PJ, Bornstein JC, Burcher E. Roles of neuronal NK1 and NK3 receptors in synaptic transmission during motility reflexes in the guinea-pig ileum. *Br J Pharmacol* 1998;124:1375–1384.
21. Tonini M, Spelta V, De Ponti F, De Giorgio R, D'Agostino G, Stanghellini V, Corinaldesi R, Sternini C, Crema F. Tachykinin-dependent and -independent components of peristalsis in the guinea pig isolated distal colon. *Gastroenterology* 2001;120:938–945.
22. Hökfelt T, Johansson O, Efendic S, Luft R, Arimura A. Are there somatostatin-containing nerves in the rat gut? Immunohistochemical evidence for a new type of peripheral nerves. *Experientia* 1975; 31:852–854.
23. Pearse AGE and Polak JM. Immunocytochemical localization of substance P in mammalian intestine. *Histochemistry* 1975;41:373–375.

24. Elde R, Hökfelt T, Johansson O, Terenius L. Immunohistochemical studies using antibodies to leucine enkephalin: initial observations on the nervous system of the rat. *Neuroscience* 1976;1:349–351.

25. Larsson LI, Fahrenkrug J, Schaffalitzky de Muckadell O, Sundler F, Håkanson R, Rehfeld JF. Localization of vasoactive intestinal polypeptide VIP to central and peripheral neurons. *Proc Natl Acad Sci USA* 1976;73:3197–3200.

26. Furness JB and Costa M. Projections of intestinal neurons showing immunoreactivity for vasoactive intestinal polypeptide are consistent with these neurons being the enteric inhibitory neurons. *Neuroscience Letters* 1979;15:199–204.

27. Costa M, Buffa R, Furness JB, Solcia E. Immunohistochemical localization of polypeptides in peripheral autonomic nerves using wholemount preparations. *Histochemistry* 1980;65:157–165.

28. Furness JB, Costa M, Morris JL, Gibbins IL. Novel neuro-transmitters and the chemical coding of neurons. In: *Advances in Physiological Research*. Plenum Press, New York, 1987;143–165.

29. Furness JB, Morris JL, Gibbins IL, Costa M. Chemical coding of neurons and plurichemical transmission. *Ann Rev Pharmacol Toxicol* 1989;29:289–306.

30. Costa M, Brookes SJH, Steele PA, Gibbins I, Burcher E, Kandiah CJ. Neurochemical classification of myenteric neurons in the guinea-pig ileum. *Neuroscience* 1996;75:949–967.

31. Bowers CW. Superfluous neurotransmitters? *Trends Neurosci* 1994;17:315–320.

32. Lundberg JM, Hökfelt T, Anggard A, Terenius L, Elde R, Markey K, Goldstein M, Kimmel J. Organization principles in the peripheral sympathetic nervous system: subdivision by coexisting peptides somatostatin-, avian pancreatic polypeptide-, and vasoactive intestinal polypeptide-like immunoreactive materials. *Proc Natl Acad Sci USA* 1982;79:1303–1307.

33. Furness JB, Young HM, Pompolo S, Bornstein JC, Kunze WAA, McConalogue K. Plurichemical transmission and chemical coding of neurons in the digestive tract. *Gastroenterology* 1995;108:554–563.

34. Surprenant A, Shen KZ, North RA, Tatsumi H. Inhibition of calcium currents by noradrenaline, somatostatin and opioids in guinea-pig submucosal neurones. *J Physiol* (Lond) 1990;431:585–608.

35. Sternini C. Receptors and transmission in the brain-gut axis: potential for novel therapies III. μ-Opioid receptors in the enteric nervous system. *Am J Physiol* 2001;281:G8–G15.

36. Furness JB, Llewellyn-Smith IJ, Bornstein JC, Costa M. Chemical neuroanatomy and the analysis of neuronal circuitry in the enteric nervous system. In: *Handbook of Chemical Neuroanatomy* Vol. 6, Ed. A. Björklund, T. Hökfelt and C. Owman. Elsevier: Amsterdam, 1988;161–218.

37. Fahrenkrug J. Vasoactive intestinal polypeptide: Measurement, distribution and putative neurotransmitter function. *Digestion* 1979;19:149–169.

38. Fahrenkrug J, Haglund U, Jodal M, Lundgren O, Olbe L, Schaffalitzky de Muckadell O. Nervous release of vasoactive intestinal polypeptide in the gastrointestinal tract of cats: possible physiological implications. *J Physiol* (Lond) 1978;284:291–305.

39. Grider JR and Makhlouf GM. Colonic peristaltic reflex: identification of vasoactive intestinal peptide as mediator of descending relaxation. *Am J Physiol* 1986;251:40–45.

40. Grider JR. Identification of neurotransmitters regulating intestinal peristaltic reflex in humans. *Gastroenterology* 1989;97:1414–1419.

41. Cooke HJ and Reddix RA. Neural regulation of intestinal electrolyte transport. In: *Physiology of the Gastrointestinal Tract*. Johnson LR (ed) Raven Press, New York, 1994;2083–2132.

42. Reddix R, Kuwahara A, Wallace L, Cooke HJ. Vasoactive intestinal polypeptide: a transmitter in submucous neurons mediating secretion in guinea pig distal colon. *J Pharmacol Exp Ther* 1994;269: 1124–1129.

43. Brunsson I, Fahrenkrug J, Jodal M, Sjöqvist A, Theodorsson E, Lundgren O. On the role of vasoactive intestinal polypeptide and tachykinins in the secretory reflex elicited by chemical peritonitis in the cat small intestine. *Acta Physiol Scand* 1990;139:63–75.

44. Schulzke JD, Riecken EO, Fromm M. Distension-induced electrogenic Cl- secretion is mediated via VIP-ergic neurons in rat rectal colon. *Am J Physiol* 1995;268:G725–G731.

45. Cooke HJ, Sidhu M, Wang YZ. Activation of 5-HT1P receptors on submucosal afferents subsequently triggers VIP neurons and chloride secretion in the guinea-pig colon. *J Autonom Nerv Syst* 1997;66:105–110.

46. Vanner S. Myenteric neurons activate submucosal vasodilator neurons in guinea pig ileum. *Am J Physiol* 2000;279:G380–G387.

47. McConalogue K, Lyster DJK, Furness JB. Electrophysiological analysis of the actions of pituitary adenylyl cyclase activating peptide in the taenia of the guinea-pig caecum. *Naunyn Schmiedeberg's Arch Pharmacol* 1995;352:538–544.

48. Murthy KS, Jin JG, Grider JR, Makhlouf GM. Characterization of PACAP receptors and signaling pathways in rabbit gastric muscle cells. *Am J Physiol* 1997;35:G1391–G1399.

49. Schubert ML, Saffouri B, Makhlouf GM. Inhibition of neurally-mediated gastrin secretion by bombesin antiserum. *Am J Physiol* 1985;248:G456–G462.

50. Lomax AEG and Furness JB. Neurochemical classification of enteric neurons in the guinea-pig distal colon. *Cell Tissue Res* 2000;302:59–73.

51. Timmermans JP, Scheuermann DW, Stach W, Adriaensen D, De Groodt Lasseel MHA. Functional morphology of the enteric nervous system with special reference to large mammals. *Eur J Morphol* 1992;30:113–122.

52. Sang Q and Young HM. Chemical coding of neurons in the myenteric plexus and external muscle of the small and large intestine of the mouse. *Cell Tissue Res* 1996;284:39–53.

53. Porter AJ, Wattchow DA, Brookes SJH, Costa M. The neurochemical coding and projections of circular muscle motor neurons in the human colon. *Gastroenterology* 1997;113:1916–1923.

54. Mann PT, Furness JB, Southwell BR. Choline acetyltransferase immunoreactivity of putative intrinsic primary afferent neurons in the rat ileum. *Cell Tissue Res* 1999;297:241–248.

55. Furness JB. Types of neurons in the enteric nervous system. *J Autonom Nerv Syst* 2000;81:87–96.

Gut-Brain Peptides in the New Millennium, edited by Y. Taché
CURE Foundation, Los Angeles, CA. © 2002

23

Mu Opioid Receptor Expression and Endocytosis in Enteric Neurons

Catia Sternini and Nicholas Brecha
*CURE/Digestive Diseases Research Center, UCLA Division of Digestive Diseases
Departments of Medicine and Neurobiology, VA Greater Los Angeles Healthcare System
Los Angeles, CA*

INTRODUCTION

The authors would like to take this opportunity to acknowledge the important intellectual contributions of Dr. John Walsh to their field of research. John has always been very interested in all aspects of peptides and peptide receptors and functions in the gut. Nick was recruited to CURE by John Walsh and Tachi Yamada in 1982 to bring his expertise in morphological approaches to study peptides and I came a year later as a fellow from Italy to work with John on peptides. Even if his major interest was on gut hormones, John was willing to be convinced that the neurons in the gut are as important as endocrine cells, and he has been continuously supportive of our research and interests to which he has contributed with his thoughtful input and comments. This chapter will briefly discuss some of the principal neurochemical features of the enteric nervous system and will focus on the μ opioid receptor (μOR), a G protein coupled receptor that is expressed by distinct enteric neuronal populations and that mediates many of the effects of opiates, potent analgesics commonly used in humans for pain control. μOR is also activated by endogenous opioids that affect several gastrointestinal functions, and it undergoes ligand-induced internalization *in vivo* and *in vitro*. Receptor endocytosis is a regulatory process that is associated with functional diminution of receptor-mediated signaling, and alterations of the mechanisms controlling cellular responses of G protein-coupled receptors to agonists might be the basis of several diseases, including gastrointestinal diseases.

THE ENTERIC NERVOUS SYSTEM (ENS)

The ENS, the neural network supplying the digestive tract, is unique for its capability of mediating reflex activity independently from the central nervous system. (1, 2). It comprises functionally distinct neuronal populations, which can be classified as primary afferent neurons, interneurons (orally and anally directed) and motor neurons (excitatory and inhibitory (1–3)). These neurons are synaptically connected to form microcircuits and they control multiple functions, including motility, blood flow, secretion and absorption. Enteric neurons contain and can release a multitude of chemical messengers, including acetylcholine, excitatory and inhibitory amino acids, serotonin, nitric oxide and an array of biologically active peptides. The chemical coding of enteric neurons, together with their morphology and projections, allows for the distinction of different classes of enteric neurons, which subserve different functions (4).

Peptides represent a major group of signaling molecules that exert multiple and profound effects in the digestive system (5). Peptides act on distinct cell types including endocrine cells, muscle cells, and enteric neurons often involving distinct receptor subtypes depending upon the target. These effects are mediated by the activation of specific receptors, many of which belong to the superfamily of seven transmembrane G protein-coupled receptors. G protein-coupled receptors represent a large and versatile class of cell surface signal transducing proteins, which activate different effector systems to induce a variety of biological functions (6). Many peptide receptors have been identified in different cell types in the gastrointestinal tract and their localization pattern has provided important insights into our understanding of the sites and modes of action of peptides. The focus of this chapter will be on the distribution and endocytosis of the μ opioid receptor (μOR), which is the main mediator of opiate side effects, and which undergoes ligand-selective endocytosis in enteric neurons *in vivo* and *in vitro* (7).

μORS IN THE ENS

μOR is the preferred receptor for alkaloids, such as morphine and fentanyl, the most efficacious and potent analgesics used in humans (8). μOR is also activated by endogenous opioids (8), including enkephalins, dynorphins, and endomorphins (9). Enkephalins and dynorphins are expressed in enteric neurons (10, 11). Enkephalins bind to μOR with much higher affinity than dynorphins (12), which preferentially activate k opioid receptors (13). Endomorphins have the highest affinity and selectivity for μOR than any other opioids (9); they directly activate μOR and induce μOR endocytosis in enteric neurons (14). However, at this time, there is no evidence for the presence of endomorphins in the gastrointestinal tract. Opioids affect a variety of functions within the digestive system, including motility, secretion, and electrolyte and fluid transport (15).

μOR is localized to enteric neurons of the rat and guinea pig gastrointestinal tract (16, 17). In the guinea pig ileum, μOR immunoreactivity is

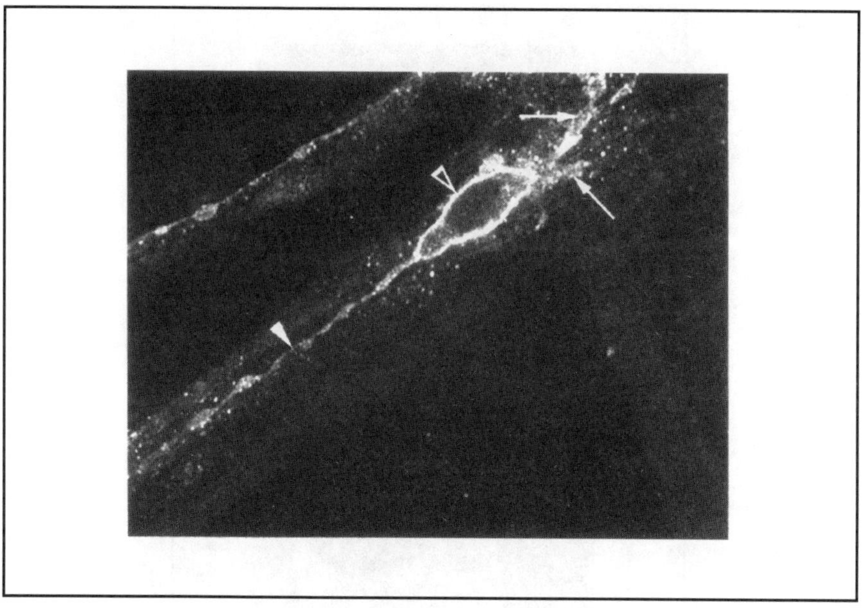

FIGURE 1. *Confocal image showing μOR immunoreactivity in a Dogiel type I myenteric neuron of the guinea pig ileum. μOR immunoreactivity is predominantly at the plasma membrane of the soma (open arrowhead) and neurites (arrows point to dendrites; closed arrowhead points to a long axonal process).*

confined to myenteric neurons (Figure 1), where it is predominantly localized at the cell surface, and to fibers distributed to the muscle layers. μOR neurons have the morphological characteristics of Dogiel type I neurons, with an oval cell body, many thick dendrites protruding from the soma and a long axonal process (17). μOR immunoreactive fibers form dense networks in the deep muscular plexus closely surrounding interstitial cells of Cajal (ICCs). This differs from what is reported in the rat, where μOR immunoreactivity has been described on the membrane of the ICCs in the rat gastrointestinal tract (16). Since two forms of μOR, μOR-1 and μOR-2 and several isoforms of μOR-1 have been reported, which can be distinguished on the basis of their pharmacological properties and anatomical distribution (18, 19), it is possible that the differences in findings between the guinea pig and rat is due to differences in antibody characteristics, which could detect different forms of μOR.

μOR enteric neurons comprise both ascending and descending neurons. About half of enteric μOR neurons are cholinergic as indicated by their expression of choline acetyltransferase (ChAT). Since cholinergic neurons of the guinea pig ileum comprise a subpopulation of tachykinergic neurons, (4) μOR/ChAT myenteric neurons can be defined as cholinergic and cholinergic/tachykinergic excitatory motor neurons to the longitudinal and

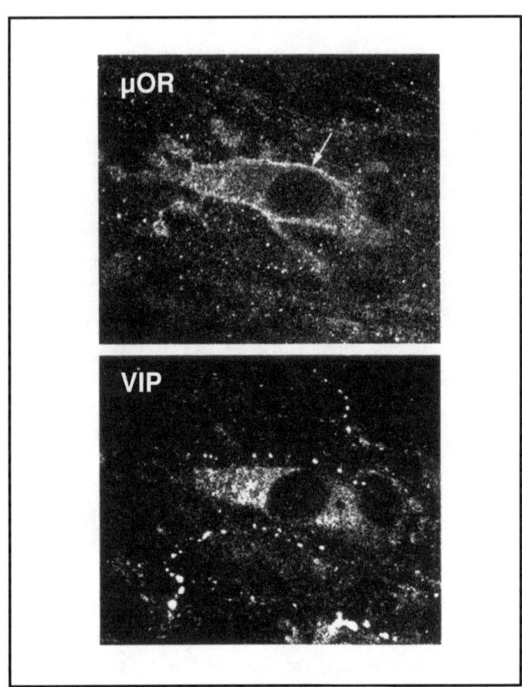

FIGURE 2. *Confocal images of a whole mount preparation showing colocalization of μOR with VIP. Note the predominant localization of μOR at the cell surface (arrow), whereas VIP immunoreactivity is localized in the cytoplasm (*).*

circular muscle. It is also likely that they comprise ascending interneurons, which also express this combination of chemical markers (ChAT and tachykinins) (4). Nearly 50% of μOR enteric neurons are descending neurons as indicated by the presence of nitric oxide synthase (NOS), the enzyme that synthesizes nitric oxide, and vasoactive intestinal polypeptide (VIP) (Figure 2), markers of inhibitory motor neurons (4, 5). Triple labeling showed that a high proportion of μOR immunoreactive neurons are ChAT/VIP neurons, indicating they are descending cholinergic interneurons (4). Finally, μORs are also expressed by myenteric neurons containing enkephalins. μOR myenteric neurons do not appear to comprise primary afferent enteric neurons as indicated by the lack of colocalization of μOR and calcium binding protein, a marker for primary afferent neurons in the guinea pig ileum (20). This is not surprising since μOR neurons have a typical morphology of Dogiel type I neurons, whereas primary afferent neurons are characterized by Dogiel type II morphology.

The presence of μOR on cholinergic ascending excitatory neurons to the muscle is in agreement with the functional evidence of opioid inhibition of electrically-induced release of acetylcholine by acting on enteric neurons primarily via the inhibitory receptor μOR, (15) thus resulting in inhibition of muscle contraction. On the other hand, the presence of μOR in the descending pathway is consistent with the described effect of μOR agonists in reducing compliance of the intestinal wall during the preparatory phase of peristalsis in intact segments of the guinea pig ileum (21). Since there is no evidence for a direct effect of μORs on smooth muscle of the guinea pig small intestine (22), whereas they inhibit enteric neurons (23), the μOR-induced inhibitory effect on compliance can be the result of a direct activation of inhibitory neurons to the circular muscle. A reduction of the excitability of interneurons located in the reflex pathway may also be involved. The presence of μOR in descending interneurons is in agreement with the latter possibility. Activation of the inhibitory μOR on descending motor neurons could result in inhibition of VIP release and NO production thus suppressing descending relaxation and consequently interfering with intestinal propulsion.

The presence of enkephalin in a subpopulation of μOR neurons suggests a possible autocrine mechanism for the regulation of endogenous opioids. Enkephalins might have a negative feedback on the neuronal activity by activating μOR. Enkephalins are capable of activating μOR (23) and of triggering μOR endocytosis in enteric neurons *in vitro* (Sternini, unpublished) and they are likely to be the endogenous opioids that primarily activate neuronal μOR in the gut.

μOR ENDOCYTOSIS IN ENTERIC NEURONS

μOR is an inhibitory G protein-coupled receptor functionally coupled to several effector pathways, including inhibition of adenylyl cyclase and of cyclic AMP formation, mediation of ion currents, modulation of inositol triphosphate turnover, and activation of mitogen-activated protein (24, 25). Coupling of the μOR to these effector systems attenuates neuronal activity by inhibiting neurotransmitter release and changing neuronal excitability by pre- and post-synaptic mechanisms. G protein-coupled receptors are modified by ligand-receptor interaction to allow coupling to G proteins and activation of second messenger system to induce signal transduction (26). They undergo desensitization and resensitization in response to agonist treatment, events that regulate cellular responsiveness to receptor activation and result from receptor-mediated processes, including phosphorylation, receptor endocytosis, intracellular sorting and recycling. Receptor internalization is not responsible for rapid cellular desensitization, but it is important in late desensitization and in resensitization. Interestingly, opioid agonists with similar abilities to activate μOR signaling have remarkably different abilities in functionally desensitizing the μOR

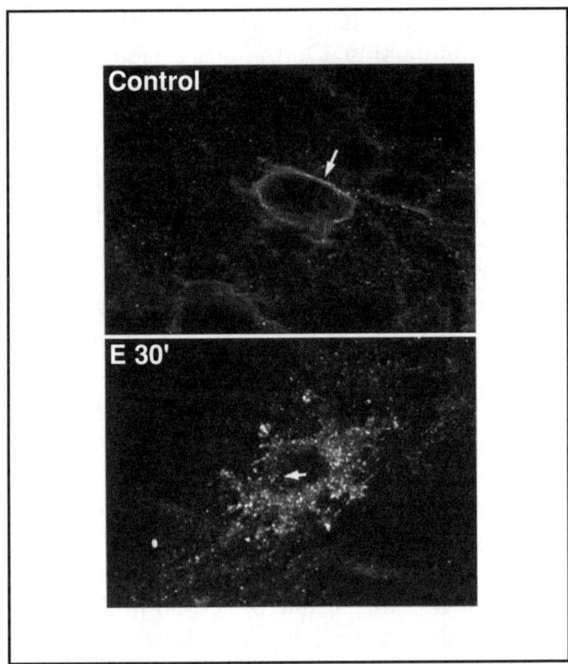

FIGURE 3. *Confocal images showing μOR at the cell surface of a neuron from a control animal (Control) and in endosomes 30 min following intraperitoneal injection of the μOR agonist, etorphine (0.1 mg/kg) (E 30') in guinea pig ileum. Arrows point to the cell surface in control and to endosomes following etorphine (E 30').*

and inducing μOR internalization (7, 14, 17, 27–32). Etorphine, fentanyl and opioid peptides induce rapid μOR internalization (Figure 3) and desensitization, whereas morphine, a high affinity μOR agonist and the prototype of opiate analgesics, fails to induce either internalization or desensitization acutely. Etorphine induces robust μOR phosphorylation followed by plasma membrane translocation of β arrestins and dynamin-dependent receptor internalization (32). By contrast, morphine's failure to induce desensitization is accompanied by a lack of μOR phosphorylation, translocation of β arrestins and dynamin-dependent receptor internalization. Furthermore, morphine induces μOR phosphorylation with β arrestin translocation and receptor sequestration when G protein kinase 2 (GRK2) is overexpressed (32). Changes in the trafficking machinery might affect cellular responsiveness by altering ligand ability to induce receptor endocytosis and desensitization. In addition, alternative splicing of the intracellular carboxy terminus of μOR-1 can influence the selectivity of ligand-induced μOR endocytosis. The novel μOR-1C splice variant, which has a distinct distribution in the brain compared to the cloned μOR-1, undergoes internalization in neurons in response to morphine, whereas the cloned μOR-1 does not undergo morphine-induced internalization (18, 33).

ROLE OF μOR ENDOCYTOSIS IN THE REGULATION OF NEURONAL RESPONSIVENESS

Ligand-induced μOR endocytosis in enteric neurons occurs predominantly via a clathrin-mediated mechanism and it is concentration-dependent (7). Following appropriate intracellular sorting requiring endosomal acidification, μOR recycles to the cell surface at about 6 hours. μOR internalization occurs both in the soma and neuronal processes and it is prevented by the opioid receptor antagonists. μOR also undergoes endocytosis in enteric neurons in response to electrical stimulation of longitudinal muscle myenteric plexus preparations with frequencies within the range that have been shown to induce enkephalin release (29). The level of receptor internalization appears to correlate to the stimulus intensity, since low frequency induces low levels of internalization in a few neurons, whereas high frequency results in high level of internalization in many neurons (29). These findings clearly indicate that native μORs in enteric neurons endocytose following their activation by endogenously released opioids. Thus, μOR endocytosis can serve as an indication of opioid release and also can be used as a means to visualize neuronal pathways activated by endogenous opioids.

Cellular sensitivity to opioids and opiates depends upon their different properties in inducing receptor desensitization and internalization, which might reflect different physiological effects on μ receptor bearing neurons, and can be modulated by the magnitude of the opioid receptor reserve (34). The existence of spare receptors, which are defined as functional receptors that can be activated, implies that an agonist can exert its full effect by activating only a fraction of the total receptor population on the cell surface. The greater the excess of functional receptors present in a system, the lower the concentration of agonist required for a cellular action. We have investigated the role of receptor endocytosis and opioid receptor reserve in regulating cellular responsiveness. These studies have used organotypic cultures of the guinea pig ileum and the nerve-mediated response of longitudinal muscle-myenteric plexus preparations (29). These investigations have shown that ligand-induced μOR endocytosis in enteric neurons reduces the nerve-mediated response (i.e. electrically induced muscle twitch contraction and acetylcholine release) *in vitro* in neuromuscular preparations of the small intestine in which μOR spare receptors have been inactivated by pretreatment with an alkylating agent, β chlornatrexamine at concentrations that irreversibly inactivate opioid receptor reserve (29). These studies clearly indicate that both receptor endocytosis and reduction of spare receptor fraction contribute to the diminution of neuronal responsiveness to opioids.

CONCLUSIONS

The molecular cloning of peptide receptors and the availability of peptide receptor antibodies and probes have been major breakthroughs in the understanding of peptide function in the ENS. First of all, they have allowed for the definition of the cellular sites expressing peptide receptors, which is essential to elucidate peptide modes of action and the circuits that control the activity of effectors (e.g. smooth muscles, neurons and endocrine cells) in response to peptide release. Furthermore, they have provided a valuable tool to establish whether these receptors are functional by visualizing their translocation from the cell surface to the cytoplasm following agonist stimulation. Release of peptides and activation of their receptors influence several functions in the gastrointestinal tract under both physiological and pathophysiological conditions. The ability to observe and quantify ligand-induced receptor endocytosis in enteric neurons and other targets in the gastrointestinal tract provides a tool to visualize neuronal pathways activated by endogenously released peptides and a means to quantify the magnitude of peptide release (29, 35). Finally, our findings that ligand-induced μOR endocytosis contributes to the reduction of the neurogenic response of intestinal neuromuscular preparations in which μOR spare fraction has been inactivated, provide evidence for a role of receptor endocytosis in the regulation of neuronal responsiveness to stimuli and opens a new area of research in the field of G protein coupled receptors function and regulation.

ACKNOWLEDGMENTS

The studies reported here have been supported by NIH grant DK54155 (CS) and DK41301 (Morphology Core, CS and NB). The authors would like to thank Sean Kohlmeier for his assistance in preparing the figures.

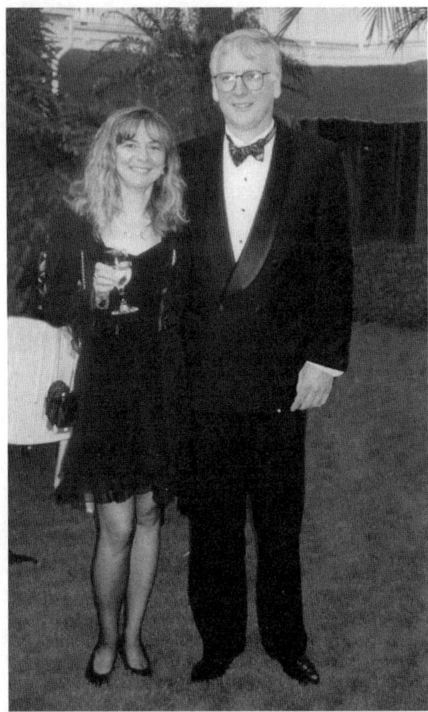

*Catia Sternini and John Walsh at the reception for the
AGA Presidential Dinner in San Diego, May 1995.*

REFERENCES

1. Furness JB, Costa M. *The Enteric Nervous System.* Churchill Livingstone, 1987.
2. Costa M, Brookes SJ. The enteric nervous system. *Am J Gastroenterol* 1994;89:S129–37.
3. Furness JB, Kunze WAA, Bertrand PP, Clerc N, Bornstein JC. Intrinsic primary afferent neurons of the intestine. *Prog Neurobiol* 1998;54:1–18.
4. Costa M, Brookes SJH, Steele PA, Gibbins I, Burcher E, Kandiah CJ. Neurochemical classification of myenteric neurons in the guinea pig ileum. *Neuroscience* 1996;75:949–967.
5. Furness JB, Bornstein JC, Murphy R, Pompolo S. Roles of peptides in transmission in the enteric nervous system. *Trends Neurosci* 1992;15:66–71.
6. Watson S, Arkinstall S. *The G-Protein Linked Receptor Facts Book.* Academic Press, 1994.
7. Sternini C. Receptors and transmission in the brain-gut axis: potential for novel therapies. III. μ opioid receptors in the enteric nervous system. *Am J Physiol* 2001;281:G8–G15.
8. Reisine T, Bell GI. Molecular biology of opioid receptors. *Trends Neurosci* 1993;16:506–510.
9. Zadina JE, Hackler L, Ge L-J, Kastin A. A potent and selective endogenous agonist for the μ-opiate receptor. *Nature* 1997;386:499–502.
10. Furness JB, Costa M, Miller RJ. Distribution and projections of nerves with enkephalin-like immunoreactivity in the guinea-pig small intestine. *Neuroscience* 1983;8:644–653.
11. Steele PA, Costa M. Opioid-like immunoreactive neurons in secretomotor pathways of the guinea-pig ileum. *Neuroscience* 1990;38:771–786.
12. Corbett AD, Paterson SJ, Kosterlitz HW. Selectivity of ligands for opioid receptors. In: *Handbook of Experimental Pharmacology, Opioids I.* Herz A, Ed. New York: Springer, 1993:645–679.

13. Chavkin C, Goldstein A. Demonstration of a specific dynorphin receptor in guinea pig ileum myenteric plexus. *Nature* 1981;291:591–593.

14. McConalogue K, Grady EF, Minnis J, Balestra B, Tonini M, Brecha NC, Bunnett NW, Sternini C. Activation and internalization of the μ opioid receptor by the newly described endogenous agonists, endomorphin-1 and endomorphin-2. *Neuroscience* 1999;90:1051–1059.

15. Kromer W. Endogenous and exogenous opioids in the control of gastrointestinal motility and secretion. *Pharmacol Rev* 1988;40:121–62.

16. Bagnol D, Mansour A, Akil H, Watson SJ. Cellular localization and distribution of the cloned mu and kappa opioid receptors in rat gastrointestinal tract. *Neuroscience* 1997;81:579–591.

17. Sternini C, Spann M, Anton B, Keith DE, Jr., Bunnett NW, von Zastrow M, Evans C, Brecha NC. Agonist-selective endocytosis of μ opioid receptor by neurons *in vivo*. *Proc Natl Acad Sci USA* 1996;93: 9241–9246.

18. Abbadie C, Pan YX, Pasternak GW. Differential distribution in rat brain of mu opioid receptor carboxy terminal splice variants MOR-1C-like and MOR-1-like immunoreactivity: evidence for region-specific processing. *J Comp Neurol* 2000;419:244–56.

19. Pan YX, Xu J, Bolan E, Abbadie C, Chang A, Zuckerman A, Rossi G, Pasternak GW. Identification and characterization of three new alternatively spliced mu-opioid receptor isoforms. *Mol Pharmacol* 1999;56:396–403.

20. Quinson N, Robbins HL, Clark MJ, Furness JB. Calbindin immunoreactivity of enteric neurons in the guinea-pig ileum. *Cell Tissue Res* 2001;305:3–9.

21. Waterman SA, Costa M, Tonini M. Modulation of peristalsis in the guinea-pig isolated small intestine by exogenous and endogenous opioids. *Br J Pharmacol* 1992;106:1004–10.

22. Johnson SM, Costa M, Humphreys CM, Shearman R. Inhibitory effects of opioids in a circular muscle-myenteric plexus preparation of guinea-pig ileum. *Naunyn Schmiedebergs Arch Pharmacol* 1987; 336:419–24.

23. North RA, Egan TM. Actions and distributions of opioid peptides in peripheral tissues. *Br Med Bull* 1983;39:71–75.

24. Dhawan BN, Cesselin F, Raghubir R, Reisine T, Bradley PB, Portoghese PS, Hamon M. International Union of Pharmacology. XII. Classification of opioid receptors. *Pharmacol Rev* 1996;48:567–592.

25. North R. Opioid actions on membrane ion channels. In: *Opioids I*. Herz A, Ed. Volume 104. Berlin: Springer-Verlag, 1993:773–797.

26. Bohm S, Grady EF, Bunnett NW. Mechanisms attenuating signaling by G protein-coupled receptors. *Biochem J* 1997;322:1–18.

27. Keith DE, Anton B, Murray SR, Zaki PA, Chu PC, Liissin DV, Monteillet-Agius G, Stewart PL, Evans CJ, von Zastrow M. μ-opioid receptor internalization: opiate drugs have differential effects on a conserved endocytic mechanism *in vitro* and in mammalian brain. *Mol Pharmacol* 1998;53:377–384.

28. Keith DE, Murray SR, Zaki PA, Chu PC, Lissin DV, Kag L, Evans CJ, von Zastrow M. Morphine activates opioid receptors without causing their rapid internalization. *J Biol Chem* 1996;271:19021–19024.

29. Sternini C, Brecha NC, Minnis J, D'Agostino G, Balestra B, Fiori E, Tonini M. Role of agonist-dependent receptor internalization in the regulation of μ opioid receptors. *Neuroscience* 2000;98: 233–241.

30. Whistler JL, Chuang H-H, Chu P, Jan LY, von Zastrow M. Functional dissociation of μ opioid receptor signaling and endocytosis: implications for the biology of opiate tolerance and addiction. *Neuron* 1999;23:737–746.

31. Whistler JL, von Zastrow M. Morphine-activated opioid receptors elude desensitization by β-arrestin. *Proc Natl Acad Sci USA* 1998;95:9914–9919.

32. Zhang J, Ferguson SSG, Barak LS, Bodduluri SB, Laporte SA, Law P-Y, Caron MG. Role of G protein-coupled receptor kinase in agonist-specific regulation of μ-opioid receptor responsiveness. *Proc Natl Acad Sci USA* 1998;95:7157–7162.

33. Abbadie C, Pasternak GW. Differential *in vivo* internalization of MOR-1 and MOR-1C by morphine. *Neuroreport* 2001;12:3069–72.

34. Chavkin C, Goldstein A. Opioid receptor reserve in normal and morphine-tolerant guinea pig ileum myenteric plexus. *Proc Natl Acad Sci USA* 1984;81:7253–7257.

35. Southwell BR, Seybold VS, Woodman HL, Jenkinson KM, Furness JH. Quantitation of neurokinin 1 receptor internalization and recycling in guinea-pig myenteric neurons. *Neuroscience* 1998;87:925–931.

Gut-Brain Peptides in the New Millennium, edited by Y. Taché
CURE Foundation, Los Angeles, CA. © 2002

24

Sensory Neurons in Gastrointestinal Function

Peter Holzer
Department of Experimental and Clinical Pharmacology, University of Graz, Austria

INTRODUCTION

Although it is now firmly established that the gastrointestinal (GI) tract contains the largest collection of neurons outside the brain (1), it took a long time until gastroenterology recognized the GI innervation as an important factor for the understanding and management of bowel disorders. It was already in the 1980s, though, that John Walsh conjured that the exploration of neural control mechanisms may provide important new insights into the regulation of gut function in health and disease. His wide-ranging interests related to both the efferent brain-gut connections as well as to the afferent gut-brain pathways and thus foresaw the dawn of neurogastroenterology. It is with deep gratitude that I record the enthusiasm and assurance with which John Walsh encouraged my studies into the role of sensory neurons in GI function. Although covering only part of the many roles which extrinsic afferent neurons play in the gut, this chapter has been written in an attempt to pay tribute to the uniquely integrated perspective of gastroenterology that was so characteristic of John Walsh.

THE GASTROINTESTINAL TRACT
IN NEED OF A SENSORY INNERVATION

The necessity of an extensive sensory innervation in the gut is evident both from a structural and functional point of view. Just consider that the GI mucosa covers the enormous area of 200–300 m^2, which is in keeping with the digestive and absorptive function of the GI tract. At the same time, the gut needs to eliminate useless material and to recognize harmful food constituents, antigens and pathogens in order to neutralize or expel them via emesis and diarrhea (2). In the upper gut, even the secretions of the stomach such as acid and pepsin can be deleterious if the self-defense of the mucosa is failing. These seemingly conflicting tasks of the alimentary canal require a careful analysis of the luminal contents and of the milieu within the GI wall so that the appropriate effector programs can be selected. To this end, the digestive system is endowed with an elaborate network of surveillance systems that comprise intrinsic and extrinsic sensory neurons (2, 3).

While the intrinsic primary afferent neurons (4) provide the enteric nervous system with the kind of information that this "brain of the gut" requires for its autonomic control of digestion, the extrinsic sensory neurons originating from the nodose ganglia (vagal afferents) and dorsal root ganglia (spinal afferents) convey information from the gut to the brain (5–7). As they supply mucosa, submucosa (particularly arterioles), muscle, enteric nerve plexuses and serosa, extrinsic sensory nerve fibers respond to changes of the chemical environment in the lumen, interstitial space and vasculature and to mechanical stimuli such as distortion of the villi, distension of the gut wall and contraction or relaxation of the muscle (5, 8–10). By notifying the brain about processes and conditions that are relevant to energy and fluid homeostasis of the body, extrinsic afferents participate in autonomic and neuroendocrine reflex circuits, but the information which they convey to the brain is rarely perceived as a conscious sensation, at least under physiological conditions (11). In a number of functional bowel disorders, however, patients suffer from GI pain and discomfort, and there is now ample evidence that hypersensitivity of the extrinsic afferent system is an important factor in the complaints of these patients (12).

In addition, some of the spinal afferents serve an efferent-like function by releasing calcitonin gene-related peptide (CGRP) and tachykinins (substance P, neurokinin A) from their peripheral endings, these transmitters in turn influencing the activity of enteric neurons and GI effector systems (13). Many of the functional implications of extrinsic afferents in the GI tract have been discovered with the help of the vanilloid compound capsaicin, the pungent ingredient of red pepper, with which the activity of a discrete population of spinal and vagal afferents expressing vanilloid receptor type 1 (VR1) can be manipulated (13–17).

NETWORK OF SENSORY NEURONS WITH OTHER GASTROINTESTINAL SURVEILLANCE SYSTEMS

Besides sensory neurons, the GI surveillance systems comprise enteroendocrine cells (EECCs) and immune cells which are strategically positioned in the GI mucosa to analyze the luminal contents. Following exposure to food and gastric secretions, EECCs release their messengers in order to coordinate various digestive processes (18) but also have the capacity to react to toxins, antigens and pathogens, although detection of these threats is the domain of the GI immune system which in anticipation of the continuous threats from the lumen is the largest in the body (3). These monitoring systems communicate with afferent neurons that send their axon terminals into the lamina propria of the GI mucosa. Through this input from EECCs and immune cells, the sensory repertoire of afferent neurons is extended to luminal stimuli that otherwise could not be encoded by their peripheral axons.

Particularly worth noting among the mediators released from EECCs are 5-hydroxytryptamine (5-HT), which stimulates vagal and spinal afferents via activation of $5\text{-}HT_3$ receptors (19), and cholecystokinin (CCK) which stimulates vagal afferents through activation of CCK_1 (CCK_A) receptors (18, 20). Furthermore, secretin (21, 22) and corticotropin-releasing factor (23) released from EECCs also lead to sensory neuron stimulation, whereas somatostatin attenuates the excitability of extrinsic afferent neurons (24, 25). Whenever the gut is affected by microbial infection, allergen exposure, inflammation or other types of injury, the GI immune system is called into operation and releases a host of neuroactive mediators. Among them are cytokines, prostaglandins, leukotrienes, bradykinin, histamine, 5-HT and serine proteases, all of which can either excite extrinsic afferent nerve fibers, in the short term, or alter their sensitivity, in the long term (2, 3, 24, 26).

SENSORY NEURONS AS AN ALARM SYSTEM IN GASTROINTESTINAL MUCOSAL INJURY

Experimentally induced injury activates afferent neurons which through their efferent-like function signal for local protective measures in the mucosa or through their afferent function activate autonomic and neuroendocrine mechanisms of homeostasis (2, 7, 13). These processes are initiated, for instance, when hydrochloric acid (HCl) and pepsin overwhelm the epithelial barrier of the gastroduodenal mucosa and attack the lamina propria, as may happen after exposure of the stomach to alcohol, nonsteroidal anti-inflammatory drugs or refluxing bile. HCl intrusion leads to an increase of mucosal blood flow and stimulation of other defense mechanisms such as bicarbonate and mucus secretion (13). These responses are brought about by spinal afferents that express VR1 (27) at which H^+ ions behave as agonists (28). Following stimulation, acid-sensitive afferent neurons evoke a peripheral vasodilator reflex (Figure 1) that depends on intact pathways through the celiac ganglion and involves CGRP, acetylcholine acting via nicotinic receptors and nitric oxide as mediators (13).

Extrinsic afferents thus represent a neural emergency system that helps protecting the GI mucosa from injury (13). This function is portrayed by the findings that GI damage due to a variety of injurious factors is attenuated by concomitant stimulation of capsaicin-sensitive afferents and exacerbated if these neurons have been defunctionalized (13, 29). The same alarm system operates in the human gastroduodenal mucosa (30) and throughout the

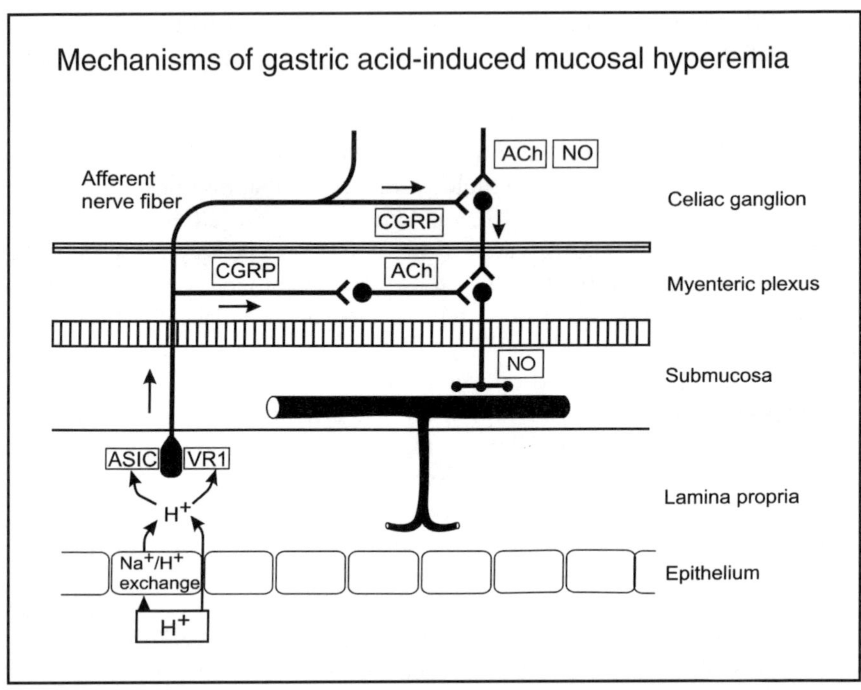

FIGURE 1. *Hypothetical neural pathways underlying the mucosal hyperemic response to acid back-diffusion in the rat stomach. Acidification of the interstitial space stimulates spinal afferent nerve fibers which by releasing calcitonin gene-related peptide (CGRP) activate a peripheral vasodilator circuit that involves neuronal structures passing through the celiac ganglion and, most likely, enteric neurons. Besides CGRP, acetylcholine (ACh) acting via nicotinic receptors and nitric oxide (NO) also play an important mediator role.*

small and large intestine of experimental animals (31). Consequently, the role of sensory neurons as a signaling system in GI mucosal homeostasis has important implications for the diagnosis, management and pharmacotherapy of GI mucosal disease. First, there is evidence that sensory nerve-mediated protection of the GI mucosa may be impaired under several pathological conditions including diabetes (13, 29). Second, any therapeutic intervention should be designed such that the neural alarm system is maintained or facilitated. The feasibility of this concept is corroborated by the observations that the mucosa protective effect of several endogenous factors (e.g., cholecystokinin/gastrin, epidermal growth factor and prostaglandin I_2) and anti-ulcer drugs (e.g., ecabet and lafutidine) involves capsaicin-sensitive afferent neurons (13, 29, 32).

While local protective measures in the rat gastric mucosa are initiated by spinal afferents (13), it is vagal afferents that signal an acute acid challenge of the rat gastric mucosa to the central nervous system (33, 34). It hence appears as if vagal and spinal afferents are specialized to mediate different homeostatic reactions to a noxious acid insult of the gastric mucosa. Although vagal afferents in the stomach have long been known to discharge action potentials upon exposure to acid, their molecular detector of H^+ ions remains unknown. Since the acid-evoked afferent signaling is not altered by pretreatment with capsaicin (33), it is improbable that acid transduction is accomplished by VR1. Whether acid-sensing ion channels (35) or $P2X_3/P2X_{2/3}$ purinoceptor cation channels (36) are involved has not yet been explored.

The involvement of vagal afferents in the central signaling of a gastric mucosal acid challenge (33, 34) and peripheral immune challenge (37) is of obvious relevance to understanding visceral sensation in health and disease. There is now growing awareness that vagal afferent neurons make a distinct contribution to the subconscious, non-perceptive aspects of GI nociception (5, 6, 38). This view is corroborated by the central processing of a gastric mucosal acid challenge in subcortical brain nuclei that are involved in emotional, behavioral, autonomic and neuroendocrine reactions to a noxious stimulus (34). There is, however, no activation of the insular cortex, the major cerebral representation area of afferent input from the stomach, which indicates that vagal afferent signaling of an acute mucosal acid insult does not give rise to perception of pain.

GASTROINTESTINAL HYPERSENSITIVITY IN FUNCTIONAL BOWEL DISORDERS

In keeping with their emergency function, sensory neurons display a high degree of plasticity which enables these cells to adapt to significant changes in their environment. However, sensory neurons may also fall victim of their adaptability, particularly if alterations of their function do not reverse once the initiating stimuli have abated. Such a scenario may underlie many cases of functional bowel disorders such as non-ulcer (functional) dyspepsia and irritable bowel syndrome, which are characterized by abdominal discomfort and pain in the absence of an identifiable organic cause. There is now good reason to hypothesize that preceding infection or inflammation has caused afferent pathways to undergo sensitization that outlasts the acute insult (12, 39, 40). GI hypersensitivity may arise from sensitization of peripheral afferent nerve fibers, sensitization of central pathways (41) as well as a distorted processing and representation of the incoming information in the brain. In analogy with somatic hyperalgesia it is hypothesized that afferent neuron hypersensitivity arises from long-lasting changes in the number, composition and properties of receptors, ion channels and transmitters or in the structure, connectivity and survival of afferent neurons (42, 43). The peripheral messengers for these persistent adaptations include nerve growth factor acting on spinal afferents, brain-derived neurotrophic factor acting on vagal afferents and cytokines (3, 42, 43).

SENSORY NEURONS IN THE THERAPY OF FUNCTIONAL BOWEL DISORDERS

The concept that hypersensitivity of primary afferent neurons contributes to the pain and discomfort associated with functional bowel disorders (12) identifies these neurons as prime targets at which novel therapies may be aimed (19, 43). Ideally, such drugs should block the exaggerated signaling of hypersensitive afferents, which implies that they hit molecular targets that are upregulated in functional bowel disorders. Although the complex innervation of the GI tract by intrinsic enteric and extrinsic autonomic neurons complicates the search for specific traits on extrinsic sensory neurons, there is ample evidence from preclinical studies that such attributes may indeed be found and utilized (43). Acid-sensing ion channels (35), $P2X_3$ purinoceptors (36), tetrodotoxin-resistant $Na_v1.8$ channels (44) and VR1 (15, 28) are of particular relevance because these excitatory ion channels are selectively expressed by extrinsic afferents (43).

While previously VR1 activated by capsaicin has served primarily as a means to discover sensory neuron implications, this receptor channel is now considered to be a potentially important target of gastroenterological pharmacotherapy. Analysis of its molecular regulation has shown that VR1 operates as a polymodal detector of potentially harmful stimuli including noxious heat, H^+ ions and lipoxygenase products (15, 28, 43, 45). Importantly, VR1 activity is regulated by several intracellular signaling cascades including protein kinase C, and VR1 function is enhanced by sensory neuron stimulants that activate protein kinase C (e.g., bradykinin) but are inactive or weakly active agonists at VR1 (43, 45). With these properties, VR1 may encode a variety of chemical stimuli that themselves are unable to directly gate VR1. Genetic deletion of VR1 results in attenuation of the inflammatory hypersensitivity to heat (46, 47), but visceral sensitivity has not yet been tested in VR1-deficient mice. It is important to note, however, that painful inflammatory bowel disease is associated with a rise of VR1 in nerve fibers of the human gut (48), which is in keeping with the regulation of VR1 by nerve growth factor and other mediators whose production is enhanced under inflammatory conditions (43, 45).

Since activation of VR1 by intraluminal capsaicin gives rise to jejunal pain in healthy volunteers (49), blockade of VR1 may be an efficacious way to suppress visceral hyperalgesia, and VR1 antagonists are worth developing and exploring for their utility in GI pain. In this context the question needs

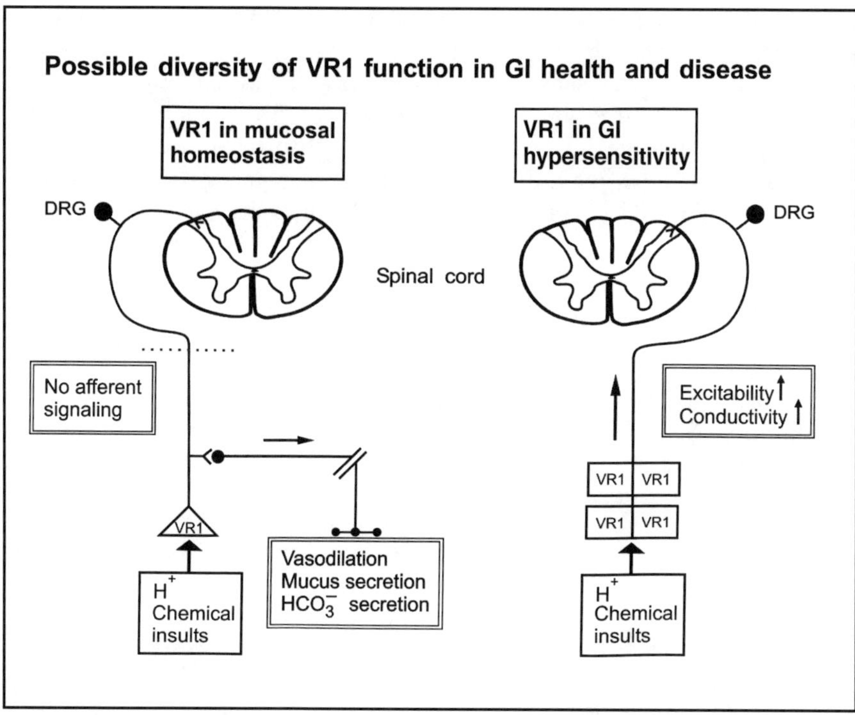

FIGURE 2. *Diverse function of VR1 as a polymodal sensor of injurious chemicals in the GI mucosa in health and disease. Physiologically, VR1 expressed by spinal afferents is involved in the alarm of local homeostatic responses to mucosal insults. Pathologically, there is an upregulation of VR1 in sensory nerve fibers that signal to the central nervous system. Under these conditions, VR1 may make an important contribution to GI hypersensitivity characteristic of functional bowel disorders.*

to be addressed, however, as to whether GI pain treatment with VR1 antagonists will spare the local alarm function of afferent neurons in the gut (Figure 2). Since VR1 appears to be involved in the monitoring of acid backdiffusion in the gastroduodenal region (27), it has to be borne in mind that blockade of this VR1 function could make the upper GI tract more vulnerable to acid-related damage. It needs to be considered, though, that the exacerbation of experimental mucosal injury observed in rats pretreated with a neurotoxic dose of capsaicin only indicates that sensory neuron-mediated mucosal protection involves capsaicin-sensitive (VR1-expressing) afferent neurons but does not necessarily reflect an implication of VR1 itself. In addition, there is room to speculate that the VR1 involved in the peripheral alarm function within the GI mucosa can pharmacologically be differentiated from the VR1 mediating GI pain. Thus, the mucosal defense reactions to acid backdiffusion and the afferent signaling of gastric acid challenge (Figure 2) are brought about by different afferent neurons (33, 34, 50).

Many other targets on sensory neurons such as 5-HT receptors, protease-activated receptors, cholecystokinin receptors, somatostatin receptors, prostaglandin receptors, cannabinoid receptors and γ-aminobutyric acid receptors (19, 24, 26, 43) are also worth exploring. In developing drugs for these targets it will be important to assess which quantitative contribution these molecular traits make to the induction of hyperalgesia and whether modulation of a single target is therapeutically efficacious (43).

ACKNOWLEDGMENTS

Work in the authors' laboratory is currently supported by the Austrian Research Funds (FWF grant P14295-MED) and the Austrian Federal Ministry of Education, Science and Culture (grants GZ 70.058/2-Pr/4/99 and GZ 70.065/2-Pr/4/2000). Thanks are due to Dr. Ulrike Holzer-Petsche and Evelin Painsipp for drawing the graphs.

REFERENCES

1. Furness JB, Costa M. *The Enteric Nervous System*. Edinburgh, Churchill Livingstone, 1987.
2. Holzer P. Inflammation and gut hypersensitivity: peripheral mechanisms. *Gastroenterol Int* 2001, in press.
3. Furness JB, Clerc N. Responses of afferent neurons to the contents of the digestive tract, and their relation to endocrine and immune responses. *Prog Brain Res* 2000;122:159–172.
4. Furness JB, Kunze WAA, Bertrand PP, Clerc N, Bornstein JC. Intrinsic primary afferent neurons of the intestine. *Prog Neurobiol* 1998;54:1–18.
5. Berthoud H-R, Neuhuber WL. Functional and chemical anatomy of the afferent vagal system. *Auton Neurosci* 2000;85:1–17.
6. Gebhart GF. Pathobiology of visceral pain: molecular mechanisms and therapeutic implications. IV. Visceral afferent contributions to the pathobiology of visceral pain. *Am J Physiol* 2000;278:G834-G838.
7. Holzer P, Schicho R, Holzer-Petsche U, Lippe IT. The gut as a neurological organ. *Wien Klin Wochenschr* 2001;113:647–660.
8. Grundy D, Scratcherd T. Sensory afferents from the gastrointestinal tract. In: *Handbook of Physiology*, Section 6, The Gastrointestinal System, Volume I, Motility and Circulation, Part 1, Schultz SG (ed). Bethesda, Maryland, American Physiological Society, 1989, pp 593–620.
9. Cervero F. Sensory innervation of the viscera: peripheral basis of visceral pain. *Physiol Rev* 1994;74:95–138.
10. Sengupta JN, Gebhart GF. Gastrointestinal afferent fibers and sensation. In: *Physiology of the Gastrointestinal Tract*, Third Edition, Johnson LR (ed). New York, Raven Press, 1994, pp 483–519.
11. Mayer EA. Gut feelings: what turns them on? *Gastroenterology* 1995;108:927–931.
12. Drossman DA, Corazziari E, Talley NJ, Thompson WG, Whitehead WE (eds). Rome II. *The Functional Gastrointestinal Disorders*. Second Edition. McLean, Virginia, USA, Degnon Associates, 2000.
13. Holzer P. Neural emergency system in the stomach. *Gastroenterology* 1998;114:823–839.
14. Holzer P. Capsaicin: cellular targets, mechanisms of action, and selectivity for thin sensory neurons. *Pharmacol Rev* 1991;43:143–201.
15. Caterina MJ, Schumacher MA, Tominaga M, Rosen TA, Levine JD, Julius D. The capsaicin receptor: a heat-activated ion channel in the pain pathway. *Nature* 1997;389:816–824.

16. Guo A, Vulchanova L, Wang J, Li X, Elde R. Immunocytochemical localization of the vanilloid receptor 1 (VR1): relationship to neuropeptides, the P2X3 purinoceptor and IB4 binding sites. *Eur J Neurosci* 1999;11:946–958.

17. Szallasi A, Blumberg PM. Vanilloid (capsaicin) receptors and mechanisms. *Pharmacol Rev* 1999;51:159–212.

18. Raybould HE. Nutrient tasting and signaling mechanisms in the gut I. Sensing of lipid by the intestinal mucosa. *Am J Physiol* 1999:277:G751-G755.

19. Kirkup AJ, Brunsden AM, Grundy D. Receptors and transmission in the brain-gut axis: potential for novel therapies. I. Receptors on visceral afferents. *Am J Physiol* 2001;280:G787-G794.

20. Sternini C, Wong H, Pham T, De Giorgio R, Miller LJ, Kuntz SM, Reeve JR, Walsh JH, Raybould HE. Expression of cholecystokinin A receptors in neurons innervating the rat stomach and intestine. *Gastroenterology* 1999;117:1136–1146.

21. Raybould HE, Hölzer H. Secretin inhibits gastric emptying in rats via a capsaicin-sensitive vagal afferent pathway. *Eur J Pharmacol* 1993;250:165–167.

22. Lu YX, Owyang C. Duodenal acid-induced gastric relaxation is mediated by multiple pathways. *Am J Physiol* 1999;276:G1501-G1506.

23. Lembo T, Plourde V, Shui Z, Fullerton S, Mertz H, Taché Y, Sytnik B, Munakata J, Mayer E. Effects of the corticotropin-releasing factor (CRF) on rectal afferent nerves in humans. *Neurogastroenterol Motil* 1996;8:9–18.

24. Buéno L, Fioramonti J, Delvaux M, Frexinos J. Mediators and pharmacology of visceral sensitivity: from basic to clinical investigations. *Gastroenterology* 1997:112:1714–1743.

25. Booth EC, Kirkup AJ, Hicks GA, Humphrey PA, Grundy D. Somatostatin sst$_2$ receptor-mediated inhibition of mesenteric afferent nerves of the jejunum in the anesthetized rat. *Gastroenterology* 2001;121:358–369.

26. Vergnolle N, Wallace JL, Bunnett NW, Hollenberg MD. Protease-activated receptors in inflammation, neuronal signaling and pain. *Trends Pharmacol Sci* 2001;22:146–152.

27. Akiba Y, Guth PH, Engel E, Nastaskin I, Kaunitz JD. Acid-sensing pathways of rat duodenum. *Am J Physiol* 1999;277:G268-G274.

28. Tominaga M, Caterina M, Malmberg AB, Rosen TA, Gilbert H, Skinner K, Raumann BE, Basbaum AI, Julius D. The cloned capsaicin receptor integrates multiple pain-producing stimuli. *Neuron* 1998;21:531–543.

29. Holzer P. Gastric mucosal protection signaled by peptidergic afferent neurons. *Drug News Perspect* 1999;12:463–472.

30. Yeoh KG, Kang JY, Yap I, Guan R, Tan CC, Wee A, Teng CH. Chili protects against aspirin-induced gastroduodenal mucosal injury in humans. *Digest Dis Sci* 1995;40:580–583.

31. Holzer P, Barthó L. Sensory neurons in the intestine. In: *Neurogenic Inflammation,* Geppetti P, Holzer P (eds). Boca Raton, CRC Press, 1996, pp 153–167.

32. Holzer P. Gastroduodenal mucosal defense. *Curr Opin Gastroenterol* 2000;16:469–478.

33. Schuligoi R, Jocic M, Heinemann A, Schöninkle E, Pabst MA, Holzer P. Gastric acid-evoked c-fos messenger RNA expression in rat brainstem is signaled by capsaicin-resistant vagal afferents. *Gastroenterology* 1998;115:649–660.

34. Michl T, Jocic M, Heinemann A, Schuligoi R, Holzer P. Vagal afferent signaling of a gastric mucosal acid insult to medullary, pontine, thalamic, hypothalamic and limbic, but not cortical, nuclei of the rat brain. *Pain* 2001;92:19–27.

35. Waldmann R, Champigny G, Lingueglia E, De Weille JR, Heurteaux C, Lazdunski M. H$^+$-gated cation channels. *Ann New York Acad Sci* 1999;868:67–76.

36. Burnstock G. Purine-mediated signalling in pain and visceral perception. *Trends Pharmacol Sci* 2001;22:182–188.

37. Maier SF, Goehler LE, Fleshner M, Watkins LR. The role of the vagus nerve in cytokine-to-brain communication. *Ann New York Acad Sci* 1998;840:289–300.

38. Traub RJ, Sengupta JN, Gebhart GF. Differential c-fos expression in the nucleus of the solitary tract and spinal cord following noxious gastric distention in the rat. *Neuroscience* 1996;74:873–884.

39. Al-Chaer ED, Kawasaki M, Pasricha PJ. A new model of chronic visceral hypersensitivity in adult rats induced by colon irritation during postnatal development. *Gastroenterology* 2000;119:1276–1285.

40. Spiller RC, Jenkins D, Thornley JP, Hebden JM, Wright T, Skinner M, Neal KR. Increased rectal mucosal enteroendocrine cells, T lymphocytes, and increased gut permeability following acute *Campylobacter enteritis* and in post-dysenteric irritable bowel syndrome. *Gut* 2000;47:804–811.
41. Cervero F, Laird JMA. Visceral pain. *Lancet* 1999;353:2145–2148.
42. Woolf CJ, Salter MW. Neuronal plasticity: increasing the gain in pain. *Science* 2000;288:1765–1768.
43. Holzer P. Gastrointestinal afferents as targets of novel drugs for the treatment of functional bowel disorders and visceral pain. *Eur J Pharmacol* 2001, in press.
44. Baker MD, Wood JN. Involvement of Na^+ channels in pain pathways. *Trends Pharmacol Sci* 2001;22:27–31.
45. Premkumar LS, Ahern GP. Induction of vanilloid receptor channel activity by protein kinase C. *Nature* 2000;408:985–990.
46. Caterina MJ, Leffler A, Malmberg AB, Martin WJ, Trafton J, Petersen-Zeitz KR, Koltzenburg M, Basbaum AI, Julius D. Impaired nociception and pain sensation in mice lacking the capsaicin receptor. *Science* 2000;288:306–313.
47. Davis JB, Gray J, Gunthorpe MJ, Hatcher JP, Davey PT, Overend P, Harries MH, Latcham J, Clapham C, Atkinson K, Hughes SA, Rance K, Grau E, Harper AJ, Pugh PL, Rogers DC, Bingham S, Randall A, Sheardown SA. Vanilloid receptor-1 is essential for inflammatory thermal hyperalgesia. *Nature* 2000;405:183–187.
48. Yiangou Y, Facer P, Dyer NH, Chan CL, Knowles C, Williams NS, Anand P. Vanilloid receptor 1 immunoreactivity in inflamed human bowel. *Lancet* 2001;357:1338–1339.
49. Hammer J, Hammer HF, Eherer AJ, Petritsch W, Holzer P, Krejs GJ. Intraluminal capsaicin does not affect fluid and electrolyte absorption in the human jejunum but does cause pain. *Gut* 1998;43:252–255.
50. Holzer P. Neural injury, repair, and adaptation in the GI tract. II. The elusive action of capsaicin on the vagus nerve. *Am J Physiol* 1999;275:G8-G13.

Gut-Brain Peptides in the New Millennium, edited by Y. Taché
CURE Foundation, Los Angeles, CA. © 2002

25

The Role of the Capsaicin Receptor (VR1) in an Animal Model of Intestinal Inflammation

Douglas C. McVey and Steven R. Vigna
*Departments of Cell Biology and Medicine, Duke University Medical Center
and Durham Veterans Administration Medical Center, Durham, NC*

INTRODUCTION

Although my original collaborations with John Walsh were in the field of gastrin-releasing peptide (GRP) biology, I am sure that he would be interested in the results of our current research into the role of sensory nerves and neuropeptides in intestinal inflammation. There isn't any aspect of regulatory peptide biology in which John was not keenly interested. John's breadth of knowledge in gastrointestinal biology in general was immense. He also had the uncanny knack of being able to see instantly the ramifications of any laboratory finding. Some of my fondest memories of working with John are of those late afternoons when he would wander into the lab, rapidly consume whatever junk food was available, ask to see the day's new data, and then sit back with his feet up on the desk or bench and proceed to outline several dozen new experiments based on those findings. Today, some 25 years later, we are still trying to finish some of those projects!

The gastrointestinal tract is subject to a wide variety of inflammations including transient acute conditions and prolonged chronic disease states. In the case of certain acute gut inflammations the cause is an infectious agent that either invades the mucosa or elaborates a toxin that initiates the inflammatory cascade. In other cases, such as the human inflammatory bowel diseases (Crohn's disease and ulcerative colitis) the causative agent is unknown. However, in both acute and chronic gastrointestinal inflammation, the exact mechanisms that link the proximal cause to the resulting tissue inflammation are not well understood.

One approach that can be taken to increase our understanding of the mechanisms of gastrointestinal inflammation is to exploit an animal model of enteritis that is convenient, highly reproducible, amenable to manipulation, and that exhibits a rapid, fulminant form of intestinal inflammation that is relevant to human disease. One model that satisfies these criteria consists of administering pure toxin A from *Clostridium difficile* to isolated segments of the rat ileum for three hours under general anesthesia. *C. difficile* toxin A administration in rats causes intestinal inflammation that is very similar to *C. difficile* colitis in people (17). The inflammatory response consists of intraluminal fluid accumulation, neutrophil infiltration, and epithelial cell destruction. We have been interested in testing the hypothesis that neurogenic mechanisms play a key role in toxin A-induced intestinal inflammation. Neurogenic inflammation is defined as the ability of a subpopulation of primary sensory neurons to invoke inflammatory responses at the site of their peripheral endings. Neurogenic mechanisms have been shown to play important roles in such inflammatory states as airway diseases, lower urinary tract conditions, arthritis, migraine, eye diseases, and skin conditions (1). Treatments aimed at disrupting the neurogenic mechanisms of intestinal inflammation are attractive candidates as new therapies because they would presumably act at a very early step in the inflammatory cascade and thus efficiently block all limbs of the subsequent pathological sequelae, both immune and other.

Early hints that neurogenic mechanisms may be involved in intestinal inflammation came from studies showing that application of the local anesthetic lidocaine or administration of the ganglionic blocker hexamethonium inhibited toxin A-induced intestinal inflammation (4). This concept was further supported by the observation that functional ablation of primary sensory neurons by subcutaneous injection of high doses of the excitotoxin, capsaicin, for 3 consecutive days in adult rats strongly inhibited the inflammatory effects of toxin A (4). Substance P (SP) and calcitonin gene-related peptide (CGRP) are two major neurotransmitters of primary sensory neurons and so it was important to determine if these peptides are involved in the intestinal effects of toxin A. Pretreatment of rats with either SP or CGRP antagonists greatly reduced luminal fluid accumulation, mucosal permeability, release of proinflammatory cytokines, structural damage, and neutrophil infiltration in response to toxin A (12, 13, 16). In addition, toxin A causes increases in intestinal SP and CGRP mRNAs and peptides in dorsal root ganglia neurons followed by increased SP and CGRP expression (3) and release (13) in the intestinal mucosa. Finally, an important role for SP and its cognate receptor (neurokinin-1, NK-1) in mediating the enterotoxic effects of toxin A is suggested by the observation that mice lacking NK-1 receptors are largely protected from the intestinal inflammatory effects of toxin A (5). The mechanisms by which SP causes intestinal inflammation probably include stimulation of NK-1 receptors expressed by enteric nerves, endothelial cells, and immune system cells such as macrophages and leukocytes (3, 8, 13).

Taken together, these findings show that intraluminal toxin A stimulates primary sensory neurons to release SP ultimately resulting in intestinal inflammation. However, the mechanism by which intraluminal toxin A stimulates SP release from primary sensory neurons in the intestinal mucosa is unknown. The first step in toxin A action is binding to mucosal enterocytes at their apical microvilli (15). It has been shown that toxin A binds to villous but not crypt enterocytes and also does not bind to goblet cells (24). These observations suggest that toxin A exerts its effects at the level of the intestinal enterocyte and does not penetrate deeper into the intestinal mucosa. This is consistent with the observations that when toxin A binds to cells it is rapidly internalized, causes glucosylation of Rho proteins, decreased protein synthesis, and finally cellular necrosis (17). Thus, the pathway by which the inflammatory effects of intraluminal toxin A are conducted from the enterocyte to SP-containing primary sensory neurons in deeper layers of the mucosa and lamina propria is unknown.

Primary sensory neurons are multimodal and thus can be activated by a variety of chemical messengers, acid, mechanical stimulation, and heat (25). For example, bradykinin, histamine, serotonin, norepinephrine, ATP, prostaglandins, NGF, and TNFα have all been shown to stimulate sensory neurons. In addition, a new mechanism has recently been identified that may be involved in the signaling pathway connecting intraluminal toxin A and primary sensory neuron SP release. A cDNA encoding a non–selective cation channel expressed in primary sensory neurons and named the Vanilloid Receptor subtype 1 (VR1) has recently been cloned (6). VR1 is stimulated by increased temperature, protons, and by capsaicin (22), a vanilloid compound that is the pungent ingredient in red peppers of the genus *Capsicum*. The specific expression of VR1 by primary sensory neurons thus explains the excitotoxic effect of capsaicin administration—low capsaicin concentrations or short exposure times activate VR1 transiently leading to increased cytoplasmic calcium concentrations and subsequent peptide (e.g., SP) release, whereas high capsaicin concentrations or prolonged exposure times result in cell necrosis due to the excessive cytoplasmic concentrations of calcium or sodium ions resulting from prolonged VR1 activation (11). The recent demonstration that VR1 is required for inflammatory sensitization to noxious thermal stimuli (7) suggests the possibility that VR1 may be involved in many if not all forms of inflammation.

These observations suggested that the capsaicin VR1 receptor may mediate substance P release and the ensuing intestinal inflammation in the *C. difficile* toxin A rat model. We tested this hypothesis by pretreating rats systemically with capsazepine before administering toxin A intraluminally. We found that capsazepine pretreatment significantly inhibited endogenous SP release as indicated by endocytosis of the NK-1 receptor (14). Capsazepine alone had no effect. Since it had previously been shown that toxin A-induced SP release results in inflammation in this model, we also tested the effects of capsazepine pretreatment on toxin A-induced enteritis. Capsazepine alone had no effect on the histological structure of the ileum but strongly preserved the villus architecture that toxin A destroys. Pretreatment with capsazepine also significantly inhibited toxin A-induced luminal fluid accumulation and tissue myeloperoxidase (MPO) activity, a biochemical index of neutrophil infiltration into the tissue. The protective effects of capsazepine were specific because it had no effect on fluid secretion caused by cholera toxin, which is noninflammatory. As discussed above, the plant vanilloid molecule, capsaicin, is highly specific for VR1 and has been shown to cause SP release (10). We reasoned therefore, that intraluminal capsaicin should cause SP release and subsequent intestinal inflammation, and these effects should also be inhibited by capsazepine pretreatment. Indeed, intraluminal administration of the hydrophobic capsaicin molecule caused structural damage to the ileum that was similar to that caused by toxin A, including complete loss of villi. Capsazepine pretreatment almost completely abolished the damaging effects of capsaicin (14). These findings provide strong support for the hypothesis that toxin A causes SP release and intestinal inflammation at least in part via activation of the VR1 receptor expressed by primary sensory neurons.

There are other reports of the intraluminal administration of capsaicin, but inflammatory end points were apparently not examined (9, 21, 26). Interestingly, intrajejunal perfusion of low concentrations of capsaicin in human volunteers did not cause fluid secretion (9), but this result is difficult to compare with the pro-secretory effect of capsaicin in the rat intestine (14) because capsaicin was administered differently in the two studies. However, the observation that the highest dose of capsaicin used in the human study caused crampy abdominal pain that persisted until the end of the 60 minute test period suggests that intraluminal capsaicin stimulates primary sensory neurons in people as it does in rats.

These findings raise the question of the mechanism by which intraluminal toxin A activates VR1. One possible mechanism to explain this is the generation of a VR1 stimulant after binding to mucosal enterocytes. In addition to capsaicin (a plant compound), heat and protons can directly activate the VR1 receptor (6, 22). While it is highly unlikely that toxin A causes an increase in intestinal temperature, it has been shown that protons decrease the temperature threshold for VR1 activation such that even moderately acidic conditions (pH < 6.4) activate VR1 at 37°C. It has been shown that high proton concentrations (pH < 6) can be generated during various forms of tissue injury including inflammation (2). Thus, if the mucosal epithelial necrosis induced by intraluminal toxin A results in acidification of the underlying mucosal tissue where primary sensory neuronal endings are located, this may be sufficient to activate the VR1 cation channel leading to SP release and subsequent inflammation. In addition, in the presence of extracellular ATP, the temperature threshold for VR1 activation is reduced from 42°C to 35°C indicating that VR1 can be activated at normal body temperature in the presence of ATP released from damaged cells (23). The possible contributions of acidification or ATP to VR1 stimulation in intestinal inflammation have not been examined.

Another possibility is that the interaction of toxin A with mucosal enterocytes results in the synthesis or release of a VR1 agonist molecule, analogous to capsaicin, that then diffuses from the mucosal epithelium to adjacent primary sensory nerve endings to bind to and activate VR1 (20). The existence of such an endogenous VR1 agonist ligand was confirmed with the demonstration that the endogenous cannabinoid agonist, anandamide (arachidonylethanolamide), acts as a vasodilator via VR1 in rat and guinea pig blood vessels (27). Other endogenous and synthetic cannabinoid receptor agonists did not duplicate the actions of anandamide. In addition, the selective VR1 antagonist, capsazepine, inhibited anandamide-induced vasodilatation whereas cannabinoid CB1 and CB2 receptor antagonists had no effect. Finally, in patch clamp experiments on *Xenopus* oocytes and mammalian cells expressing VR1, anandamide induced a capsazepine-sensitive current (27). It was subsequently shown that anandamide is also a full agonist at the human VR1 receptor (19).

These observations suggested the possibility that endogenous anandamide may mediate toxin A-induced SP release via VR1 receptors expressed by primary sensory afferent nerves in the intestinal mucosa. That is, anandamide may be synthesized or released by villous enterocytes in response to toxin A binding and the anandamide thus generated may diffuse to adjacent VR1-expressing nerve fibers in the mucosa or lamina propria. We tested this hypothesis by administering anandamide and other cannabinoids to isolated segments of the rat ileum by the same techniques previously used in studies of toxin A. We found that intraluminal injection of anandamide caused intense inflammation in the rat ileum (D. C. McVey and S. R. Vigna, manuscript submitted for publication). The effects of anandamide were similar to the effects of toxin A in terms of histological damage, luminal fluid accumulation, and increased MPO activity. Pretreatment of the rats with capsazepine had no effect when given alone but significantly inhibited anandamide-induced inflammatory measures. Another endocannabinoid, palmitylethanolamide, and two synthetic cannabinoid agonists, WIN 55,212 and HU 210, had no effects. To determine the specificity of the effects of anandamide we tested the effect of pretreating the rats with specific cannabinoid-1 (CB-1) and cannabinoid-2 (CB-2) receptor antagonists. CB-1 and CB-2 receptor antagonists had no effects on the ileum when given alone and neither antagonist inhibited the effects of intraluminal anandamide. Since intraluminal toxin A has been shown to cause SP release in the intestine (13), we tested the effects of intraluminal administration of anandamide on SP release. Anandamide caused an increase in NK-1 receptor endocytosis, an index of endogenous

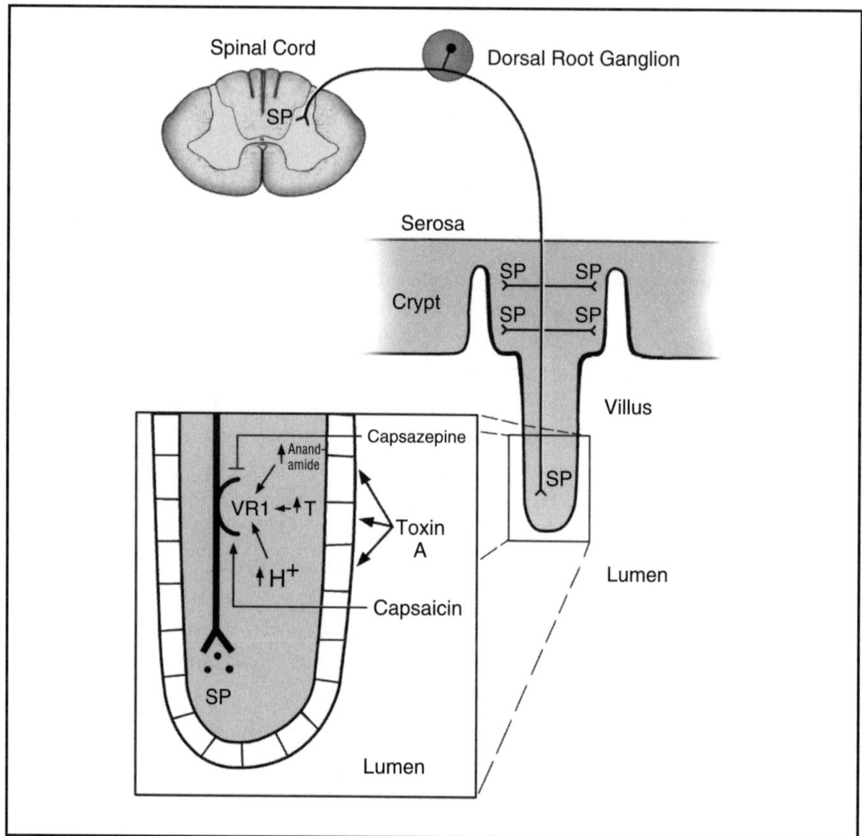

FIGURE 1. *A schematic illustration of the proposed mechanisms of action of intraluminal toxin A and capsaicin in causing intestinal inflammation in the rat. Primary sensory neurons, with their cell bodies in the dorsal root ganglia, express the VR1 receptor which is stimulated directly by capsaicin and indirectly by toxin A. Toxin A may stimulate VR1 by causing tissue acidification ($\uparrow H^+$), increased tissue temperature ($\uparrow T$), or by releasing anandamide ($\uparrow$ Anandamide). The possible role of extracellular ATP is not shown (see text). VR1 stimulation results in SP release orthodromically in the spinal cord in laminae I and II to contribute to the transmission of pain signals in the spinal cord and antidromically in the intestine to cause inflammation. Capsazepine is a VR1 antagonist that blocks VR1 activation by all pathways and thus inhibits toxin A-, capsaicin-, and anandamide-induced inflammation.*

SP release, and this effect was blocked by pretreatment with the specific capsaicin VR1 antagonist, capsazepine. In addition, if anandamide stimulates SP release then anandamide-induced intestinal inflammation should be blocked by SP receptor antagonist pretreatment. Indeed, pretreatment of the rats with the specific NK-1 receptor antagonist, L-733,060, had no effect when tested alone but significantly inhibited anandamide-stimulated inflammation. The inactive enantiomer of L-733,060, L-733,061, had no effect, demonstrating that the effects of L-733,060 were specific for the NK-1 receptor and not due to nonspecific effects of these drugs (18). These results demonstrate that the endocannabinoid anandamide stimulates intestinal primary sensory neurons via the VR1 receptor causing SP release and resulting in enteritis. This in turn suggests that perhaps endogenous anandamide mediates the effects of toxin A in intestinal inflammation. The possible role of the capsaicin VR1 receptor in mediating the neurogenic component of *C. difficile* toxin A-induced intestinal inflammation is summarized in Figure 1. It remains for future studies to measure the levels of endogenous anandamide in the intestine in response to toxin A and other inflammatory agents in order to test the hypothesis that anandamide mediates toxin A-induced enteritis.

ACKNOWLEDGMENTS

This work was supported by a VA Merit Review grant and by NIH grant DK-50265.

REFERENCES

1. Geppetti P and Holzer P, Eds. In: *Neurogenic Inflammation,* Boca Raton, CRC Press, 1996.
2. Bevan S and Geppetti P. Protons: small stimulants of capsaicin-sensitive sensory nerves. *Trends Neurosci* 1994;17:509–512.
3. Castagliuolo IA, Keates C, Qiu B, Kelly CP, Nikulasson S, Leeman SE, and Pothoulakis C. Increased substance P responses in dorsal root ganglia and intestinal macrophages during *Clostridium difficile* toxin A enteritis in rats. *Proc Natl Acad Sci USA* 1997;94:4788–4793.
4. Castagliuolo IJ, LaMont T, Letourneau R, Kelly C, O'Keane JC, Jaffer A, Theoharides TC, and Pothoulakis C. Neuronal involvement in the intestinal effects of *Clostridium difficile* toxin A and *Vibrio cholerae* enterotoxin in rat ileum. *Gastroenterology* 1994;107:657–665.
5. Castagliuolo I, Riegler M, Pasha A, Nikulasson S, Lu B, Gerard C, and Gerard NP. Neurokinin-1 (NK-1) receptor is required in *Clostridium difficile*-induced enteritis. *J Clin Invest* 1998;101:1547–1550.
6. Caterina MJ, Schumacher MA, Tominaga M, Rosen TA, Levine JD, and Julius D. The capsaicin receptor: a heat-activated ion channel in the pain pathway. *Nature* 1997;389:816–824.
7. Davis JB, Gray J, Gunthorpe MJ, Hatcher JP, Davey PT, Overend P, Harries MH, Latcham J, Clapham C, Atkinson K, Hughes SA, Rance K, Grau E, Harper AJ, Pugh PL, Rogers DC, Bingham S, Randall A, and Sheardown SA. Vanilloid receptor-1 is essential for inflammatory thermal hyperalgesia. *Nature* 2000;405:183–187.
8. Figini M, Emanueli C, Grady EF, Kirkwood K, Payan DG, Ansel J, Gerard C, Geppetti P, Bunnett NW. Substance P and bradykinin stimulate plasma extravasation in the mouse gastrointestinal tract and pancreas. *Am J Physiol* 1997;272:G785–G793.
9. Hammer J, Hammer HF, Eherer AJ, Petritsch W, Holzer P, Krejs GJ. Intraluminal capsaicin does not affect fluid and electrolyte absorption in the human jejunum but does cause pain. *Gut* 1998;43:252–255.
10. Holzer P. Capsaicin: cellular targets, mechanisms of action, and selectivity for thin sensory neurons. *Pharmacol Rev* 1991;43:143–201.
11. Holzer P. Neural injury, repair, and adaptation in the GI tract II. The elusive action of capsaicin on the vagus nerve. *Am J Physiol* 1998;275:G8–G13.

12. Keates AC, Castagliuolo I, Qiu B, Nikulasson S, Sengupta A, Pothoulakis C. CGRP upregulation in dorsal root ganglia and ileal mucosa during *Clostridium difficile* toxin A-induced enteritis. *Am J Physiol* 1998;37:G196–G202,.

13. Mantyh CR, Pappas TN, Lapp JA, Washington MK, Neville LM, Ghilardi JR, Rogers SD, Mantyh PW, Vigna SR. Substance P activation of enteric neurons in response to intraluminal *Clostridium difficile* toxin A in the rat ileum. *Gastroenterology* 1996;111:1272–1280,.

14. McVey DC, and Vigna SR. The capsaicin VR1 receptor mediates substance P release in toxin A-induced interitis in rats. *Peptides* 2001;22:1439–1446.

15. Pothoulakis C. Pathogenesis of *Clostridium difficile*-associated diarrhoea. *Eur J Gastroenterol Hepatol* 1996;8:1041–1047.

16. Pothoulakis C, Castagliuolo I, LaMont JT, Jaffer A, O'Keane JC, Snider RM, Leeman SE. CP-96,345, a substance P antagonist, inhibits rat intestinal responses to *Clostridium difficile* toxin A but not cholera toxin. *Proc Natl Acad Sci USA* 1994;91:947–951.

17. Pothoulakis C and LaMont JT. Microbes and microbial toxins: Paradigms for microbial-mucosal interactions II. The integrated response of the intestine to *Clostridium cifficile* toxins. *Am J Physiol* 2001;280:G178–G183.

18. Rupniak NMJ and Kramer MS. Discovery of the anti-depressant and anti-emetic efficacy of substance P receptor (NK$_1$) antagonists. *Trends Pharmacol Sci* 1999;20:485–490.

19. Smart D, Gunthorpe MJ, Jerman JC, Nasir S, Gray J, Muir AI, Chambers JK, Randall AD, and Davis JB. The endogenous lipid anandamide is a full agonist at the human vanilloid receptor (hVR1). *Br J Pharmacol* 2000;129:227–230.

20. Szallasi A and DiMarzo V. New perspectives on enigmatic vanilloid receptors. *Trends Neurosci* 2000;23:491–497.

21. Tamura CS and Ritter RC. Intraintestinal capsaicin transiently reduces CGRP-like immunoreactivity in rat submucosal plexus. *Brain Res* 1997;770:248–255.

22. Tominaga M, Caterina MJ, Malmberg AB, Rosen TA Gilbert H, Skinner K, Raumann BE, Basbaum AI, and Julius D. The cloned capsaicin receptor integrates multiple pain-producing stimuli. *Neuron* 1998;21:531–543.

23. Tominaga M, Wada M, Masu M. Potentiation of capsaicin receptor activity by metabotropic ATP receptors as a possible mechanism for ATP-evoked pain and hyperalgesia. *Proc Natl Acad Sci USA* 2001;98:6951–6956.

24. Torres J, Jennische E, Lange S, Lönnroth I. Enterotoxins from *Clostridium difficile;* diarrhoeogenic potency and morphological effects in the rat intestine. *Gut* 1990;31:781–785.

25. Wood JN. Pathobiology of visceral pain: Molecular mechanisms and therapeutic implications II. Genetic approaches to pain therapy. *Am J Physiol* 2000;278:G507–G512.

26. Zittel TT, Meyer JH, Raybould HE. Small intestinal capsaicin-sensitive afferents mediate feedback inhibition of gastric emptying in rats. *Am J Physiol* 1994;267:G1142–G1145.

27. Zygmunt PM, Petersson J, Andersson DA, Chuang H, Di Marzo V, Julius D, Högestätt D. Vanilloid receptors on sensory nerves mediate the vasodilator action of anandamide. *Nature* 1999;400:452–457.

Gut-Brain Peptides in the New Millennium, edited by Y. Taché
CURE Foundation, Los Angeles, CA. © 2002

26

Turning Off the Signal: Mechanisms that Terminate the Biological Responses to Neuropeptides

Nigel W. Bunnett

Departments of Surgery and Physiology, University of California, San Francisco

INTRODUCTION

Signaling by neuropeptides must be tightly regulated to ensure the appropriate physiological response. The steps that initiate signaling by neuropeptides have been thoroughly investigated. Nerve fibers and endocrine cells respond to appropriate stimuli by releasing peptides into the interstitial fluid. Peptides diffuse through the interstitial fluid or the circulation to interact with high affinity with receptors at surface of target cells. The receptors engage the machinery of signal transduction to alter the function of the target cell, causing it to secrete, contract, move, divide or die. As important as the processes that initiate signaling by peptides are those which terminate their responses. These processes serve to restrict the sphere of influence of a peptide and to limit the duration of its biological effects on the target cell. Broadly speaking, they can be divided into processes that act at the level of the peptide and its G-protein coupled receptor (Figure 1). Peptidases that are soluble in the interstitial fluid, anchored to the plasma membrane, or in intracellular compartments degrade neuropeptides and thereby terminate their capacity to signal. Interaction of the peptide with its receptor triggers a cascade of events that uncouples the receptor from down-stream signaling proteins, which effectively switches off the signal. These processes prevent the uncontrolled stimulation of target cells, which may otherwise result in exaggerated signaling and disease.

This brief chapter summarizes my research over the past twenty years into the mechanisms that switch off signaling by neuropeptides and their receptors. I am deeply indebted to John H. Walsh for his support of my endeavors. Some of the work I will discuss was in direct collaboration with John. All of it was influenced by our frequent discussions. These discussions were most beneficial to my research; I remember them most fondly.

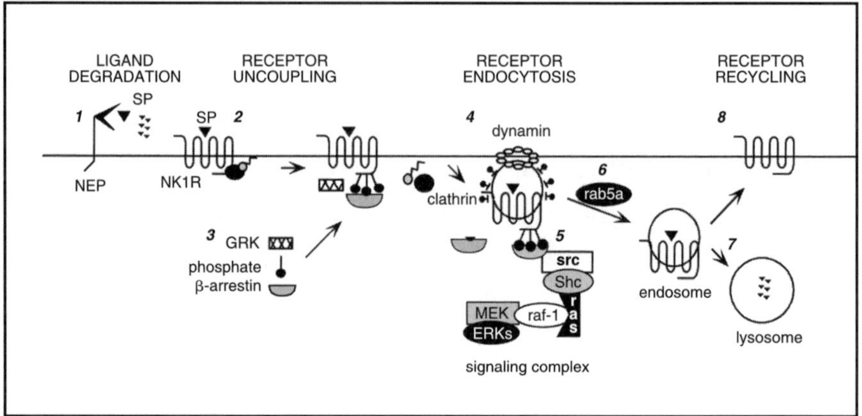

FIGURE 1. *Mechanisms that regulate responses to SP and the NK1R. (1) NEP degrades SP at the plasma membrane. (2) SP binding to the NK1R triggers membrane trafficking of G-protein receptors kinases (GRK) and β-arrestins (3), which disrupts the NK1R from heterotrimeric G-proteins and terminates the signal. (4) β-arrestins are clathrin adaptors for receptor endocytosis and also recruit components of the MAP kinase cascade to endosomes (5). (6) rab5a mediates trafficking of endosomes to a perinuclear compartment, where SP dissociates and is degraded in lysosomes (7). (8) NK1R recycling mediates resensitization.*

MECHANISMS OF NEUROPEPTIDE DEGRADATION

Peptides are Rapidly Degraded in Interstitial Fluid

Peptides are rapidly cleared from the circulation by a combination of degradation by circulating proteases or clearance by the kidney. The half–life of a peptide in the circulation can be readily determined by sequential blood sampling. Although such studies are valid for hormonal peptides, they are of little use for neuropeptides that act locally within tissues. Thus, an early challenge was to develop methods to permit the sampling of interstitial fluid and the assay of neuropeptides. The technique of microdialysis was devised for this purpose (1). By implanting dialysis fibers of a few micrometers diameter into the wall of the intestine, and perfusing them with physiological solution, it is possible to sample a dialysate of the interstitial fluid bathing nerve endings in which peptides can be measured. Radiolabeled peptides can also be introduced into the interstitial fluid through dialysis fibers or fine catheters. Labeled metabolites may be collected into adjacent fibers and separated by high pressure liquid chromatography. In this manner, we found that bombesin (2), neurotensin (3), substance P (SP) (4, 5) and enkephalins (6) are degraded in the gastric submucosa with half lives of minutes. By using specific inhibitors of proteases, we reported that aminopeptidases, angiotensin converting enzyme and neutral endopeptidase (NEP, EC3.4.24.11) contribute to this degradation.

Cell Surface Peptidases Degrade Neuropeptides

We characterized membrane-associated peptidases that can degrade neuropeptides using selective inhibitors. In this manner, we found that membrane preparations of gastric muscle rapidly degrade SP and gastrin releasing peptide (GRP) by action of NEP (Figure 1) (7). The role of NEP in peptide degradation in the stomach was confirmed by isolation of the gastric protease and demonstration that gastric NEP degrades and inactivates SP, GRP, enkephalins, gastrin and cholecystokinin 8 (8, 9). We subsequently localized NEP to epithelial and muscle layers of the stomach and intestine, where it may degrade many different neuropeptides (10).

NEP is a cell-surface peptidase; it is anchored to the plasma membrane of cells with a single hydrophobic domain, and the bulk of the enzyme, including its active site, projects into the interstitial fluid where it is well placed to degrade extracellular peptides. Although NEP degrades several neuropeptides, it prefers short peptides and SP is the most favorable substrate from a kinetic standpoint. There are extended forms of many neuropeptides, which may be more resistant to peptidases than shorter forms. To examine this possibility, we compared the ability of NEP to degrade the long and short forms of somatostatin and GRP (Figure 2). Under conditions in which NEP completely degraded somatostatin-14 and GRP-10, somatostatin-28 and GRP-27 were completely resistant to hydrolysis (Bunnett and Walsh, unpublished observations). These results indicate that the longer forms of neuropeptides are more resistant to peptidases and, may therefore, have a longer half life in the interstitial fluid and a greater sphere of influence than short peptides.

NEP Plays a Physiological Role in Terminating the Effects of Peptides.

Several strategies have been used to elucidate the physiological role of NEP, including use of selective inhibitors, expression of NEP in heterologous systems, and deletion of the NEP gene. We evaluated the effects of inhibitors on the contractile actions of neuropeptides on isolated gastric muscle cells. Inhibitors of a variety of peptidases, including NEP, potentiated the biological actions of enkephalins (11), GRP (12) and somatostatin (13). Notably, a combination of NEP and aminopeptidase inhibitors increased the potency of somatostatin-14 for inhibiting contraction of gastric myocytes by >1,000 fold. In contrast, peptidase inhibitors do not alter the contractile effects of somatostatin-28, which is resistant to degradation.

The role of NEP was further evaluated in heterologous expression systems. Although the affinity of SP for the neurokinin 1 receptor (NK1R) (Kd 3.5 nM) is ~1,000-fold higher than its affinity for NEP (Km 32 μM),

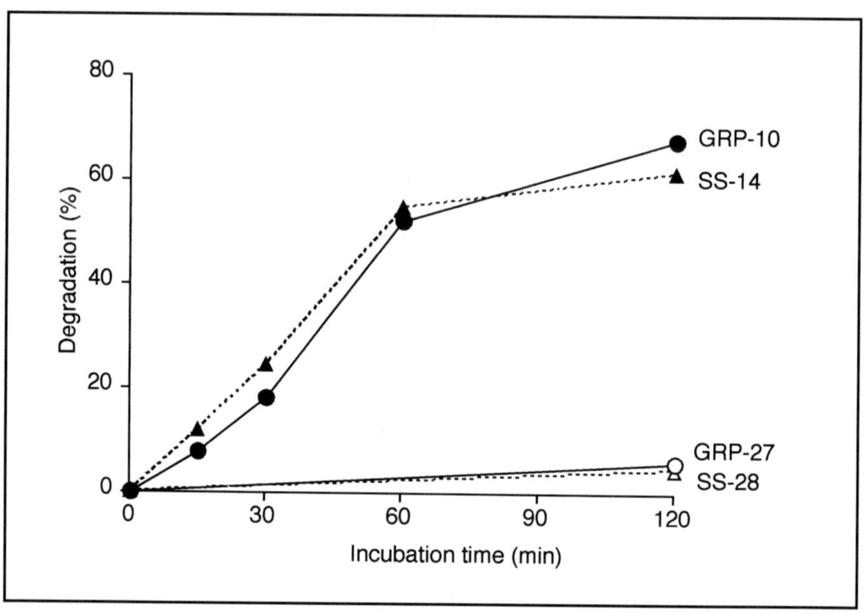

FIGURE 2. *Degradation of GRP and somatostatin by NEP. Peptides were incubated with recombinant human NEP under identical conditions. Metabolites were separated by high pressure liquid chromatography to assess degradation. Note that whereas the shorter peptides are rapidly degraded, the longer forms are resistant to hydrolysis by NEP.*

the co-expression of NEP in the same cell as the NK1R accelerates SP degradation, diminishes the ability of SP to bind its receptor, and markedly attenuates signaling to low concentrations of the peptide (14). These findings contributed to the large body of work that indicates that NEP plays a major role in terminating signaling by tachykinins such as SP.

The physiological role of NEP was unequivocally demonstrated by genetic deletion of this enzyme. SP is a major mediator of neurogenic inflammation, a form of inflammation that is regulated by sensory nerves and characterized by elevated extravasation of plasma proteins and neutrophils from post-capillary venules (15–17). Mice lacking NEP exhibited a 3–5 fold elevated extravasation of plasma proteins in all gastrointestinal tissues, the pancreas, trachea and skin compared to wild-type mice (18). Administration of recombinant NEP, or antagonists of the NK1R abolished this response, suggesting that absence of NEP results in the diminished degradation of SP and consequent activation of the NK1R, leading to plasma extravasation. Indeed, deletion of NEP is associated with diminished SP degradation and elevated SP levels in gastrointestinal tissues (18, 19) (Bunnett, unpublished observation). These findings suggested that mice lacking NEP would be more sensitive to inflammatory challenges, which proved to be the case.

Thus, the deletion of NEP exacerbates hapten-induced colitis (19), ileitis induced by toxin A from *Clostridium difficile* (20), and allergic dermatitis (21). In all cases, inflammation is attenuated with recombinant NEP or by antagonists of the NK1R. NEP is down-regulated during intestinal inflammation (22), which may exacerbate the inflammatory response.

MECHANISMS OF RECEPTOR DESENSITIZATION

Peptide degradation is the first and earliest step that shuts off signaling by a neuropeptide. Other mechanisms operate at the level of the receptor.

Biological Responses to Neuropeptides are Transient and Rapidly Desensitize

Peptide binding to its receptor alters the receptor conformation to facilitate coupling to heterotrimeric G-proteins which engage the machinery of signal transduction. Soon thereafter, a series of highly coordinated events serve to terminate the signal (Figure 1). These events include uncoupling the receptor from G-proteins and removal of the receptor from the cell surface so that it can no longer interact with peptides in the extracellular fluid.

It is well established that biological responses to neuropeptides are usually transient and desensitize to repeated stimulation. For example, responses to SP rapidly desensitize and slowly resensitize in transfected cells, primary cultures of enteric neurons, and in the intact animal (23–27). This desensitization is principally mediated by uncoupling of the activated receptor from heterotrimeric G-proteins. Agonists trigger the translocation of G-protein receptor kinases (GRKs) and second messenger kinases (protein kinase A and C) from the cytosol to the plasma membrane, where they can phosphorylate receptors (28, 29). β-arrestins also translocate to the cell surface where they interact with GRK-phosphorylated receptors to disrupt their association with heterotrimeric G-proteins and thereby mediate uncoupling and desensitization (25, 26).

Neuropeptides Trigger Redistribution of Receptors and Associated Signaling Molecules

Agonist-induced redistribution of receptors and associated signaling molecules plays a major role in regulation of signal transduction. The examination of receptor trafficking was facilitated by the availability of reagents that enabled the direct observation of receptors in tissue sections and living cells, namely specific receptor antibodies and fluorescently tagged peptides and their receptors. By using antibodies to the three neurokinin receptors in

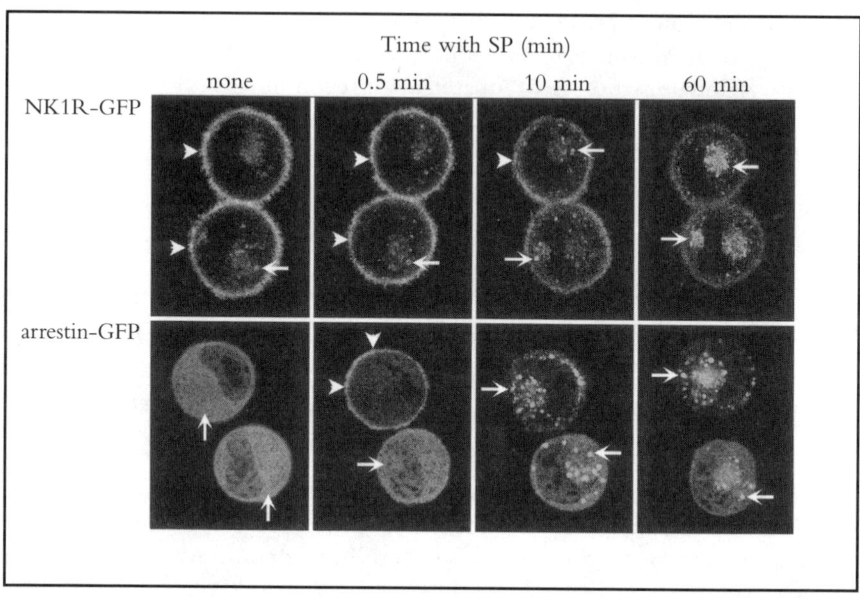

FIGURE 3. *SP-induced trafficking of the NK1R and β-arrestin1 tagged with green fluorescent protein and expressed in KNRK cells. In the unstimulated state the NK1R is at the cell surface and β-arrestins are in the cytosol. After 30 s with SP, β-arrestins move to the plasma membrane. At later times the NK1R and β-arrestins internalize into endosomes.*

combination with fluorescent agonists it was possible, for the first time, to localize receptors with high resolution in tissues, primary cell cultures and neurons (30–33), and to directly observe trafficking of receptors in living cells in real time (25, 32, 34–37). Similar fluorescent probes also permitted examination of trafficking of GRP receptors (35).

The pathway, mechanism and possible functions of agonist-induced trafficking of several neuropeptide receptors have been delineated. SP induces endocytosis of the NK1R by a mechanism that is disrupted by potassium depletion and hyper-osmolar sucrose, and which is thus dependent on clathrin (34, 36). SP also induces rapid trafficking of β-arrestins from the cytosol to the plasma membrane (28, 29) (Figure 3). In addition to their role in uncoupling, β-arrestins are also clathrin adaptor proteins. Expression of dominant negative mutants of β-arrestin, to disrupt the function of endogenous proteins, inhibits SP-induced endocytosis of the NK1R, indicating a role for β-arrestins in receptor internalization (26). Small GTPases such as dynamin and rab proteins play important roles in many steps of vesicular trafficking that have been delineated by expressing dominant negative mutants. For example, a dominant negative mutant of dynamin prevents SP-induced endocytosis of the NK1R, confirming a role for dynamin in the pinching off of clathrin coated pits (38). Dominant negative rab5a slows endocytosis and causes retention of the NK1R in vesicles close to the plasma membrane that fail to progress to a perinuclear region, indicating a role for rab5a in early stages of vesicular transport (38).

Receptor Trafficking is Required for Signal Transduction

Recent evidence indicates that receptor endocytosis has many roles other than simply to remove receptors from the cell surface and thereby contribute to desensitization. For receptors that recycle to the plasma membrane, such as the NK1R, endocytosis is required for resensitization of signaling. Thus, inhibition of endocytosis by expression of dominant negative dynamin or rab5a impedes resensitization of SP-induced Ca^{2+} mobilization (38). The explanation of this effect is probably that resensitization requires ligand dissociation in acidified endosomes, and dephosphorylation of the receptor by endosomal phosphatases followed by dissociation of β-arrestins. In support of this explanation is the finding that bafilomycin, which inhibits vacuolar H^+-ATPases, and the phosphatase inhibitor okadaic acid suppress resensitization of the NK1R (24).

In addition to their role in uncoupling and endocytosis, β-arrestins are also molecular scaffolds for various components of the MAP kinase pathway (Figure 1). Thus, β-arrestin-dependent endocytosis mediates mitogenic signaling and activation of extracellular signal regulated kinases 1 and 2 (ERKs) by certain receptors, including the NK1R and proteinase-activated receptor 2 (PAR2). Expression of dominant negative mutants of β-arrestin and dynamin, but not rab5a, inhibits SP-induced activation of ERK1/2 (38, 39). Moreover, SP does not fully activate ERK1/2 in cells expressing a naturally occurring truncated form of the NK1R, which fails to interact efficiently with β-arrestin and is thus resistant to endocytosis and desensitization (29, 40). SP stimulates the formation of a complex containing NK1R, β-arrestin and src (39). ERKs activated in this manner translocate to the nucleus to induce proliferation. Similarly, dominant negative β-arrestin inhibits agonist-induced endocytosis of PAR2 and reduces ERK1/2 activation (41). PAR2 agonists stimulate the formation of complex comprising PAR2, β-arrestin, raf-1 and activated ERK1/2 in cells expressing the PAR2 (41). Thus, β-arrestins are scaffolds that recruit and organize components of the mitogen activated protein kinase cascade into endosomes, although the make up of the complex depends on the receptor in question.

Neuropeptide Receptors Compete for β-arrestins: Novel Mechanisms of Receptor Interactions

A common theme of signaling by neuropeptides is that a single peptide can interact with different receptors. For example, the tachykinins SP, neurokinin A (NKA) and NKB bind the three neurokinin receptors with graded affinities. Thus, one agonist could regulate a cell though distinct receptors once the optimal concentration is achieved. Furthermore, different agonists may simultaneously or sequentially activate distinct receptors on the same cell. Recent observations indicate that one receptor can influence trafficking and signaling of another receptor by virtue of competing for a limited intracellular store of β-arrestins (42). β-arrestins mediate endocytosis of both the NK1R and NK3R, since dominant negative β-arrestin inhibits endocytosis of both receptors. However, whereas an NK1R agonist causes sequestration of NK1R with β-arrestins in the same endosomes, thereby depleting them from the cytosol, β-arrestins do not prominently sequester with the activated NK3R and rapidly return to the cytosol. In cells coexpressing both receptors, prior activation of the NK1R inhibits endocytosis and homologous desensitization of the NK3R, which is reversed by overexpression of β-arrestins. Similar results are obtained in enteric neurons that naturally co-express the NK1R and NK3R. In contrast, activation of the NK3R does not affect NK1R endocytosis or desensitization. Thus, the high affinity and prolonged interaction of the NK1R with β-arrestins depletes β-arrestins from the cytosol and limits their role in desensitization and endocytosis of the NK3R. Since β-arrestins are critical for desensitization, endocytosis and mitogenic signaling of many receptors, this sequestration is likely to have important and widespread implications.

CONCLUSIONS

In common with most important biological processes, there is apparent redundancy in the mechanisms that terminate signaling by neuropeptides and their receptors. Ligand degradation by a host of cell surface and soluble peptidases is a first line of defense, that serves to confine neuropeptides to defined regions within a tissue. Extended forms of a peptide, that may be more resistant to degradation, could thus influence more distant target cells. Receptor phosphorylation by G-protein receptor kinases and association with β-arrestins effectively uncouples receptors from signaling proteins and terminate their capacity to signal. Endocytosis of receptors could also contribute to desensitization, by depleting receptors from the surface of the cell and thereby preventing access to peptides in the extracellular fluid. Recent evidence also indicates that this endocytosis is important for resensitization of signaling and for mitogenic signaling of some receptors.

Despite the importance of these regulatory mechanisms, little is known about how they are themselves controlled. For example, what factors regulate the expression and activity of proteases and β-arrestins? Does activation of one receptor alter the trafficking of another, and if so by what means? Are there abnormalities in expression and activity of critical regulatory proteins in disease states that contribute to dysfunction? In view of the importance of mechanisms that terminate signaling by peptides and their receptors, these questions merit further investigation.

My research in this area has been enormously influenced by John H. Walsh. John was the most intellectually generous scientist. He read and critiqued all of my papers and grant proposals, gave me unrestricted access to antibodies, peptides and cell lines, and provided me with many of my best ideas. For these reasons, I am enormously indebted to John; I count myself most fortunate to have known him as a mentor, colleague and friend.

ACKNOWLEDGMENTS

The research discussed in this chapter was funded by NIH grants DK39957, DK43207 and DK57840.

REFERENCES

1. Bunnett NW, Walsh JH, Debas HT, Kauffman GL, Jr., Golanska EM. Measurement of prostaglandin E2 in interstitial fluid from the dog stomach after feeding and indomethacin. *Gastroenterology* 1983; 85:1391–1398.

2. Bunnett NW, Reeve JR, Jr., Walsh JH. Catabolism of bombesin in the interstitial fluid of the rat stomach. *Neuropeptides* 1983;4:55–64.

3. Bunnett NW, Mogard M, Orloff MS, Corbet HJ, Reeve JR, Jr., Walsh JH. Catabolism of neurotensin in interstitial fluid of the rat stomach. *Am J Physiol* 1984;246:G675–682.

4. Bunnett NW, Orloff MS, Turner AJ. Catabolism of substance P in the stomach wall of the rat. *Life Sci* 1985;37:599–606.

5. Orloff MS, Turner AJ, Bunnett NW. Catabolism of substance P and neurotensin in the rat stomach wall is susceptible to inhibitors of angiotensin converting enzyme. *Regul Pept* 1986;14:21–31.

6. Bunnett NW, Walsh JH, Debas HT. Metabolism of enkephalin in stomach wall of rats. *Am J Physiol* 1990;258:G143–151.

7. Bunnett NW, Kobayashi R, Orloff MS, Reeve JR, Turner AJ, Walsh JH. Catabolism of gastrin releasing peptide and substance P by gastric membrane-bound peptidases. *Peptides* 1985;6:277–283.

8. Bunnett NW, Debas HT, Turner AJ, Kobayashi R, Walsh JH. Metabolism of gastrin and cholecystokinin by endopeptidase 24.11 from the pig stomach. *Am J Physiol* 1988;255:G676–684.

9. Bunnett NW, Turner AJ, Hryszko J, Kobayashi R, Walsh JH. Isolation of endopeptidase-24.11 (EC 3.4.24.11, "enkephalinase") from the pig stomach. Hydrolysis of substance P, gastrin-releasing peptide 10, [Leu5] enkephalin, and [Met5] enkephalin. *Gastroenterology* 1988;95:952–957.

10. Bunnett NW, Wu V, Sternini C, Klinger J, Shimomaya E, Payan D, Kobayashi R, Walsh JH. Distribution and abundance of neutral endopeptidase (EC 3.4.24.11) in the alimentary tract of the rat. *Am J Physiol* 1993;264:G497–508.

11. Menozzi D, Gu ZF, Maton PN, Bunnett NW. Inhibition of peptidases potentiates enkephalin-stimulated contraction of gastric muscle cells. *Am J Physiol* 1991;261:G476–484.

12. Gu ZF, Menozzi D, Okamoto A, Maton PN, Bunnett NW. Neutral endopeptidase (EC 3.4.24.11) modulates the contractile effects of neuropeptides on muscle cells from the guinea-pig stomach. *Exp Physiol* 1993;78:35–48.

13. Gu ZF, Pradhan T, Coy DH, Mantey S, Bunnett NW, Jensen RT, Maton PN. Actions of somatostatins on gastric smooth muscle cells. *Am J Physiol* 1992;262:G432–438.

14. Okamoto A, Lovett M, Payan DG, Bunnett NW. Interactions between neutral endopeptidase (EC 3.4.24.11) and the substance P (NK1) receptor expressed in mammalian cells. *Biochem J* 1994;299: 683–693.

15. McDonald DM, Bowden JJ, Baluk P, Bunnett NW. Neurogenic inflammation. A model for studying efferent actions of sensory nerves. *Adv Exp Med Biol* 1996;410:453–462.

16. Figini M, Emanueli C, Grady EF, Kirkwood K, Payan DG, Ansel J, Gerard C, Geppetti P, Bunnett N. Substance P and bradykinin stimulate plasma extravasation in the mouse gastrointestinal tract and pancreas. *Am J Physiol* 1997;272:G785–793.

17. Steinhoff M, Vergnolle N, Young SH, Tognetto M, Amadesi S, Ennes HS, Trevisani M, Hollenberg MD, Wallace JL, Caughey GH, Mitchell SE, Williams LM, Geppetti P, Mayer EA, Bunnett NW. Agonists of proteinase-activated receptor 2 induce inflammation by a neurogenic mechanism. *Nat Med* 2000;6:151–158.

18. Lu B, Figini M, Emanueli C, Geppetti P, Grady EF, Gerard NP, Ansell J, Payan DG, Gerard C, Bunnett N. The control of microvascular permeability and blood pressure by neutral endopeptidase. *Nat Med* 1997;3:904–907.

19. Sturiale S, Barbara G, Qiu B, Figini M, Geppetti P, Gerard N, Gerard C, Grady EF, Bunnett NW, Collins SM. Neutral endopeptidase (EC 3.4.24.11) terminates colitis by degrading substance P. *Proc Natl Acad Sci USA* 1999;96:11653–11658.

20. Kirkwood KS, Kim EH, He XD, Calaustro EQ, Domush C, Yoshimi SK, Grady EF, Maa J, Bunnett NW, Debas HT. Substance P inhibits pancreatic exocrine secretion via a neural mechanism. *Am J Physiol* 1999;277:G314–320.

21. Scholzen TE, Steinhoff M, Bonaccorsi P, Klein R, Amadesi S, Geppetti P, Lu B, Gerard NP, Olerud JE, Luger TA, Bunnett NW, Grady EF, Armstrong CA, Ansel JC. Neutral endopeptidase terminates substance P-induced inflammation in allergic contact dermatitis. *J Immunol* 2001;166:1285–1291.

22. Hwang L, Leichter R, Okamoto A, Payan D, Collins SM, Bunnett NW. Downregulation of neutral endopeptidase (EC 3.4.24.11) in the inflamed rat intestine. *Am J Physiol* 1993;264:G735–743.

23. Bowden JJ, Garland AM, Baluk P, Lefevre P, Grady EF, Vigna SR, Bunnett NW, McDonald DM. Direct observation of substance P-induced internalization of neurokinin 1 (NK1) receptors at sites of inflammation. *Proc Natl Acad Sci USA* 1994;91:8964–8968.

24. Garland AM, Grady EF, Lovett M, Vigna SR, Frucht MM, Krause JE, Bunnett NW. Mechanisms of desensitization and resensitization of G protein-coupled neurokinin1 and neurokinin2 receptors. *Mol Pharmacol* 1996;49:438–446.

25. McConalogue K, Corvera CU, Gamp PD, Grady EF, Bunnett NW. Desensitization of the neurokinin-1 receptor (NK1-R) in neurons: effects of substance P on the distribution of NK1-R, Galphaq/11, G- protein receptor kinase-2/3, and beta-arrestin-1/2. *Mol Biol Cell* 1998;9:2305–2324.

26. McConalogue K, Dery O, Lovett M, Wong H, Walsh JH, Grady EF, Bunnett NW. Substance P-induced trafficking of beta-arrestins. The role of beta-arrestins in endocytosis of the neurokinin-1 receptor. *J Biol Chem* 1999;274:16257–16268.

27. Maa J, Grady EF, Kim EH, Yoshimi SK, Hutter MM, Bunnett NW, Kirkwood KS. NK-1 receptor desensitization and neutral endopeptidase terminate SP-induced pancreatic plasma extravasation. *Am J Physiol Gastrointest Liver Physiol* 2000;279:G726–732.

28. McConalogue K, Bunnett NW. G protein-coupled receptors in gastrointestinal physiology. II. Regulation of neuropeptide receptors in enteric neurons. *Am J Physiol* 1998;274:G792–796.

29. Dery O, Defea KA, Bunnett NW. Protein kinase C-mediated desensitization of the neurokinin 1 receptor. *Am J Physiol Cell Physiol* 2001;280:C1097–1106.

30. Vigna SR, Bowden JJ, McDonald DM, Fisher J, Okamoto A, McVey DC, Payan DG, Bunnett NW. Characterization of antibodies to the rat substance P (NK-1) receptor and to a chimeric substance P receptor expressed in mammalian cells. *J Neurosci* 1994;14:834–845.

31. Sternini C, Su D, Gamp PD, Bunnett NW. Cellular sites of expression of the neurokinin-1 receptor in the rat gastrointestinal tract. *J Comp Neurol* 1995;358:531–540.

32. Bunnett NW, Dazin PF, Payan DG, Grady EF. Characterization of receptors using cyanine 3-labeled neuropeptides. *Peptides* 1995;16:733–740.

33. Grady EF, Baluk P, Böhm S, Gamp P, Wong H, Payan DG, Ansel J, Portbury AL, Furness JB, McDonald DM, Bunnett NW. Characterization of antisera specific to NK1, NK2 and NK3 neurokinin receptors and their utilization to localize receptors in the rat gastrointestinal tract. *J Neurosci* 1996;16: 6975–6986.

34. Grady EF, Garland AM, Gamp PD, Lovett M, Payan DG, Bunnett NW. Delineation of the endocytic pathway of substance P and its seven- transmembrane domain NK1 receptor. *Mol Biol Cell* 1995;6:509–524.

35. Grady EF, Slice LW, Brant WO, Walsh JH, Payan DG, Bunnett NW. Direct observation of endocytosis of gastrin releasing peptide and its receptor. *J Biol Chem* 1995;270:4603–4611.

36. Grady EF, Gamp PD, Baluk P, McDonald DM, Payan DG, Bunnett NW. Endocytosis and recycling of NK1 tachykinin receptors in enteric neurons. *Neuroscience* 1996;16:1239–1254.

37. Grady EF, Gamp PD, Jones E, Baluk P, McDonald DM, Payan DG, Bunnett NW. Endocytosis and recycling of neurokinin 1 receptors in enteric neurons. *Neuroscience* 1996;75:1239–1254.

38. Schmidlin F, Dery O, DeFea KO, Slice L, Patierno S, Sternini C, Grady EF, Bunnett NW. Dynamin and Rab5a-dependent trafficking and signaling of the neurokinin 1 receptor. *J Biol Chem* 2001;276: 25427–25437.

39. DeFea KA, Vaughn ZD, O'Bryan EM, Nishijima D, Dery O, Bunnett NW. The proliferative and antiapoptotic effects of substance P are facilitated by formation of a beta-arrestin-dependent scaffolding complex. *Proc Natl Acad Sci USA* 2000;97:11086–11091.

40. Böhm SK, Khitin L, Smeekens SP, Grady EF, Payan DG, Bunnett NW. Identification of potential tyrosine-containing endocytic motifs in the carboxyl-tail and seventh transmembrane domain domain of the neurokinin 1 receptor. *J Biol Chem* 1997;272:2363–2372.

41. DeFea KA, Zalevsky J, Thoma MS, Dery O, Mullins RD, Bunnett NW. Beta-arrestin-dependent endocytosis of proteinase-activated receptor 2 is required for intracellular targeting of activated ERK1/2. *J Cell Biol* 2000;148:1267–1281.

42. Schmidlin F, Dery O, Bunnett N, Grady E. Heterologous regulation of signaling and trafficking of G-protein coupled receptors: interactions between the neurokinin 1 and 3 receptors. *Proc Natl Acad Sci USA* 2002;99:3324–3329.

Gut-Brain Peptides in the New Millennium, edited by Y. Taché
CURE Foundation, Los Angeles, CA. © 2002

27

Sensory Transduction in Visceral Afferents: Role of CCK and Serotonin

Helen E Raybould

Department of Anatomy, Physiology and Cell Biology, UC Davis School of Veterinary Medicine, Davis, California

During the intestinal phase of the meal, signals generated by the presence of nutrients in the intestinal lumen results in inhibition of gastric motility and secretion, together with stimulation of pancreatic secretion, gallbladder contraction and relaxation of the Sphincter of Oddi. These processes are regulated to match the digestive and absorptive capacity of the intestine with the entry of food from the stomach and secretions from the pancreas and gallbladder. These observations imply the existence of "sensors" that can detect the presence of nutrients in the intestine. When John wrote the chapter entitled "Gastrointestinal Hormones" in the *Physiology of the Digestive Tract* (1), he described how the entero-endocrine cells localized in the epithelial cell layer of the intestinal wall release their secretory products when nutrients are present in the intestinal lumen. However, our concepts of how the products of EC cells are released by nutrients and initiate alterations in gastrointestinal function have changed over the last 10 to 15 years since John wrote that chapter. Rather than act as hormones, it is evident that an important pathway of action is to act on specific receptors expressed on the terminals of extrinsic primary afferent neurons. This chapter will discuss the role of cholecystokinin (CCK) and serotonin in mediating the effects of nutrients to stimulate extrinsic primary afferent neurons and thereby produce reflex changes in gastrointestinal function.

Our recent understanding of detection of nutrients in the intestine relies largely on data generated in functional experiments measuring inhibition of gastric motility or acid secretion, or food intake as a measure of activation of intestinal sensors. This approach has yielded useful information about the nature of the mechanisms by which nutrients are detected. It is clear that nutrients act separately from any osmotic or mechanical effects, that all macronutrient groups alter gastric secretion, motor function and food intake, and that each macronutrient group acts via activation of separate and distinct pathways and mechanisms.

The first observation that led to the change in thinking with regard to "brain-gut" peptides was that peripherally administered cholecystokinin could influence behavior, in this case inhibition of food intake, and that this effect was dependent on an intake vagal pathway from the subdiaphragmatic viscera to the brain (1). A direct involvement of extrinsic primary afferents in mediating inhibition of gastric emptying, secretion and food intake in response to chemical stimulation of the gut wall has been demonstrated using the sensory neurotoxin capsaicin to produce a functional ablation of visceral afferents (2, 3). Intraluminal application of capsaicin has shown a role for mucosal afferent terminal fields in mediating feedback responses of the stomach and pancreas (4, 5). Direct application to vagal nerve trunks or the celiac ganglion (to selectively denervate either vagal or spinal afferents, respectively), has shown that a vagal afferent pathway mediates inhibition of gastric emptying and gastric acid secretion in response to intestinal lipid (6, 7). In contrast, inhibition of gastric emptying in response to monosaccharides is dependent on both a vagal and spinal capsaicin sensitive pathway (8).

Thus, the response to intestinal nutrients is not only dependent on the release of peptides and hormones from entero-endocrine cells, but also on intact extrinsic, specifically afferent, neural pathways from the gut to the brain. The concept evolved that these hormones released by nutrients may not act as hormones at all but may act locally to stimulate peptide receptors on the peripheral terminals of extrinsic afferent fibers.

LIPID AND CCK

It was well established from the early work of Hunt and Knox and later from James Meyer working at CURE, that hydrolysis of triglyceride is required in order for lipids to inhibit gastric emptying or stimulate pancreatic secretion (1), effects that are associated with the release of CCK. Moreover, only fatty acids of chain length of C10 and above were effective. Later work from a number of investigators confirmed that increases in plasma levels of CCK induced by intestinal lipid have the same requirements.

The absorption of lipid in the intestine requires a number of different steps. After lipolysis of ingested triglyceride into long chain fatty acids and monoglycerides, these molecules diffuse into the enterocyte and are resynthesized to triglyceride by the endoplasmic reticulum (9). Apolipoproteins are transferred to the newly synthesized lipids, chylomicrons are formed and released by exocytosis from the basolateral membrane of the enterocyte. Chylomicrons diffuse through the lamina propria and enter lymph lacteals. Fatty acids greater than C10-C12 are absorbed via chylomicron formation into the lymph, while fatty acids less than C10 diffuse predominately into the portal blood and are carried bound to albumin to the liver. Inhibition of gastric emptying or food intake by fat is induced by free fatty acids, and only by long chain fatty acids (>C12). Likewise, it is long chain fatty acids that are effective to release CCK. It has recently been shown that there is a good correlation between increasing plasma levels of CCK and inhibition of gastric motility in humans by fatty acids of chain length above but not below C10 (10). The question remains as to what it is about the long chain triglyceride that determines release of CCK and activation of intestinal feedback responses?

We were interested in determining whether lipid acts lumenally (for example on the lumenal aspect of endocrine cells) or whether absorption is required, and whether it is sufficient for the lipid to enter an epithelial cell or whether a cellular event downstream is required. We have obtained evidence that chylomicron formation is required for lipid to inhibit gastric emptying (11). The role of chylomicron formation in this sensory transduction pathway has been investigated using the surfactant Pluronic L-81 (L-81) that inhibits chylomicron formation. In awake rats, lipid-induced inhibition of gastric emptying is abolished when lipid is infused together with L-81. This demonstrates that the ability of intestinal lipid to produce feedback inhibition of gastric emptying depends on chylomicron formation, which blocks the appearance of postabsorptive chylomicrons in the lamina propria and mesenteric lymph. However, it is not clear if it is the triglyceride content of the chylomicrons or some other component that is signaling to either the endocrine cells or extrinsic primary afferent neurons.

More recently, we have obtained evidence that it is a constituent of chylous lymph that initiates feedback (12). We hypothesized that inhibition of gastric motor function is dependent on the post absorptive components of intestinal lipid digestion and absorption, possibly chylomicrons and/or chylomicron components, for example apo A-IV, rather than the products of lipid absorption (triglyceride) itself. The effect of post absorptive chylomicron products was studied by measuring the ability of chylous lymph given intra-arterially to inhibit gastric motility. Lymph was collected from awake lymph-fistula donor rats, during intestinal infusion with either a glucose-saline maintenance solution or lipid. The effect of lymph, injected intra arterially close to the upper GI tract, on gastric motility was determined in anesthetized recipient rats. Injection of lymph collected during intestinal lipid infusion significantly inhibited gastric motility compared to injection of equivalent amounts of triglyceride. Additionally, inhibition of gastric motility was significantly reduced after injection of lymph collected from rats during lipid infusion with pluronic L-81, (an inhibitor of chylomicron formation and apolipoprotein (apo) A-IV secretion), compared to lymph injection from donor animals treated with Pluronic L-63 (a non-inhibitory control for pluronic L-81). These data suggest that it is not the lipid content of chylous lymph that is effective, but other chylomicron components. Injection of purified recombinant apo A-IV significantly inhibited gastric motility. Taken together, this data suggests that products of lipid digestion and absorption, other than fatty acids or TG, released by the intestine during lipid digestion likely serve as signals to initiate intestinal feedback regulation of GI function. Most likely, apo A-IV is one of the signals involved. Apolipoprotein (apo) A-IV is synthesized by enterocytes in response to lipid absorption in the intestine (13). Apo A-IV synthesis and release into the mesenteric lymph depends upon the transport of lipid via chylomicrons, and therefore, the secretion and release of apo A-IV is dependent on chain length of the absorbed fatty acid (14). Formation of chylomicrons and synthesis of one of these apolipoproteins can be rapid and has been proposed to be involved in signaling intestinal lipid content to other organs (15, 16). For example, intraperitoneal injection of exogenous apo A-IV has been shown to inhibit gastric emptying, gastric acid secretion and food intake in rats.

It is interesting to note that, since CCK mediates inhibition of gastric emptying in response to triglyceride, this data implies that chylomicron formation may be necessary for release of CCK. Initial studies from our laboratory suggest that this is indeed the case. Perfusion of triglyceride into the intestine of awake rats increases plasma levels of CCK rapidly, within the first 10 minutes of perfusion. The rise in plasma CCK is not seen when triglyceride is perused with Pluronic L81 to inhibit chylomicron formation (11). Thus at this point it is unclear at to whether the effect of lipid under physiological condition to release CCK is directly on endocrine cells or whether an interaction occurs between enterocytes and endocrine cells. It is not known whether endocrine cells express the intracellular machinery required to form chylomicron or to handle significant levels of fatty acid in the cell. These interesting issues are presently under investigation.

CARBOHYDRATES AND 5-HT

Dietary carbohydrates release a number of different substances from enteroendocrine cells in the small intestine including glucagon-like peptide (GLP), gastric inhibitory peptide (GIP), and serotonin (5-HT) which may be involved in mediating carbohydrate induced changes in gastric function and food intake (17). We have obtained good evidence indicating that 5-HT has a role in mediating dietary carbohydrate-induced intestinal feedback inhibition of gastric motor function. The evidence comes from release studies, electrophysiological recordings of visceral afferents, and functional studies using 5-HT receptor antagonists, in particular for the 5-HT$_3$ receptor subtype.

Release of 5-HT from the intestinal mucosa is under neural, paracrine and direct control and is secreted from EC cells in response to changes in lumenal contents. Evidence from both *in vivo* and *in vitro* studies suggests that 5-HT can be released by intestinal perfusion of hyperosmotic glucose solutions or acid (18). The exact mechanism by which lumenal glucose or acid stimulates 5-HT secretion and the physiological importance of these observations is not known. However, 5-HT is capable of producing changes in activity of extrinsic and intrinsic neurons. Electrophysiological recordings of vagal afferents with terminal fields in the intestine of the ferret and rat are extremely sensitive to exogenously administered 5-HT (19, 20). This seems to be a 5-HT$_3$-mediated response since it was antagonized by a specific antagonist, granisetron or tropisteron. Further support for this model comes from evidence that vagal afferents express 5-HT$_3$ receptors. A direct role for 5-HT acting via 5-HT$_3$ receptors has been demonstrated in mediating inhibition of gastric emptying and pancreatic secretion in response to glucose (Raybould, unpublished observations, 20). Taken together, this evidence clearly supports a role for 5-HT and 5-HT$_3$ receptors and extrinsic primary afferent neurons in the intestinal feedback inhibition induced by glucose in the intestinal lumen.

Only monosaccharides are absorbed across the gut epithelium (21). Ingested complex carbohydrates are digested in the lumen and by brush border enzymes to generate monosaccharides glucose, galactose or fructose. Glucose and galactose enter the enterocyte via the sodium/glucose co-transporter SGLT-1 located on the apical surface of enterocytes. They exit the cell by facilitated diffusion via the basolaterally-located GLUT-2. Fructose is absorbed by facilitated diffusion via GLUT-5. We have obtained preliminary evidence that SGLT-1 is critical to produce glucose-induced inhibition of gastric emptying (22). Perfusion of the intestine with an analogue of glucose, α-methyl glucose, a substrate of SGLT-1 inhibits gastric emptying; analogues of glucose that are not substrates of SGLT-1 do not inhibit gastric emptying.

Since we have established a role for 5-HT, the question arises as to the mechanism by which glucose, possibly acting via SGLT-1, releases 5-HT from enterochromaffin cells in the intestinal mucosa. Previous studies on 5-HT release from the intestinal mucosa have used *in vitro* preparations including isolated loops of intestine, sheets of mucosa or impure preparations of EC cells. Enterocytes express SGLT-1 and, therefore, it is important to discriminate between a direct effect of glucose on EC cells or an indirect effect mediated by enterocytes, both mechanisms are possible. In order to help address this question, we have used a human tumor cell line, BON cells, that release 5-HT in response to a number of different stimuli (23). BON cells release glucose in response to D-glucose. Glucose-evoked release of 5-HT was mimicked by a non-metabolizable substrate of SGLT-1 but not GLUT-2, α-methyl glucose, but not by mannitol or fructose. Glucose-evoked release of 5-HT was also phloridzin-sensitive, which is a blocker of SGLT-1. These results suggest that SGLT-1 is involved in initiating feedback responses to glucose in the intestine and that this process may involve release of 5-HT from enterochromaffin cells by a mechanism involving SGLT-1.

CONCLUSIONS

The term "brain-gut" peptide was originally coined to describe those peptides and hormones, originally isolated from the gastrointestinal tract, that were later found to be located in neurons in the central nervous system. It is now clear that a number of these "brain-gut" transmitters, such as CCK and 5-HT, act on the "brain-gut" axis to produce well-characterized changes in gastrointestinal function that were initially thought to be mediated via humoral pathways (1). We have gained a better understanding of the neural pathways by which these agents act, but interestingly, we are now turning back to examine some fundamental questions about the mechanism of release from entero-endocrine cells in the intestinal wall.

ACKNOWLEDGMENTS

The work of the author is supported by NIH DK 41004. The authors would like to thank the many investigators who have contributed to the work described in this manuscript, in particular Helen Cooke, Patrick Tso, James Meyer, Ted Kalogeris, and Jorg Glatzle.

REFERENCES

1. Walsh J. Gastrointestinal Hormones. In: Johnson LR, Ed. *Physiology of the Gastrointestinal Tract.* Volume 1. 2nd ed. New York: Raven Press 1987:181–253.
2. Raybould HE, Lloyd KC. Integration of postprandial function in the proximal gastrointestinal tract. Role of CCK and sensory pathways. *Ann NY Acad Sci* 1994;713:143–156.
3. Ritter R, Brenner L, Yox D. Participation of vagal sensory neurons in putative satiety signals from the upper gastrointestinal tract. In: Ritter S, Ritter R, and Barnes C, Eds. *Neuroanatomy and Physiology of Abdominal Vagal Afferents.* Boca Raton: CRC Press 1992:221–248.
4. Zittel TT, Rothenhofer I, Meyer JH, Raybould HE. Small intestinal capsaicin-sensitive afferents mediate feedback inhibition of gastric emptying in rats. *Am J Physiol* 1994;267:G1142-G1145.
5. Li Y, Owyang C. Pancreatic secretion evoked by cholecystokinin and non-cholecystokinin- dependent duodenal stimuli via vagal afferent fibres in the rat. *J Physiol* 1996;494 (Pt 3):773–782.
6. Lloyd KC, Holzer HH, Zittel TT, Raybould HE. Duodenal lipid inhibits gastric acid secretion by vagal, capsaicin- sensitive afferent pathways in rats. *Am J Physiol* 1993;264:G659-G663.
7. Holzer HH, Turkelson CM, Solomon TE, Raybould HE. Intestinal lipid inhibits gastric emptying via CCK and a vagal capsaicin-sensitive afferent pathway in rats. *Am J Physiol* 1994;267:G625–G629.
8. Raybould HE, Holzer H. Dual capsaicin-sensitive afferent pathways mediate inhibition of gastric emptying in rat induced by intestinal carbohydrate. *Neurosci Lett* 1992;141:236–238.
9. Tso P, Balint JA. Formation and transport of chylomicrons by enterocytes to the lymphatics. *Am J Physiol* 1986;250:G715-G726.
10. McLaughlin J, Grazia LM, Jones MN, D'Amato M, Dockray GJ, Thompson DG. Fatty acid chain length determines cholecystokinin secretion and effect on human gastric motility. *Gastroenterology* 1999;116:46–53.

11. Raybould HE, Meyer JH, Tabrizi Y, Liddle RA, Tso P. Inhibition of gastric emptying in response to intestinal lipid is dependent on chylomicron formation. *Am J Physiol* 1998;274:R1834–R1838.

12. Glatzle J, Kalogeris TJ, Zittel TT, Guerrini S, Tso P, Raybould HE. Chylomicron components mediate intestinal lipid-induced inhibition of gastric motor function. *Am J Physiol Gastrointest Liver Physiol* 2002;282:G86–G91.

13. Hayashi H, Nutting DF, Fujimoto K, Cardelli JA, Black D, Tso P. Transport of lipid and apolipoproteins A-I and A-IV in intestinal lymph of the rat. *J Lipid Res* 1990;31:1613–1625.

14. Kalogeris TJ, Monroe F, Demichele SJ, Tso P. Intestinal synthesis and lymphatic secretion of apolipoprotein A-IV vary with chain length of intestinally infused fatty acids in rats. *J Nutr* 1996;126: 2720–2729.

15. Okumura T, Taylor IL, Fukagawa K, Tso P, Pappas TN. Apolipoprotein A-IV acts centrally in the brain to reduce the severity of gastric ulceration in the rat. *Brain Res* 1995;673:153–156.

16. Okumura T, Fukagawa K, Tso P, Taylor IL, Pappas TN. Intracisternal injection of apolipoprotein A-IV inhibits gastric secretion in pylorus-ligated conscious rats. *Gastroenterology* 1994;107:1861–1864.

17. Buchan AM. Nutrient Tasting and Signaling Mechanisms in the Gut III. Endocrine cell recognition of luminal nutrients. *Am J Physiol* 1999;277:G1103–G1107.

18. Drapanas T, McDonald JC, Stewart JD. Serotonin release following instillation of hypertonic glucose into the proximal intestine. *Ann Surg* 1969;156:528–536.

19. Hillsley K, Kirkup AJ, Grundy D. Direct and indirect actions of 5-hydroxytryptamine on the discharge of mesenteric afferent fibres innervating the rat jejunum. *J Physiol* 1998;506 (Pt 2):551–561.

20. Zhu J, Zhu X, Owyang C, Li Y. Intestinal serotonin acts as a paracrine substance to mediate vagal signal transmission evoked by luminal factors in the rat. *J Physiol* 2001;530:431–442.

21. Levin RJ. Digestion and absorption of carbohydrates—from molecules and membranes to humans. *Am J Clin Nutr* 1994;59:690S–698S.

22. Raybould HE, Zittel TT. Inhibition of gastric motility induced by intestinal glucose in awake rats: role of Na(+)-glucose co-transporter. *Neurogastroenterol Motil* 1995;7:9–14.

23. Kim M, Cooke HJ, Javed NH, Carey HV, Christofi F, Raybould HE. D-Glucose Releases 5-Hydroxytryptamine from Human BON Cells as a Model of Enterochromaffin Cells. *Gastroenterology* 2001;121:1400–1406.

Gut-Brain Peptides in the New Millennium, edited by Y. Taché
CURE Foundation, Los Angeles, CA. © 2002

28

Leptin Improves Rat Gastric Vagal Afferents Responsiveness to CCK Regardless the Change of Circulating CCK Level: An *in vitro* Study

Jen Yu Wei and Yu Hua Wang
*CURE/Digestive Diseases Research Center, UCLA Division of Digestive Diseases
Department of Medicine and VA Greater Los Angeles Healthcare System
Los Angeles, CA*

INTRODUCTION

The binding of a ligand to its receptor to induce the physiological manifestation of an effector is one of the fundamental mechanisms governing the body functions. It has been well documented that, in human plasma, cholecystokinin (CCK) level is elevated about 10 fold post-prandially (1). In rats, the CCK circulating level increases from 0.31 ± 0.5 pmol during fasting to 6.2 ± 1.8 pmol after feeding (2). A report suggests that circulating CCK could aim directly at the brain target and act as a physiological satiety factor (3). The majority of findings, however, is consistent with the notion that the secreted CCK excites gastric vagal afferents (GVA) terminals, whose afferent signal, in turn, reaches central targets controlling the short-term food intake related behavior (4–6). It is generally agreed that the circulating CCK activates GVAs is mediated by CCK-A receptor (7–9). However, how the pre-existing CCK concentration in the interstitial fluid (i.e., the ambient milieu of GVAs terminals) might influence the CCK-sensitivity of the GVAs has not been investigated.

In the *in vitro* isolated stomach-vagus nerve preparation there is no circulating blood. Pre- and post-prandial circulating CCK levels can be precisely mimicked by intra-arterial (ia) injection of appropriate doses of CCK-8. Therefore, the blood-borne interference (10, 11) can be completely prevented. We have recently reported in this *in vitro* preparation that the CCK-sensitivity of GVAs was suppressed when the circulating CCK level was elevated from 0.1 to 10 pmol (9). Consequently, the CCK responsiveness of the GVAs was markedly reduced. This result indicates that vagal afferent signaling depends on the prior state of the terminal microenvironment, i.e., the history of exposure of the GVA to CCK, and most probably, to other ligands as well. In this particular case, ambient CCK can inhibit GVA signaling. However, other evidence suggests that the CCK-responsiveness of GVAs can be maintained under physiological conditions, despite pre-existing CCK (4–6). *Thus there must be a yet unknown mechanism to compensate the inhibitory effect of pre-existing ambient CCK.*

Leptin and CCK are known to influence food intake, however they have, until recently, been considered to act independently via distinct pathways. In contrast to CCK, leptin is an adipocyte-derived circulating hormone, secreted in direct proportion to the degree of adiposity (12, 13). Circulating leptin is currently thought to cross the blood-brain barrier (14) and acts at hypothalamic area to regulate long-term food intake and body weight (15, 16). However, growing evidence indicates that the peripheral effects of leptin on vagus afferent signaling, and specifically the synergistic interactions between peripheral leptin and CCK is taking place at the level of vagal afferent terminals (16).

Four years ago it was unknown whether leptin, like CCK, is capable of activating primary afferent neurons. Our previous report indicates that a population of GVAs did respond to leptin (17). Based on the difference in their initial leptin sensitivity, leptin-responsive GVAs were sub-grouped into two types. Type 1 units demonstrated leptin sensitivity in their "naive" state and their responses to leptin were unaltered following CCK-8 stimulation. In contrast, Type 2 units did not exhibit leptin sensitivity initially at doses to be tested, but did respond to leptin following CCK-8 application. Because the experiment was conducted in the *in vitro* isolated stomach-vagus nerve preparation, the possible involvement of the central nervous system and/or systemic responses was completely eliminated, demonstrating an unequivocally peripherally mediated action. Therefore, we showed that in addition to an effect mediated via the hormonal pathway to the brain, leptin is also capable of acting via a peripheral neuronal pathway at GVAs, and that CCK may interact with leptin to alter vagal afferent signaling.

Our finding has prompted other investigators to study the implications and further aspects of such an interaction, since vagal afferent signaling is known to be important in the regulation of food intake (18–23). Convergent findings indicate that leptin may potentiate the suppressing action of CCK on food intake (18, 20). Current understanding of the synergistic interaction between leptin and CCK has been summarized in a recently published review article (16). Leptin-mediated effect on hepatic and gastric vagal afferent has also been reported by other investigators (22, 23).

These advances have triggered new investigations on the presence of leptin receptors on gastric or hepatic vagal afferent terminals. Recent studies using reverse transcription-polymerase chain reaction, showed mRNAs encoding long (Ob-Rb) and short (Ob-Ra) leptin receptor isoforms in the rat nodose ganglion. Western blot analysis confirmed the presence of leptin receptor-immunoreactive proteins in extracts from the vagus nerve trunk. In addition, immunohistochemistry showed the presence of leptin receptors and leptin induced transcription factor STAT3 in the cytoplasm of nodose ganglion cells (24).

These observations provide neuroanatomical support for the vagus nerve being a site of leptin's peripheral action to influence vagal afferent signaling. Although CCK pretreatment has been shown to increase the sensitivity of type 2 leptin-responsive GVAs, it remains unknown whether leptin pretreatment could have any influence on CCK-responsive GVAs.

In this chapter, we will present an unexpected finding, which may reveal mechanisms by which the CCK sensitivity of GVAs can be improved and optimized regardless of the alterations in the ambient CCK level.

EXPERIMENTAL DESIGN AND METHODS

Preparation and Setup

Experiments were conducted in an *in vitro* isolated stomach preparation. The detailed methods for the preparation, the recording technique, data acquisition and analysis have been described in detail in our previous reports (9, 17).

In brief, the stomach and subdiaphragmatic vagus nerves were removed from overnight fasted urethane anesthetized Sprague-Dawley rats (male 250–300g) and transferred into an organ bath. The bath was perfused with oxygenated Ringer's solution containing D-glucose (9) at a flow rate of 3.0 ± 0.5 ml/min. The left gastric artery was catheterized for intra-arterial (ia) injections of vehicle or reagents. The bath temperature was kept at $33 \pm 1°C$. Unit action potentials were recorded from the distal cut end of ventral gastric vagal nerve filaments via a bipolar recording electrode. A quotient (Q) was used to present the response magnitude (Q = 5-minute spike counts after a treatment / counts before a treatment). Data are presented as means $\pm$ SEM. Statistical significance ($p < 0.05$) was assessed with t-test or ANOVA followed by Dunnett's multiple comparison test. For discrete data (the case numbers) analysis, χ^2 and contingency coefficient were used.

Drugs and Solutions

Modified Ringer's solution was made as previously described (9). Recombinant murine leptin [1 µg/ml in phosphate-buffered saline (PBS), Amgen, Thousand Oaks, CA] and CCK fragment 26–33 sulfated CCK-8 [24 ng/µl (20 pmol/µl) in distilled water; Research Biochemicals, International, Natick, MA] were stored at -70 and $-20°C$, respectively, until used. To prevent nonspecific absorption, the solutions were diluted immediately before use with vehicle: 0.1% fetal bovine serum (Sigma, St. Louis, MO) in PBS, pH

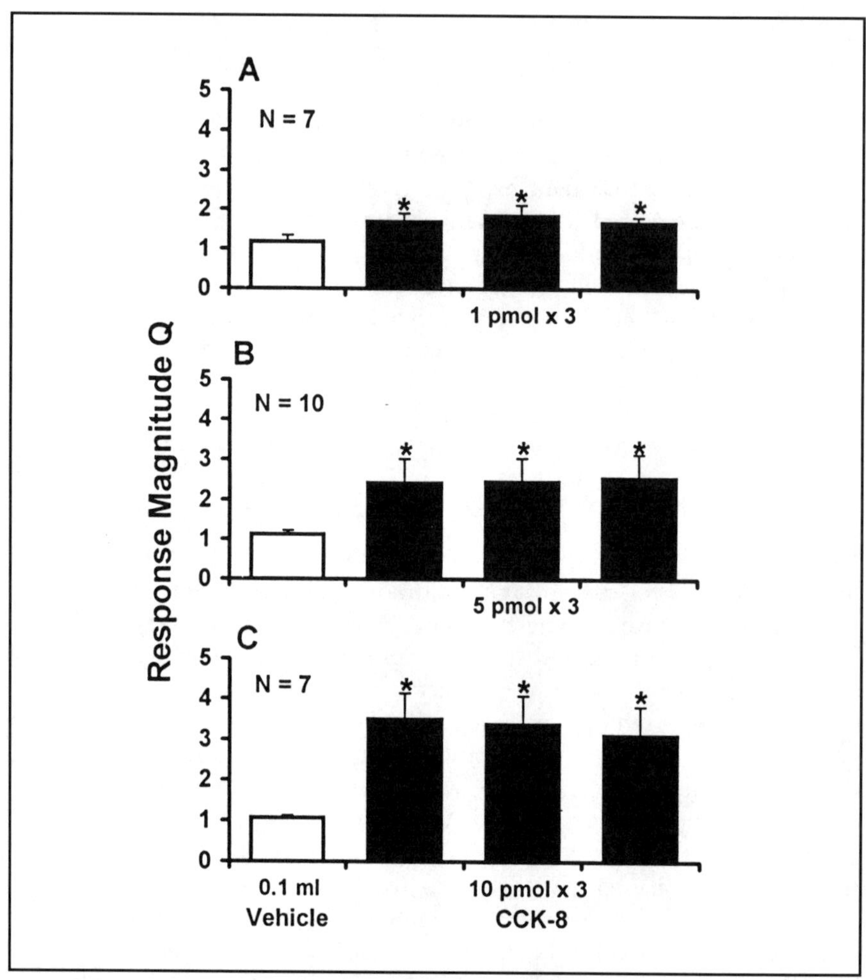

FIGURE 1. *Panel (A) shows the responses of GVAs to ia injections of vehicle and 1 pmol of CCK-8 ×3. The dose was increased to 5 and 10 pmol in Panels (B) and (C). The response to CCK activation is reproducible and dose-dependent, and the response magnitude (Q) to CCK is significantly higher than that to vehicle (p < 0.05, ANOVA, indicated by the asterisks).*

7.4 (GIBCO BRL, Grand island, NY). The appropriate volume of vehicle was given to the control trials.

RESULTS

A total of 64 GVAs were isolated and studied from six separate groups of experiments (3 control and 3 experimental, N = 29).

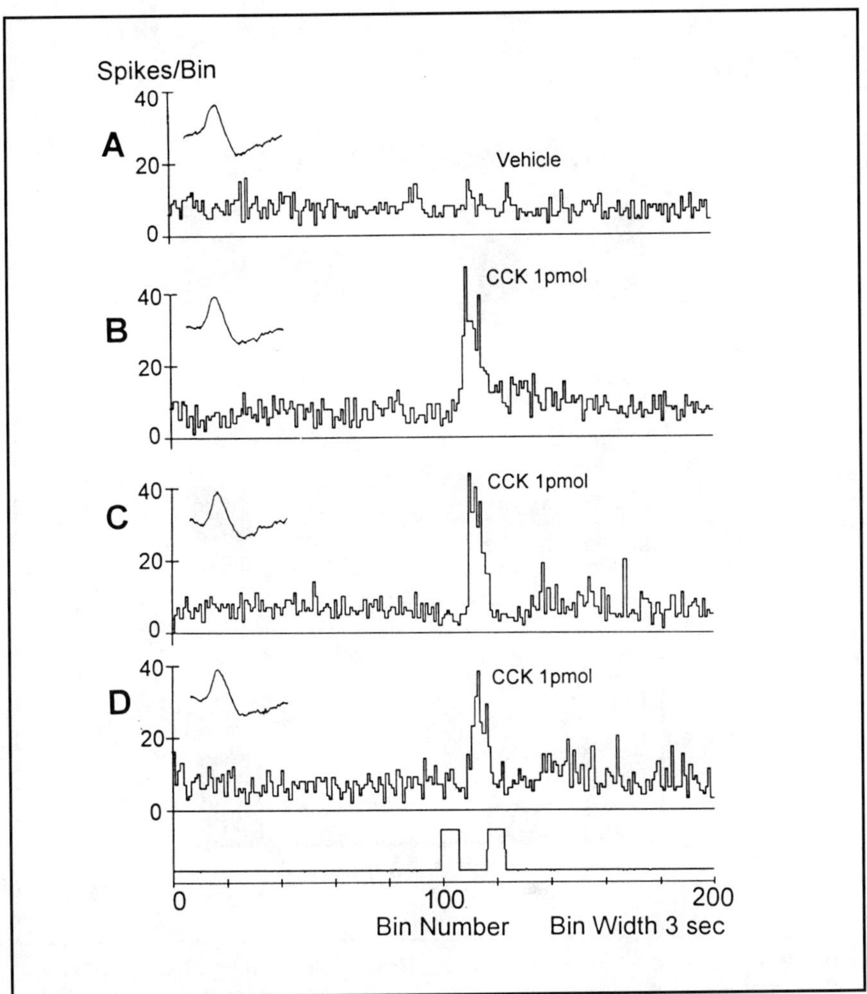

FIGURE 2. *A presentation of spike counts per bin vs bin number histogram to show the response pattern of a GVA fiber in response to ia injection of vehicle (A) and of 3 consecutive injections of 1 pmol of CCK-8 (B–D). The inset shows the waveforms of the unit action potential. The total time span of the waveform trace is 6 msec. The first stimulation mark on the lower trace of (D) indicates the time for the onset and termination of a treatment, the second indicates the time span for flushing the catheter with PBS.*

Figure 1 shows the reproducible response of GVAs to 3 consecutive ia injections of CCK-8 at doses of 1, 5, and 10 pmol in 3 separate control experiments. The GVAs magnitude (Q) response to CCK-8 ia injection was dose–dependent and was significantly higher than that of vehicle. An example of a GVA responding to 3 consecutive ia injections of vehicle and low dose (1 pmol) CCK-8 is illustrated in Figure 2.

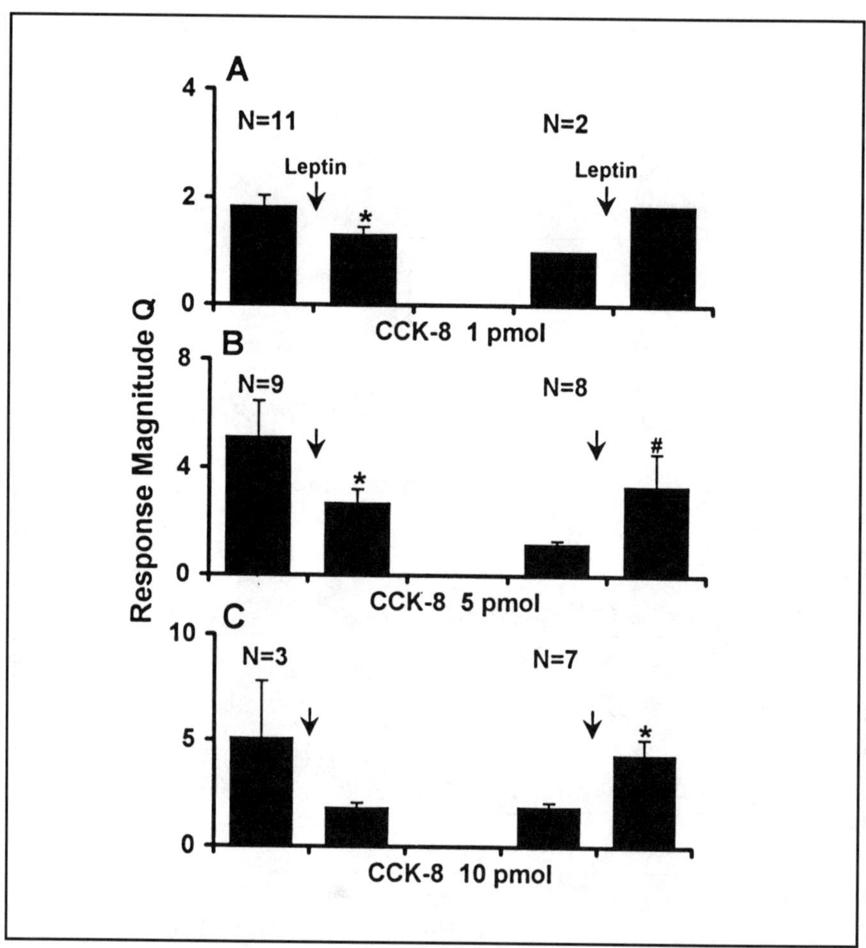

FIGURE 3. *(A) shows the responses of 13 GVAs (from 5 experiments) to ia injections of low dose (1 pmol) CCK-8, before and after leptin (5 μg) pretreatment. Leptin suppressed the CCK responsiveness of 11/13 GVAs from 1.81 ± 0.22 to 1.29 ± 0.16 (means ± SEM, p < 0.05, t-test), whereas enhanced 2/13 from 0.96 to 1.83. In separate 6 experiments, to mimic the post-prandial elevated circulating CCK level, the dose of CCK-8 was increased to 10 pmol (high dose). By contrast, leptin only suppressed 3/10 GVAs from 5.02 ± 2.75 to 1.75 ± 0.28 (p > 0.05), but enhanced 7/10 from 1.80 ± 0.27 to 4.25 ± 0.80 (p < 0.05, (C). The intermediate dose (5 pmol) of CCK-8 was used in additional 5 experiments, leptin suppressed 9/17 GVAs from 5.07 ± 1.39 to 2.66 ± 0.55 (p < 0.05), while enhanced almost equal number (8/17) of GVAs from 1.14 ± 0.17 to 3.31 ± 1.24 (p = 0.056, (B).*

Figure 3 shows the responsiveness of GVAs to low (A), high (C) and intermediate (B) doses of CCK-8 ia injection before vs after leptin pretreatment to illustrate the effect of leptin on the CCK responsiveness of GVAs is a contrasting one. When terminals of GVAs were pre-exposed to and activated by a low dose of CCK-8 (1 pmol), leptin pretreatment tends to suppress the responsiveness of the majority of GVAs (11/13) to a subsequent repeated dose of CCK activation (Figure 3A). In contrast, leptin tends to enhance the CCK responsiveness if a high dose (10 pmol) of CCK-8 was employed (Figure 3C). Figure 3B shows that the suppressing vs enhancing action is almost evenly distributed when the intermediate dose of CCK-8 was used (Figure 3B). The CCK dose and the direction of the contrasting effect were fit into a 3×2 contingency table. It was significantly correlated ($\chi^2 = 7.15$, $p < 0.05$ two-tailed, Contingency Coefficient P = 0.39, n = 40).

DISCUSSION

Our new finding presents an example (with possible broad implication) on how a peptide may exert a contrasting effects on another peptide both being known to influence food intake and body weight. Although the detailed mechanism remains unknown, it seems likely that leptin binding is specific and did not cross-react with CCK (25). However, it is possible that the contrasting effect might be related to two sub-populations of CCK-A receptor with low and high states of affinity (26).

The doses of CCK-8 that we used in the current study are within the range of that reported in the literature (2). For leptin, the doses used for intracerebroventricular (icv) administration are in the a range of 0.35–3.5 µg/per rat (27–28), while for intravenous injections they reached 0.25–1.0 mg/rat (29) or 3 µg/mouse (30). For instance an icv bolus of leptin (0.15 to 36 µg/rat) dose-dependent reduced body weight (31). In our current study, a bolus of 5 µg/0.1 ml leptin solution was injected into the left gastric artery of an *in vitro* isolated rat stomach. Because the total volume of purfusate in the organ bath is 50 ml, the injected leptin will finally be diluted 500-fold. Considering the reported gastric leptin is released in a rapid and large scale in fundic epithelium of rat (32), and biologically active doses in the literature, it seems the dose we used is reasonable.

We have previously reported that acutely elevating the ambient CCK level results in the reduction of CCK sensitivity of GVAs (9). However, convergent evidence indicates the reduction did not occur under physiological conditions. Thus, there must be a yet unknown mechanism to compensate for the suppressing effect.

One of the possible physiological implications of current finding is that leptin may improve the slope of dose-response curve by shifting the low dose portion of the curve to the right, while shifting the high dose portion to the left as represented in Figure 4. Consequently, the direction of leptin's

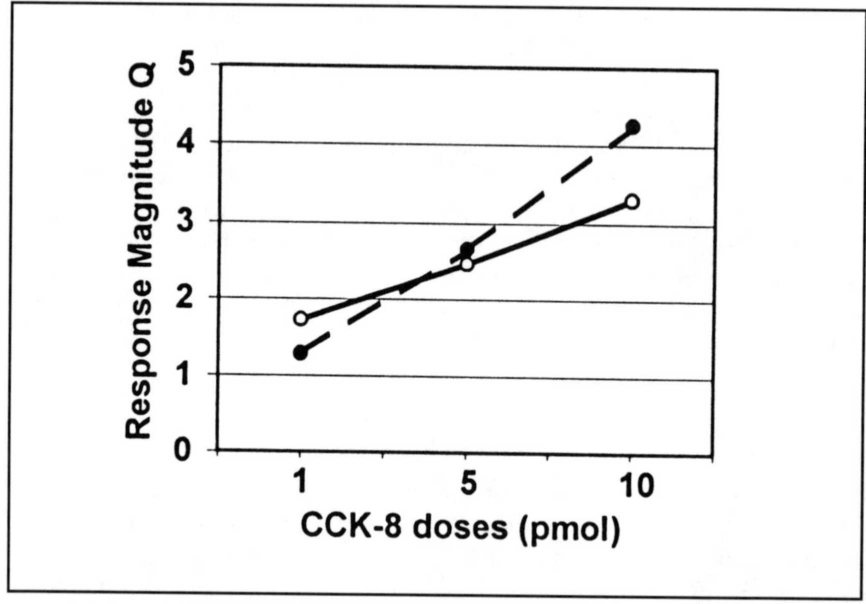

FIGURE 4. *A schematic illustration of the possible implications of current findings. The solid-line with open circuit is the CCK-dose-dependent response curve of GVAs based on the data presented in Figure 1. The broken line with filled circuit is plotted based on the bars (with *) presented in Figure 3. Leptin shifts the low dose portion of the dose-response line to the right and shifts the high dose to the left. Consequently the slope is elevated, i.e., the contrast is increased.*

contrasting effect counteracts the suppressing effect of ambient CCK level. It seems reasonable to speculate that the contrasting effects may be one of undefined mechanisms, which may help to maintain the CCK sensitivity of GVAs regardless of the alterations in the ambient CCK level.

Because gastric leptin (32) and CCK are prandially released, it will be important to assess whether the contrasting effects of leptin may play a role in the regulation of food intake and may be involved in the development of eating disorders, such as anorexia (no appetite) and bulimia (no satiation) nervosa.

ACKNOWLEDGMENTS

We thank Amgen Inc for the generous donation of recombinant mouse leptin. This study was supported by the National Institute of Diabetes and Digestive and Kidney Diseases, Grant DK48476 (JYW) and Central Grant DK-43301 (JH Walsh).

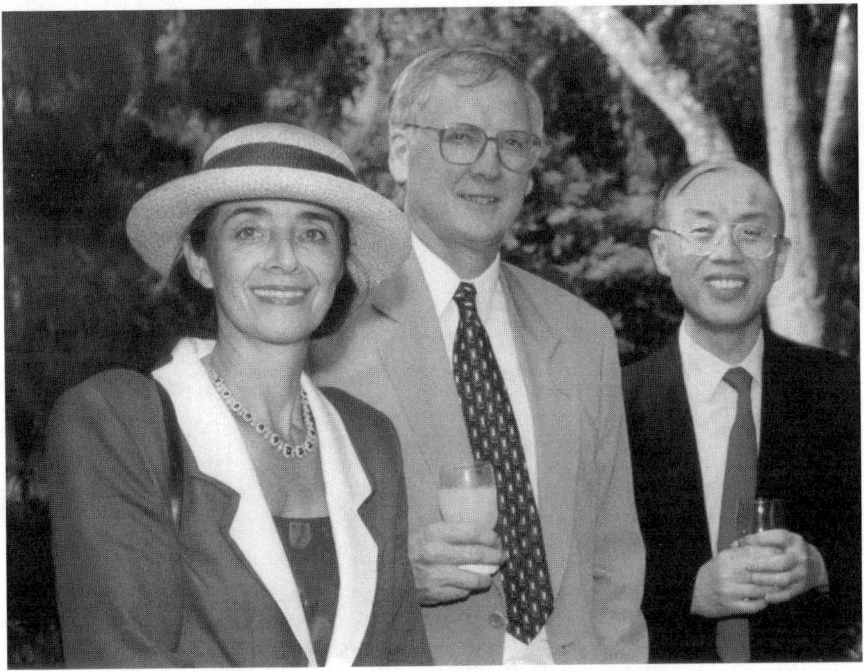

June 25, 1995 at the UCLA Faculty Center, left to right:
Drs. Yvette Taché, John Walsh and Jen Yu Wei.

REFERENCES

1. Liddle RA, Goldfine ID, Rosen MS, Taplitz RA, Williams JA. Cholecystokinin bioactivity in human plasma: molecular forms, responses to feeding, and relationship to gallbladder contraction. *J Clin Invest* 1985;75:1144–52.
2. Liddle RA, Goldfine ID, Williams JA. Bioassay of plasma cholecystokinin in rats: effects of food, trypsin inhibitor, and alcohol. *Gastroenterology* 1984;87:542–9.
3. Baldwin BA, Parrott RF, Ebenezer IS. Food for thought: a critique on the hypothesis that endogenous cholecystokinin act as a physiological satiety factor. *Progress in Neurobiology* 1995;55:477–507.
4. Gibbs J, Smith GP. Cholecystokinin and satiety in rats and rhesus monkeys. *Am J Clin Nutr* 1977;30: 758–61.
5. Gibbs J, Smith GP, Geary N. The brain-gut axis in the regulation of food intake. *The Regulatory Peptide Letter* 1992;4:14–9.
6. Lieverse RJ, Jansen JB, Masclee AM, Lamers CB. Satiety effects of cholecystokinin in Humans. *Gastroenterology* 1994;106:1451–4.
7. Dourish CT, Ruckert AC, Tattersall FD, Iversen SD. Evidence that decreased feeding induced by systemic injection of cholecystokinin is mediated by CCK-A receptors. *Eur J Pharmacol* 1989;173: 233–4.
8. Moran TH, Ameglio PH, Schwartz GJ, McHugh PR. Blockade of type A, not type B, CCK receptors attenuates satiety action of exogenous and endogenous CCK. *Am J Physiol* 1992;262:R46–R50.
9. Wei JY, Wang YH. Effect of CCK pretreatment on the CCK sensitivity of rat polymodal gastric vagal afferent *in vitro. Am J Physiol* (Endocrinol. Metab.) 2000;279:E695–706.
10. Huang SC, Talkad VD, Fortune KP, Jonnalagadda S, Severi C, Fave GD, Gardner JD. Modulation of cholecystokinin activity by albumin. *Proc Natl Acad Sci USA* 1995;92:10312–6.

11. Koulischer D, Moroder L, Deschodt-Lanckman M. Degradation of cholecystokinin octapeptide, related fragments and analogs by human and rat plasma *in vitro*. *Regul Pept* 1982;4:127–39.

12. Loftus TM. An adepocyte-central nervous system regulatory loop in the control of adipose homeostasis. *Semin Cell Dev Biol* 1999;10:11–8.

13. Zhang YY, Proenca R, Maffei M, Barone M, Leopold L, Friedman JM. Positional cloning of the mouse obese gene and its human homologue. *Nature* 1994;372:425–32.

14. Banks WA, Kastin AJ, Huang WT, Jaspan JB, Maness LM. Leptin enters the brain by a saturable system independent of insulin. *Peptides* 1996;17:305–11.

15. Satoh N, Ogawa Y, Katsuura G, Hayase M, Tsuji T, Imagawa K, Yoshimasa Y, Nishi S, Hosoda K, Nakao K. The arcuate nucleus as a primary site of satiety effect of leptin in rats. *Neurosci Lett* 1997;224:149–52.

16. Wang L, Barachina MD, Martines V, Wei JY, Taché Y. Synergistic interaction between CCK and leptin to regulate food intake. *Regul Pept* 2000;92:79–85.

17. Wang YH, Taché Y, Scheibel AB, Go VLW, Wei JY. Two types of leptin-responsive gastric vagal afferent terminals: an *in vitro* single-unit study in rats. *Am J Physiol* 1997;273:R833–7.

18. Barrachina MD, Martinez V, Wang L, Wei JY, Taché Y. Synergistic interaction between leptin and cholecystokinin to reduce short-term food intake in lean mice. *Proc Natl Acad Sci USA* 1997;94:10455–60.

19. Matson CA, Ritter RC. Long-term CCK-Leptin synergy suggests a role for CCK in the regulation of body weight. *Am J Physiol* 1999;276:R1038–1045.

20. Matson CA, Wiater MF, Kuijer JL, Weigle DS. Synergy between leptin and cholecystokinin (CCK) to control daily caloric intake. *Peptides* 1997;18:1275–1278.

21. Barrachina MD, Martines V, Wei JY, Taché Y. Leptin-induced decrease in food intake is not associated with changes in gastric emptying in lean mice. *Am J Physiol* 1997;272:R1007–11.

22. Shiraishi T, Sasaki K, Niijima A, Oomura Y. Leptin effects on feeding-related hypothalamic and peripheral neuronal activities in normal and obese rats. *Nutrition* 1999;15:576–579.

23. Yuan CS, Attele AS, Wu JA, Zhang L, Shi ZQ. Peripheral gastric leptin modulates brain stem neuronal activity in neonates. *Am J Physiol* 1999;277:G626–30.

24. Buyse M, Ovesjo ML, Goiot H, Guilmeau S, Peranzi G, Moiza L, Walker F, Lewin MJM, Meister B, Bado A. Expression and regulation of leptin receptor proteins in afferent and efferent neurons of the vagus nerve. *Euro J Neurosci* 2001;14:64–72.

25. Harris DM, Flannigan KL Go VLW, Wu SV. Regulation of cholecystokinin-mediated amylase secretion by leptin in rat pancreatic acinar tumor cell line AR42J. *Pancreas* 1999:19:224–30.

26. Asin KE, Bednarz L. Differential effects of CCK-JMV-180 on food intake in rats and mice. *Pharmacol Biochem Behav* 1992;42:291–295.

27. Sindelar DK, Havel PJ, Seeley RJ, Wilkinson CW, Woods SC, Schwartz MW. Low plasma leptin levels contribute to diabetic hyperphagia in rats. *Diabetes* 1999;48:1275–80.

28. Van Dijk G, Seeley RJ, Thiele TE, Friedman MI, Wilkinson CW, Burn P, Campfield LA, Tenenbaum R, Baskin DG, et al. Metabolic, gastrointestinal, and CNS neuropeptide effects of brain leptin administration in the rat. *Am J Physiol* 1999;276:R1425–33.

29. Satoh N, Ogawa Y, Katsssssuura G, Numata Y, Tsuji T, Hayase M, Ebihara K, Masuzaki H, Hosoda K, Yoshimasa Y, Nakao K. Sympathetic activation of leptin via ventromedial hypothalamus: leptin-induced increase in catacholamine secretion. *Diabetes* 1999;48:1787–93.

30. Camfield LA, Smith FJ, Guisez Y, Devos R, Burn P. Recombinant mouse OB protein:evidence for a periphral signal linking adiposity and central neural network. *Science* 1995;269:546–9.

31. Cusin I, Rohner-Jeanrenaud F, Stricker-Krongrad A, Jeanrenaud B. The weight-reducing effect of an intracerebroventricular bolus injection of leptin in genetically obese fa/fa rats. *Diabetes* 1996;45:1446–50.

32. Bado A, Levasseur S, Attoub S, Kermorgant S, Laigneau JP, Bortoluzzi MN, Moizo L, Lehy T, Guerre-Millo M, Marchand-Brustel Y, Lewin MJ. The stomach is a source of leptin. *Nature* 1998;390:790–3.

Gut-Brain Peptides in the New Millennium, edited by Y. Taché
CURE Foundation, Los Angeles, CA. © 2002

29

Behavioral Effects of Gastrointestinal Hormones

John E. Morley
*GRECC, VA Medical Center and Division of Geriatric Medicine
Saint Louis University School of Medicine, St. Louis, MO*

INTRODUCTION

It is now well recognized that the majority of the autonomic nervous system carries messages from the periphery to the central nervous system, while only about 20% of the autonomic nervous system actually produces the peripheral effects classically associated with this system. Thus, the autonomic nervous system is a conduit by which alterations in visceral sensations can lead to alterations in the central nervous system function and thus behavior. The behavior in which this role has been best studied is appetite and food ingestion. Alterations in cognition, including delirium, can also be affected by this mechanism.

The majority of the effects of gastrointestinal hormones on behavior are mediated indirectly through stimulation of the ascending fibers in the vagus nerve. In addition, both peptide hormones and cytokines have been demonstrated to cross the blood-brain barrier and produce some of their effects by direct actions on the brain (1). This chapter will discuss the role of gastrointestinal hormones on two behaviors viz. the regulation of food intake and cognition.

THE GUT, THE BRAIN, AND FOOD INTAKE

Historical Aspects

Studies in the 1940s and 1950s showed that lesions and stimulation of the hypothalamus demonstrated an important role of the hypothalamus in the regulation of food intake. Stimulation of the ventromedial hypothalamus leads to decreased food intake and lesions lead to hyperphagia. Opposite effects were seen when these interventions were applied to the lateral hypothalamus. This led to the postulate that within the hypothalamus there was a dual center regulation of feeding (Figure 1). Subsequently, numerous other areas in the brain were demonstrated to alter food intake after they were lesioned or stimulated.

Obviously, the demonstration of the role of the central nervous system in the regulation of food intake led to the question: "What changes within the body are capable of producing signals to the hypothalamus?" The first studies concentrated on the role of nutrients. This led to the discovery that the hypothalamus monitors circulating glucose levels and eats or fasts in order to maintain the circulating levels of glucose constant. This theory is known as the glucostatic theory of Mayer. Body fat stores appeared to be monitored by the circulating levels of free fatty acids. This concept has required revision since the recognition that adipose cells produce leptin, an anorectic peptide. Other nutrients that appear to play a role in the regulation of appetite include amino acids and perrines (Figure 1). Alterations in body temperature also appear capable of modulating food intake.

Cholecystokinin (CCK)

In 1937 Maclagan found that a partially purified preparation from the gastrointestinal tract, known as enterogastrone, reduced feeding when administered peripherally (2). In the 1960s Davis, et al. (3) using cross-perfusion techniques showed that a circulating substance played a role in producing satiation. In 1967, Schally et al. (4) reported that enterogastrone, a substance rich in CCK, inhibited food intake, thus confirming the results from the 1930's. In 1972 Lars Sjoden (5) found that a side effect of CCK was to decrease feeding in dogs. In the following year Gibbs et al. (6) reported that CCK reduced feeding in rats. In 1976 Sturdevant and Goetz (7) showed that CCK both stimulates and inhibits feeding in humans. In the early 1980s, CCK was clearly demonstrated to inhibit feeding in lean and obese humans (8, 9).

Numerous studies have now established that CCK is a true satiety agent (10). CCK antagonists increase feeding (11). CCK produces its effect predominantly by stimulating the ascending fibers of the vagus. Fibers pass from the vagus through the nucleus tractus solitarius to the paraventricular nucleus of the hypothalamus, carrying the satiating signal produced by CCK (12). The effects of CCK on satiation are mediated through the CCK-A receptor (13). The Otsuka Long-Evans Tokushima Fatty (OLETF) rats do not express CCK-A receptors and become obese (14).

While studies in humans have been controversial, on the whole, it appears that CCK decreases food intake (15). CCK appears to be a more effective satiating agent when there is food in the stomach (16). L-phenylalanine increases CCK and decreases food intake in humans (17). CCK does not decrease food intake in vagotomized humans (18). In humans, the CCK-A antagonist, loxiglumide, has minimal effects on food intake after a mixed meal (19). Intraduodenal fat infusion produces satiation (20) which is medi-

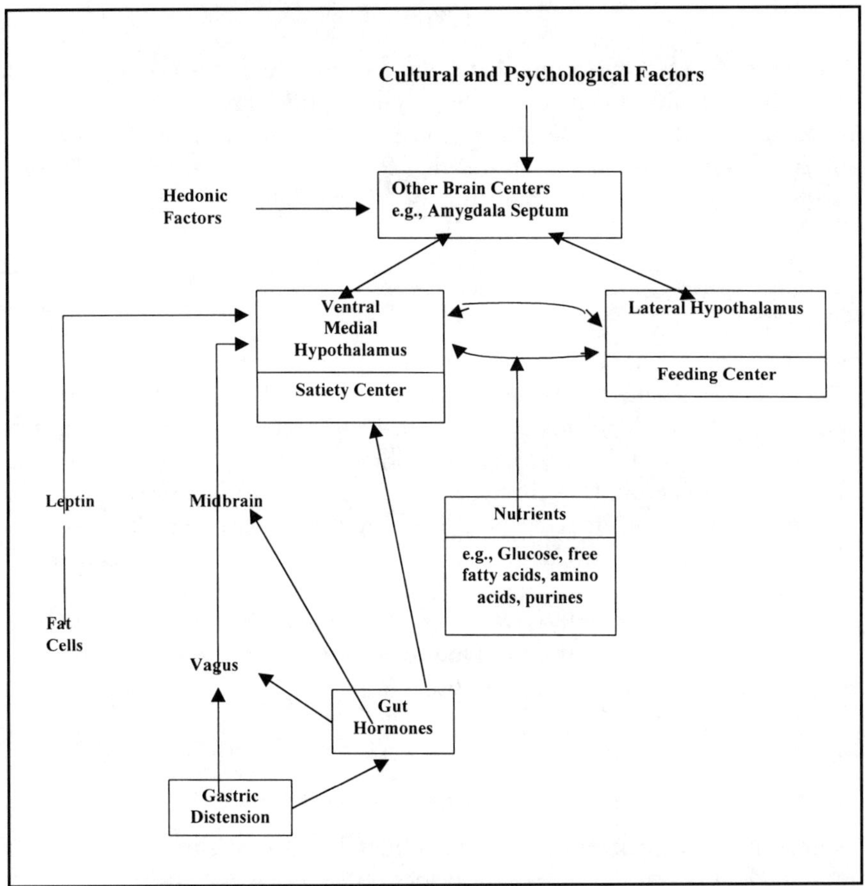

FIGURE 1. *Overview of the mutiple factors involved in the peripheral regulation of food intake.*

ated by long chain, but not short chain, fatty acids and CCK-A receptor, since loxiglumide, reverses the satiating effect of intraduodenal lipid (21).

It is now well established that with aging there is a physiological anorexia (22). There seems to be predominantly mediated through early satiation produced by alterations in the gastrointestinal tract. The predominant effect appears to be a loss of gastric fundal compliance, resulting in more rapid antral filling. Antral stretch then occurs sooner producing early satiation. In addition, older persons have increased levels of circulating CCK, especially in response to intraduodenal fat infusions (23). CCK infusions produce increased satiation in older compared to younger persons (24). This is, in part, due to decreased clearance of CCK with aging. Thus CCK appears to play a role in the pathophysiology of the anorexia of aging.

Ghrelin

Ghrelin is a peptide hormone that is produced in the fundus of the stomach and is structurally similar to motilin, a gut peptide that also increases food intake (25, 26, 27). Both peripheral and central administration of ghrelin result in obesity in rodents by stimulating food intake and decreasing fat oxidation (28). In rodents, the most potent effect of ghrelin on feeding is after direct injection into the arcuate nucleus (29). Ghrelin increases arcuate NPY expression (25). Ghrelin has prokinetic effects on the stomach and decreased gastric vagal afferent activity in rodents (25).

In humans, ghrelin at a dose of 5 pmol/kg/min increased food consumption and increased appetite (26). While having no effect on gastric emptying. Ghrelin levels decline following a meal and increased by 30% following a 12 hour fast (30, 31). As in rodents, in humans the most abundant amounts of ghrelin are found in the stomach (30). Ghrelin levels are elevated in patients with anorexia nervosa (30) and decreased in persons with obesity (32). Pima Indians, a population in which obesity is epidemic, have very low levels of ghrelin. Patients with cardiac cachexia have very high levels of ghrelin which are correlated positively with the elevated levels of tumor necrosis factor alpha.

Ghrelin releases growth hormone (GH) and has been successfully used to treat the anorexia of aging (33). Due to its potent releasing and orexigenic properties, analogs of ghrelin may prove to be excellent candidates to treat the anorexia of aging.

Other Gastrointestinal Hormones

Numerous other gastrointestinal hormones have been shown to decrease food intake in a variety of animal species (10) (Figure 2).

Glucagon-like peptide I (GLP-I) is a peptide hormone produced in the gastrointestinal tract. It is released from the gut in response to a carbohydrate meal. GLP-I stimulates insulin release from the pancreas and is thought to be a major incretin. GLP-I also produced a dose dependent reduction in food and calorie intake in humans with a maximum effect at a dose of 1.5 pmol/kg/min (34). Besides reducing food intake, GLP-I also enhanced satiety and increased fullness (35) and inhibits gastrointestinal motility. Flint et al. (36) found that not only did GLP-I reduce hunger ratings but it also reduced resting metabolic rate, and carbohydrate oxidation and slowed gastric emptying (37). Naslund et al. (38) reported a similar reduction in hunger ratings during GLP-I infusions. In a meta-analysis of the effects of GLP-I (7–36) amide on food intake, Verdich et al. (39) found that 4 of the 7 studies decreased food intake. However when all available data was combined there was a significant reduction of food intake (11.7%) by GLP-1. Lean subjects had a greater decrease in food intake than did obese subjects. Overall, GLP-I

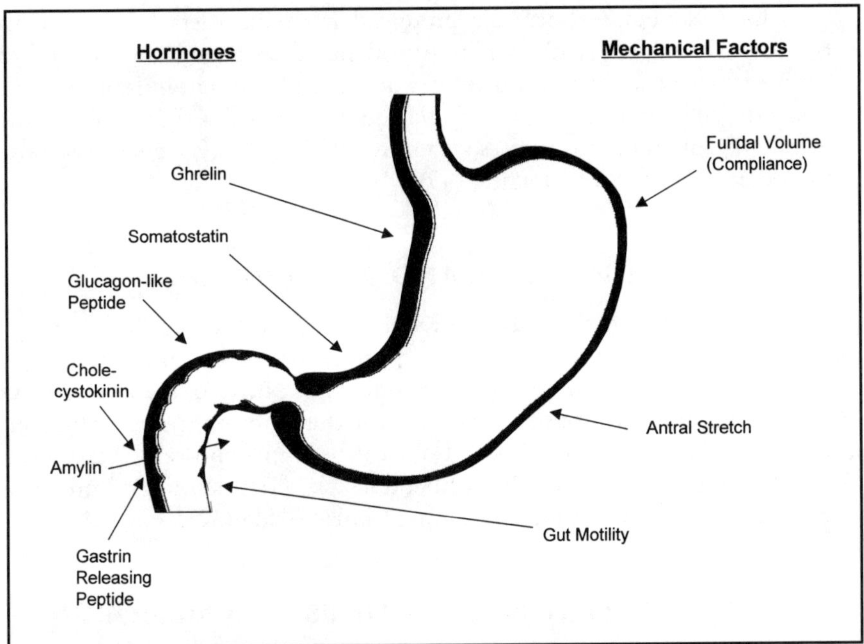

FIGURE 2. *Gastrointestinal factors involved in the regulation of appetite.*

appears to be an important satiating agent in humans. Some of the effect of GLP-I on reducing food intake is related to its ability to slow gastric empty-ing. Recently we have shown that miglitol, an antidiabetic drug, increased GLP-I and this increase was associated with a decrease in food intake. There is no difference in the release of GLP-I between young and older persons, suggesting that GLP-I does not play a role in the anorexia of aging.

Muurahainen et al. (40) showed that the frog skin peptide, bombesin, re-duced food intake in humans. Lieverse et al. (41) reported a similar decrease in food intake with a reduction in the subjective feeling of fullness. This ef-fect was not blocked by the CCK antagonist, loxiglumide. In addition, they could show no effect of bombesin on food intake in obese women (42). Bombesin is more effective at reducing food intake after a preload (43). Gas-trin-releasing peptide, the mammalian analog of bombesin, reduced calorie intake in humans without altering fluid intake. Gastrin releasing peptide produced a reduction in the feeling of hunger and early fullness.

Somatostatin is a peptide that suppresses the release of many gastrointesti-nal hormones and reduces gastrointestinal motility. In rodents somatostatin has a biphasic effect on food intake, both suppressing and increasing food intake (44). This effect is produced through activation of ascending vagal fibers. In humans, somatostatin decreased feelings of hunger (45).

Amylin is a peptide hormone produced from the islets of Langerhans (46). It is co-produced with insulin. In rodents it has been demonstrated to decrease food intake after both central and peripheral administration (47). Pramaltide, an amylin analog, has been shown to reduce weight in obese diabetics (48). Amylin levels increase from middle to old age suggesting a possible role in the anorexia of aging (49).

NITRIC OXIDE AND FOOD INTAKE

Inhibition of nitric oxide leads to a reduction in food intake (50). This appears to include inhibition of the nitric oxide production in the fundus of the stomach as well as in the hypothalamus (51). Nitric oxide release plays an important role in adaptive relaxation of the stomach. Mice with their brain nitric oxide synthase knocked out eat least in response to starvation. There is evidence that a number of peptides viz. NPY, leptin and orexin A produced their effects on feeding through nitric oxide (52).

GASTROINTESTINAL PEPTIDES AND MEMORY

When mice are fed immediately following training in an aversive T-maze, they remember the task better than when access to food is delayed (53). Similarly in humans feeding improves short-term memory (54).

We hypothesized that this effect of food on memory was mediated by gastrointestinal hormones. We then demonstrated that CCK-octapeptide increased memory retention when administered intraperitoneally (53). This effect was more potent when CCK was administered intraperitoneally compared to subcutaneously suggesting that the effect is produced within the abdominal cavity. CCK-8 reversed the amnesia produced by the anticholinergic drug, scopolamine, and by the protein synthesis inhibitor, anisomycin. The CCK-A receptor antagonist, L-364,718, was shown to attenuate then enhanced memory associated with a meal (55).

Stimulation of the vagus produces an increase of electrical activity in the central nucleus of the amygdala (56). CCK receptors are present in the nucleus tractus solitarius (57). The amygdala is a central area involved in the laying down of memories (58). We thus, hypothesized that CCK produced its memory enhancing effects by stimulating the vagus which activates fibers in the nucleus tractus solitarius which pass to the amygdala. We then showed that the CCK effects on memory were blocked by vagotomy (53). Beta-endorphin an endogenous opioid, is a potent amnestic agent. When beta-endorphin was administered directly into the amygdala, it blocked the memory enhancing effects of peripherally administered CCK (59). The stria-terminalis carries fibers coursing to the amygdala. A knife cut through

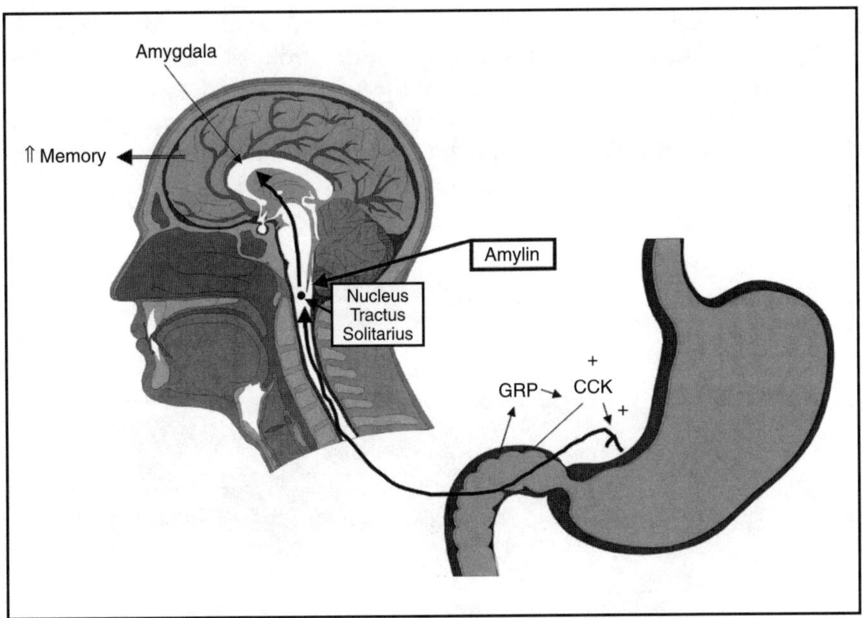

FIGURE 3. *Effects of gut peptides on memory CCK = Cholecystokinin; GRP = Gastrin Releasing Peptide.*

the stria terminalis abolished the ability of peripherally administered CCK to enhance memory (60).

A number of other gastrointestinal hormones have also been shown to modulate memory. These include bombesin and gastrin releasing peptide (61). The bombesin effect on memory was an inhibited by a CCK-A antagonist suggesting that its effects on memory are mediated through CCK release. Pancreastatin enhanced memory in time-dependent manner (61). Amylin also enhances memory after peripheral administration (62). Amylin is amnestic when administered directly into the central nervous system.

These studies confirm that the enhanced memory related to food ingestion occurs secondarily to the release of gastropancreatic hormones. CCK produces its memory enhancing effects by stimulating ascending vagal fibers which carry the message to the nucleus tractus solitarius and from there fibers course through the stria terminalis to the amygdala (Figure 3).

CONCLUSION

This brief overview demonstrates the importance of gastrointestinal hormones in the short-term regulation of satiation in humans. CCK appears to play an important role in the pathogenesis of the early satiation seen in many older persons. In addition, there is emerging evidence that gastrointestinal hormones play an important role in the modulation of memory.

I knew John when I was an Endocrine fellow at UCLA. John was extremely helpful to me early in my career and we collaborated on a number of studies involving the development of gut peptide radioimmunoassays. John was a wonderful person and an intellectual giant.

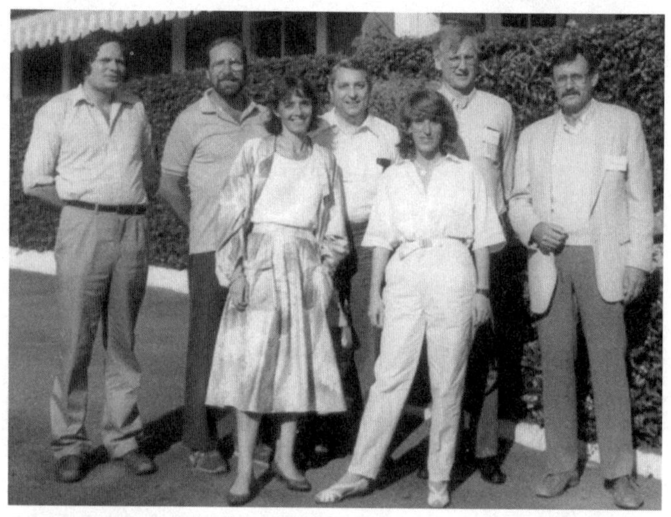

Back row (from left): John Morley, M. Barry Sterman, Carmine Clemente, John Walsh, Donald Novin. Front row (from left): Yvette Taché and Joyce M. Fried.

REFERENCES

1. Kastin AJ, Pan W, Maness LM, Banks WA. Peptides crossing the blood-brain barrier: some unusual observations. *Brain Research* 1999;848:96–100.
2. Morley JE. Neuropeptide regulation of appetite and weight. *Endocrine Reviews* 1987;8:256–287.
3. Silver AJ, Flood JF, Song AM, Morley JE. Evidence for a physiological role for CCK in the regulation of food intake in mice. *Am J Physiol* 1989;256:R646–652.
4. Morley JE, Levine AS, Bartness TJ, Nizielski SE, Shaw MJ, Hughes JJ. Species differences in the response to cholecystokinin. *Ann New York Acad Sci* 1985;448:413–416.
5. Morley JE. Anorexia of aging: physiologic and patholic. *Am J Clin Nutr* 1997;66:760–773
6. MacIntosh CG, Andrews JM, Jones KL, Wishart JM, Morris HA, Jansen JB, Morley JE, Horowitz M, Chapman IM. Effects of age on concentrations of plasma cholecystokinin, glucagons-like peptide 1, and peptide YY and their relation to appetite and pyloric motility. *Am J Clin Nutr* 1999;69:999–1006.
7. Sturdevant R, Goetz H. Cholecystokinin both stimulates and inhibits human food intake. *Nature (Lond)* 1976;261:713–715.
8. Kissileff HR, Pi-Sunyer FX, Thornton J, Smith GP. C-terminal octapeptide of cholecystokinin decreases food intake in man. *Am J Clin Nutr* 1981;34:154–160.
9. Pi-Sunyer FX, Kissilef HR, Thornton J, Smith GP. C-terminal octapeptide of cholecystokinin decreases food intake in man. *Am J Clin Nutr* 1981;34:154–160.
10. Silver AJ, Morley JE. Role of CCK in regulation of food intake. *Progress in Neurobiology* 1991;36:23–34.
11. Silver AJ, Flood JF, Song Am, Morley JE. Evidence for a physiological role for CCK in the regulation of food intake in mice. *Am J Physiol* 1989;256:R646–652.
12. Broberger C, Hokfelt T. Hypothalamic and vagal neuropeptide circuitries regulating food intake. *Physiol and Behav* 2001;74:669–682.
13. Patterson LM, Zheng HY, Berthoud HR. Vagal afferents innervating the gastrointestinal tract and CCKA-receptor immunoreactivity. *Anatomical Record* 2002;266:10–20.
14. Covasa M, Ritter RL. Attenuated satiation response to intestinal nutrients in rats that do not express CCK-A receptors. *Peptides* 2001;22:1339–1348.
15. Degen L, Matzinger D, Drewe J, Beglinger C. The effect of cholecystokinin in controlling appetite and food intake in humans. *Peptides* 2001;22:1265–1269.
16. Muurahainen NE, Kissileff HR, Lachaussee J, Pi-Sunyer FX. Effect of a soup preload on reduction of food intake by cholecystokinin in humans. *Am J Physiol* 1991;260:R672–680.
17. Ballinger AB, Clark ML. L-phenylalanine releases cholecystokinin (CCK) and is associated with reduced food intake in humans: evidence for a physiological role of CCK in control of eating. *Metabolism:Clinical and Experimental* 1994;43:735–738.
18. Morley JE, Levine AS, Bartness TJ, Nizielski SE, Shaw MJ, Hughes JJ. Species differences in the response to cholecystokinin. *Ann New York Academy of Sciences* 1985;448:413–416.
19. French SJ, Bergin A, Sepple CP, Read NW, Rovati L. The effects of loxiglumide on food intake in normal weight volunteers. *Int J Obesity and Related Metab Disorders* 1994;18:738–741.
20. Matzinger D, Degen L, Drewe J, Meuli J, Duebendorfer R, Ruckstuhl N, D'Amato M, Rovati L, Beglinger C. The role of long chain fatty acids in regulating food intake and cholecystokinin release in humans. *Gut* 2000;46:688–693.
21. Gutzwiller JP, Drewe J, Ketterer S, Hildbrand P, Krautheim A, Beglinger C. Interaction between CCK and a preload on reduction of food intake is mediated by CCK-A receptors in humans. *Am J Physiol-Reg Integr and Compar Physiol* 2000;279:R189–195.
22. Morley JE. Anorexia of aging: physiologic and patholic. *Am J Clin Nutr* 1997;66:760–773.
23. MacIntosh CG, Andrews JM, Jones KL, Wishart JM, Morris HA, Jansen JB, Morley JE, Horowitz M, Chapman IM. Effects of age on concentrations of plasma cholecystokinin, glucagons-like peptide 1, and peptide YY and their relation to appetite and pyloric motility. *Am J Clin Nutr* 1999;69:999–1006.
24. MacIntosh CG, Morley JE, Wishart J, Morris H, Jansen JBMJ, Horowitz M, Chapman IM. Effect of exogenous cholecystokinin (CCK)-8 on food intake and plasma CCK, leptin, and insulin concentrations in older and young adults: Evidence for increased CCK activity as a cause of the anorexia of aging. *J Clin Endocrin and Metab* 2001;86:5830–5837.

25. Asakawa A, Inui A, Kaga T, Yuzuriha H, Nagata T, Ueno N, Makino S, Fujimiya M, Niijima A, Fujino MA, Kasuga M. Ghrelin is an appetite-stimulatory signal from stomach with structural resemblance to motilin. *Gastroenterology* 2001;120:337–345.

26. Wren AM, Seal LJ, Cohen MA, Brynes AE, Frost GS, Murphy KG, Dhillo WS, Ghatei MA, Bloom SR. Ghrelin enhances appetite and increases food intake in humans. *J Clin Endocrin and Metab* 2001; 86:5992–5995.

27. Asakawa A, Inui A, Momose K, Ueno N, Fujino MA, Kasuga M. Motilin increases food intake in mice. *Peptides* 1998;19:987–990.

28. Ravussin E, Tschop M, Morales S, Bouchard C, Heiman ML. Plasma ghrelin concentration and energy balance: overfeeding and negative energy balance studies in twins. *J Clin Endocrin and Metab* 2001; 86:4547–4551.

29. Wren AM, Small CJ, Abbott CR, Dhillo WS, Seal LJ, Cohen MA, Batterham RL, Taheri S, Stanley SA, Ghatei MA, Bloom SR. Ghrelin causes hyperphagia and obesity in rats. *Diabetes* 2001;50:2540–2547.

30. Ariyasu H, Takaya K, Tagami T, Ogawa Y, Hosoda K, Akamizu T, Suda M, Koh T, Natsui K, Troyooka S, Shirakami G, Usui T, Simatsu A, Doi K, Hosoda H, Kojima M, Kangawa K, Nakao K. Stomach is a major source of circulating ghrelin, and feeding state determines plasma ghrelin-like immunoreactivity levels in humans. *J Clin Endocrin and Metab* 2001;86:4753–4758.

31. Otto B, Cuntz U, Fruehauf E, Wawarta R, Folwaczny C, Riepl RL, Heiman ML, Lehnert P, Fichter M, Tschop M. Weight gain decreases elevated plasma ghrelin concentrations of patients with anorexia nervosa. *Euro J Endocrin* 2001;145:R5–R9.

32. Tschop M, Weyer C, Tataranni PA, Devanarayan V, Ravussin E, Heiman ML. Circulating ghrelin levels are decreased in human obesity. *Diabetes* 2001;50:707–709.

33. Kaiser FE, Silver Aj, Morley JE. The effect of recombinant human growth hormone on malnourished older individuals. *J Am Geriat Soc* 1991;39:235–240.

34. Gutzwiller JP, Goke B, Drewe J, Hildebrand P, Ketterer S, Handschin D, Winterhalder R, Conen D, Beglinger C. Glucagon-like peptide-1: a potent regulator of food intake in humans. *Gut* 1999;44: 81–86.

35. Gutzwiller JP, Drewe J, Goke B, Schmidt H, Rohrer B, Lareida J, Beglinger C. Glucagon-like peptide-1 promotes satiety and reduces food intake in patients with diabetes mellitus type 2. *Am J Physiol* 1999;276:R1541–1544.

36. Naslund E, Barkeling B, King N, Gutniak M, Blundell JE, Holst JJ, Rossner S, Hellstom PM. Energy intake and appetite are suppressed by glucagons-like peptide-1 (GLP-1) in obese men. *Int J Obesity and Related Metabolic Disorders* 1999;23:304–311.

37. Flint A, Raben A, Ersboll AK, Holst JJ, Astrup A. The effect of physiological levels of glucagons-like peptide-1 on appetite, gastric emptying, energy and substrate metabolism in obesity. *Int J Obesity* 2001; 25:781–792.

38. Naslund E, Gutniak M, Skogar S, Rosssner S, Hellstrom PM. Glucagon-like peptide 1 increases the period of postprandial satiety and slows gastric emptying in obese men. *Am J Clin Nutr* 1998;68: 525–530.

39. Verdich C, Flint A, Gutzwiller JP, Naslund E, Beglinger C, Hellstrom PM, Long SJ, Morgan LM, Holst JJ, Astrup A. A meta-analysis of the effect of glucagons-like peptide-1 (7-36) amide on ad libitum energy intake in humans. *J Clin Endocrin and Metab* 2001;86:4382–4389.

40. Muurahainen NE, Kissileff HR, Pi-Sunyer FX. Intravenous infusion of bombesin reduces food intake in humans. *Am J Physiol* 1993;264:R350–354.

41. Lieverse RJ, Jansen JB, van de Zwan A, Samson L, Masclee AA, Rovati LC, Lamers CB. Bombesin reduces food intake in lean man by a cholecystokin-independent mechanism. *J Clin Endocrin and Metab* 1993;76:1495–1498.

42. Lieverse RJ, Jansen JB, Masclee AA, Lamers CB. Significant satiety effect of bombesin in lean but not in obese subjects. *Int J Obesity and Related Metabolic Disorders* 1994;18:579–583.

43. Gutzwiller JP, Drewe J, Hildebrand P, Rossi L, Lauper JZ, Beglinger C. Effect of intravenous human gastrin-releasing peptide on food intake in humans. *Gastroenterology* 1994;106:1168–1173.

44. Levine AS, Morley JE. Peripherally administered somatostatin reduces feeding by a vagal mediated mechanism. *Pharmacology, Biochemistry and Behavior* 1982;16:897–902.

45. Lieverse RJ, Jansen JB, Masclee AM, Lamers CB. Effects of somatostain on human satiety. *Neuroendocrinology* 1995;61:112–116.

46. Morley JE, Suarez MD, Mattamal M, Flood JF. Amylin and food intake in mice: effects on motivation to eat and mechanism of action. *Pharmacol Biochem and Behav* 1997;56:123–129.

47. Morley JE, Flood JF, Horowitz M, Morley PM, Walter MJ. Modulation of food intake by peripherally administered amylin. *Am J Physiol* 1994;267:R178–184.

48. Weyer C, Maggs DG, Young AA, Kolterman OG. Amylin replacement with pramlintide as an adjunct to insulin therapy in type 1 and type 2 diabetes mellitus: a physiological approach toward improved metabolic control. *Current Pharmaceutical Design* 2001;7:1353–1373.

49. Edwards BJ, Perry HM, Kaiser FE, Morley JE, Kraenzle D, Kreutter DK, Stevenson RW. Age-related changes in amylin secretion. *Mech Aging and Develop* 1996;86:39–51.

50. Morley JE, Mattammal MB. Nitric oxide synthase levels in obese Zucker rats. *Neuroscience Letters* 1996;209:137–139.

51. Morley JE, Kumar VB, Mattammal MB, Farr S, Morley PM, Flood JF. Inhibition of feeding by a nitric oxide synthase inhibitor: effects of aging. *Euro J Pharmacol* 1996;311:15–19.

52. Morley JE, Alshaher MM, Farr SA, Flood JF, Kumar VB. Leptin and neuropeptide Y (NPY) modulate nitric oxide synthase: further evidence for a role of nitric oxide in feeding. *Peptides* 1999;20:595–600.

53. Flood JF, Smith GE, Morley JE. Modulation of memory processing by cholecystokinin on the vagus nerve. *Science* 1987;236:832–834.

54. Kaplan RJ, Greenwood CE, Winocur G, Wolever TM. Dietary protein, carbohydrate, and fat enhance memory performance in the healthy elderly. *Am J Clin Nutr* 2001;74:687–693.

55. Flood JF, Morley JE. Cholecystokinin receptors mediate enhanced memory retention by feeding and gastrointestinal peptides. *Peptides* 1989;10:809–813.

56. Dell P, Olson R. Projections thalamiques corticules et cerebelleuses des afferences visceralls vagales. *CR Soc Biol (Paris)* 1951;145:1084–1088.

57. Zarbin MA, Wamsley JK, Innis RB. Cholecystokinin receptors: presence and axonal flow in rat vagus nerve. *Life Sci* 1981;29:697–701.

58. Introini-Collison IB, McGaugh JL. Interaction of hormones and neurotransmitter systems in the modulation of memory storage. In: *Peripheral Signaling of the Brain.* Frederickson RCA, McGaugh JL, Felten DL (Ed.), Hoegrefe and Haber, Toronto, 275–302, 1991.

59. Flood JF, Garland JS, Morley JE. Evidence that cholecystokinin-enhanced retention is mediated by changes in opioid activity in the amygdala. *Brain Research* 1992;585:94–104.

60. Flood JF, Merbaum MO, Morley JE. The memory enhancing effects of cholecystokinin octapeptide are dependent on an intact stria terminalis. *Neurobiol of Learning and Memory* 1995;64:139–145.

61. Flood JF, Morley JE. Effects of bombesin and gastrin-releasing peptide on memory processing. *Brain Research* 1988;460:314–322.

62. Morley JE, Flood JF, Farr SA, Perry HJ III, Kaiser FE, Morley PM. Effects of amylin on appetite regulation and memory. *Can J Physiol and Pharmacol* 1995;73:1043–1046.

Gut-Brain Peptides in the New Millennium, edited by Y. Taché
CURE Foundation, Los Angeles, CA. © 2002

30

Enhanced Efficiency of Nutrient Absorption May Play a Role in Obesity: Role of Peptide YY

Ian L. Taylor
Tulane University School of Medicine
New Orleans, LA

James Croom
Department of Poultry Science
North Carolina State University

INTRODUCTION

I first met John Walsh when he visited Rod Gregory and Graham Dockray in the Physiology Laboratories at Liverpool University's School of Medicine. I'd been working on a G17 specific radioimmunoassay in Liverpool after which I was invited out to join John and Mort Grossman in Los Angeles. I remember the day John picked me up from LAX. It was sunny and warm in sharp contrast to the cold and dampness that characterized a Liverpool summer. I started to work on the Pancreatic Polypeptide (PP) family after I arrived at CURE. John played a key role in my career and was coauthor on the initial papers examining the mechanisms of release of PP. He played a particularly important role in the early studies on the role of the vagal-cholinergic system in PP release. In addition he was a coauthor on the studies to examine the biological effects of PP on the stomach and pancreas. I will always remember John as one of the brightest people I have ever known; he was always full of novel ideas. He was also a great friend and it is this special friendship that I will miss most of all. Gastroenterology has sadly lost one of the truly innovative thinkers and one of the very best mentors of young scientists.

A goal of limiting the prevalence of overweight US adults to no more than 20% was set in *Healthy People 2000*. Unfortunately, while 26% of adults were overweight in the 1980's, one third of US citizens were categorized (1) as overweight in the 1990's and over 50% will be overweight in this decade. The incidence of obesity is increasing at an alarming rate, particularly in adolescents and certain minority populations, a trend that has obvious implications for the future of health care in this country.

The ultimate cause of obesity is the over consumption of calories in relationship to physiological need (2). The specific physiological variables associated with the development of obesity can be partitioned into two separate, but highly integrated, systems. The first are those associated with satiety and include both central and peripheral neurohormonal elements. The second involves the efficiency with which nutrients are absorbed from the gastrointestinal tract and then metabolized by the body. The following is a brief consideration of the role that regulation of intestinal absorption plays in the development of obesity.

ENERGETIC COSTS OF ABSORPTION: IMPACT ON GROWTH AND BODY COMPOSITION

One variable that has received little attention is how the energetic costs of absorptive function impact on body weight and composition (3). We have developed (4) a scalar for estimating changes in the energetic efficiency of nutrient uptake in the intestinal mucosa termed "Apparent Energy Efficiency" of absorption (the ratio of ATP expended [ηmol min- mg intestinal tissue] to intestinal glucose uptake [ηmol min- mg intestinal tissue]). The intestinal tract accounts for approximately 17–20% of whole body gross energy expenditure in ruminants and domestic animals (5). Cant, et al. (3) used a mathematical model to demonstrate that the energy demands of the gastrointestinal tract dictate the overall efficiency of growth and an optimum for growth efficiency was reached when the gastrointestinal tract accounted for 15–20% of whole animal energy use. A significant proportion (29–62%) of the energy demands of the gastrointestinal (GI) tract are associated with Na^+, K^+-ATPase which maintains the electrochemical gradient essential for the functioning of a variety of Na^+-dependent cotransporters of glucose and amino acids. Any improvement in the energetic efficiency of nutrient absorption is likely to have significant effects on body weight.

Diamond (6) had proposed that the absorptive capacity of the small intestine is tied to the needs of the body as a whole which is an extension of the concept of "symmorphosis" first proposed by Taylor and Weibel in 1981 (7) in regards to the respiratory system. This theory was based on the assumption (7) that "animals are built reasonably—no more structure is formed and maintained than is required to satisfy functional needs." In contrast, other studies (8, 9, 10) suggest that upregulation of intestinal absorptive capacity may be necessary to sustain maximum growth or performance in some species of domestic animals genetically selected for enhanced growth. In an extension of these concepts we have proposed that the intestine is able to adapt during periods of real or perceived nutrient stress to increase the energetic efficiency of nutrient absorption, significantly impacting body mass and composition.

The following example serves to show how small changes in gut energetic efficiency can have profound effects on long-term energy balance and body weight. If we assume that a 40 year-old non–obese person requires 2000 calories (C) per day to maintain their body weight, approximately 400 C, or 20% of these calories are partitioned to maintain the GI. If the intestinal Na^+, K^+-ATPase, which is essential for glucose and amino acid absorption, accounts for 60% of the energy expended in the GI tract, then this would equal 240 C or 12% of whole body energy. If we maintained the daily calorie intake at 2000 C and increased the efficiency of glucose and amino acid transport by 10% that would mean that the energy exenditure to maintain the gastrointestinal ATPase function would drop by 43 calories per day. These calories would be partitioned to fat synthesis at the rate of 4.8 g per day. This would result in the deposition of 1.7 kg or 3.9 lbs of body fat per year. If this person did not change their dietary status, activity and remained in good health, this would result in a gain of 39 pounds of extra body fat over the next decade.

PEPTIDE YY: MECHANISM OF ACTION
AND THE ILEAL BRAKE

The western "supermarket diet" is characterized by large volume, calorically dense meals (11). High carbohydrate, high fat meals are associated with the release of an ileocolonic hormone (12–15) peptide YY (PYY), which we have proposed as one of the mediators of the "ileal brake" (12, 13). The term "ileal brake" was coined to describe a phenomenon whereby perfusion of the ileum and colon with fat slows intestinal transit and delays gastric emptying (16). Undefined hormonal signals originating from the ileum and/or colon were originally proposed as mediators of the brake (16) which is engaged when nutrients pass beyond the absorptive surface of the intestine. PYY is released into the systemic circulation from endocrine cells in the ileum and colon (17, 18) and delays the rate of delivery of food to an already overburdened small intestine by slowing gastric emptying and intestinal transit. Additionally, PYY has been shown to enhance intestinal epithelial cell growth *in vitro* (19) and *in vivo* in total parenteral nutrition fed mice (20). This would lead to an increase in mucosal cell mass which coupled with the increased nutrient mucosal contact time would lead to increased nutrient digestion and absorption. This would be compatible with the statement of Hallden and Aponte (21) that "PYY seems to modify digestive processes to ensure efficient utilization of ingested food."

Peptide YY exerts its effects on gastric and intestinal function by decreasing vagal-cholinergic output to the gastrointestinal tract (22–25). Peptide YY receptors have been demonstrated in the vagal nuclear complex (DVC) of the brain of the rat (22, 23). *In vivo* radio-receptor studies with labeled PYY have extended these observations by demonstrating that circulating PYY binds to receptors in the DVC (22). *In vitro* radio-receptor studies (22) demonstrate PYY binding sites in the area postrema (AP), the nucleus tractus solitarius (NTS) and the dorsal motor nucleus of the vagus (DMNV). The AP and NTS are circumventricular organs which are discrete regions of the brain characterized by the presence of fenestrated capillaries. Most capillary beds in the brain are non-fenestrated and serve as a "blood-brain" barrier limiting access of circulating peptide hormones to brain tissue. Circumventricular organs allow the passage of peptides across the blood-brain barrier thus limiting access of these hormones to specific regions of the brain in this case the vagal nuclear complex (26). PYY has been shown to act directly on the DVC, to suppress gastric motility (27) and PYY's inhibitory effects on the stomach have been shown to be vagal-cholinergic dependent (24). Injection of PYY into the circulation or directly into the DVC alters electrical activity in the DVC (25) which is in keeping with a direct effect of PYY on the vagus.

PYY is copackaged with glicentin in the L-cell and both peptides are secreted by this cell (28, 29). Glicentin exerts trophic effects on the rat small intestine and has been postulated to be involved in the ileal brake phenomenon (29). The simultaneous release of both PYY and glicentin would result in both increased nutrient absorption and intestinal growth. This combined effect, while beneficial in the face of nutrient malabsorption, would be detrimental when eating large volume, high fat, high carbohydrate meals.

PEPTIDE YY AND THE ILEAL BRAKE: AN ETIOLOGICAL CONNECTION TO OBESITY

Although the ileal brake may have evolved as a compensatory mechanism in response to malabsorption or episodic nutrient deficiency followed by excess, it may now be playing a detrimental role in the etiology of obesity in developed countries. Recent studies (30, 31, 32) have established that PYY enhances the absorption of water, electrolytes, glucose and lipids. Bilchik, et al. (30) reported that intravenous infusion of PYY stimulates absorption of water and electrolytes in dogs. We have demonstrated that PYY treatment in mice increases jejunal glucose absorption without concomitant increases in tissue respiration (31). Figure 1 demonstrates the effects of PYY treatment [300 µg/kg/day] for 3 days on the apparent energetic efficiency of jejunal active glucose uptake in two month old Swiss-Webster mice. Glucose uptake was increased in those animals but the amount of ATP expended per ηmol glucose uptake was reduced (Figure 1). These data indicate that PYY treatment increases the energetic efficiency of active intestinal glucose transport.

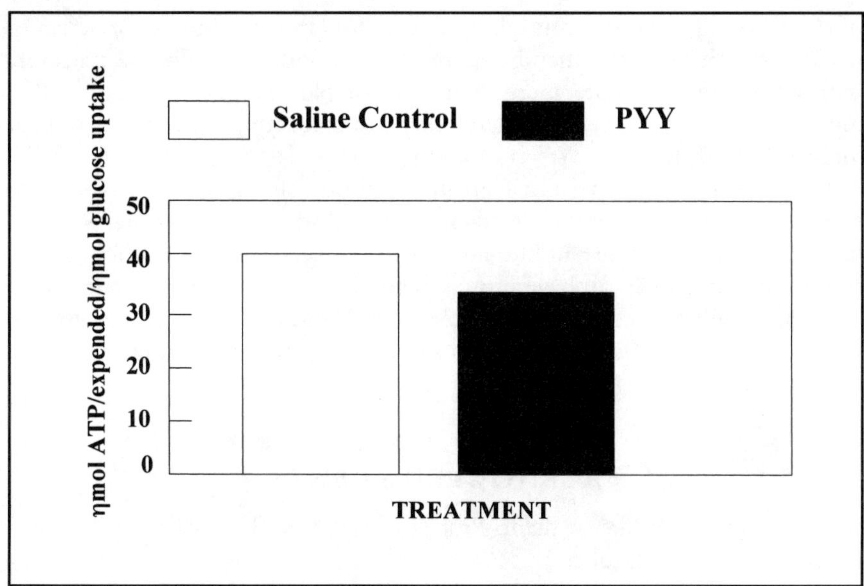

FIGURE 1. *The effects of subcutaneous injection of PYY 300 μg kg-1 per day for 3 days in male Swiss-Webster mice on the apparent energetic efficiency of active jejunal glucose transport.*

Furthermore, PYY likely enhances the absorption and intracellular transport of lipids via stimulation of apolipoprotein A-IV (32) and intestinal fatty acid binding protein (21). In humans, increased energetic efficiency of the absorptive process in subjects eating excessive calories would lead to weight gain. Experimental support for the concept that PYY's enhancement of the capacity and efficiency of intestinal absorption affects growth can be found in recent studies from our laboratory which demonstrate that in ovo administration of PYY increases glucose absorption in hatchling turkey poults (10) and enhances growth and feed efficiency of chickens and turkeys during the first week of post-hatch (33, 34).

The mechanisms by which PYY exerts these effects on fat and glucose absorption is unclear. Hallden and Aponte (21) have speculated that intestinal fatty acid binding protein is stimulated by PYY by indirect or direct action on transcription in the nucleus. In terms of glucose absorption there is an intracellular pool of glucose transporters, (SGLT1) in the enterocyte that allows regulated insertion of SGLT1 into the brush border membrane (35). We speculate that there are two populations of glucose transporters in the region of the brush border. One population is the transporters that are active and already inserted into the brush border membrane. A second population might lie just beneath the membrane or in the membrane but not in an active form. It is our hypothesis that PYY either stimulates the insertion of the second pool of nascent glucose receptors into membrane or activates inactive receptors in the membrane resulting in enhanced glucose transport without a commensurate increase in measurable energy expenditure. The involvement of the putative S2 glucose transporter (36) in the regulation of intestinal absorption by PYY is unknown.

In summary, we propose that greater attention should be focused on the energetic efficiency of nutrient digestion and absorption as another variable in the etiology of obesity in humans. Small changes in the efficiency of gastrointestinal function can have pronounced effects on long-term energy balance. Although this chapter has focused on the role of PYY in obesity, we wish to emphasize the potential importance of gastrointestinal energetic efficiency in the etiology of obesity.

ACKNOWLEDGMENTS

The authors would like to thank Professor Brian McBride of the University of Guelph for his helpful conceptual and editorial assistance during the preparation of this manuscript. The authors would like to thank Dr. Gerald Havenstein of North Carolina State University for reviewing this manuscript.

REFERENCES

1. Kuczmarski RJ, Campbell SM, Johnson CL. Increasing prevelance of overweight among U.S. adults. *JAMA* 1994;272:205–211.
2. Grundy SM. Multifactorial causation of obesity: implications for prevention. *Am J Clin Nutr* 1998;67: 5635–57215
3. Cant JP, McBride BW, Croom WJ. The regulation of intestinal metabolism and its impact on whole animal energetics. *J Anim Sci* 1996;74:2541–2553.
4. Bird AR, Croom WJ Jr., Fan YK, Daniel LR, Black BL, McBride BW, EJ Eisen, Bull LS, Taylor IL. Jejunal glucose absorption is enhanced by epidermal growth factor in mice. *J Nutr* 1994;124:231–240.
5. Kelly JM and McBride BW. The sodium pump and other mechanisms of thermogenesis in selected tissue. *Proc Nutr Soc* 1990;49:85.
6. Diamond J. Evolutionary Design of intestinal nutrient: Enough but not too much. *NIPS* 1991;6:92–96.
7. Taylor CR and Weibel ER. Design of the Mammalian respiratory system. I. Problem and strategy. *Respiration Physiol* 1981;44:41–10.
8. Obst BS and Diamond J. Ontogenesis of intestinal nutrient transport in domestic chickens (Gallus Gallus) and its relation to growth. *The Auk* 1992;109:451–464.
9. Croom WJ, Bird AR, Black BL, McBride BW. Manipulation of gastrointestinal nutrient delivery in livestock. *J Dairy Sci* 1993;76:2112–2124.
10. Croom WJ Jr, McBride BW, Bird AR, Fan YK, Odle J, Froetschel M, Taylor IL. Regulation of intestinal glucose absorption: A new issue in animal science. *Can J Anim Sci* 1998;78:1–13.
11. van Dam RM, Rimm EB, Willett WC, Stampfer MJ, Hu FB. Dietary patterns and risk for Type 2 diabetes mellitus in U.S. men. *Ann of Int Med* 2001;136: 201–209.
12. Aponte GW, Fink AS, Meyer JH, Tatemoto K, Taylor IL. Regional distribution and release of peptide YY with fatty acids of different chain length. *Am J Physiol* 1985;249:G745–G750.
13. Taylor IL and Mannon P. Gastrointestinal hormones. In: *Textbook of Gastroenterology,* eds: T Yamada, DH Alpers, C Owyang, DW Powell and FE Silverstein, Lippincott, Philadelphia. 1991;24–49.

14. Spiller RC, Trotman IF, Adrian TE, Bloom SR, Misiewicz JJ, Silk DB. Further characterization of the "ileal brake" reflex in man—effect of ileal infusion of partial digests of fat, protein and starch on jejunal motility and release of neurotensin, enteroglucagon and peptide YY. *Gut* 1988;29:1042.

15. Fu-Cheng S, Anini Y, Chariot J, Voisin T, Galmiche JP, Roze C. Peptide YY release after intraduodenal, intraileal, and intracolonic administration of nutrients in rats. *Eur J Physiol* 1995;435:66–75.

16. MacFarlane AR, Kinsman R, Read NW, Bloom SR. The ileal brake: Ileal fat slows small bowel transit and gastric emptying in man. *Gut* 1983;24:A471.

17. Aponte GW, Park K, Hess R, Garcia R, Taylor IL. Meal-induced peptide tyrosine (PYY) inhibition of pancreatic secretion in the rat. *FASAB J* 1989;3:1945–1955.

18. Rudnicki M, McFadden DW, Liwnicz BH, Balasubramaniam A, Nussbaum MS, Dayal R, Fischer, JE. Endogenous peptide YY on jejunal exposure to gastrointestinal contents. *J Surg Res*, 1990;48:485–490.

19. Mannon PJ and Mele JM. Peptide YY Y_1 receptor activates mitogen-activated protein kinase and proliferation in gut epithelial cells via the epidermal growth factor receptor. *Biochemical Journal* 2000; 250PT3:661.

20. Chance WT, Zhang X, Zuo L, Balasubramaniam A. Reduction of gut hypoplasia and cachexia in tumor-bearing rats maintained on total parenteral nutrition and treated with peptide YY and clenbuterol. *Nutrition* 1998;14:502–507.

21. Hallden G and Aponte GW. Evidence for a role of the gut hormone PYY in the regulation of intestinal fatty acid-binding protein transcripts in differentiated subpopulations of intestinal epithelial cell hybrids. *J Biol Chem* 1997;272:12591–12600.

22. Hernandez EJ, Whitcomb DC, Vigna SR, Taylor IL. Saturable binding of circulating peptide YY in the dorsal vagal complex of rats. *Am J Physiol* 1994;266:G511–G516.

23. Leslie RA, McDonald TJ, Robertson HA. Autoradiographic localization of peptide YY and neuropeptide Y binding sites in the medulla oblongata. *Peptides* 1988;9:1071–1076.

24. Pappas TN, Debas HT, Taylor IL. Enterogastrone-like effect of peptide YY is vagally mediated in the dog. *J Clin Invest* 1986;77:49–53.

25. Chen CH and Rogers RC. Central inhibitory action of peptide YY on gastric motility in rats. *Am J Physiol* 1995;269:R787–792.

26. Whitcomb DC and Taylor IL. A new twist in the brain-gut axis. *Am J Med Sci* 1992;304:334–338.

27. Fujimiya M and Inui A. Peptidergic regulation of gastrointestinal motility in rodents. *Peptides* 2000; 21:1565–1582.

28. Katschinski M. Nutritional implications of cephalic phase gastrointestinal responses. *Appetite* 2000; 34:189–196.

29. Shibata C, Naito H, Jin X-L, Ueno T, Funayama Y, Hashimoto A, Matsuno S, Sasaki I. Effect of glucagons, glicentin, glucagons-like-peptide-1 and -2 on interdigestive gastroduodenal motility in dogs with vagally denervated gastric pouch. *Scand J Gastroenterol* 2001;36:1049–1055.

30. Bilchik AJ, Hines OJ, Zinner MJ, Adrian TE, Berger JJ, Ashley SW, McFadden DW. Peptide YY augments postprandial small intestinal absorption in the conscious dog. *Am J Surg* 1994;167:570.

31. Bird AR, Croom WJ Jr, Fan Y-K, Black BL, McBride BW, Taylor IL. Peptide regulation of intestinal glucose absorption. *J Anim Sci* 1996;74:2523–2540.

32. Tso P, Liu M, Kalogeris TJ, Thomson ABR. The role of apolipoprotein A-IV in the regulation of food intake. *Ann Rev Nutr* 2001;21:231–254.

33. Coles BA, Croom WJ, Brake J, Daniel LR, Christensen VL, Phelps CP, Gore A, Taylor IL. In ovo peptide YY (PYY) administration improves growth and feed conversion ratios in week-old broiler chicks. *Poultry Science* 1999;78:1320–1322.

34. Coles BA, Croom WJ, Daniel LR, Christensen VL. In ovo peptide YY administration improves body weight at hatch and day 3 in turkey poults. *J Applied Poultry Res* 2001;10:380–384.

35. Wright EM, Hirsch JR, Loo DDF, Zampighi GA. Regulation of Na+/glucose cotransporters. *J Exp Biol* 1997;200:287–293.

36. Halaihel N, Gerbaud D, Vasseur M, Alvarado F. Heterogeneity of pig intestinal D-glucose transport. *Am J Physiol* 1999;277:C1130–C1141.

Gut-Brain Peptides in the New Millennium, edited by Y. Taché
CURE Foundation, Los Angeles, CA. © 2002

31

Pathophysiology of Diabetic Gastroparesis

Sebastian G. de la Fuente, Toku Takahashi,
and Theodore N. Pappas
Department of Surgery, Duke University Medical Center, Durham, NC

INTRODUCTION

A variety of medical conditions present with altered gastric motor activity that impairs normal emptying of gastric contents into the duodenum. Classically, gastroparesis is defined as delayed emptying of solids in the absence of mechanical obstruction. Based on the progression of the disease and duration of symptoms, gastric stasis is usually classified as either acute or chronic gastroparesis. Acute gastroparesis is commonly associated with drug therapy (i.e., opiates), electrolyte imbalances or surgery, whereas chronic gastroparesis results from metabolic diseases, neuromuscular abnormalities, idiopathic gastroparesis, or diabetic gastropathy. Regardless of the etiology, gastroparetic patients often present early satiety, nausea, vomiting, pain, fullness and bloating. Severe cases may result in life-threatening situations due to electrolyte imbalances and nutritional deficiencies.

With regards to diabetic gastropathy, gastroparesis is commonly seen in longstanding insulin-dependent diabetes though it may also affect non-insulin-independent diabetes mellitus patients. Delayed emptying in diabetic patients is primarily related to impaired phasic motor activity in the antrum; however, several other defects have been lately recognized to be altered in these patients, including abnormal fundic relaxation, increased outflow resistance, and inhibition of interdigestive migratory motor complexes. Although researchers have been investigating diabetic gastroparesis for several years now, many questions remain to be answered. This chapter examines current concepts on diabetic gastroparesis as well as the wide collection of articles published by Dr. John H. Walsh and his former collaborators in this field.

The motor function of the stomach is controlled at three different levels. First, parasympathetic pathways provide extrinsic neural control through the vagus nerves. The vagal trunks emerge from the esophageal hiatus and bifurcate throughout the gastric wall providing innervation to the entire stomach. Secondly, the enteric nervous system constituted by a vast network of ganglionic plexus serves as an integrative circuit between the extrinsic input

TABLE 1. *Major alterations in diabetic gastroparesis*

- Vagal neuropathy
- Gastric dysrhythmias
- Antral hypomotility
- Lack of antroduodenal coordination
- Pyloropasms
- Abnormal jejunal motor activity

and sensory afferents present in the gastric wall, which are stimulated by intraluminal stimulus. Multipolar cells, collectively known as interstitial cells of Cajal, form a two-dimensional network in the myenteric regions of the gastric body and antrum providing pacemaker functions that allows propulsion of ingested particles. A third level of motility control exists at the smooth muscle cells where peptides and other neurotransmitters bind, exciting receptors present in their membranes. Fine coordination at all these levels is required to guarantee emptying of the gastric contents into the duodenum.

After ingestion of a meal, regular gastric contractions begin in the body of the stomach and disperse through the antrum mixing and triturating the ingested food. Emptying of solids starts only when particles smaller than 1mm leave the stomach in a suspension known as chyme. Once evacuation begins, nutrients are emptied in a linear fashion into the duodenum. Still, undigestible particles are retained for longer periods until fasting or interdigestive motor complexes propel them through the pylorus into the intestines. Although it was believed for many years that diabetic patients experience postprandial motor abnormalities only, it is widely accepted to date that motility disarranges occur in both postprandial and fasting states.

Diabetic gastropathy encompasses a variety of pathophysiologic events all of which have been associated with poor gastric motility (Table 1). Neuropathy resulting from toxic glycemia levels has been detected in patients with long standing diabetes and gastroparesis. Early studies by Feldman and colleagues demonstrated convincing evidence that a functional derangement of vagal function occurs in diabetics after observing reduced gastric acid secretion in patients in response to sham feeding (1). However, others stated that the correlation between delayed gastric emptying and autonomic nerve dysfunction is rather weak (2). It is now recognized that acute changes in glycemia levels have major influences on gastric motor and sensory functions though, it remains to be investigated whether these effects result from direct injury to the vagus; are secondary to humoral imbalances; or are due to inhibition of the gastric pacemaker. Either way, it is usually advocated that patients maintain strict control of their blood glucose concentrations (2). Based on animal models of diabetes where endogenous levels of neuropeptides have been found to be elevated, the attention is being focused on studying the mechanisms by which hormones and peptides might alter gastric emptying.

Although few of these observations have been confirmed in humans, the odds are that inadequate levels of neuropeptides contribute to the multifactorial genesis of diabetic gastroparesis. It is worthwhile to emphasize at this point that although the pathophysiologic pathways have been divided in the present chapter for didactic purposes, most likely all these mechanisms act simultaneously in delaying gastric emptying in diabetic patients.

The Neural Pathway

Based on similarities between radiographic findings in patients with diabetic gastroparesis and gastric atony secondary to surgical vagotomy, it has been theorized for years that diabetics suffer an "autovagotomy" that excludes the stomach from vagal innervation. Further observations in patients with long standing insulin-dependent diabetes that secreted lower concentrations of acid than healthy individuals provided a credible evidence of a vagal neuropathy (1). Light- and electron-microscopy examinations of vagus nerves from patients that had undergone surgery for intractable gastroparesis demonstrate advance ultrastructural abnormalities in the vagal nerves in some patients (3, 4) but not in others (5). Nevertheless, none of these histologic studies demonstrated abnormalities in the storage or release of neuropeptides such as described in diabetic animals (6).

The association of gastroparetic symptoms and autonomic neuropathy in diabetic patients is relatively weak. Enck, et al. reported an inverse relationship between severity of symptoms and severity of neural damage in patients with diabetic gastroparesis (7). In their studies, patients with severe symptoms exhibited normal evoked potentials, while patients with minor signs of gastroparesis had significantly higher perception thresholds for electrical stimulation and in some cases no evoked potential at all.

Gastric Dysrhythmias

A gastric pacemaker situated in the upper portion of the stomach in an area along the greater curvature discharges myoelectrical activity that propagates circumferentially and distally towards the pylorus with an increasing amplitude and velocity. In humans, this gastric slow wave propagates at a frequency of approximately 3 cycles-per-minute. Some investigators have suggested that gastroparesis might be attributed to dysrthythmic rates in the gastric pacemaker. It is known that bradygastrias (1–2.4 cpm activity) and tachygastrias (3.6–9.9 cpm activity) are associated with gastric hypomotility and lack of coordinated gastric contractions. Patients with gastric dysrhythmias experience irregularities in gastric emptying rates through the entire emptying cycle (8). Although gastric dysrhythmias have been found in diabetic patients with meal-related symptoms (9), patients with insulin-dependent diabetes mellitus and autonomic neuropathy studied under euglycemic conditions do not experience disturbed gastric myoelectrical activity (10). This suggests that hyperglycemia might contribute to the induction of dysrhythmias.

Although morphological changes have not been documented in the myenteric plexus from patients with diabetes by conventional histology, specific immunohistochemical techniques revealed various abnormalities of the enteric plexus of diabetic animals. These changes include degeneration of adrenergic neurons, increments in the choline acetyltransferase activity, increase in the fluorescence intensity for VIP-like immunoreactivity and impaired nitric oxide synthase expression (11). In addition, remodeling of interstitial cells of Cajal has been found recently in a murine model of diabetic gastroparesis. The interstitial cells of Cajal play a major role in both myogenic and neurogenic aspects of gastric motility. Depletion of some of these cells was observed in the distal antrum while others showed atrophic changes. Although these observations have not been corroborated in humans, taken together they may play a major role in the pathogenesis of diabetic gastroparesis.

Effects of Hyperglycemia on Gastric Motility

Acute changes in blood glucose concentrations influence motor and sensory gastric functions as well as motility in other regions of the gastrointestinal tract. Hyperglycemia affects not only intracellular metabolic pathways but also membrane functions in neural cells. Elevated levels of glucose slow gastric emptying rates significantly in diabetic patients and healthy individuals (12). Barnett and Owyang documented disruption of normal fasting migration complexes in healthy volunteers at plasma glucose concentrations of 140 mg/dl after intravenous infusion of glucose (13). Horowitz on the other hand, observed a strong correlation between delayed gastric emptying of liquids and blood glucose levels of 270 mg/dl or higher in patients with type I and II diabetes (14). Furthermore, delayed emptying has also been reported in patients with poor glycemic control without evidence of vagal neuropathy. Nevertheless, the mechanisms responsible for the inhibitory actions of glucose in gastric motility remain obscure. It has recently been demonstrated that acute hyperglycemia impairs antral contractions and antro-pyloric coordination in rats and that the inhibitory effect of hyperglycemia on gastric emptying is mediated via impaired vagal activity (15).

In normal individuals, hyperglycemia reduces fundic tone, inhibits antral pressure waves and stimulates pyloric contractions. Additionally, it has been established in both diabetics and healthy subjects that hyperglycemia affects the gastric pacemaker by over stimulating it, which in turn provokes tachygastrias. The higher incidences of tachygastrias can be blocked by pretreatment with indomethacin, suggesting a prostaglandin-sensitive pathway related to hyperglycemic induced arrthymias (16). It is unclear whether insulin affects gastrointestinal motility. Although insulin might influence gastric motility, its effects are unlikely to be as important as hyperglycemia in slowing gastric emptying since patients with diabetes are insulin resistant or have no endogenous insulin secretion.

The Humoral Pathway

Postprandial release of hormones and neuropeptides is altered in diabetics. The importance of these hormonal changes remain uncertain; however, it is becoming apparent that hormonal abnormalities may contribute to the pathogenesis of diabetic gastroparesis. Diabetics have altered secretion of various hormones and neuropeptides including glucagon, motilin, pancreatic polypeptide (PP), neuropeptide Y (NPY), cholecystokinin (CCK) and gastrin.

Neuropeptide Y (NPY) levels are increased in certain hypothalamic nuclei after induction of diabetes in animal and have been shown to directly influence gastrointestinal motor control via myenteric neurons. Furthermore, central and peripheral injection of NPY inhibits gastrointestinal motility. However, the gastrointestinal distribution of NPY in diabetic animal models is somewhat different to that described in the central nervous system. NPY concentrations in the hypothalamus are significantly increased in diabetic rats (17), and hypoinsulinemia increases hypothalamic NPY levels (18). Alterations of hypothalamic NPY, which has potent effects on hypothalamo-pituitary, may contribute to certain neuroendocrine disturbances in diabetes mellitus. It has recently been demonstrated that acute hyperglycemia significantly elevated NPY concentrations in the hypothalamus (19). Central NPY has been shown to delay gastric emptying by inhibiting vagal efferent activity via Y2 receptors (20).

L cells, which are present throughout the entire gut mucosa, are responsible for the synthesis of enteroglucagon and other peptides derived from preproglucagon. The amino-terminal region of preproglucagon is further cleaved giving raise to glicentin and oxyntomodulin, whereas the carboxyl terminal portion produces biologically active glucagon-like peptides (GLP-1 and GLP-2). Although little is known to date about the GLP-2 functions, GLP-1 seems to be the most active glucagon gene product synthesized in the intestines. Its functions include stimulation of insulin release with an effect dependent on blood glucose levels, inhibition of glucagon discharge, inhibition of gastric acid secretion, and retardation of gastric emptying. Recently, GLP-1 has been found to impair gastric emptying in normal individuals by inhibiting antral waves, reducing transpyloric propagated antral waves and stimulating localized phasic and tonic pyloric contractions (21). Even though higher than normal postprandial plasma levels of glucagon have been documented in non-insulin-dependent diabetic subjects (22), the role of glucagon itself and glucagon-like peptides in particular in gastroparetic patients is not understood.

Motilin is a 22-amino acid peptide present in enteroendocrine cells in the upper small intestine that stimulates interdigestive antral contractions promoting gastric emptying. Despite the absence of interdigestive motor activity phase-three in gastroparetic diabetics, elevated levels of motilin have been recognized in these patients (23). Some authors attributed the hypermotilinemia to the lack of motilin action on smooth muscle cells due to cholinergic deficiency (24); most likely hypermotilinemia results from a compensatory mechanism based on the fact that motilin levels decrease with the introduction of a prokinetic (24).

Finally, several other neuroendocrine peptides have shown to be altered in animals and diabetic patients. CCK is abnormally augmented after a test meal in patients with diabetes especially in those with neuropathy. The elevated gastrin levels in diabetic patients are similar to the levels seen after vagotomy. On the other hand, somatostatin, VIP, substance P and galanin were found to be reduced in obese mice with non–insulin diabetes (25).

MOTILITY ANOMALIES

The aforementioned changes well recognized in diabetics represent factors that might contribute in the genesis of gastroparesis; however, the final endpoints are always the similar alterations in motility patterns. The antroduodenal coordination and pyloric relaxation are of vital importance for emptying of solids. Solids are retained in the stomach until the antrum ground them into particles small enough to be passed through the relaxed pyloric sphincter. If any of these phenomenons are altered, gastroparesis results.

A sensitive finding in diabetic gastropathy is the alteration of interdigestive motor migrating complexes especially phase 3 waves. Phase 3 is characterized by 5–10 min period of peristaltic waves that begins in the antrum area and migrates through to the distal ileum. The proposed function of the motor migration complex (MMC) is to sweep the stomach from solids and maintain certain gastrointestinal motility during fasting periods. Patients with diabetic gastropathy experience disruptions in phase 3 complexes characterized by prolongation or even complete absence of these patterns. Furthermore, in fasting states only a few number of antral phase 3 complexes are followed by duodenal complexes, indicating poor antro–duodenal coordination (25). Additionally, the MMC cycles are longer in these patients because of prolongation of phase 2 (26). Following a high-calorie meal fewer antral contractions and lower motility indexes are observed in diabetic patients as opposed to normal individuals, allowing the diagnosis of antral hypomotility (26).

Increments in pyloric pressure and pylorospasms are seen in more advanced states of diabetic gastroparesis. Patients have increased pyloric activity before and after meals with abnormally prolonged tonic contractions of the sphincter (27). Consequently, pyloric dysmotility probably alters gastric emptying by disturbing duodenal chyme transport.

CONCLUSIONS

Diabetic gastropathy refers to a variety of neuromuscular abnormalities suffered by patients with long standing diabetes mellitus. Approximately 50% of patients with insulin- and non-insulin dependent diabetes experience delayed emptying of solids and liquids; however, the presence of retarded gastric emptying correlates weakly with gastrointestinal dysfunctional symptoms. Most investigators believe that abnormal gastric emptying complicate diabetes of more than 10-years duration, and that generalized autonomic neuropathy plays a crucial role in the genesis of the disease. Recent data suggest that abnormal levels of glucose also contribute, thus recommending strict control of blood glucose concentrations in diabetic patients.

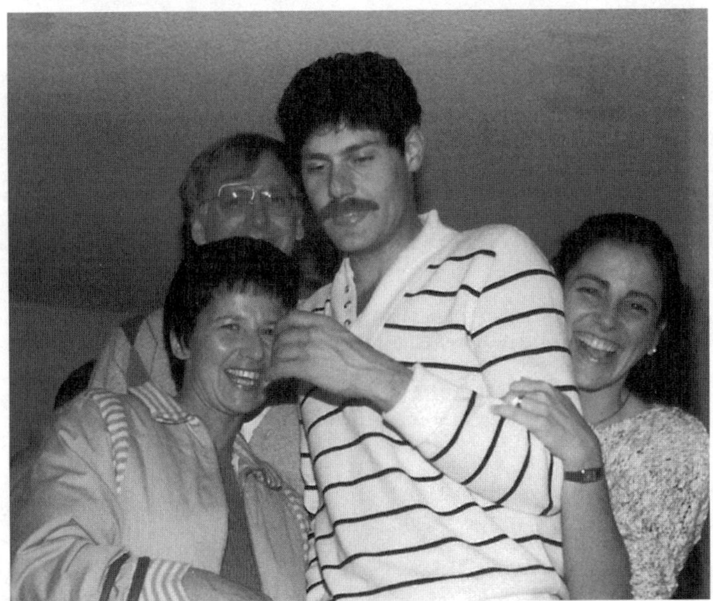

John Walsh, Mary Territo, Ted, and Theky Pappas at Pappas home in 1984, California.

REFERENCES

1. Feldman M, Corbett DB, Ramsay EJ, Walsh JH, Richardson CT. Abnormal gastric function in long-standing, insulin-dependent diabetic patients. *Gastroenterology* 1979;77:12–17.

2. Horowitz M, Wishart JM, Jones KL, Hebbard GS. Gastric emptying in diabetes: an overview. *Diabetic Med* 1996;13:S16–S22.

3. Kristensson K, Nordborg C, Olsson Y, Sourander P. Changes in the vagus nerve in diabetic mellitus. *Acta Pathol Microbiol Scand* 1971;79: 684–685

4. Guy RJ, Dawson JL, Garret JR, Laws JW, Thomas PK, Sahrma AK, Watkins PJ. Diabetic gastroparesis from autonomic neuropathy. *J Neurol Neurosurg Psychiatry* 1984;47:686–691.

5. Yoshida MM, Schuffler MD, Sumi SM. There are no morphological abnormalities of the gastric wall or abdominal vagus in patients with diabetic gastroparesis. *Gastroenterology* 1988;94:907–914.

6. Belai A, Lincoln J, Burnstock G. Lack of release of vasoactive intestinal polypeptide and calcitonin gene-related peptide during electrical stimulation of enteric nerves in streptozotocin-diabetic rats. *Gastroenterology* 1987;93:1034–1040.

7. Enck P, Frieling T. Pathophysiology of diabetic gastroparesis. *Diabetes* 1997;46: S77–S81.

8. Abell TL, Camilleri M, Hench VS, Malagelada JR. Gastric electromechanical function and gastric emptying in diabetes with gastroparesis. *Eur J Gastroenterology Hepatol* 1991;3:163–167.

9. Koch KL, Stern RM, Stewart WR, Vasey MW. Gastric emptying and gastric myoelectrical activity in patients with diabetic gastroparesis: effect of long-term domperidone treatment. *Am J Gastroenterology* 1989;84:1069–1075.

10. Jebbink HJA, Bruijs PPM, Bravemboer B, Akkermans L, vanBerge-Henegouwen G, Smout A. Gastric myoelectrical activity in patients with type I diabetes mellitus and autonomic neuropathy. *Dig Dis Sci* 1994;39:2376–2383.

11. Takahashi T, Nakamura K, Hiroshi I, Sima A, Owyang C. Impaired expression of nitric oxide synthase in the gastric myenteric plexus of spontaneous diabetic rats. *Gastroenterology* 1997;113:1535–1544.

12. Schavarcz E, Palmer M, Aman J, Horowitz M, Stridsberg M, Berne C. Physiological hyperglycemia slows gastric emptying in normal subjects and patients with insulin-dependent diabetes mellitus. *Am J Gastroenterology* 1987;82:29–35.

13. Barnett JL, Owyang C. Serum glucose concentration as a modulator of interdigestive gastric motility. *Gastroenterology* 1988;94:739.

14. Horowitz M, Harding PE, Maddox AF. Gastric and esophageal emptying in insulin-dependent diabetes mellitus. *J Gastroenterol Hepatol* 1986;97–100.

15. Ishiguchi T, Tada H, Nakagawa K, Yamamura T, Takahashi T. Hyperglycemia impair antro-pyloric co-ordination in conscious rats. *Auton Neurosci* 2002, in press.

16. Hasler WL, Soudah HC, Dulai G, Qwyang C. Mediation of hyperglycemia-induced gastric slow-wave dysrhythmias by endogenous prostaglandins. *Gastroenterology* 1995;108:727–736.

17. Williams G, Steel JH, Cardoso H, Ghatei MA, Lee YC, Gill JS, et al. Increased hypothalamic neuropeptide Y concentrations in diabetic rat. *Diabetes* 1988;37:763–72.

18. Malabu UH, McCarthy HD, McKibbin PE, Williams G. Peripheral insulin administration attenuates the increase in neuropeptide Y concentrations in the hypothalamic arcuate nucleus of fasted rats. *Peptides* 1992;13:1097–102.

19. Ishiguchi T, Nakajima M, Sone H, Kumagai AK, Takahashi T. Gastric distension-induced pyloric relaxation: central nervous system regulation and effects of acute hyperglycemia. *J Physiol* (London) 2001;533:801–813.

20. Ishiguchi T, Amano T, Matsubayashi H, Tada H, Fujita M, Takahashi T. Centrally administered neuropeptide Y delays gastric emptying via Y2 receptors in rats. *Am J Physiol* 2001;281:R1522–1530.

21. Schirra J, Houck P, Wank U, Arnold R, Goke B, Katschinski M. Effects of glucagon-like peptide-1 (7–36) amide on antro-pyloro-duodenal motility in the interdigestive state and with duodenal lipid perfusion in humans. *Gut* 2000;46:622–631.

22. Fischer H, Heideman T, Domschke W, Konturek JW. Disturbed gastric motility and pancreatic hormone release in diabetic mellitus. *J Physiol Pharmacol* 1998;49:529: 541.

23. Nakanome C, Akai H, Hongo M, Imai N, Toyota T, Goto Y, Okuguchi F, Komatsu K. Disturbances of the alimentary tract motility and hypermotilinemia in the patients with diabetes mellitus. *Tohoku J Exp Med* 1983;139:205–215.

24. Achem-Karam SR, Funakoshi A, Vinik AI, Chung O. Plasma motilin concentration and interdigestive migrating motor complex in diabetic gastroparesis: effects of metroclopramide. *Gastroenterology* 1985;88:492–499.
25. El-Salhy M. Neuroendocrine peptides of the gastrointestinal tract of an animal model of human type 2 diabetes mellitus. *Acta Diabetol* 1998;35:194–198.
26. Samsom M, Jebbink R, Akkermans L, vanBerge-Henegouwen G, Smout A. Abnormalities of antro-duodenal motility in type I diabetes. *Diabetes Care* 1996;19:21–27.
27. Mearin F, Camilleri M, Malagelada JR. Pyloric dysfunction in diabetics with recurrent nausea and vomiting. *Gastroenterology* 1986;90:1919–1925.

IV.

Processes of Gastrointestinal Injury and Repair

Gut-Brain Peptides in the New Millennium, edited by Y. Taché
CURE Foundation, Los Angeles, CA. © 2002

32

Multifactorial Regulation of Paracellular Permeability in Gastric Mucosa

Andrew H. Soll and Monica C. Chen
*CURE/Digestive Diseases Research Center, UCLA Division of Digestive Diseases
Department of Medicine and VA Greater Los Angeles Healthcare System
Los Angeles, CA*

INTRODUCTION

A reductionist approach has been developed in our laboratory for characterizing the multiple cellular elements involved in regulatory processes in the stomach. Over the years we have developed methods for the isolation, enrichment, culture and functional characterization of several cell types involved in the regulation of acid secretion and mucosal defense. Morton Grossman, John Walsh, and Jon Isenberg were key mentors, especially during the early phases of this work. The work on parietal, chief, and endocrine cell function provided insight into regulatory control by endocrine, hormonal, and local pathways. Current work utilizes monolayers of mucosal cells formed in culture to study the epithelial mechanisms underlying the gastric barrier to acid. We hypothesize that the regulation of paracellular permeability is a key element in controlling the apical barrier to acid; the regulation of paracellular permeability mirrors the theme of combinatorial control.

GASTRIC MUCOSAL DEFENSE

The gastric mucosa has a remarkable ability to defend itself against injury from the acid-peptic activity of gastric juice, and to undergo rapid repair when injury does occur. Several elements are involved in mucosal defense and repair. Primary lines of defense involve the pre-epithelial mucous and bicarbonate barrier, epithelial cell mechanisms, and sub-epithelial blood flow. Critical repair mechanisms include restitution (lateral migration of cells), replication, and wound healing (1–5).

Three categories of epithelial cell function are involved in mucosal defense: (1) the apical membrane, which is a component of the gastric barrier to acid diffusion (6–8), (2) basolateral Na^+/H^+ and Cl^-/HCO_3^- exchange, which permits mucosal cells to extrude "back-diffused" acid, and (3) intrinsic epithelial cell mechanisms, which defend against oxidative and other insults (9, 10).

THE APICAL BARRIER TO ACID

The pH gradient established by HCO_3^- secretion into a mucous layer protects the intracellular pH of surface mucosal cells (11). However, cells lining the gastric glands are not protected by a mucous layer and yet withstand apical exposure to pepsin at a pH < 1.5. Studying monolayers formed from enzyme-dispersed canine oxyntic mucosal cells in primary culture, we found that gastric epithelial cells displayed marked resistance to apical—but not basolateral—acidification. This indicated that the apical membrane was a critical component of the gastric barrier to acid (6). Further studies indicated that the paracellular pathway was the first point of injury caused by extreme or prolonged apical acidification. As the apical pH was dropped from 7 to 3.0, transepithelial resistance (TER) increased (6) and paracellular permeability—as reflected by mannitol flux—decreased (7), indicating that apical H^+ decreases permeation via the paracellular permeability. The increase in TER and monolayer integrity was sustained until an apical pH of 2 to 2.5 in Ussing chambers and to about 3.5 in Transwell inserts (which do not have a firm seal at the edge of the acid exposed area) (7, 8). With further apical acidification, TER decreased with time, and mannitol flux (3Å), but not inulin flux (11Å), increased (7) indicating a paracellular leak with preservation of size sieving (12). Despite this leak, monolayer integrity was not lost and changes remain reversible. However, when this low pH was sustained for a few hours, monolayer integrity was eventually irreversibly lost. This triphasic response to apical acidification dramatically contrasts with effects of basolateral acidification. Decreasing basolateral pH below 6 produces a rapid loss of cell viability and monolayer integrity, evident by a rapid and irreversible decrease in TER to fluid resistance (6), and parallel increases in mannitol and inulin flux.

REGULATION OF MUCOSAL DEFENSE

Several chemotransmitters endogenous to the gastric mucosal environment appear to regulate mucosal defense, repair and healing. Growth factors have received the most attention; the list includes members of the epithelial growth factor (EGF) family, as well as the mesenchymally-derived growth factors, insulin growth factor-I (IGF-I) and bFGF (basic fibroblast growth factor) (3). EGF is present in salivary glands, duodenal Brunner's glands and in mucosal epithelial cells following injury (13–15). The EGF family member tumor growth factor alpha (TGFα) is present in parietal cells (16, 17). These endogenous growth factors have a variety of effects. EGF enhances mucosal repair, healing and resistance to injury (3, 18–21). bFGF enhances ulcer healing, presumably by accelerating angiogenesis as well as stimulating fibroblast growth (22). Furthermore, we and others have shown that EGF, bFGF, and IGF-I enhanced epithelial cell growth and migration (19, 23, 24). Gastrin, prostaglandins (25), and nitric oxide (26) also enhance mucosal resistance to injury. However, the physiological importance of these pathways has been difficult to define *in vivo*, in particular because the regulatory elements are present in the gastric mucosal environment. Primary cell culture models provide a useful approach for dissecting the potential roles of individual factors. For example, we have shown that TGFα is present in our cultures and enhances cell proliferation (17), migration (23) and TER (8), thus supporting the view that EGF family members are physiological regulators of these processes *in vivo*.

ACTIONS OF APICAL EGF

Although most evidence indicates that growth factors are secreted and act at basolateral membranes, emerging evidence from several epithelial tissues suggests that EGF may also act at apical surfaces. EGF is secreted at the luminal surface in salivary and Brunner's glands and is present in milk (27, 28). However, the significance of luminal EGF is controversial, in part because the stability of EGF in gastric acid is unclear. One recent report suggests that EGF is degraded to smaller forms that retain moderate activity (29). The physiologic importance of luminal EGF is supported by observations that removing submandibular glands enhances susceptibility of the esophageal and gastric mucosa to injury (30, 31), whereas exogenous luminal EGF has some protective effects (31, 32). EGF receptors (EGFR) have been identified on the apical surface of several epithelial tissues (33–35), although their significance is controversial.

REGULATION OF JUNCTIONAL PERMEABILITY BY EGF

In studies with our primary gastric monolayers, we found that apical junctional permeability was regulated by EGF (8) and that this regulation had a major impact on the resistance of gastric monolayers to apical H^+, indicating that the regulation of paracellular permeability is critical for maintenance of mucosal integrity in the face of luminal acid. We also found consistent evidence that EGF increases TER by activating apical—as well as basolateral—receptors (8). The number of apical receptors was low, but a consistent, sustained rise in TER was produced. Furthermore, the presence of a small number of specific, apical EGFR was confirmed by binding studies with biologically active ^{125}I-EGF. Apical applications of antibody to human EGFR blocked binding to the apical, but not basolateral EGFR, indicating that the apical receptor was immunologically related to human EGFR and that apical EGFR were distinct from basolateral receptors (8). Exposure of the apical surface to EGF lead to tyrosine phosphorylation of a 225 kD moiety, identified as EGFR. Apical and basolateral EGF treatment also induced tyrosine phosphorylation of β-catenin, a component bound to E-cadherin at the zonula occludens. Of interest, apical EGFR induced a level of tyrosine phosphorylation of β-catenin that was comparable to levels produced by the much more numerous basolateral EGFR (8).

ENDOGENOUS TGFα REGULATES THE APICAL BARRIER TO ACID

Immunoneutralization of endogenous TGFα impaired the ability of monolayers to tolerate apical acidification, as reflected by an accelerated drop in TER and rise in mannitol; apical EGF treatment restored monolayer resistance to apical acidification. Immunoblockade of basolateral, but not apical, EGFR also impaired the resistance to apical acidification and enhanced mannitol in monolayers cultured in Transwell inserts. We speculate that apical EGFR regulate the barrier to apical acidification via effects on paracellular resistance. Although exogenous basolateral EGF has a lesser apparent effect on the barrier to acid in our model, endogenous ligand active at basolateral EGFR plays an important role in maintaining the barrier to apical acid (36).

OTHER REGULATORS OF PARACELLULAR PERMEABILITY

Secretin, which regulates gastric (37) chief cell function, was also found to regulate paracellular permeability. Basolateral—but not apical—secretin at concentrations from 1 to 100 nM dose-dependently increased resistance. IGF-I and FGF were also found to regulate paracellular permeability, acting at basolateral, but not apical, receptors (38).

REGULATION OF THE PARACELLULAR PATHWAY IN OTHER MODELS

The literature indicates that the synthesis, assembly, and function of the apical junctional complex are regulated by signaling elements, including hormones, growth factors, cytokines, bacteria, nutrients, and post-receptor activators. An increase in paracellular permeability in response to luminal nutrients has been clearly established and is of obvious physiological relevance (39, 40). The cytokines interferon-(INF)-γ and tumor necrosis factor (TNF)-α induce a delayed increase in paracellular permeability (40). These observations are particularly interesting because patients with inflammatory bowel disease have increased IFN-γ expression and increased intestinal permeability (40). Interleukins 4 and 13 (41) and nitrous oxide (NO) (42) also increase paracellular permeability. Hepatocyte growth factor (HGF) increases paracellular permeability in T84 cells over a 24 h period (43). In the liver, vasopressin increases paracellular permeability, as evidenced by increased biliary clearance of molecules normally restricted by the tight junction (44) and collapse of the canalicular space between liver cell couplets (45). In non-transformed mouse mammary epithelial cells, treatment for several days with corticosteroids increased TER (46) and TGFβ antagonized these effects (47); these more prolonged effects on paracellular permeability likely reflect induction of junctional protein synthesis and assembly rather than acute regulation. There are few examples of physiological regulators that increase TER (decrease paracellular permeability), such as observed in our studies with gastric epithelial cells.

MOLECULAR MECHANISMS REGULATING PARACELLULAR PERMEABILITY

The molecular mechanisms mediating paracellular permeability remain to be defined. We examined the role of the protooncogene product Src, the first identified cytoplasmic protein tyrosine kinase, because of Src's recognized involvement at the cytoskeletal-membrane interface. Tyrosine phosphorylation of Src at Tyr416 was measured with a site-specific phosphotyrosine antibody (37). PP2 (0.1 to 10 μM), a selective Src tyrosine kinase inhibitor, but not the inactive isomer PP3, abolished the increase in transepithelial resistance by secretin, but only modestly attenuated apical EGF effects. Inhibition over this dose range of PP2 is highly specific for Src-family kinase. AG1478 (100 nM), a specific EGFR tyrosine kinase inhibitor, attenuated the resistance increase to EGF but not secretin. Secretin, but not EGF, induced tyrosine phosphorylation of Src416 in a dose-dependent fashion, with the maximal response observed at 1 min. PP2, but not PP3, dramatically inhibited this tyrosine phosphorylation (37). Furthermore, secretin was found to induce tyrosine phosphorylation of three Src substrates Pyk2, FAK, and paxillin. Secretin-induced phosphorylation of these Src substrates was also blocked by PP2. Thus, we concluded that secretin increases paracellular resistance in gastric mucosa through a Src-mediated pathway, while the effect of EGF is Src-independent. Src appears to mediate the physiological effects of this Gs-coupled receptor in primary epithelial cells.

MOLECULAR MECHANISMS UNDERLYING APICAL RESISTANCE TO ACID

Studies cited above indicated that apical acidification decreased paracellular permeability. To explore the mechanisms of the acid regulation of the TER we examined the role for Src-family tyrosine kinase and Src substrates. The selective Src kinase inhibitor PP2 reduced the apical acid-induced increase in TER by about 40%. Furthermore, Western blots performed using a site-specific phosphotyrosine antibody revealed that apical acidification increased Src Tyr416 autophosphorylation. Changes were found in two Src isoforms at 62 kDa and 58 kDa. Maximal stimulation of phosphorylation was reached at 2.5 to 5 minutes and was sustained for 30 min. This Tyr416 phosphorylation was partially attenuated by pretreatment with PP2. Apical acidification also dramatically stimulated site-specific tyrosine phosphorylation of Pyk2. Detected with Pyk2(p)–Tyr402 antibody, this phosphorylation was time dependent, with maximal activation at 5 min after apical acidification, and was partially attenuated by PP2 pretreatment. Neither the inactive Src kinase inhibitor PP3 and AG1478, a highly specific EGFR tyrosine kinase inhibitor, blocked the acid-induced increase in TER nor tyrosine phosphorylation of Src or Pyk2. Thus we found that apical acidification produced parallel increases in TER and tyrosine phosphorylation of Src and its substrate Pyk2. Because the Src kinase inhibitor PP2 inhibited both the acid-induced increase in TER and phosphorylation of Src and Pyk2, we speculate that Src kinase family at least partially mediates dynamic tyrosine phosphorylation events required for the decrease in paracellular permeability in response to apical acidification. These findings indicate a novel role of Src-family tyrosine kinase in the regulation of the apical barrier to acid.

SUMMARY

We found that permeability of the tight junctions separating epithelial cells is regulated by several endogenous factors, including secretin, EGF, IGF-I, FGF. These data therefore indicate that autocrine, paracrine, and endocrine pathways regulate gastric paracellular permeability. In this primary cell model these chemotransmitters rapid regulate paracellular permeability, as evident by an increase in TER and decrease in mannitol flux. Secretin and EGF act in a synergistic fashion, suggesting utilization of distinct cell activation pathways. EGF works through apical receptors and activates classic EGF receptor tyrosine phosphorylation mechanisms. In contrast, secretin acts via Src-dependent mechanisms and induces tyrosine phosphorylation of Src and substrates of Src. These studies provide a clear example of the regulation of tight junctions by endogenous chemotransmitters and elucidate a novel mechanism by which the stomach defends itself against injury.

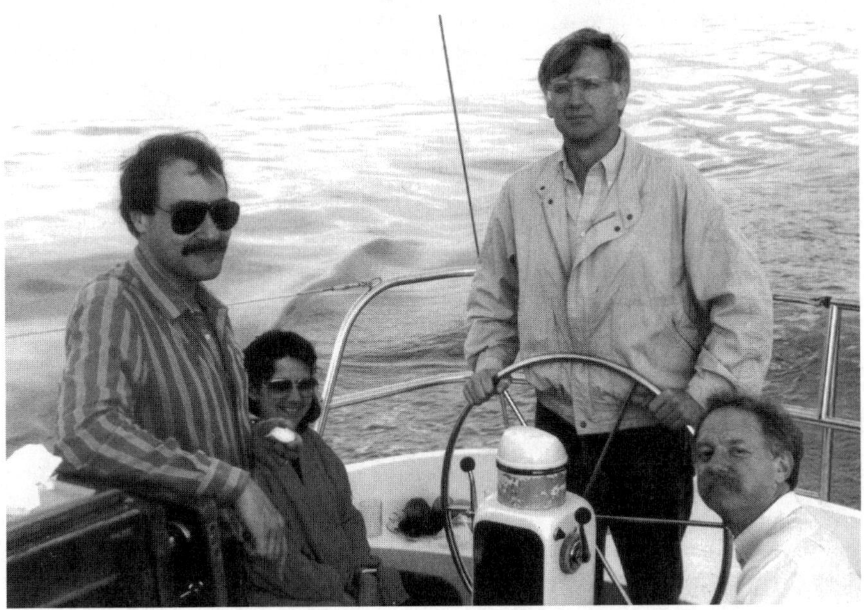

John out sailing with Drew at a meeting in Vancouver in July, 1986.
Left to right, Drs. Tom Garrick, Mary Territo, John Walsh and Gordon Kauffman.

ACKNOWLEDGMENTS

Supported by grants NIDDK 19984 and by the Medical and Research Services of the Department of Veterans Affairs

REFERENCES

1. Soll AH. Gastric, duodenal, and stress ulcer. In: *Gastrointestinal Disease,* Sleisenger M and Fordtran J, Eds. 5 Ed. Philadelphia: W.B. Saunders, 1993:580–679.
2. Allen A, Flemstrom G, Garner A, Kivilaakso E. Gastroduodenal mucosal protection. *Physiol Rev* 1993;73:823–857.
3. Jones MK, Tomikawa M, Mohajer B, Tarnawski AS. Gastrointestinal mucosal regeneration: role of growth factors. *Front Biosci* 1999;4:D303–D309.
4. Romano M, Kraus ER, Boland CR, Coffey RJ. Comparison between transforming growth factor alpha and epidermal growth factor in the protection of rat gastric mucosa against drug-induced injury. *Ital J Gastroenterol* 1994;26:223–228.
5. Wallace JL. Nonsteroidal anti-inflammatory drugs and the gastrointestinal tract. Mechanisms of protection and healing: current knowledge and future research. *Am J Med* 2001;110:19S–23S.
6. Sanders MJ, Ayalon A, Roll M, Soll AH. The apical surface of canine chief cell monolayers resists H^+ back-diffusion. *Nature* 1985;313:52–54.
7. Chen MC, Chang A, Buhl T, Tanner M, Soll AH. Apical acidification induces paracellular injury in canine gastric mucosal monolayers. *Am J Physiol* 1994;267:G1012–G1020.
8. Chen MC, Goliger J, Bunnett N, Soll AH. Apical and basolateral EGF receptors regulate gastric mucosal paracellular permeability. *Am J Physiol* 2001;280:G264–G272.

9. Nakamura K, Rokutan K, Marui N, Niki S, Aoike A, Kawai K. Induction of heat shock proteins and their implication in protection against ethanol-induced damage in cultured guinea pig gastric mucosal cells. *Gastroenterology* 1991;101:161–166.

10. Olson CE. Glutathione modulates toxic oxygen metabolite injury of canine chief cell monolayers in primary culture. *Am J Physiol* 1988;254:G49–G56.

11. Chu S, Tanaka S, Kaunitz JD, Montrose MH. Dynamic regulation of gastric surface pH by luminal pH. *J Clin Invest* 1999;103:605–612.

12. Madara JL, Stafford J, Barenberg D, Carlson S. Functional coupling of tight junctions and microfilaments in T84 monolayers. *Am J Physiol* 1988;254:G416–G423.

13. Wright NA, Pike CM, Elia G. Ulceration induces a novel epidermal growth factor-secreting cell lineage in human gastrointestinal mucosa. *Digestion* 1990;46 Suppl 2:125–133.

14. Barnard JA, Beauchamp RD, Russell WE, Dubois RN, Coffey RJ. Epidermal growth factor-related peptides and their relevance to gastrointestinal pathophysiology. *Gastroenterology* 1995;108:564–580.

15. Sarraf CE, Alison MR, Ansari TW, Wright NA. Subcellular distribution of peptides associated with gastric mucosal healing and neoplasia. *Microsc Res Tech* 1995;31:234–247.

16. Beauchamp RD, Barnard JA, McCuthen CM, Cherner JA, Coffey RJ. Localization of transforming growth factor alpha and its receptor in gastric mucosal cells. Implications for a regulatory role in acid secretion and mucosal renewal. *J Clin Invest* 1989;83:1017–1023.

17. Chen MC, Lee AT, Karnes WE, Avedian D, Martin M, Sorvillo JM, Soll AH. Paracrine control of gastric epithelial cell growth in primary culture by transforming growth factor-α. *Am J Physiol* 1993;264:G390–G396.

18. Romano M, Polk WH, Awad JA, Arteaga CL, Nanney LB, Wargovich MJ, Kraus ER, Boland CR, Coffey RJ. Transforming growth factor alpha protection against drug-induced injury to the rat gastric mucosa *in vivo*. *J Clin Invest* 1992;90:2409–2421.

19. Chen MC, Lee AT, Soll AH. Mitogenic response of canine fundic epithelial cells in short-term culture to transforming growth factor α and insulinlike growth factor 1. *J Clin Invest* 1991;87:1716–1723.

20. Cook PW, Mattox PA, Keeble WW, Pittelkow MR, Plowman GD, Shoyab M, Adelman JP, Shipley GD. A heparin sulfate-regulated human keratinocyte autocrine factor is similar or identical to amphiregulin. *Mol Cell Biol* 1991;11:2547–2557.

21. Li J, Aderem A. MacMARCKS, a novel member of the MARCKS family of protein kinase C substrates. *Cell* 1992;70:791–801.

22. Szabo S, Folkman J, Vattay P, Morales RE, Pinkus GS, Kato K. Accelerated healing of duodenal ulcers by oral administration of a mutein of basic fibroblast growth factor in rats. *Gastroenterology* 1994;106:1106–1111.

23. Kato K, Chen MC, Nguyen M, Lehmann FS, Podolsky DK, Soll AH. Effects Of growth factors and trefoil peptides on migration and replication in primary oxyntic cultures. *Am J Physiol* 1999;276:G1105–G1116.

24. Dignass AU, Tsunekawa S, Podolsky DK. Fibroblast growth factors modulate intestinal epithelial cell growth and migration. *Gastroenterology* 1994;106:1254–62.

25. Atay S, Tarnawski AS, Dubois A. Eicosanoids and the stomach. *Prostaglandins Other Lipid Mediat* 2000;61:105–124.

26. Lopez-Belmonte J, Whittle BJ, Moncada S. The actions of nitric oxide donors in the prevention or induction of injury to the rat gastric mucosa. *Br J Pharmacol* 1993;108:73–78.

27. Goodlad RA, Wright NA. Epidermal growth factor and transforming growth factor-alpha actions on the gut. *Eur J Gastroenterol Hepatol* 1995;7:928–932.

28. Berseth CL. Enhancement of intestinal growth in neonatal rats by epidermal growth factor in milk. *Am J Physiol* 1987;253:G662–G665.

29. Playford RJ. Peptides and gastrointestinal mucosal integrity. *Gut* 1995;37:595–597.

30. Konturek PK, Brzozowski T, Konturek SJ, Dembinski A. Role of epidermal growth factor, prostaglandin, and sulfhydryls in stress-induced gastric lesions. *Gastroenterology* 1990;99:1607–1615.

31. Sarosiek J, Marshall BJ, Peura DA, Hoffman S, Feng T, McCallum RW. Gastroduodenal mucus gel thickness in patients with helicobacter pylori: a method for assessment of biopsy specimens. *Am J Gastroenterol* 1991;86:729–734.

32. Riegler M, Sautner T, Wenzl E. The effect of nutrition on intestinal epithelial barrier function. *Ann Surg* 1996;223:447–448.

33. Thompson JF. Specific receptors for epidermal growth factor in rat intestinal microvillus membranes. *Am J Physiol* 1988;254:G429–G435.

34. Gonnella PA, Siminoski K, Murphy RA, Neutra MR. Transepithelial transport of epidermal growth factor by absorptive cells of suckling rat ileum. *J Clin Invest* 1987;80:22–32.

35. Taylor TB, Ramsdell JS. Transforming growth factor-alpha and its receptor are expressed in the epithelium of the rat prostate gland. *Endocrinology* 1993;133:1306–1311.

36. Chen MC, Solomon TE, Kui R, Soll AH. Apical EGF receptors regulate the epithelial barrier to gastric acid: endogenous TGF-alpha is an essential facilitator. *Am J Physiol Gastrointest Liver Physiol* 2002, resubmitted.

37. Chen MC, Solomon TE, Salazar EP, Kui R, Rozengurt E, Soll AH. Secretin Regulates Paracellular Permeability in Canine Gastric Monolayers by a Src kinase-dependent Pathway. *Am J Physiol Gastrointest Liver Physiol* 2002, resubmitted.

38. Chen MC, Goliger J, Soll AH. Regulation of paracellular permeability by growth factors in canine gastric mucosa monolayers. *Gastroenterology* (Philadelphia PA) 112, A86. 1997.

39. Turner JR, Rill BK, Carlson SL, Carnes D, Kerner R, Mrsny RJ, Madara JL. Physiological regulation of epithelial tight junctions is associated with myosin light-chain phosphorylation. *Am J Physiol* 1997;273:C1378–C1385.

40. Nusrat A, Turner JR, Madara JL. Molecular physiology and pathophysiology of tight junctions. IV. Regulation of tight junctions by extracellular stimuli: nutrients, cytokines, and immune cells. *Am J Physiol Gastrointest Liver Physiol* 2000;279:G851–G857.

41. Ceponis PJ, Botelho F, Richards CD, McKay DM. Interleukins 4 and 13 increase intestinal epithelial permeability by a phosphatidylinositol 3-kinase pathway. Lack of evidence for STAT 6 involvement. *J Biol Chem* 2000;275:29132–29137.

42. Gorodeski GI. NO increases permeability of cultured human cervical epithelia by cGMP-mediated increase in G-actin. *Am J Physiol Cell Physiol* 2000;278:C942–C952.

43. Hollande F, Blanc EM, Bali JP, Whitehead RH, Pelegrin A, Baldwin GS, Choquet A. HGF regulates tight junctions in new nontumorigenic gastric epithelial cell line. *Am J Physiol Gastrointest Liver Physiol* 2001;280:G910–G921.

44. Lowe PJ, Miyai K, Steinbach JH, Hardison WG. Hormonal regulation of hepatocyte tight junctional permeability. *Am J Physiol* 1988;255:G454–G461.

45. Nathanson MH, Gautam A, Ng OC, Bruck R, Boyer JL. Hormonal regulation of paracellular permeability in isolated rat hepatocyte couplets. *Am J Physiol* 1992;262:G1079–G1086.

46. Zettl KS, Sjaastad MD, Riskin PM, Parry G, Machen TE, Firestone GL. Glucocorticoid-induced formation of tight junctions in mouse mammary epithelial cells *in vitro*. *Proc Natl Acad Sci USA* 1992;89:9069–9073.

47. Woo PL, Cha HH, Singer KL, Firestone GL. Antagonistic regulation of tight junction dynamics by glucocorticoids and transforming growth factor-β in mouse mammary epithelial cells. *J Biol Chem* 1996;271:404–412.

Gut-Brain Peptides in the New Millennium, edited by Y. Taché
CURE Foundation, Los Angeles, CA. © 2002

33

Duodenal Mucosal Defense Mechanisms

Jonathan D. Kaunitz
*CURE/Digestive Diseases Research Center, UCLA Division of Digestive Diseases
Department of Medicine and VA Greater Los Angeles Healthcare System
Los Angeles, CA*

Yasutada Akiba
Keio University School of Medicine, Shinjuku-ku, Tokyo, Japan

INTRODUCTION

The location of the duodenal epithelium just distal to the gastric antrum, and proximal to the pancreaticobiliary ducts uniquely exposes it to a highly variable pH environment due to peristaltically conveyed pulses of concentrated gastric acid combining with secreted bicarbonate. Since the duodenum does not have the inherent acid protective structural properties of the stomach and esophagus, whose tight intercellular junctions severely curtail transepithelial ionic permeation (1, 2), the duodenum, being leaky, has evolved alternate means for defense against acid (Figure 1).

In this chapter, we will systematically describe the current knowledge concerning duodenal defense mechanisms, ending with a scheme that integrates these mechanisms into a coherent protective response to luminal acid. Moreover, we will discuss how these mechanisms might be altered in the disease cystic fibrosis, in which the duodenum appears to be highly resistant to damage due to luminal acid (3–5).

DUODENAL LUMINAL PH

Gastric acid secretion, antral peristalsis, and duodenal and pancreatic bicarbonate secretion expose the proximal duodenum to cyclical and rapid variations of luminal pH. These cycles are more pronounced post-prandially, and induce variation in luminal pH between two and seven on a scale of minutes (6–8). Furthermore, the constant mixture of strong mineral acid with bicarbonate produces extraordinarily high $p\mathrm{CO}_2$ levels, which can be in excess of 400 mm Hg (9). In contrast, gastric luminal pH is sustained on

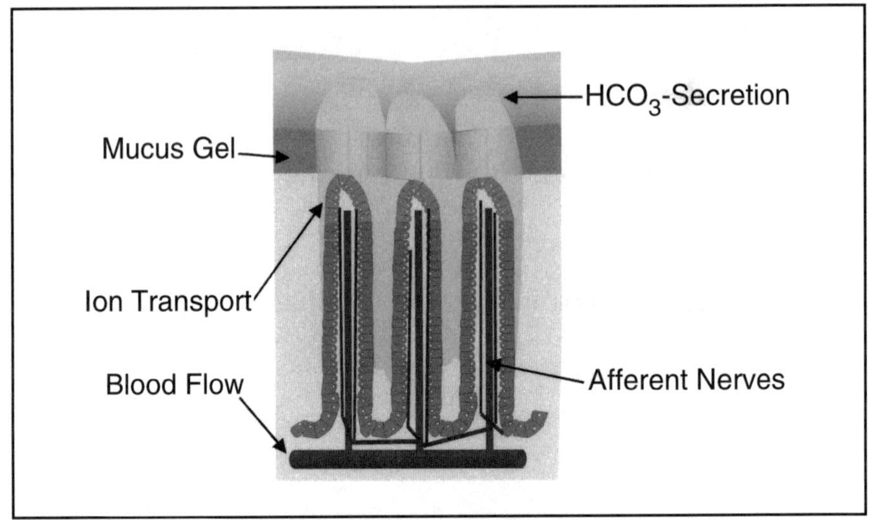

FIGURE 1. Duodenal defense mechanisms. *All of these mechanisms are believed to defend the mucosa against luminal acid, although bicarbonate secretion is the most accepted.*

a minute-to-minute scale, although it does of course vary over a 24 hr period. Rapid shifts of duodenal pH are likely to create intense stress on the epithelial cells to maintain constant intracellular pH (pH_i) in order to maintain function and prevent necrosis due to irreversible intracellular acidification. Thus, a potent defensive system must be in place to prevent cellular acidification during mucosal acid challenge.

DEFENSE MECHANISMS

The most studied duodenal defense mechanism is epithelial bicarbonate secretion. Other potential defense mechanisms include the mucus gel and mucosal blood flow. Reparative processes such as restitution from injury are beyond the scope of this chapter and will not be addressed further.

Bicarbonate Secretion

Bicarbonate secretion is a logical duodenal defense mechanism for the following reasons: 1) Duodenal bicarbonate secretion/cm^2 epithelium is much greater than gastric bicarbonate secretion (2, 10–12); 2) pH electrode studies suggest that epithelial bicarbonate secretion creates a layer of neutral pH next to the mucosa (13–15); 3) *Helicobacter pylori* infection complicated by duodenal ulcers is associated with diminished bicarbonate secretion, and eradication of helicobacter infection restores duodenal bicarbonate secretory capacity (16, 17); and 4) bicarbonate neutralizes duodenal luminal pH, clearly serving as an initial defense against gastric acid. The mechanism by which bicarbonate is secreted from the epithelial cell is controversial. Formerly, it was thought that CO_2 diffusing into the cell was converted to bicarbonate and protons by cellular carbonic hydrase. Bicarbonate was then secreted across the apical membrane by anion exchange. More recent studies, including molecular immunolocalization and studies of pH_i, suggest that this mechanism is supplemented by transport of bicarbonate from the blood across the basolateral membrane by the pancreatic variant of the sodium-bicarbonate cotransporter (NBC), NBC1, in response to decreased pH_i resulting from exposure to luminal acid (18–21). Since inhibiting or eliminating the apical membrane chloride channel cystic fibrosis transmembrane regulator (CFTR) greatly attenuates bicarbonate secretion (22, 23), the CFTR has been implicated in the mechanism of bicarbonate secretion. However, it is unknown whether it serves directly as a bicarbonate channel, or indirectly to preserve transmembrane electrical or ion gradients. Recent data is consistent with the CFTR directly regulating other bicarbonate transporting apical proteins, such as the DRA anion exchanger, (24, 25), providing a logical explanation of deficient bicarbonate secretion in the presence of CFTR dysfunction.

Role of Alkali Loading

We have re-examined the role of bicarbonate secretion in overall duodenal defense from acid, and in doing so, have formulated a novel hypothesis with regard to the role of bicarbonate transport. To test these possibilities, we developed a technique for the measurement of pH_i, blood flow, and mucus gel thickness in the duodenum of anesthetized rats (26, 28). With this system, we could perfuse solutions of varying pH through a chamber placed over the exposed duodenal mucosa, thereby simulating changes in luminal pH. We found that exposing the mucosa to a brief pulse of acid, promptly decreased pH_i. This fall of pH_i, even with mildly acidic perfusates, suggested that acid could readily penetrate the overlying mucus gel and the mucosa, therefore calling into question the role of pre-epithelial bicarbonate neutralization in duodenal mucosal defense. With removal of the acid challenge, pH_i was elevated to supernormal values, which indicated that cellular buffering power has increased, not decreased, during acid challenge. Furthermore, a second acid challenge acidified pH_i less than the first; further confirming that acid exposure was associated with cellular alkali loading and increased cellular buffering power. This somewhat surprising finding was confirmed by comparison with prior studies conducted in a variety of systems, in which acid pulses were followed by pH_i overshoot, indicative of cellular alkali loading in cells containing a plasma membrane alkali-loading mechanism such as sodium-bicarbonate cotransport (27).

Further studies indicated that this alkali loading was inhibited by the stilbene anion transport inhibitor DIDS (4,4′diisothiocyanostilbene-2,2′-disulfonic acid). When exposed to two short acid pulses, pH_i decreased less during the second challenge; again strongly suggestive that cellular buffering power was increased during acid exposure. Again, DIDS inhibited this adaptive effect (28). Our studies were thus consistent with alkali loading being induced by luminal acid exposure by a DIDS-inhibitable mechanism. This finding was expected insofar as primary isolated duodenal epithelial cells recovered from acid exposure by a mechanism consistent with the activity of an NBC (29), and that bicarbonate-secreting pancreatic duct cells have a basolateral membrane NBC (30). Recently, our laboratory, in collaboration with Dr. Ira Kurtz, have confirmed the presence of the pancreatic-type isoform of NBC1 (pNBC1) in the basolateral membrane of rodent proximal duodenal epithelial cells using immunohistochemistry (18, 31).

Alkali loading during acid challenge, which increases cellular buffering power and attenuates the fall of pH_i, is an attractive means of defending the epithelium from acid challenge. To address how bicarbonate secretion is related to this observation, we performed parallel experiments in which bicarbonate secretion was measured in a perfused duodenal loop exposed to the same pH perfusion sequence as the measurements of pH_i. Bicarbonate secretion was measured by the conventional acid back-titration technique, but also by measurement of total dissolved CO_2 content of the effluent collected from the perfusion with a CO_2 electrode. We found that titratable alkalinity increased substantially during acid perfusion. Surprisingly, total CO_2 content decreased somewhat at the same time (28). To account for the large discrepancy between the back-titration experiments and the measurement of effluent CO_2 content, we performed control experiments in which we measured total CO_2 content in the perfusates and effluent of perfused duodena. We found that there was a finite loss of CO_2 during duodenal perfusion, in agreement with prior studies (32) but inadequate to explain the discrepancy.

To help interpret the data, we postulated three means by which acid can disappear from the lumen: back-diffusion of acid, back-diffusion of CO_2, and neutralization by secreted bicarbonate. If all of the acid disappearance measured by back-titration occurred by bicarbonate neutralization, the effluent CO_2 content should increase to the same extent as did titratable acidity, which was not the case. If the perfusate bicarbonate was converted into CO_2, which then back-diffused into the epithelium, we would still predict a large increase of effluent CO_2 content. Hence, the best means of explaining the discrepancy between effluent CO_2 content and acid disappearance is by postulating that most of the acid loss during perfusion with pH 2 solution is due to acid back-diffusion. In that case, bicarbonate secretion must have been unchanged or perhaps decreased during acid challenge. The implications of these data, combined with our measurements of pH_i, support our hypothesis that increased cellular buffering, and not bicarbonate secretion, was the primary duodenal defense mechanism from acid. Acid was not neutralized at the duodenal surface, since cellular pH_i clearly decreased during acid challenge, and since acid back-diffusion was the major means of acid loss when perfused over the mucosa. Furthermore, since bicarbonate secretion was unchanged during acid perfusion, and only increased after acid removal, secreted bicarbonate is unlikely to be protective, since its increased secretion is present only when it is not needed i.e., when luminal acid is no longer present. Supporting the concept that bicarbonate secretion is not enhanced during luminal acid stress are the observations that lowered pH_i deceases cellular bicarbonate concentration, inhibiting bicarbonate exit, and that CFTR permeability to the related anion chloride is diminished at acidic pH_i due to lack of CFTR phosphorylation (33).

We further tested this hypothesis by measuring epithelial injury under conditions in which alkali loading is either inhibited or enhanced, in order to confirm that bicarbonate loading, and not secretion is the primary defensive mechanism. To accomplish this, DIDS, and the anion channel inhibitor NPPB (5-nitro-2-(3-phenylpropylamino) benzoic acid), added to the perfusate, respectively either decreased or increased pH_i. Changes of pH_i also correlated with mucosal injury susceptibility. The most striking finding was that NPPB inhibited bicarbonate secretion but increased pH_i and decreased injury susceptibility. Thus, NPPB 'uncoupled' bicarbonate secretion from mucosal protection, a novel finding that casts further doubt on the primacy of bicarbonate secretion on mucosal protection (18). In this proposed mechanism, shown in Figure 2, bicarbonate secretion occurs to remove excess alkali from the cell when excess intracellular bicarbonate is no longer needed after acid challenge.

Blood Flow

Mucosal blood flow is an accepted component of upper gastrointestinal barrier function. In the stomach, for example, interventions that attenuate the hyperemic response to acid perfusion increase mucosal injury (34–36). The data derived from studies of duodenum are less conclusive, however. One potential confounder is that bicarbonate secretion and blood flow are co-regulated by stimuli, making it difficult to determine the relative importance of blood flow in terms of overall barrier function.

With our technique, we were able to measure blood flow, pH_i, and mucus gel thickness simultaneously. This technique enabled us to formulate novel conclusions about the relative contribution of blood flow to overall barrier

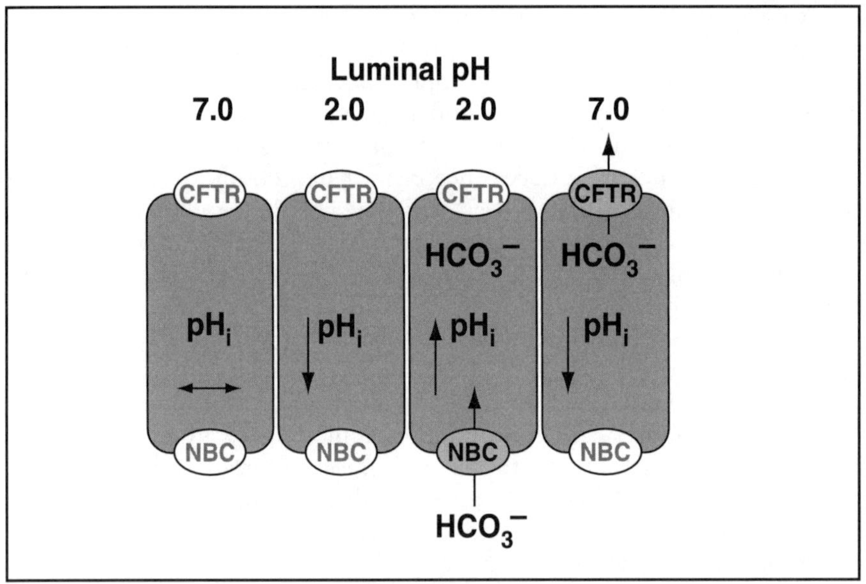

FIGURE 2. Sequential response of duodenal epithelial cells to luminal acid. *In the left panel, steady-state pH_i = ~7.1 when no acid is present. In the succeeding panels to the right, luminal acid rapidly acidifies the epithelial cells. Low pH_i decreases CFTR conductance and intracellular $[HCO_3^-]$, suppressing HCO_3^- secretion. Low pH_i also increases the activity of the basolateral sodium-bicarbonate cotransporter (pNBC1), which in turn increases cellular bicarbonate concentration. When luminal pH returns to neutrality, acid diffuses out of the cell while. The excess intracellular alkali raises pH_i over baseline (overshoot), which activates CFTR and DRA, which then increases bicarbonate secretion. In the disease cystic fibrosis, a dysfunctional CFTR and DRA limit apical HCO_3^- exit, which raises pH_i.*

function. Mucosal blood flow, as measured by laser-Doppler flowmetry, increased in response to acid perfusion (26, 37). This response differs from the gastric mucosa, which must be either injured or pre-treated with gastrin or other compound in order to induce this acid response (38, 39). Our studies revealed some novel observations about the nature of duodenal blood flow and its regulation. For example, inhibition of sodium-proton exchange (NHE) with the potent amiloride analog dimethylamiloride inhibited the hyperemic acid response. Interestingly, acidification of the cytoplasm by alternate means such as with ammonium pre-pulse or valinomycin increased blood flow (26). These studies suggested that acid must pass through the epithelial cell and exit via NHE prior to eliciting a hyperemic response. In further studies, we examined the sensing mechanisms underlying the hyperemic response. Capsazepine, an antagonist to the recently cloned vanilloid receptor, abolished the hyperemic response to acid, confirming the involvement of vanilloid receptors in the acid response. Further studies also confirmed that the hyperemic response was mediated by a well-known pathway that in-

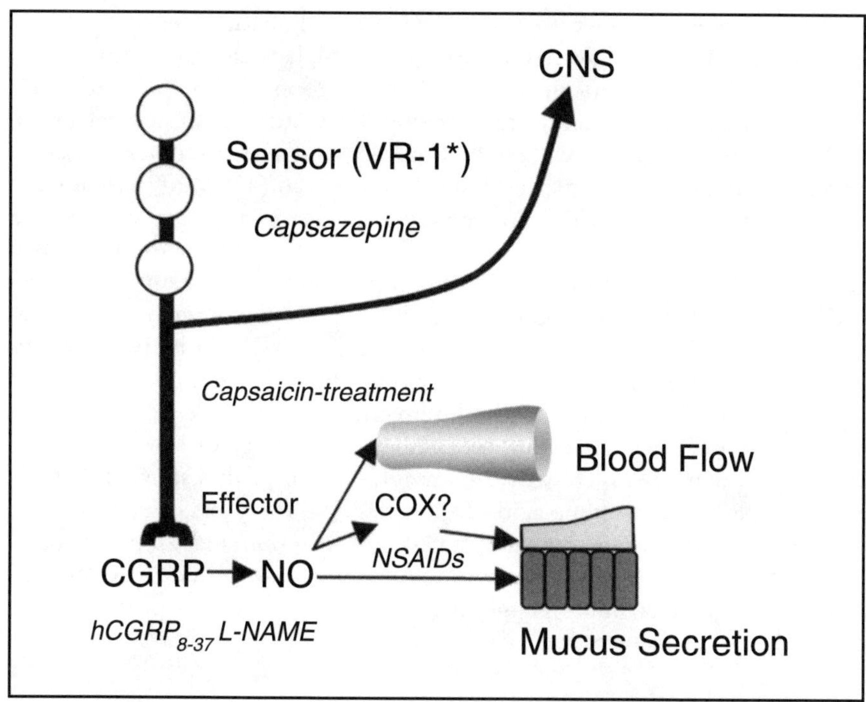

FIGURE 3. The capsaicin pathway. *Mucosal responses to luminal acid are mediated by this pathway, which includes an acid sensor, which is a vanilloid receptor, afferent nerves, and an effectors mechanism dependent on the secretion of calcitonin gene-related peptide (CGRP) and nitric oxide synthase (NOS). Prostaglandin synthesis is also involved in the regulation of mucus gel thickness. Italics denote inhibitors of each component.*

cludes afferent sensory nerves, nitric oxide release, the neuropeptide calcitonin gene–related peptide (CGRP), but was not inhibited by indomethacin, a non–selective inhibitor of cyclooxygenase. These studies provided data supporting our proposed mechanism of duodenal acid–induced hyperemia, including acid diffusion into the epithelial cell, basolateral extrusion via NHE, activation of vanilloid receptors on afferent nerves, CGRP release, with activation of endothelial nitric oxide synthesis, with production of vasodilatory nitric oxide. A scheme of proposed regulatory mechanisms for blood flow is shown in Figure 3.

Mucus Secretion

The role of mucus in duodenal mucosal defense is the subject of only a few studies. The most accepted hypothesis is that mucus stabilizes the pre-epithelial pH gradient, with neutral pH measured near the mucosa, preventing acid from entering the epithelial cells (13, 40–42). Mucus secretion is also co-regulated by the same neurohormonal and pharmacologic stimuli that increase other defense mechanisms such as bicarbonate secretion and blood flow, making it a likely candidate for being a secondary defense mechanism.

With our technique, we could optically and non-invasively measure mucus gel thickness in our anesthetized preparation (43). We found, for example, that mucus gel thickness rapidly increases in response to perfused acid, but equally rapidly decreases in thickness when the acid challenge is removed. Measurement of effluent mucus glycoprotein content was consistent with increased sloughing of mucus into the perfusate when mucus was rapidly secreted, indicating that there is a dynamic relation between mucus secretion and erosion, as has been previously hypothesized (44). When the secretion slowed, the rapid sloughing remained, thinning the gel until a new steady state occurred. A scheme depicting our concept of how mucus gel thickness is regulated is shown in Figure 4. Further studies showed that the capsaicin pathway, involving acid-sensing vanilloid receptors, afferent nerves, CGRP, and nitric oxide, regulates mucus gel secretion and that non-selective COX inhibition with indomethacin abolishes the mucus secretory response to all secretagogues, suggesting a fundamental role of prostaglandins in duodenal mucus secretion (45).

CLINICAL CORRELATE

We have formulated the "CF paradox" (18), in which we pose the question: why are duodenal ulcers not increased in patients with CF? Patients with CF, for example, have high normal acid secretion (46), and hence must take anti-secretory medications in order to diminish esophageal acid reflux and to prevent acid-mediated inactivation of pancreatic enzymes (47, 48). Furthermore, pancreatic and duodenal bicarbonate secretion are presumably impaired by the disease (23), and duodenal pH is lower than normal (49). Combined with the frequent prevalence of chronic lung disease, these patients have substantial risk for peptic ulceration. Clinical experience, and the literature, however, does not support an increased incidence of peptic ulceration in this population, but rather, it appears that the prevalence of peptic ulceration may actually be diminished (5). Our hypothesis that elevated cellular buffering power is present when the CFTR is dysfunctional and is supported by independent observations: 1) resting pH_i is elevated in cells derived from individuals with a dysfunctional CFTR (50) and 2) the apical anion exchanger DRA, the only other known apical exit pathway for bicarbonate, is downregulated when the CFTR is dysfunctional (24, 25), which would support the concept that bicarbonate is 'trapped' in the cell in CF, raising pH_i and increasing cellular buffering power. Furthermore, pH_i dysregulation in CF may influence

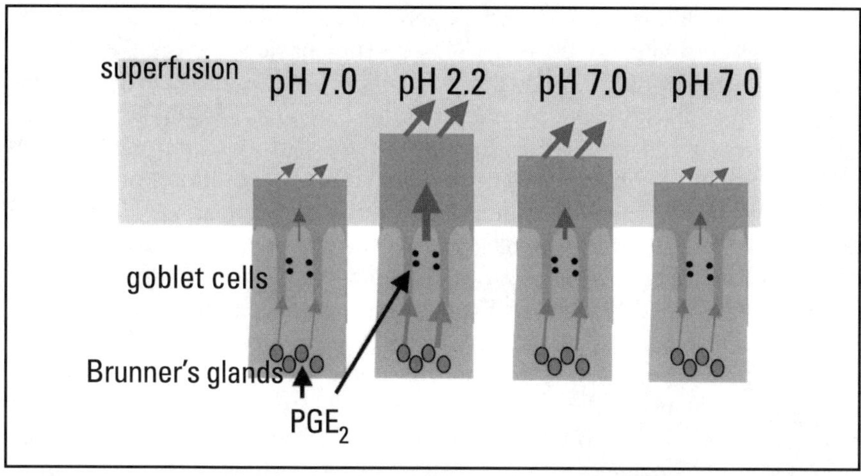

FIGURE 4. Dynamic regulation of mucus gel thickness in response to luminal acid. *In the left panel, alkaline mucus secretion and the rate of sloughing into the lumen are balanced. Luminal acid creates a sudden exocytotic burst of mucus secretion from goblet cells and Brunner's glands, which thickens the gel. The newly secreted mucus sloughs into the lumen at a higher rate, resulting in a new steady-state gel thickness. Removal of luminal acid decreases mucus secretion, decreasing gel thickness, and also initiates synthesis of new mucus granules.*

organellar pH, which in turn may mis-process secreted mucin glycoproteins (51), producing part of the CF phenotype.

We propose that the impairment of duodenal bicarbonate secretion in the disease may explain why this population may be protected from peptic ulceration. If the cells can alkali load normally via a basolateral NBC1, and by in-diffusing CO_2 converted to HCO_3^- by carbonic anhydrase, but cannot secrete bicarbonate across the apical membrane due to defective functioning of CFTR and DRA, cellular buffering may be abnormally high due to the dysfunction of the two major apical bicarbonate exit pathways. This increased cellular buffering power may then protect the epithelial cells from undue acidification due to low luminal pH.

SUMMARY AND CONCLUSIONS

Study of the duodenal response to acid has yielded novel insights into how mucosal surfaces protect themselves from a hostile environment. Exposure of the mucosa to physiologic acid solutions promptly lowered pH_i, followed by recovery after acid was removed, indicating that acid at physiologic concentrations readily diffuses into, but does not damage duodenal epithelial cells. Cellular acid then exits the cell via an amiloride-inhibitable process, presumably sodium-proton exchange (NHE1). MGT and blood flow increase promptly during acid perfusion; both decrease after acid challenge and are inhibited by vanilloid receptor antagonists or by sensory afferent denervation. Bicarbonate secretion increases following, but not during luminal acid challenge. Inhibition of cellular alkali uptake by anion transport inhibitors lowers pH_i, and increases mucosal injury, whereas inhibition of apical alkali secretion alkalinizes pH_i and diminishes injury. We propose that luminal acid diffuses into the epithelial cells, lowering pH_i. Acidic pH_i increases the activity of a basolateral NHE, acidifying the submucosal space and increasing cellular alkali loading. The acidic submucosal space activates capsaicin receptors on afferent nerves, increasing MGT and blood flow. With continued acid exposure, a new steady state with thickened mucus gel, increased blood flow, and a higher cellular buffering power protects the mucosa from acid injury. After acid challenge, mucus secretion, blood flow and pH_i return to normal, while bicarbonate secretion increases. Through these integrated mechanisms, the epithelial cells are protected from damage due to repeated pulses of concentrated gastric acid.

Cellular alkali loading in response to acid is plausible and fits well with the existing body of data correlating ulcer disease with bicarbonate secretion, in that bicarbonate secretion is the end result of cellular alkali loading, although it may not, in and of itself, be protective against acid. The alkali-loading hypothesis also fits well with the clinical observation of the sparing of CF patients from ulcer disease. Although the signal for alkali loading may be decreased pH_i, enhanced blood flow and mucus secretion in response to acid challenge rely on well-described pathways that are present in may tissues (52–54), and serve as a useful paradigm for epithelial responses to environmental stimuli.

ACKNOWLEDGMENTS

We would like to thank Drs. Eli Engel and Paul Guth for their helpful advice, and Drs. Kotaro Kaneko, Yasu Nishizaki, and Shin Tanaka for developing the experimental system used in these studies and for their invaluable intellectual contributions. Supported by Department of Veterans Affairs Merit Review Funding and National Institutes of Health, Digestive Diseases and Kidney Institute RO1 DK 54221.

REFERENCES

1. Orlando RC, Lacy ER, Tobey NA, Cowart K. Barriers to paracellular permeability in rabbit esophageal epithelium. *Gastroenterology* 1992;102:910–923.
2. Allen A, Flemström G, Garner A, Kivilaakso E. Gastroduodenal mucosal protection. *Physiol Rev* 1993; 73:823–857.
3. Aterman K. Duodenal Ulceration and Fibrocystic Pancreas Disease. *Am J Dis Child* 1961;101:210–215.

4. Fiedorek SC, Shulman RJ, Klish WJ. Endoscopic detection of peptic ulcer disease in cystic fibrosis. *Clin Pediatr (Phila)* 1986;25:243–246.

5. Rosenstein BJ, Perman JA, Kramer SS. Peptic ulcer disease in cystic fibrosis: an unusual occurrence in black adolescents [letter]. *Am J Dis Child* 1986;140:966–969.

6. Ovesen L, Bendtsen F, Tage-Jensen U, Pedersen NT, Gram BR, Rune SJ. Intraluminal pH in the stomach, duodenum, and proximal jejunum in normal subjects and patients with exocrine pancreatic insufficiency. *Gastroenterology* 1986;90:958–962.

7. Rune SJ, Viskum K. Duodenal pH values in normal controls and in patients with duodenal ulcer. *Gut* 1969;10:569–571.

8. Rhodes J, Apsimon HT, Lawrie JH. pH of the contents of the duodenal bulb in relation to duodenal ulcer. *Gut* 1966;7:502–508.

9. Rune SJ, Henriksen FW. Carbon dioxide tensions in the proximal part of the canine gastrointestinal tract. *Gastroenterology* 1969;56:758–762.

10. Hogan DL, Ainsworth MA, Isenberg JI. Review article: gastroduodenal bicarbonate secretion. *Aliment Pharm Ther* 1994;8:475–488.

11. Miller TA. Gastroduodenal mucosal defense: factors responsible for the ability of the stomach and duodenum to resist injury. *Surgery* 1988;103:389–397.

12. Säfsten B. Duodenal bicarbonate secretion and mucosal protection. *Acta Physiol Scand* 1993;Supplementum 613:1–41.

13. Flemström G, Kivilaakso E. Demonstration of a pH gradient at the luminal surface of rat duodenum *in vivo* and its dependence on mucosal alkaline secretion. *Gastroenterology* 1983;84:787–794.

14. Kiviluoto T, Ahonen M, Bäck N, Häppölä O, Mustonen H, Paimele H, Kivilaakso E. Preepithelial mucus-HCO_3^- layer protectes against intracellular acidosis in acid-exposed gastric mucosa. *Am J Physiol* 1993;264:G57–G63.

15. Quigley EM, Turnberg LA. pH of the microclimate lining human gastric and duodenal mucosa *in vivo*. Studies in control subjects and in duodenal ulcer patients. *Gastroenterology* 1987;92:1876–1884.

16. Aceti A, Celestino D, Caferro M, Casale V, Citarda F, Conti EM, Grassi A, Grilli A, Pennica A, Sciarretta F, Leri O, Ameglio F, Sebastiani A. Basophil-bound and serum immunoglobulin E directed against *Helicobacter pylori* in patients with chronic gastritis. *Gastroenterology* 1991;101:131–137.

17. Hogan DL, Rapier RC, Dreilinger A, Koss MA, Basuk PM, Weinstein WM, Nyberg LM, Isenberg J I. Duodenal bicarbonate secretion: eradication of *Helicobacter pylori* and duodenal structure and function in humans. *Gastroenterology* 1996;110:705–716.

18. Akiba Y, Furukawa O, Guth PH, Engel E, Nastaskin I, Sassani P, Dukkipatis R, Pushkin A, Kurtz I, Kaunitz JD. Cellular bicarbonate protects rat duodenal mucosa from acid-induced injury. *J Clin Invest* 2001;108:1807–1816.

19. Caroppo R, Debellis L, Valenti G, Alper S, Fromter E, Curci S. Is resting state HCO_3^- secretion in frog gastric fundus mucosa mediated by apical Cl^-–HCO_3^- exchange? *J Physiol (Lond)* 1997;499:763–771.

20. Alper SL, Rossmann H, Wilhelm S, Stuart-Tilley AK, Shmukler BE, Seidler U. Expression of AE2 anion exchanger in mouse intestine. *Am J Physiol* 1999;277:G321-G332.

21. Stuarttilley A, Sardet C, Pouyssegur J, Schwartz MA, Brown D, Alper SL. Immunolocalization of anion exchanger AE2 and cation exchanger NHE-1 in distinct adjacent cells of gastric mucosa. *Am J Physiol* 1994;266:C559-C568.

22. Hogan DL, Crombie DL, Isenberg JI, Svendsen P, Schaffalitzky dM, Ainsworth MA. Acid-stimulated duodenal bicarbonate secretion involves a CFTR-mediated transport pathway in mice. *Gastroenterology* 1997;113:533–541.

23. Pratha VS, Hogan DL, Martensson BA, Bernard J, Zhou R, Isenberg JI. Identification of transport abnormalities in duodenal mucosa and duodenal enterocytes from patients with cystic fibrosis *Gastroenterology* 2000;118:1051–1060.

24. Elgavish A, Meezan E. Altered sulfate transport via anion exchange in CFPAC is corrected by retrovirus-mediated CFTR gene transfer. *Am J Physiol* 1992;263:C176-C186.

25. Wheat VJ, Shumaker H, Burnham C, Shull GE, Yankaskas JR, Soleimani M. CFTR induces the expression of DRA along with Cl^-/HCO_3^- exchange activity in tracheal epithelial cells. *Am J Physiol* 2000;279:C62-C71.

26. Akiba Y, Kaunitz JD. Regulation of intracellular pH and blood flow in rat duodenal epithelium *in vivo. Am J Physiol* 1999;276:G293-G302.

27. Boron WF. Intracellular pH transients in giant barnacle muscle fibers. *Am J Physiol* 1977;233:C61–C73.

28. Akiba Y, Furukawa O, Guth PH, Engel E, Nastaskin I, Kaunitz JD. Acute adaptive cellular base uptake in rat duodenal epithelium. *Am J Physiol* 2001;280:G1083-G1092.

29. Ainsworth MA, Amelsberg M, Hogan DL, Isenberg JI. Acid-base transport in isolated rabbit duodenal villus and crypt cells. *Scand J Gastroenterol* 1996;31:1069–1077.

30. Shumaker H, Amlal H, Frizzell R, Ulrich CD, Soleimani M. CFTR drives Na^+-$nHCO_3^-$ cotransport in pancreatic duct cells: a basis for defective HCO_3^- secretion in CF. *Am J Physiol* 1999;276:C16–C25.

31. Praetorius J, Hager H, Nielsen S, Aalkjaer C, Friis UG, Ainsworth MA, Johansen T. Molecular and functional evidence for electrogenic and electroneutral Na^+-HCO_3^- cotransporters in murine duodenum. *Am J Physiol* 2001;280:G332-G343.

32. Feitelberg SP, Hogan DL, Koss MA, Isenberg JI. pH threshold for human duodenal bicarbonate secretion and diffusion of CO_2. *Gastroenterology* 1992;102:1252–1258.

33. Reddy MM, Kopito RR, Quinton PM. Cytosolic pH regulates GCl through control of phosphorylation states of CFTR. *Am J Physiol* 1998;275:C1040-C1047.

34. Li DS, Raybould H, Quintero E, Guth PH. Calcitonin gene-related peptide mediates the gastric hyperemic response to acid back-diffusion. *Gastroenterology* 1992;102:1124–1128.

35. Merchant NB, Dempsey DT, Grabowski MW, Rizzo M, Ritchie WPJ. Capsaicin-induced gastric mucosal hyperemia and protection: the role of calcitonin gene-related peptide. *Surgery* 1994;116:419–425.

36. Svanes K, Gislason H, Guttu K, Herfjord JK, Fevang J, Gronbech JE. Role of blood flow in adaptive protection of the cat gastric mucosa. *Gastroenterology* 1991;100:1249–1258.

37. Akiba Y, Guth PH, Engel E, Nastaskin I, Kaunitz JD. Acid-sensing pathways of rat duodenum. *Am J Physiol* 1999;277:G268-G274.

38. Holzer P. Chemosensitive afferent nerves in the regulation of gastric blood flow and protection. *Adv Exp Med Biol* 1995;371B:891–895.

39. Tanaka S, Akiba Y, Kaunitz JD. Pentagastrin gastroprotection against acid is related to H_2 receptor activation but not acid secretion. *Gut* 1998;43:334–341.

40. Allen A, Hutton D, McQueen S, Garner A. Dimensions of gastroduodenal surface pH gradients exceed those of adherent mucus gel layers. *Gastroenterology* 1983;85:463–476.

41. Kivilaakso E, Flemström G. Surface pH gradient in gastroduodenal mucosa. *Scand J Gastroenterol* 1984;105:49–52.

42. Turnberg LA. Gastric mucus, bicarbonate and pH gradients in mucosal protection. *Clin Invest Med* 1987;10:178–180.

43. Akiba Y, Guth PH, Engel E, Nastaskin I, Kaunitz JD. Dynamic regulation of mucus gel thickness in rat duodenum. *Am J Physiol* 2000;279:G437-G447.

44. Keogh JP, Allen A, Garner A. Relationship between gastric mucus synthesis, secretion and surface gel erosion measured in amphibian stomach *in vitro. Clin Exp Pharmacol Physiol* 1997;24:844–849.

45. Akiba Y, Furukawa O, Guth PH, Engel E, Nastaskin I, Kaunitz JD. Sensory pathways and cyclooxygenase regulate mucus gel thickness in rat duodenum. *Am J Physiol* 2001;280:G470-G474.

46. Cox KL, Isenberg JN, Ament ME. Gastric acid hypersecretion in cystic fibrosis. *J Pediatr Gastroenterol Nutr* 1982;1:559–565.

47. Youngberg CA, Berardi RR, Howatt WF, Hyneck ML, Amidon GL, Meyer JH, Dressman JB. Comparison of gastrointestinal pH in cystic fibrosis and healthy subjects. *Dig Dis Sci* 1987;32:472–480.

48. Robinson PJ, Smith AL, Sly PD. Duodenal pH in cystic fibrosis and its relationship to fat malabsorption. *Dig Dis Sci* 1990;35:1299–1304.

49. Barraclough M, Taylor CJ. Twenty-four hour ambulatory gastric and duodenal pH profiles in cystic fibrosis: effect of duodenal hyperacidity on pancreatic enzyme function and fat absorption. *J Pediatr Gastroenterol Nutr* 1996;23:45–50.

50. Elgavish A. High intracellular pH in CFPAC: a pancreas cell line from a patient with cystic fibrosis is lowered by retrovirus-mediated CFTR gene transfer. *Biochem Biophys Res Commun* 1991;180:342–348.

51. Poschet JF, Boucher JC, Tatterson L, Skidmore J, Van Dyke RW, Deretic V. Molecular basis for defective glycosylation and Pseudomonas pathogenesis in cystic fibrosis lung. *Proc Natl Acad Sci USA* 2001; 98:13972–13977.
52. Hua XY, Wong S, Jinno S, Yaksh TL. Pharmacology of calcitonin gene related peptide release from sensory terminals in the rat trachea. *Can J Physiol Pharmacol* 1995;73:999–1006.
53. Rybarova S, Kocisova M, Mirossay L. Role of afferent sensory neurones in gastric injury/protection. *Physiol Res* 1994;43:347–354.
54. Li DS, Raybould HE, Quintero E, Guth PH. Role of calcitonin gene-related peptide in gastric hyperemic response to intragastric capsaicin. *Am J Physiol* 1991;261:G657-G661.

Gut-Brain Peptides in the New Millennium, edited by Y. Taché
CURE Foundation, Los Angeles, CA. © 2002

34

Topography of Cell Proliferation in the Gastric Ulcer Margin of the Rat

Herbert F. Helander
Discovery, AstraZeneca AB, Mölndal, Sweden

INTRODUCTION

During the early phase of gastric ulcer healing, the epithelial cells of the ulcer margin divide at a high rate and start to migrate across the ulcer bed, which is eventually covered by these cells. Previous investigations on experimental ulcers of the rat oxyntic mucosa have demonstrated profound changes in the structure and function of the epithelial cells of the ulcer margin. Thus, parietal cells were largely absent within a few hundred microns from the ulcer edge, and those few remaining appeared to be very immature (1). In the bottom of the glands, immature mucous neck cells showing frequent mitotic figures replaced the zymogen cells. These changes were interpreted as signs of dedifferentiation, but it was uncertain whether these immature cells arose from pre-existing mature cells, or if they were formed by mitosis after ulcer induction.

Subsequent studies by in situ hybridization on the ulcer margin demonstrated that the mRNA levels for the H^+, K^+-ATPase (2) and pepsinogen C (3) were below the limit of detection, indicating that the production of hydrochloric acid (1) and pepsinogen C was severely depressed. In contrast, the mRNA levels for carbonic anhydrase II in the ulcer margin appeared to be elevated (4).

The present study extends these investigations by focusing on the topography of cell division in the ulcer margin. Particular attention is paid to the hypertrophic portion of the ulcer margin, which bulges into the ulcer area.

MATERIAL AND METHODS

Animals

Forty-two female Sprague-Dawley rats (Möllegård, Skensved, Denmark) weighing about 200–220 g were used in this study. Before surgery, two

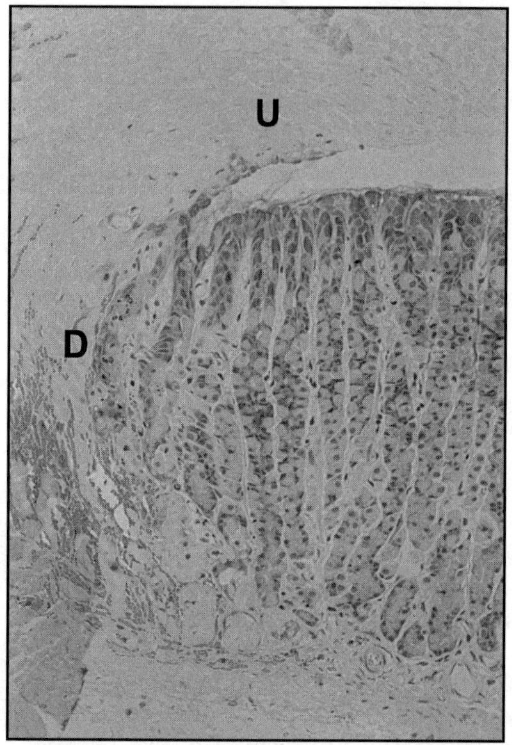

FIGURE 1. *Ulcer margin from rat after 1 day of healing. Part of the ulcer bed (U) is already covered by a few flat epithelial cells. There is a clear demarcation (D) between the ulcer margin and the necrotic tissues. × 100.*

animals were kept in each cage; after surgery they were kept in individual cages. The room was regulated with respect to temperature (18–22°C), humidity (about 55%) and light/dark cycle (12/12 h). The rats had free access to R–3 food (Lactamin AB, Stockholm, Sweden) and to drinking water. They were allowed at least one week of acclimatization before surgery. Surgical procedures, as well as sacrifice, were carried out between 9 and 11 a.m. The Ethical Committee of Gothenburg University approved of the study.

Study Design

On the first day of the study, the rats were anesthetized with isoflurane and an ulcer about 7 mm in diameter, was produced in the oxyntic mucosa by exposing the serosa of the gastric corpus to 80% acetic acid for 60 sec, as previously described (1). This operation was carried out in 4 groups each comprising 6 rats; these rats were killed after 1, 2 or 6 (2 groups) days. Another 2 groups with 6 non-ulcer control animals in each were killed after 1 or 6

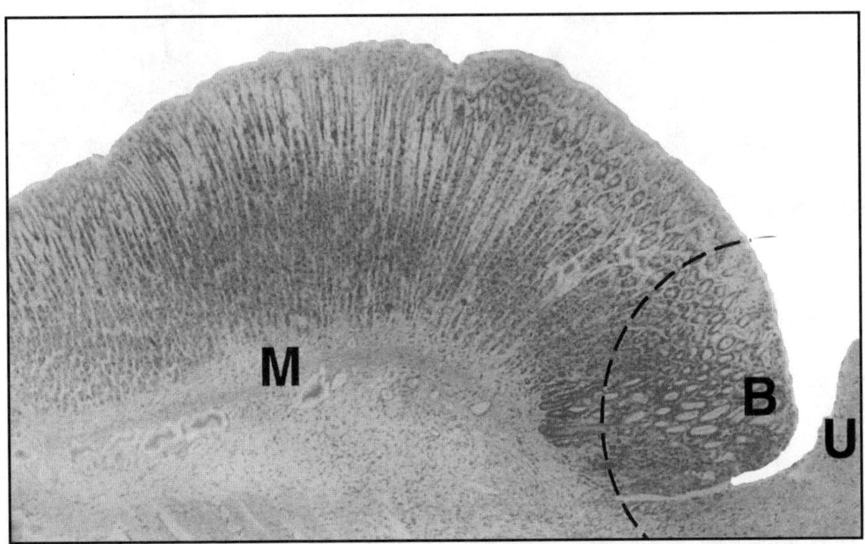

FIGURE 2. *Ulcer margin from rat after 6 days of healing. Close to the ulcer (U) the glands are tilted and the mucosa bulges into the ulcer (B). M, muscularis mucosae. The area within $^1/2$-mm from the ulcer is limited by the circle. × 55.*

days. Six sham-operated rats were also killed after 6 days. All rats were equipped with an osmotic minipump (model 2ML1; Alzet, Palo Alto, CA, USA) implanted subcutaneously in the back of the rats. The insertion of pumps took place on the first day of study, except for one group of 6-day ulcer rats, in which the pumps were put in place on day 5. The pumps contained (methyl-^{3}H)-thymidine, which was released continuously; the 24-hr dose was calculated to 0.1 µCi/g body weight. Before insertion, the pumps were kept in saline at 37°C overnight. After surgery, the animals were immediately provided with food and water.

After 1, 2 or 6 days, following an over-night fast with free access to drinking water, the animals were anesthetized with isoflurane. Vascular perfusion with 4% buffered formaldehyde was carried out as previously described (1). The stomach was then removed and the ulcer margin excised. The tissues were postfixed in formaldehyde and embedded in Historesin® (Heraeus Kulzer GmbH, Heidelberg, Germany). Two-micron thick sections were cut perpendicularly to the mucosal surface, picked up on glass slides, dried and dipped in RPN40 nuclear emulsion (Amersham Pharmacia Biotech AB, Uppsala, Sweden) for autoradiography. After exposure for about 3 months in the dark, the preparations were developed according to the recommendations of the manufacturer, and stained with hematoxylin and eosin. All sections were cover slipped, coded and examined in the light microscope using an ×40 oil immersion objective lens.

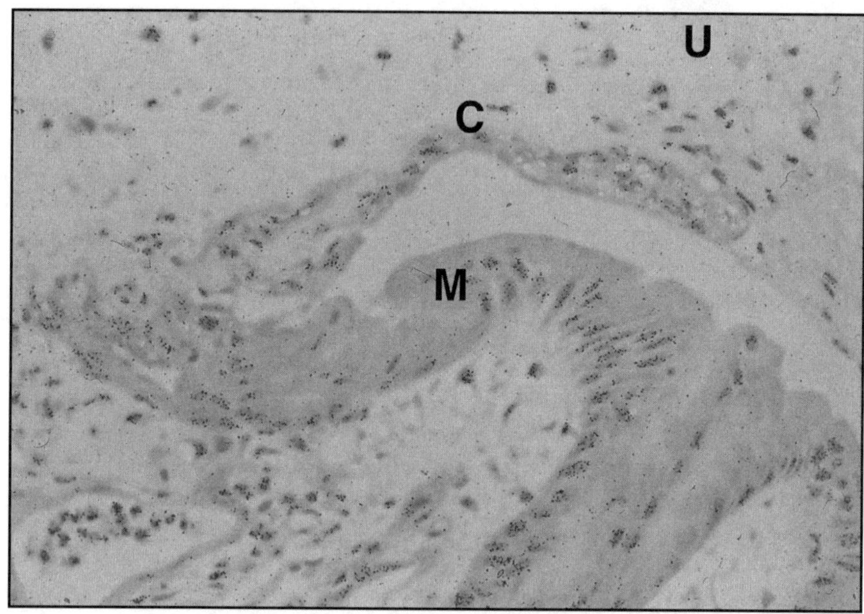

FIGURE 3. *Micrograph of ulcer margin bordering on the ulcer bed after 6 days of healing. Small dense silver grains indicate cell divisions. A monolayer of labeled cuboidal or flat epithelial cells covers the peripheral portion of the ulcer bed. These cells most probably have migrated from the ulcer margin. × 300.*

Cells were considered labeled if more than 4 silver grains were found over, or close to, the nucleus. The counting of nuclei was carried out in numerous fields (usually 173×173 μm or 200×200 μm) of the ulcer margin, covering the area within $1/2$-mm from the ulcer edge or more. Within this area, the mean total number of cell nuclei counted per rat ranged between 820 (in the 1-day ulcer rats) and 1250 (in the 2-day ulcer rats). In undamaged oxyntic mucosa, counting was carried out in 5 swaths (173 or 200 μm wide) each comprising 5 equally thick layers of the mucosa parallel to the mucosal surface; the total number of cell nuclei counted per rat averaged about 2700. The results were averaged for each level.

Labeling index (LI) is expressed as percentage (means ± SEM) of labeled cells, i.e., the number of labeled nuclei divided by the total number of nuclei.

RESULTS

Microscopic Survey

After 1 day of healing, the ulcer margin was well demarcated from the ulcer bed (Figure 1). After 6 days, the mucosa of the ulcer margin often appeared

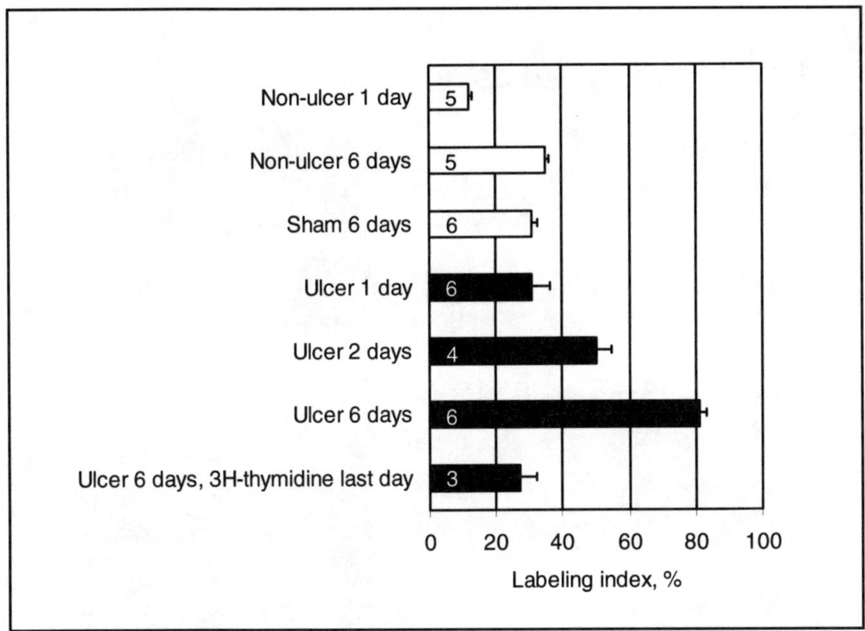

FIGURE 4. *Labeling index of epithelial cells (excluding the parietal cells) in non-ulcer control rats and in ulcer rats (means + SEM). The data were calculated from normal ventral, oxyntic mucosa in the non-ulcer rats. In the ulcer rats the data were obtained from the ulcer margin within 1/2-mm from the ulcer. Numbers within bars indicate number of rats.*

thicker than normal and its middle and upper portions bulged into the ulcer (Figure 2). A deep groove, extending down to the bottom of the glands, now formed a clear demarcation between the ulcer margin and the ulcer bed. From the gland epithelium closest to the ulcer a single layer of cuboidal or flat cells was often seen to extend for a few hundred microns covering the peripheral portion of the ulcer bed (Figures 1 and 3). The glands closest to the ulcer edge were tilted towards the ulcer and their lumen was frequently dilated.

Labeling of Epithelial Cells

Non-ulcer Controls

After 1 and 6 days of continuous administration of ^{3}H-thymidine the LI of the normal oxyntic mucosa was 12 ± 1.1% and 35 ± 1.2%, respectively (Figure 4). In the sham operated controls given ^{3}H-thymidine for 6 days, the LI averaged 31 ± 1.7%. The great majority of the labeled cells were found in the superficial regions of the epithelium (Figure 5). No parietal cells were labeled.

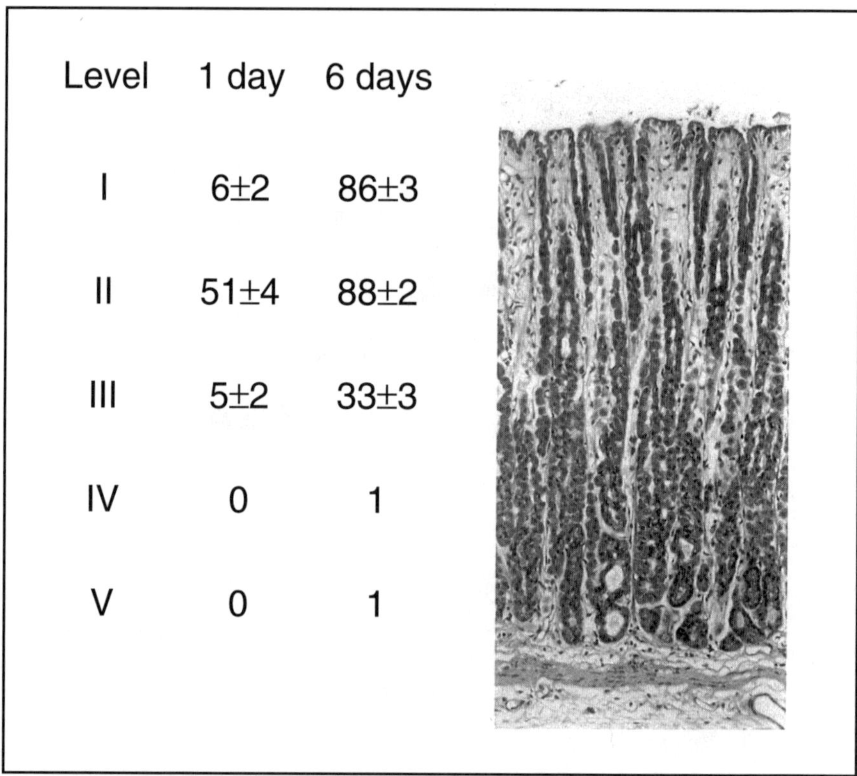

FIGURE 5. *LI's of oxyntic mucosa from non-ulcer control rats given 1 day or 6 days infusion of ^{3}H-thymidine. The oxyntic mucosa has been divided into 5 equally thick layers (I–V), parallel to the mucosal surface. × 140.*

Ulcer Rats

The LI's were increased above control values in an area within 1/2-mm from the ulcer edge (Figure 4). Parietal cells were hardly ever labeled, and therefore, the LI's were calculated for non-parietal epithelial cells. The highest LI's were generally observed in the cells close to the ulcer bed (Figure 6). At 1 mm from the ulcer edge the labeling patterns (i.e., the percentage labeled cells and their distribution in the various layers of the mucosa) were similar to that of normal oxyntic mucosa. After 1 and 6 days of healing, the LI's within 1/2-mm from the ulcer were about 2 1/2 times those of the corresponding non-ulcer controls (Figure 4). After 6 days of healing the LI was above 90% in 6 of the 8 regions found within 1/2-mm from the ulcer edge. The LI in the 6-day ulcer rats given ^{3}H-thymidine only during the last 24 hrs averaged 27 ± 5.4%.

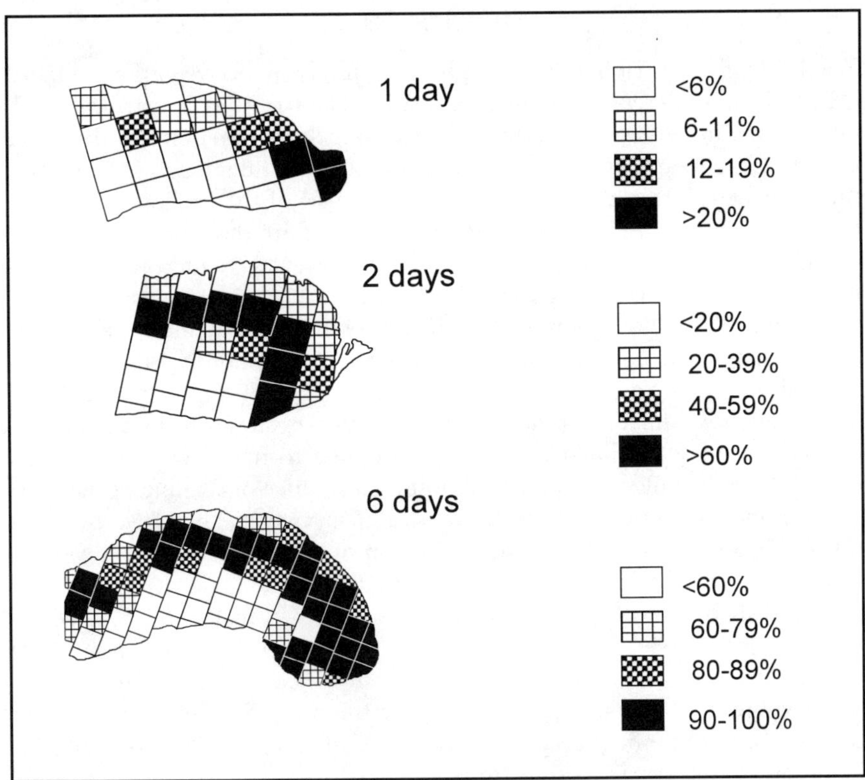

FIGURE 6. *Schematic representation of the labeling index topography in rat ulcer margins after 1, 2 and 6 days of healing. The data from the 6-day ulcer margin were obtained from the section in Figure 2. The LI's have been determined separately in each region, as indicated. The ulcer bed is to the right; 1 and 2 days $\times$ 30; six days $\times$ 25.*

Cells in the Lamina Propria

In comparison with the epithelial cells, the number of cell nuclei in the lamina propria was low. In the 6-day ulcer margin the epithelial cells were 4 times as many, and in the 6-day non-ulcer controls almost 7 times as many, as the lamina propria cells. About $1/4$ of the lamina propria cells were vessels and the rest were mainly inflammatory cells and smooth muscle cells. No attempts were carried out to identify other types of cells.

In the 6-day ulcer rats, the LI for both vessels and non-vessel cells was around 50%, a significant increase from the LI in the non-ulcer control rats and the 1-day ulcer rats, where LI's were only a few percent. Many of the labeled non-vessel cells were eosinophilic leukocytes. It should be pointed out that the calculations of LI's are based on a comparatively small number of cells.

DISCUSSION

The healing of gastric ulcers depends on an interplay between the epithelial cells and the underlying granulation tissue orchestrated by a host of growth factors and hormones. After the acute phase, the epithelium in the ulcer margin starts to provide epithelial cells destined to migrate over and cover the ulcer bed. This is reflected by an increased LI of the mucosa which extends up to 600 μm from the injury; lasting for more than 14 days (6).

In the ulcer margin, the present study shows a successive increase of the epithelial cell LI (not counting parietal cells) from 31% after 1 day to 81% after 6 days of healing. Twenty-seven % of the nuclei in the 6-day ulcer rats became labeled during the last 24 hours before sacrifice. This indicates that many of the cells in the ulcer margin divide more than once during the 6 days after ulcer induction, and/or that the rate of cell division varies during the healing period. The LI was highest in the regions closest to the ulcer, more specifically, the middle bulge region. The almost total absence of labeling of the parietal cells in this region indicates that these are "survivors". They have, thus, not formed by mitosis in cells after the induction of the ulcers.

It is concluded that 6 days after ulcer induction, the great majority of epithelial cells of the ulcer margin, within 1/2-mm from the ulcer, have divided at least once. An exception was the parietal cells, which did not divide. The rate of epithelial cell proliferation was highest closest to the ulcer where the hypertrophic mucosa faces the ulcer. Studies are under way to determine the influence of various agents, including gastrin, on cell proliferation in the gastric ulcer margin.

ACKNOWLEDGMENTS

Ms. Ulrika Hallin provided skilled technical assistance.

REFERENCES

1. Helander HF. Morphological studies on the margin of the gastric corpus ulcer in the rat. *J Submicroscop Cytol* 1983;15:627–643.

2. Bamberg K, Nylander S, Helander KG, Lundberg LG, Sachs G, Helander HF. In situ hybridization of mRNA for the gastric H^+K^+-ATPase in rat oxyntic mucosa. *Biochim Biophys Acta* 1994;1190: 355–359.

3. Helander HF, Weijdegård B, Bamberg K. The expression of pepsinogen mRNA in normal gastroduodenal mucosa and the gastric ulcer margin of the rat. *Histochem and Cell Biol* 1996;105:163–169.

4. Helander HF, Weijdegård B, Bamberg K. Localization of mRNA for carbonic anhydrase II (CAII) in rat gastro-duodenal mucosa. *Molec Biol of the Cell* 1995;6:310a.

5. Li H, Helander HF. Hypergastrinemia increases the proliferation of gastro-duodenal epithelium during gastric ulcer healing in rats. *Dig Dis Sci* 1996;41:40–48.

6. Helpap B, Hattori T, Gedigk P. Repair of gastric ulcer. A cell kinetic study. *Virchows Arch [Pathol Anat]* 1981;392:159–170.

7. Håkanson R, Blom H, Carlsson E, Larsson H, Ryberg B, Sundler F. Hypergastrinemia produces trophic effects in stomach but not in pancreas and intestines. *Gastroenterology* 1986;96:723–729.

Gut-Brain Peptides in the New Millennium, edited by Y. Taché
CURE Foundation, Los Angeles, CA. © 2002

35

Prospective Therapeutic Applications of Cholecystokinin–B/Gastrin Receptor Antagonists for Gastrointestinal Disorders: Preclinical Studies

Yoshiaki Goto,[1] Atsushi Maeda,[2] and Katsuko Yamashita[2]
[1] *Clinical Research Division, Nippon Colin Co., Ltd.*
[2] *Institute of Geriatrics, Tokyo Women's Medical College*
[1] *2700-1 Hayashi, Komaki 485-8501, Japan*
[2] *2-15, Shibuya, Shibuya-ku, Tokyo 150-0002, Japan*

INTRODUCTION

The site of action of gastrointestinal hormones potentially provides novel therapeutic targets with respect to drug discovery for digestive diseases therapy. In particular, modulation of the trophic actions of gastrin may have therapeutic application for digestive diseases. The development of potential selective CCK–B/gastrin (G) receptor antagonists has been under extensive investigation over the last decade and resulted in the development of novel non-peptide CCK–B/G antagonists (1–15). It is, however, difficult to predict the structure-activity relations among the newly synthesized compounds and chemical moieties of active compounds (1–15).

Non-peptide ureidoacetamides, originally developed by Rhone–Poulenc Rorer, are potent and selective ligands for CCK–B/G (16–18). The lead candidates of their compounds, display a high affinity for CCK–B/G receptors with a 100 - 1000 fold preferential selectivity compared with CCK–A receptors. In the present study, we describe our recent progress to develop a prototype of non-peptide CCK–B/G antagonists. We also discuss the acid rebound phenomena after long-term treatment with omeprazole (OMP) and CCK–B/G antagonists in relation with the hypergastrinemia (HG) during achlorhydria.

Materials and Experimental Methods

Receptor Binding Assays to Human CCK-B/G and CCK-A Receptors
A stable transformed Chinese hamster ovary cell line (CHO) was established according to a standard procedure; briefly, the coding region of human

CCK-B/G and CCK-A receptors was subcloned to give an expression vector carrying a neomycin-resistant gene. A binding assay was conducted with [^{125}I]Tyr-gastrin or [^{125}I]BH–CCK-8 at pH 7.4. The specific binding was determined as the difference between the total and the non-specific binding in the presence of human gastrin-17(hG-17) or CCK-8.

Gastric Acid Response to Secretagogues in the Anesthetized Rats

Acid output was determined according to the previously described method (19) in anesthetized male Sprague-Dawley rats. A tracheostomy was performed and the esophagus and the pylorus were ligated. Then, a double lumen plastic gastric cannula was inserted into the forestomach. The gastric lumen was rinsed once every 10 min and each effluent was titrated to pH 7.0. After the basal period, the acid output was stimulated by intravenous infusion of pentagastrin (PG) at 16 µg/kg/h for 120 min, human gastrin-17 (hG-17) at the doses of 1 and 4 µg/kg/h for 30 min each dose, or by subcutaneous administration of histamine. Acid output response was compared as 10 min time course response (µEq.H$^+$/10min) or integrated acid response (net increase in acid output) for 120 min after each secretagogue. Test compounds and CCK-B/G antagonists were administered intraduodenally or intravenously, respectively before the onset of the secretagogue challenge.

Long-term Treatment with Omeprazole

There is a paucity of experimental models established to study the acid-rebound after long-term achlorhydria. Rats were treated with OMP orally for one day up to 4 weeks. Three or 10 days after the onset of OMP treatment, rats were subjected to acid secretory responses to graded doses of hG-17 followed by histamine. Histological examination of enterochromoffin-like (ECL) cells hyperplasia was undertaken by counting the numbers of chromogranin staining cells 4 weeks after OMP treatment. Serum gastrin levels were also radioimmunologically determined with and without concomitant administration of CCK-B/G antagonists. Gastric histidine decarboxylase (HDC) activity was also determined by *ex vivo* production of $^{14}CO_2$ from the labeled histidine.

RESULTS

1. Antisecretory Activity of CCK-B/G receptor Antagonists

The influence of prototypes of CCK-B/G antagonists such as DA-4161, D51-9927 and D61-1608, as well as DA-4161 and YM-022 (chemical structures illustrated in Figure 1), was examined by intraduodenal or intravenous administration 30 or 10 min prior to PG infusion, respectively. In rats with an acid secretory response to PG and its complete inhibition

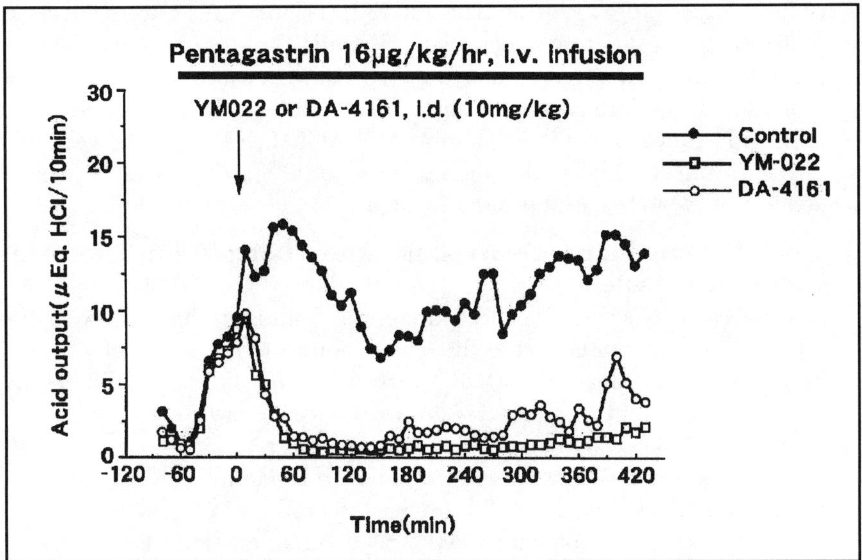

FIGURE 1. *Chemical structure of CCK-B/G antagonists: YM-022 and ureidoacetamide compound, DA-4161.*

FIGURE 2. *Effects of DA-4161 and YM-022 on acid secretory response to PG. DA-4161 and YM-022 were intraduodenally administered 30 min after intravenous PG infusion. Each dot represents the mean ± SEM of 6–9 experiments.*

by CCK-B/G antagonists were confirmed, as shown in Figure 2. Continuous intravenous infusion of PG (16 µg/kg/hr) resulted in a plateau acid output levels approximately 90 min after the administration. Intraduodenal or intravenous administration of prototype compounds such as DA-4161, D51-4984, D51-9927 and D61-1608, dose-dependently inhibited the acid output evoked by PG (Figure 2). Both of DA-4161 and YM-022, (10 mg/kg) completely abolished the acid response to PG. The integrated 120 min acid output was calculated with and without CCK-B/G antagonists. The parenteral (oral) ED_{50s} of D51-9927 and D61-1608 were estimated for both as 0.5 mg/kg while the systemic (i.v.) ED_{50s} were 4 µg/kg, and 2.3 µg/kg, respectively. The corresponding oral and systemic ED_{50s} for YM-022 were 1.9 mg/kg and 1.3 µg/kg, respectively. The ratio of the oral and intravenous i.v. ED_{50s} of D51-9927, D61-1608 and YM-022 were 125, 220, and 145, respectively. Both D51-9927 and D61-1608 were ineffective to antagonize the acid responses to histamine and bethanechol at doses 10 time higher than the ED_{50} inhibiting PG stimulation. In fact, D61-1608 and its ester compound D51-9927, showed remarkable *in situ* intestinal bioavailability improvement compared with the mother compound, whilst the absorption rate of YM-022 was demonstrated to be extremely limited.

2. Antiulcer Activities

Acute gastric mucosal lesions (AGML) were developed by oral administration of 300 mg/kg of aspirin. CCK-B/G antagonists were given as pretreatment at different doses (3, 10, 30 and 100 mg/kg, orally) 30 min prior to aspirin dosing. Aspirin induced AGML within 5 h with ulcer index of 50–74 mm in total length. D51-9927 and D61-1608 dose-dependently prevented the development of AGML. YM-022 showed prophylactic effect only at the highest dose (100 mg/kg). The anti-ulcer activity of DA-4161 is illustrated in Figure 3.

3. Acid Rebound and Hyperplasia After Long-Term Treatment with Omeprazole

Acid Rebound Response. The most interesting finding in this study was that CCK-B/G antagonists restore the acid rebound responses to hG-17 and histamine after long-term OMP treatment. HG-17 dose-dependently stimulated acid output in control group. Acid secretory response to 4 µg/kg/hr of hG-17 was markedly augmented after 2 and 4 weeks OMP treatment (Figure 4). Gastric acid response to histamine was also potentiated in OMP-treated group. The hypersusceptibility of acid production after 4 weeks treatment with OMP was maintained for at least ten days after the last treatment. Acid rebound responses developed after long-term treatment with OMP were clearly prevented by CCK-B/G antagonists including YM-022.

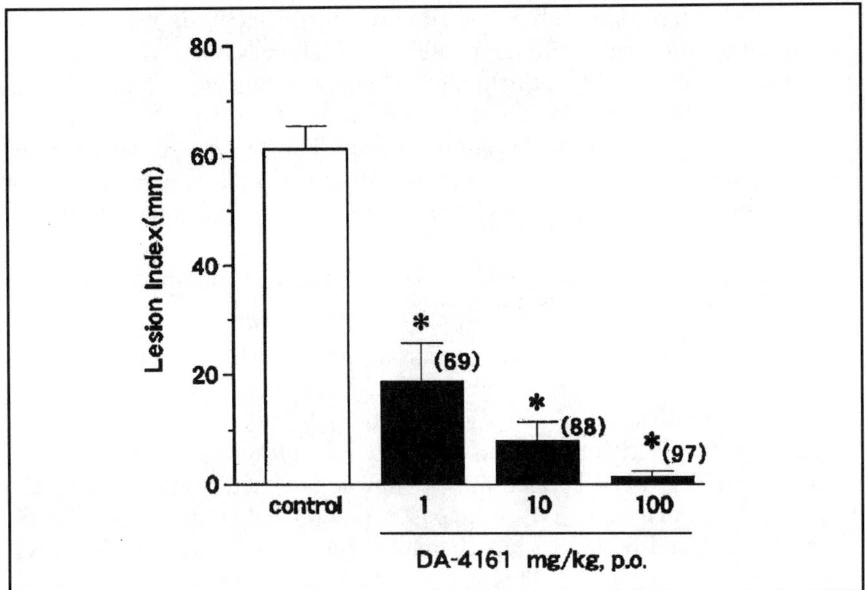

FIGURE 3. *Anti-ulcer activity of DA-4161 in rats. Gastric ulcers were induced by oral administration of aspirin (300 mg/kg). Five hours after aspirin ingestion, rodents were euthanized and the gastric mucosal lesions determined. All data indicate the mean±SEM. Statistically significant from control at ★: P < 0.05. Figures in the parenthesis indicate % inhibition.*

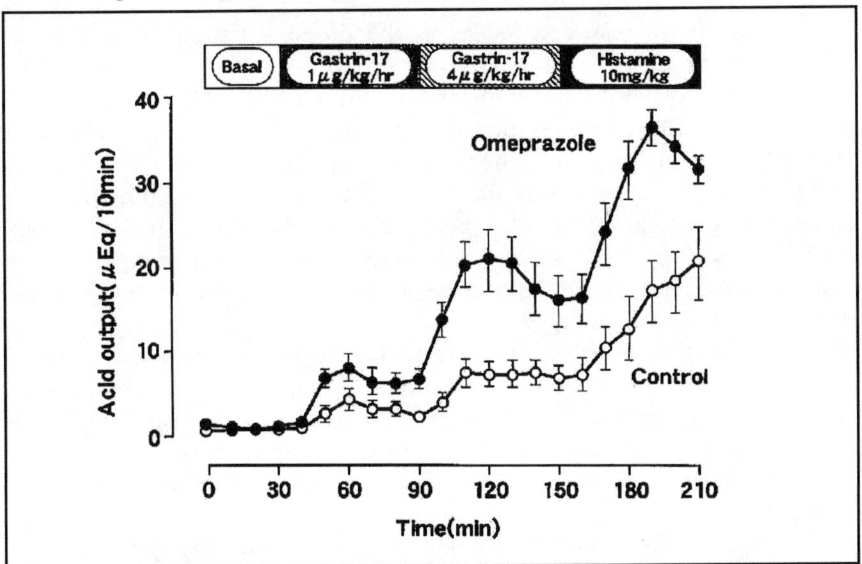

FIGURE 4. *Gastric acid rebound responses to 4 weeks treatment with omeprazole in rats. Three days after the final omeprazole administration, gastric secretory responses were examined in the anesthetized rat. Each dot represents the mean ± SEM of 5 animal studies.*

ECL-Cell Hyperplasia. Hypergastrinemia during achlorhydria has been postulated to cause a mitogenic effect on ECL cells. This was confirmed in our present study. The thickness of the gastric mucosa and the number of ECL cells were significantly increased in the OMP treated group, compared with those in the control group. The hyperplasia of gastrointestinal mucosa caused by OMP was restored by concomitant treatment with the various CCK-B/G antagonists. Serum gastrin levels in the OMP-treated group were elevated but none of CCK-B/G antagonists affect gastrin levels, though CCK-B/G antagonists alone resulted in a slight increment of circulating gastrin values.

Gastric Mucosal HDC. In order to gain insight into the mechanisms of action of ureidoacetamides, we examined the influence of CCK-B/G compounds on gastric HDC activity. D61-1608, did not cause any significant effect on basal activity of gastric HDC *ex vivo*. However, the activation of gastric HDC evoked by feeding was almost completely abolished by the CCK-B/G antagonist. By contrast, D61-1608 failed to suppress HDC activity induced by PG or hG-17 whilst the acid response to gastrin was completely antagonized. This suggests that gastric HDC activity is not implicated in the acid response to PG or hG-17.

DISCUSSION

Long term HG in man and rodent has been demonstrated to cause ECL-cell hyperplasia (20–27). There are large proportions of gastrin receptors on pancreatic tumors and colon cancers (28–36). Direct trophic effects of gastrin and CCK on gastrointestinal and pancreatic tumor cells *in vitro* have currently been investigated. The possible implication of gastrin in tumor growth has been supported by anti-tumor activity of newly synthesized gastrin receptor antagonists. Evidence strongly suggests that gastrin plays substantial roles in gastrointestinal and pancreatic tumor cell growth and also that gastrin receptor antagonists may provide a novel pharmacological approach to anti-cancer therapy.

The CCK-B/G receptors are located principally on histamine secreting ECL cells, parietal cells and somatostatin-secreting D cells of the stomach and widely throughout the central nervous system. Both gastrin and CCK can activate this receptor equivalently. In the periphery, gastrin is the predominant hormone acting on CCK-B/G receptors, while in the brain it is mainly CCK.

Gastrin is one of the classic peptide hormones regulating gastric acid secretion and mucosal cell function (21, 26, 30). Hypergastrinemia thus leads to ECL cell hyperplasia evolving into ECL carcinoid tumors as well as parietal cell hyperplasia in rats. Certain gastrointestinal and lung tumor cell lines express CCK-B/G receptors. It is likely that gastrin may play a role in normal colon proliferation and that HG can act as a tumor promoting factor. Effects of gastrin can be blocked by specific CCK-B/G antagonists or by use of monoclonal antibodies to neutralize circulating gastrin. The principal acute effects of gastrin neutralization or receptor blockage are presumed to inhibit acid secretion and to suppress histamine release and HDC activity in ECL cells (37–39). The chronic prolonged neutralization of gastrin may result in preventing hyperplasia of ECL cells and parietal cells. These effects are consistent with the absence of acid secretion and decreased numbers of ECL cells and parietal cells found in transgenic mice in which either gastrin or CCK receptors have been eliminated by recombinant technology.

The most widely prescribed drugs in the United States and Europe are proton pump inhibitors (PPIs). A major adverse effect of PPIs is that they cause HG due to achlorhydria, resulting in parietal cell hyperplasia and acid rebound. These effects are reproducible and it is possible to design experimental trials to assess gastrin receptor antagonists. A major potential clinical feature for CCK-B/G antagonists will be whether these antagonists can reverse parietal cell hyperplasia and acid rebound. Ideally, such agents may evoke parietal cell hypoplasia and counteract acid rebound during long-term treatment of reflux esophagitis. Alternatively, CCK-B/G antagonists may be clinically useful for treatment of severe reflux esophagitis.

Since gastrin is the major regulator of HDC, CCK-B/G antagonists may lead to depletion of ECL cell histamine and extend the period of time in which the stomach is refractory to acid stimulation. Combined with the antitrophic action on parietal cells, CCK-B/G antagonists may emerge as one of the best drugs to manage acid secretion including for long-term use. Although HG-induced ECL cell hyperplasia in humans is less pronounced than in rats, ECL-cell carcinoid tumors occur in some patients with atrophic gastritis.

Potential antitumor effects of gastrin antagonists in humans are less predictable from current available data. There are no tumors other than ECL cell carcinoids that uniformly express growth-stimulating gastrin receptors. However, the use of gastrin receptor antagonists as adjunctive treatment in gastrointestinal and lung cancers would be a possible area for research once an agent has been approved for human use as a gastric antisecretory agent.

The only well-recognized effects of gastrin in humans are the stimulation of gastric acid secretion and cell proliferation of parietal cells and, to a lesser extent, ECL. Reversal of the effects of induced HG seems attractive for initial drug evaluation. The antisecretory effects can be tested against gastrin infusion and protein meals in animals and in humans. The antitrophic effects should be tested in the model system of PPI-induced HG, preferably in patients with chronic severe reflux esophagitis. The effects can be monitored regularly by biopsy of gastric corpus mucosa and morphometric analysis of parietal cell and ECL cell density and by measurement of intragastric acid responses to PPI treatment. After a prolonged treatment with PPI, whether CCK–B/G antagonists can prevent acid rebound should be tested. All of these measurements may be combined with other parameters such as symptom relief and improved quality of life in patients with severe symptomatic reflux.

CONCLUSION

Gastrin has well defined to possess secretory and trophic actions in the stomach that are mediated by CCK–B/G (also known as CCK-2) receptors. Gastrin also has possible trophic actions on normal colon and on gastrointestinal neoplasms. The use of CCK–B/G receptor antagonists may have clinical utility as gastric antisecretory agents, but it is more likely that their antitrophic actions on gastric mucosa will be more valuable clinically.

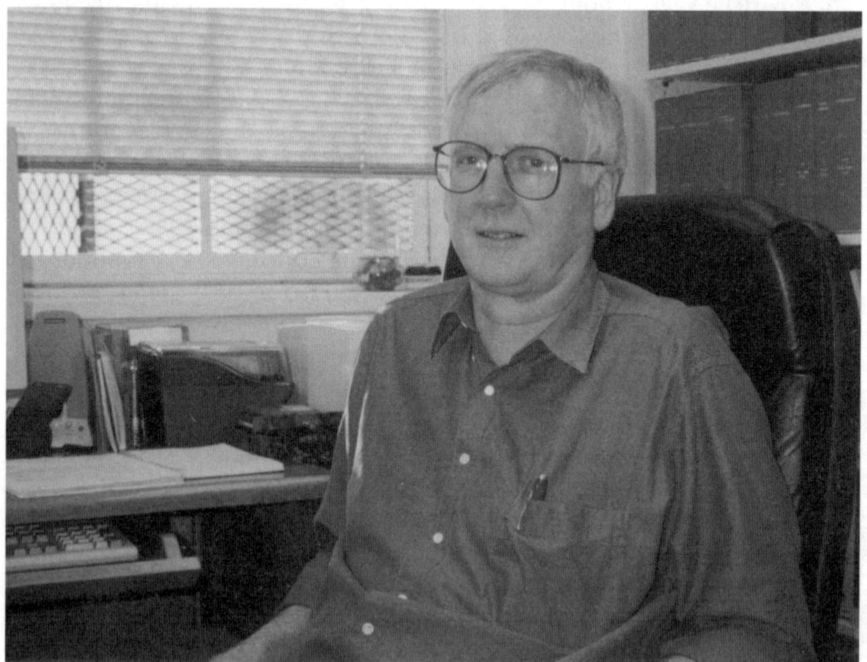

John relaxed in his office at CURE a couple weeks prior to his trip to Kyoto, Japan, December of 1999.

REFERENCES

1. Hayward NJ, Harding M, Lloyd SA, McKnight AT, Hughes J, Woodruff GN. The effect of CCKb/gastrin antagonists on stimulated gastric acid secretion in the anesthetized rat. *Br J Pharmacol* 1991;104:973–977.

2. Chang RSL and Lotti VJ. Biochemical and pharmacological characterization of an extremely potent and selective nonpeptide cholecystokinin antagonists. *Proc Natl Acad Sci USA* 1986;83:4923–4926.

3. Chang RSL and Lotti VK. A potent nonpeptide cholecystokinin antagonistic selective for peripheral tissues isolated from Aspergillus alliaceus. *Science* 1985;230:177–179.

4. Hughes J, Boden P, Costall D, Domeney A, Kelly E, Horwell DC, Hunter JC, Pinnock RD, Woodruff GN. Development of a class of selective cholecystokinin type B receptor antagonists having potent anxiolytic activity. *Proc Natl Acad Sci USA* 1990;87:6728–6732.

5. Nishida A, Yuki H, Tsutsumi R, Miyata K, Kamato T, Ito H, Yamano M, Honda K. L-365,260, a potent CCK-B/gastrin receptor antagonist, suppresses gastric acid secretion induced by histamine and bethanechol as well as pentagastrin in rats. *Jpn J Pharmacol* 1992;58:137–145.

6. Nishida A, Kobayashi-Uchida A, Akuzawa S, Takinami Y, Shishido T, Kamato T, Ito H, Yamano, Yuki H, Nagakura Y, Honda K, Miyata K. Gastrin receptor antagonist YM022 prevents hypersecretion after long-term acid suppression. *Am J Physiol* 1995;269:G699–G705.

7. Nishida A, Miyata K, Tsutsumi R, Yuki H, Akuzawa S, Kobayashi A, Kamato T, Ito H, Yamano M, Katsuyama Y. Pharmacological profile of (R)-1-[2,3-dihydro-1-(2'-methyphenacy)-2-oxo-5-phenyl-1H-1,4-benzo-diazepin-3-yl]-3-(3-methylphenyl)urea (YM022), a new potent and selective gastrincholecystokinin-B receptor antagonist, *in vitro* and *in vivo*. *J Pharmacol Exp Ther* 1994;269:725–731.

8. Nishida A, Takinami Y, Yuki H, Kobayashi A, Akuzawa S, Kamato T, Ito H, Yamano M, Nagakura Y, Miyata K. YM022, {(R)-1-[2,3-dihydro-1-(2'-methyphenacy)-2-oxo-5-phenyl-1H-1,4-benzo-diazepin-3-yl]-3-(3-methylphenyl)urea}, a potent and selective gastrin/cholecystokinin-B receptor antagonists, prevents gastric and duodenal lesions in rats. *J Pharmacol Exp Ther* 1994;270:1256–1261.

9. Shiosaki K, Lin CW, Kopecka H, Craig R, Wagenaar FL, Bianchi B, Miller T, WitteD, Nadzan AM. Development of CCK-tetrapeptide analogues as potent and selective CCK-A receptor agonists. *J Med Chem* 1990;33:2950–2.

10. Kerwin JF, Jr. Further developments in cholecystokinin antagonist research. *Drugs Future* 1991;16:1111–1119.

11. Evans BE. Recent developments in cholecystokinin antagonist research. *Drugs Future* 1989;14:971–979.

12. Bock MG. Development of non-peptide cholecystokinin type B receptor antagonsists. *Drugs Future* 1991;631–640.

13. Hagishita S, Murakami Y, Seno K, Kamata S, Haga N, Monoike T, Kanda Y, Kiyama R, Shiota T, Ishihara Y, Ishikawa M, Shimamura M, Abe K, Yoshimura K. Synthesis and pharmacological properties of ureidomethylcarbomoyl-phenylketone derivatives. A new potent and subtype-selective nonpeptide CCK-B/gastrin receptor antagonist, S-0509. *Bioorg Med Chem* 1997;5:1695–1714.

14. Makovec F. CCK-B/gastrin receptor antagonists. *Drugs Future* 1993;18:919–931.

15. Takeuchi K, Hirata T, Yamamoto H, Kunikata T, Ishikawa M, Ishihara Y. Effects of S-0509, a novel CCKb/gastrin receptor antagonist, on acid secretion and experimental duodenal ulcers in rats. *Aliment Pharmacol Ther* 1999;13:87–96.

16. Pendley CE, Fitzpatrick LR, Capolino AJ, Davis MA, Esterline NJ, Jakubowska A, Bertrand P, Guyon C, Dubroeucq MC, Martin GE. RP73870, a gastrin/cholecystokinin-B receptor antagonist with potent anti-ulcer activity in the rat. *J Pharmacol Exp Ther* 1995;273:1015–1022.

17. Bertrand P, Böhme GA, Durieux C, Guyon C, Jeantaud B, Boudeau P, Ducos B, Pendley CE, Martin GE. Pharmacological properties of ureidoacetamides, new potent and selective non-peptide CCKB/gastrin receptor antagonists. *Eur J Pharmacol* 1994;262:233–245.

18. Böhme GA, Bertrand P, Guyon C Capet M, Pendley C, Stutzmann JM, Doble A, Dubroeucq MC, Martin G, Blanchard JC. The ureidoacetamides, a novel family of non-peptide CCK-B/gastrin antagonists. *Ann NY Acad Sci* 1994;713:118–120.

19. Goto Y and Debas HT. GABA-mimetic effect on gastric acid secretion; possible significance in central mechanisms. *Dig Dis Sci* 1983;28:56–60.

20. Brenna E, Håkanson R, Sundler F, Sandvik AK, Waldum HL. The effect of omeprazole-induced hypergastrinemia on the oxyntic mucosa of Mastomys. *Scand J Gastroenterol* 1991;26:667–672.

21. Larsson H, Carlsson E, Mattsson H, Lundell L, Sundler G, Wallmark B, Watanabe T, Håkanson R. Plasma gastrin and gastric enterochromaffin-like cell activation and proliferation: studies with omeprazole and ranitidine in intact and antrectomized rats. *Gastroenterology* 1986;90:391–396.

22. Larsson H, Carlsson E, Håkanson R, Mattsson H, Nilsson G, Seensalu R, Wallmark B, Sundler F. Time-course of development and reversal of gastric endocrine cell hyperplasia after inhibition of acid secretion; studies with omeprazole and ranitidine in intact and antrectomized rats. *Gastroenterology* 1988;95:1477–1486.

23. Larsson H, Carlsson E, Ryberg B, Fryklund J, Wallmark B. Rat parietal cell function after prolonged inhibition of gastric acid secretion. *Am J Gastroenterol* 1988;254:G33–G39.

24. Dockray GJ, Hamer C, Evans D, Varro A, Dimaline R. The secretory kinetics of the G cell in omeprazole-treated rats. *Gastroenterology* 1991;100:1187–1194.

25. Håkanson R, Tielemans Y, Chen D, Andersson K, Mattsson H, Sundler F. Time-dependent changes in enterochromaffin-like cell kinetics in stomach of hypergastrinemic rats. *Gastroenterology* 1993; 105:15–21.

26. Walsh JH. Role of gastrin as a trophic hormone. *Digestion* 1990:47(suppl):11–16.

27. Seva C, Dickinson CJ, Yamada T. Growth-promoting effects of glycine-extended progastrin. *Science* 1994;265:410–412.

28. Blackmore M and Hirst BG. Autocrine stimulation of growth of AR4-2J rat pancreatic tumour cells by gastrin. *Br J Cancer* 1992;66:32–38.

29. Ryberg B, Axelson J, Håkanson R, Sundler F, Mattsson H. Trophic effect of continuous infusion of [Leu15]-gastrin-17 in the rat. *Gastroenterology* 1990;98:33–38.

30. Eissele R, Patberg H, Koop H, Krack W, Lorenz W, McNight AT. Effect of gastrin receptor blockade on endocrine cells in rats. *Gastroenterology* 1992;103:1596–1601.

31. Singh P, Owlia A, Espeijo R, Dai B. Novel gastrin receptors mediate mitogenic effects of gastrin and processing intermediates of gastrin on Swiss 3T3 fibroblasts. *J Biol Chem* 1995;270:8429–8438.

32. Bold RJ, Ishizuka J, Townsend M Jr, Thompson JC. Gastrin stimulates growth of human colon cancer cells via a receptor other than CCK-A or CCK-B. *Biochem Biophys Res Commun* 1994;202: 1222–1226.

33. Singh P, Xu Z, Dai B, Rajaraman S, Rubin N, Dhruva B. Incomplete processing of progastrin expressed by human colon cancer cells: role of noncarboxy-amidated gastrins. *Am J Physiol* 1995;266: G459–G468.

34. Dickinson C. Relationship of gastrin processing to colon cancer. *Gastroenterology* 1995;109: 1384–1388.

35. Sobhani I, Lehy T, Laurent-Puig P, Cadiot G, Ruszniewski P, Mignon M. Chronic endogenous hypergastrinemia in human: evidence for a mitogenic effect on the colonic mucosa. *Gastroenterology* 1993;105:22–30.

36. Ogihara Y and Takeuchi K. Current topics on gastrin/CCK receptors. *GI Research* (in Japanese) 1996;4:298–302.

37. Chowdhury R, Zhang Z, Hocker M, Wang TC. Activation of human histidine decarboxylase gene promoter activity by gastrin is mediated by two distinct nuclear factors. *J Biol Chem* 1999;274: 20961–20969.

38. Chen D, Zhao CM, Yamada H, Norlen P, Håkanson R. Novel aspects of gastrin-induced activation of histidine decarboxylase in rat stomach ECL cells. *Regul Pept* 1998;77:169–175.

39. Russel DH and Durie BGM. Ornithine decarboxylase—a key enzyme in growth. *Prog Cancer Res Ther* 1978;4:43.

Gut-Brain Peptides in the New Millennium, edited by Y. Taché
CURE Foundation, Los Angeles, CA. © 2002

36

Long-Term Studies of *Helicobacter pylori* Infection in Mongolian Gerbils: Effects of Eradication Timing on Prevention of Malignant Gastric Changes

Misako Ebata, Yoshihiro Keto, and Susumu Okabe
Department of Applied Pharmacology, Kyoto Pharmaceutical University
Misasagi, Yamashina, Kyoto, Japan

INTRODUCTION

Many epidemiological investigations have demonstrated that *Helicobacter pylori (H. pylori)* infection directly and indirectly induces neoplasms, including gastric carcinoma and MALT lymphoma (1–4). It has been previously reported that *H. pylori* infection induces atrophic gastritis, ulcers, and intestinal metaplasia in Mongolian gerbils (M. gerbils) (5–8). In general, atrophic gastritis and intestinal metaplasia are considered to be the origin of gastric adenocarcinoma (9, 10). In prior studies, Tatematsu, et al. (11) and Sugiyama, et al. (12) reported that *H. pylori* infection enhances N-methyl-N'nitro-N-nitrosoguanidine (MNNG)- or N-methyl-N-nitrosourea (MNU)-induced gastric carcinogenesis in M. gerbils, resulting in both intestinal-type and diffuse-type adenocarcinoma. In 1998, Watanabe, et al. (13) demonstrated that *H. pylori* infection induced intestinal-type gastric adenocarcinoma 62 wks following inoculation in M. gerbils. Our groups (14) have also confirmed that intestinal-type adenocarcinoma developed 18 months after *H. pylori* inoculation in M. gerbils. As gastric adenocarcinoma was induced without carcinogen administration, Watanabe and our group concluded that *H. pylori* might represent a gastric carcinogenic agent. Eradication of *H. pylori* in patients with various gastric diseases is the most important therapy, to prevent both relapse of healed ulcers and potential progression to gastric carcinoma.

Crabtree and Figura (15) issued the following statement, "The key current questions are whether the long-term consequences of mucosal damage, such as atrophy and intestinal metaplasia, can be reversed after elimination of infection and whether, with the development of a simple 1-wk therapeutic regimen for eradicating *H. pylori,* large-scale treatment of infected patients will have a beneficial effect on the incidence of gastric cancer."

In the present study, M. gerbils were used to examine whether or not: 1) *H. pylori* infection for up to 24 months results in a much higher incidence and severity of carcinoma having metastases and vascular invasion; and 2) eradication of *H. pylori* infection can prevent the development of grossly visible and histological gastric changes.

MATERIALS AND METHODS

Animals

Male Mongolian gerbils (6-wk-old, 40–50 g) were purchased from Seac Yoshitomi (Fukuoka, Japan). The animals were kept in an isolated clean room with regulated temperature (approximately 20–22°C), humidity (approximately 55%), and light/dark cycle (12/12 hr). The gerbils were deprived of food for 24 hr before and 4 hr after *H. pylori* inoculation, but otherwise had free access to food and tap water. The animals were killed either 21 or 24 months after *H. pylori* inoculation. The maintenance of the animals and the experimental procedures were carried out in accordance with the guidelines of the Ethics Committee of Kyoto Pharmaceutical University.

H. pylori *Preparation and Inoculation*

TN2GF4 strain, cag A- and vac A-positive *H. pylori,* isolated from a patient with a gastric ulcer, was kindly provided by Takeda Chemical Industries Ltd. (Osaka, Japan). The bacteria was incubated overnight in a brain–heart infusion broth (Difco Laboratories, Detroit, MI) containing 10% fetal bovine serum (Gibco BRL, Grand Island, NY) at 37°C under a microaerophilic atmosphere; the bacteria was allowed to grow to a concentration of approximately 2.0×10^8 colony-forming units (CFU)/mL. *H. pylori* $(2.0 \times 10^8$ CFU/mL) was orally inoculated into each animal at a dosage of 1.0 mL/animal.

Macroscopical Studies

The animals were killed with an overdose of ether. The stomach of each animal was removed, opened along the greater curvature, and then spread upon a cork board. The lesion area (mm^2) was promptly measured under a dissecting microscope ($\times 10$; Olympus, Tokyo, Japan). The author (S.O.) who determined the ulcer size was blinded as to the treatment to which any given animal was subjected.

Drugs

Omeprazole (Astra Japan, Osaka) and clarithromycin (Taisho Pharmaceutical Co., Tokyo) were suspended in 0.5% carboxymethylcellulose and administered at a concentration of 1.0 mL/100 g body weight.

Histological and Serological Studies

Thirty gerbils were divided into three groups. Group 1 did not receive *H. pylori* eradication treatment. Eradication treatment was performed in Groups 2 and 3 either 4 or 8 months after *H. pylori* inoculation, respectively. All animals were killed either 21 or 24 months after *H. pylori* inoculation. Before gastric removal, a blood sample was extracted with a capillary tube from one orbital plexus of any given animal. After centrifuging each blood sample at 3,000 rpm for 15 min, the serum was isolated and utilized for determination of serum gastrin levels. Serum gastrin was quantified by a radioimmunoassay (Mitsubishi Kagaku Bio-Clinical Laboratories, Inc., Tokyo, Japan).

Following gross observation of the stomachs, animal tissue samples were fixed in 10% formalin and embedded in paraffin for histology. Four-μm sections were prepared and subsequently stained both with hematoxylin and eosin and with alcian blue (pH 2.5)-periodic acid Schiff, in order to detect mucin-containing cells. The gastric sampling area is demonstrated in our previous report (14).

Statistical Analysis

Data are presented as means ± SEM. Statistical differences were evaluated using the Student's t-test or Dunnett's multiple comparison test, with a P value of < 0.05 regarded as significant.

RESULTS

Pathological Changes of the Gastric Mucosa in H. pylori-*infected M. gerbils*

Twenty-one or 24 months post-inoculation, the stomachs of *H. pylori*-infected gerbils exhibited several large hyperplastic polyps characterized by hyperplasia of the tall columnar surface epithelium and severe edema. The stomach weights of these gerbils were 3.3 ± 0.4 g and 3.7 ± 0.4 g at 21 and 24 months, respectively (Figures 1, 2). Certain hyperplastic polyps displayed a small apical erosion; the areas for these erosions were 3.9 ± 1.1 mm^2 and 2.9 ± 0.8 mm^2 per animal at 21 and 24 months, respectively (Figure 3). Clearly demarcated ulcers in the oxyntic glandular area, in the

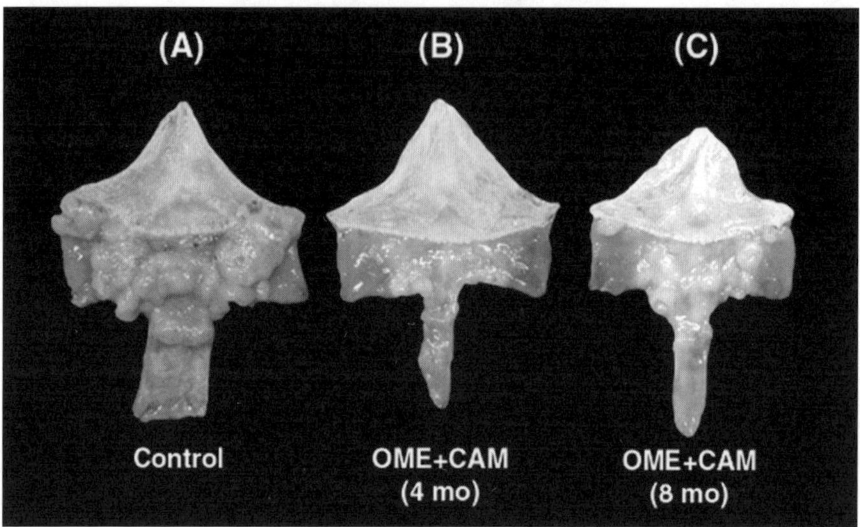

FIGURE 1. *Gross appearances of M. gerbil stomachs 21 months after* H. pylori *inoculation. Several large hyperplastic polyps with small apical erosions were observed in the gastric glandular area of the control stomachs (A). Only a few visible lesions were observed in the gastric mucosa of gerbils treated with omeprazole (OME) and clarithromycin (CAM) beginning either 4 (B) or 8 months (C) post-inoculation.*

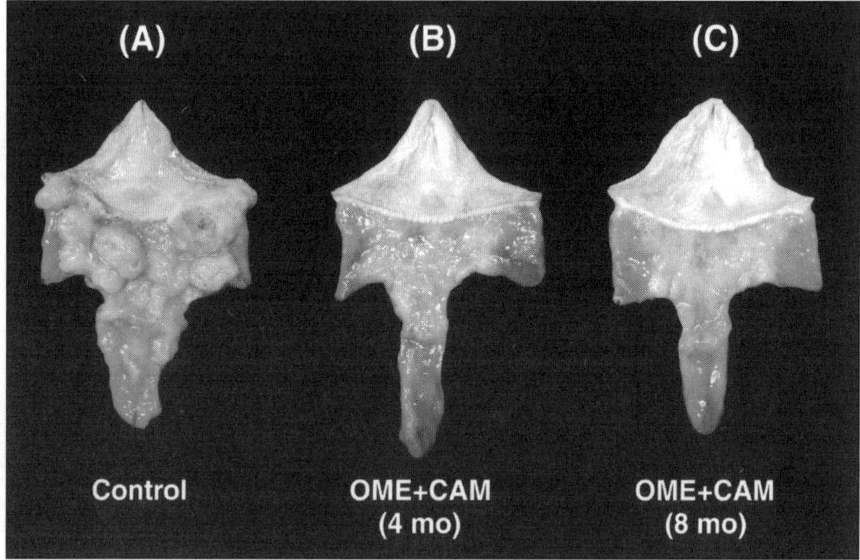

FIGURE 2. *Gross appearances of M. gerbil stomachs 24 months after* H. pylori *inoculation. As in the case of 21 months post-inoculation, several large hyperplastic polyps with small erosions were observed in the gastric glandular area of the control stomachs (A). However no visible lesions were observed in the gastric mucosa of gerbils treated with omeprazole (OME) and clarithromycin (CAM) beginning either 4 (B) or 8 months post-infection (C).*

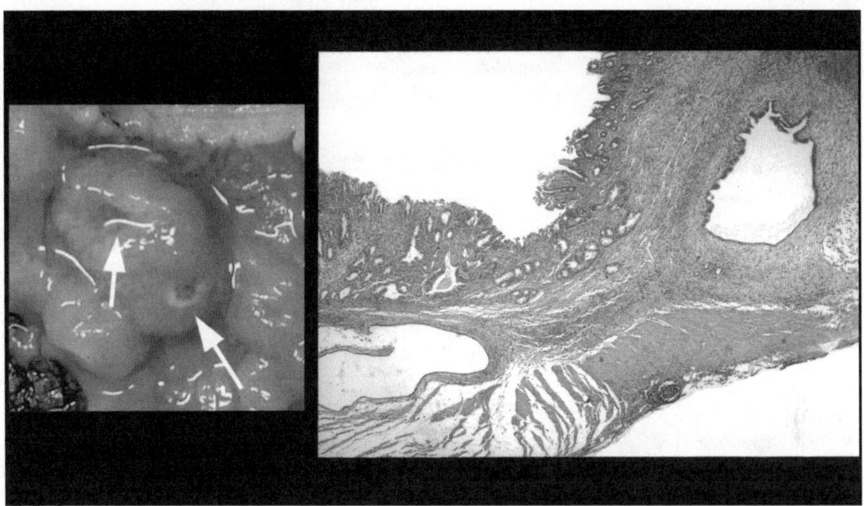

FIGURE 3. *Gross and microscopic appearances of a M. gerbil stomach 24 months after* H. pylori *inoculation. Note the apical erosions on the hyperplastic polyps. Gastric atrophy, intestinal metaplasia, and large cysts were observed in the submucosal area.*

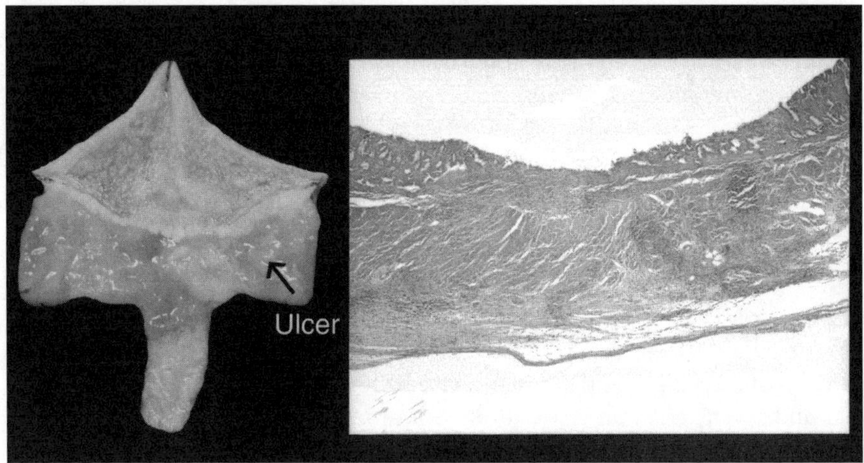

FIGURE 4. *Gross and microscopic appearances of a M. gerbil stomach 21 months after* H. pylori *inoculation. Note the development of an ulcer in the oxyntic gland area, without the appearance of a single hyperplastic polyp in the entire stomach.*

absence of hyperplastic polyps, were demonstrated in one gerbil 21 months post-inoculation and in two gerbils 24 months post-inoculation (Figure 4).

Histologically, atrophic gastritis, intestinal metaplasia, ulcers, and hyperproliferation in the submucosal layer were all observed at >50% incidences

TABLE 1. *Incidence of histopathological changes observed in the* H. pylori-*infected* M. *gerbil stomachs examined 21 or 24 months post-inoculation.*

	Control		Eradication at 4 mo		Eradication at 8 mo	
	21 mo	24 mo	21 mo	24 mo	21 mo	24 mo
Atrophic gastritis	9 / 9	8 / 8	1 / 7	0 / 5	8 / 10	5 / 8
Ulcer	5 / 9	5 / 8	0 / 7	0 / 5	0 / 10	0 / 8
Intestinal metaplasia	9 / 9	8 / 8	1 / 7	0 / 5	6 / 10	2 / 8
Hyperproliferation in the submocosal layer	4 / 9	4 / 8	1 / 7	0 / 5	0 / 10	0 / 8
Carcinoids	4 / 9	6 / 8	0 / 7	0 / 5	0/ 10	0 / 8
Adenocarcinoma	1 / 9	1 / 8	0 / 7	0 / 5	0 / 10	0 / 8

(Table 1). Moreover, carcinoid tumors and adenocarcinoma developed at incidences of 4/9 and 1/9 in animals 21 months post-inoculation and 6/8 and 1/8 in animals 24 months post-inoculation (Figures 5–7).

The adenocarcinomas, consisting of well differentiated intestinal-type epithelium containing a plethora of sialomucin-producing goblet cells, penetrated into the lamina muscularis and serosa. Nonetheless, metastatic disease and vascular invasion was not observed in any gerbils.

Effects of H. pylori *Eradication on Gastric Mucosal Changes*

Twenty-one or 24 months post-inoculation, the stomach weights of gerbils that underwent *H. pylori* eradication with omeprazole and clarithromycin, regardless of whether eradication was executed 4 or 8 months after inoculation, were approximately one third of those in the control groups. The gastric mucosal surface of animals that underwent eradication treatment grossly appeared to approximate that of the normal gerbil without *H. pylori* infection (Figures 1, 2). Histologically, the gastric mucosa of gerbils that underwent eradication treatment 4 months post-inoculation exhibited normal architecture. Nonetheless, the stomachs of gerbils that underwent eradication treatment 8 months post-inoculation exhibited gastric atrophy with intestinal metaplasia, infiltration of inflammatory cells, and submucosal edema (Figure 8). Carcinoid tumors and adenocarinoma were not found in these stomachs.

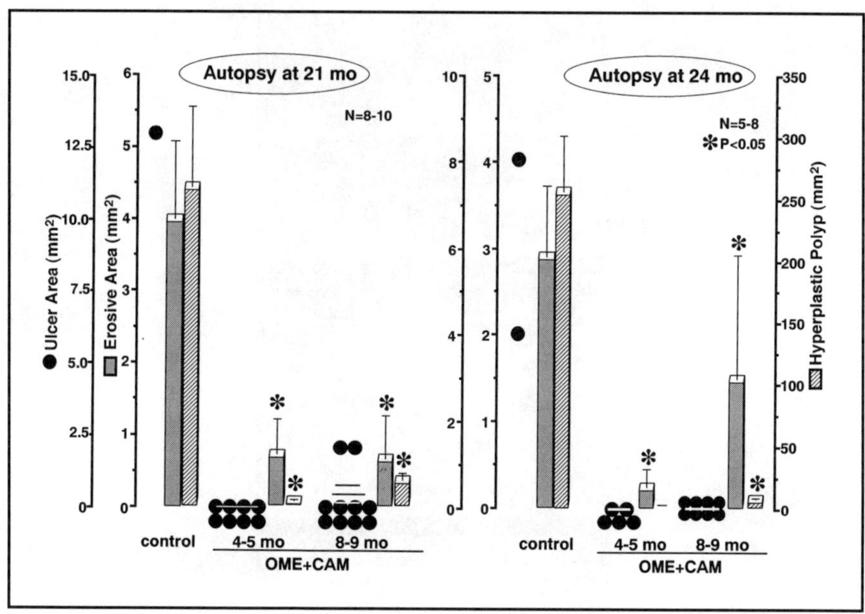

FIGURE 5. *Effects of* H. pylori *eradication with omeprazole (OME) and clarithromycin (CAM) on gastric mucosal changes in* H. pylori-*infected M. gerbils. OME (60 mg/kg, 4 wks) and CAM (100 mg/kg, 2 wks) were orally administered beginning 4 or 8 months post-inoculation; stomachs were examined 21 or 24 months post-inoculation. Data are presented as means ± SE for 5–10 animals. * Significantly different from the control animals, P < 0.05.*

Serum Gastrin Levels

Serum gastrin levels in the control group were 294.0 ± 52.3 and 266.0 ± 34.4 pg/ml at 21 and 24 months post-inoculation, respectively. In the animals that underwent eradication 4 months after inoculation, serum gastrin levels were significantly reduced to 69.1 ± 9.3 and 136.4 ± 45.0 pg/ml at 21 and 24 months post-inoculation, respectively. In the animals that underwent eradication treatment 8 months after inoculation, serum gastrin levels were 78.7 ± 9.8 and 230.5 ± 12.3 pg/ml at 21 and 24 months post-infection, respectively. The gastrin levels measured at 21 months were significantly reduced compared with the corresponding control animals.

DISCUSSION

This study demonstrated that *H. pylori* infection in M. gerbils for up to 24 months resulted in development of hyperplastic polyps, ulceration, atrophic gastritis with intestinal metaplasia, and submucosal hyperplasia. Moreover,

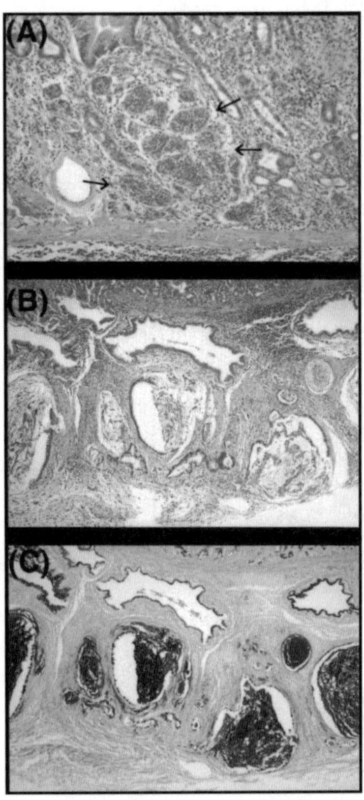

FIGURE 6. *Histological changes of M. gerbil gastric mucosa 21 months after* H. pylori *inoculation. Note the well-developed carcinoid tumor (a) and adenocarcinoma (b). The adenocarcinoma penetrated into the lamina muscularis and serosa in the proximal pyloric region. Well-differentiated intestinal-type epithelium in the adenocarcinoma exhibited a large number of sialomucin-producing goblet cells (c). [(a) ×100, (b) ×50, (c) ×50].*

H. pylori infection resulted in both carcinoid tumor and gastric adenocarcinoma development, although the incidence of the latter was low. Such findings correspond well with those reported by both Watanabe, et al. (13) and our group (14), who examined M. gerbil stomachs 62 wks and 18 months post-inoculation, respectively. In contrast to the study's expectations, however, prolonged infection for 24 months did not result in an increased incidence and severity of gastric damage, to include metastatic disease and vascular invasion. The only observed difference was that of the size of hyperplastic polyps, which became slightly enlarged due to progression of hyperplasia. As was expected, eradication of *H. pylori* at both earlier and later timeframes resulted in normal-appearing gastric surfaces both 21 and 24 months post-inoculation, i.e., no hyperplastic polyps or ulcers were observed. Although the study did not examine *H. pylori* viability, it appears that

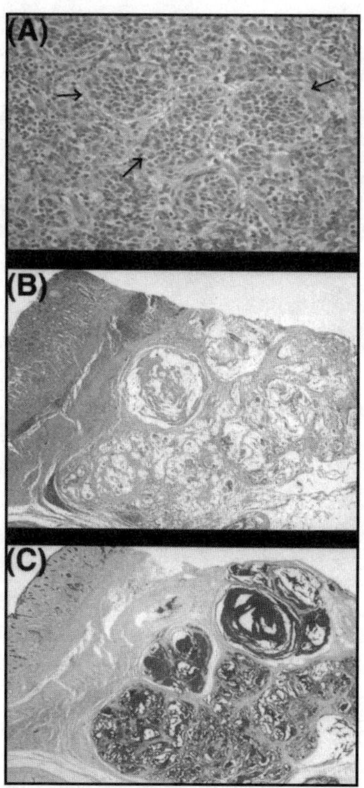

FIGURE 7. *Histological changes of M. gerbil gastric mucosa 24 months after* H. pylori *inoculation. Note the development of a carcinoid tumor (a) and adenocarcinoma (b). The adenocarcinoma penetrated into the lamina muscularis and serosa in the distal pyloric region. Well-differentiated intestinal-type epithelium in the adenocarcinoma exhibited a large number of sialomucin-producing goblet cells (c). [(a) ×100, (b) ×50, (c) ×50].*

eradication treatment with omeprazole and clarithromycin persisted for the duration of each study arm, i.e., up to 15 months.

It remains of note that visible changes in the stomach surfaces of *H. pylori*-infected gerbils were clearly differentiated into two types, i.e., hyperplastic polyps and ulcers. Although the overall incidence of the former appeared to be higher than that of the latter, the findings of the study strongly suggest that the pathogenesis of such polyps and ulcers remains distinct. As was previously reported (7), the present study confirmed that clearly demarcated deep ulcers are first found in the oxyntic mucosa of gerbil stomachs 4 to 6 months post-inoculation at an incidence of >81%, followed by hyperplastic polyps, which can be observed even 12 months post-inoculation. It accordingly remains possible that stomach ulceration which persist for much longer time precludes the development of mucosal hyperplasia by some mechanism. Our

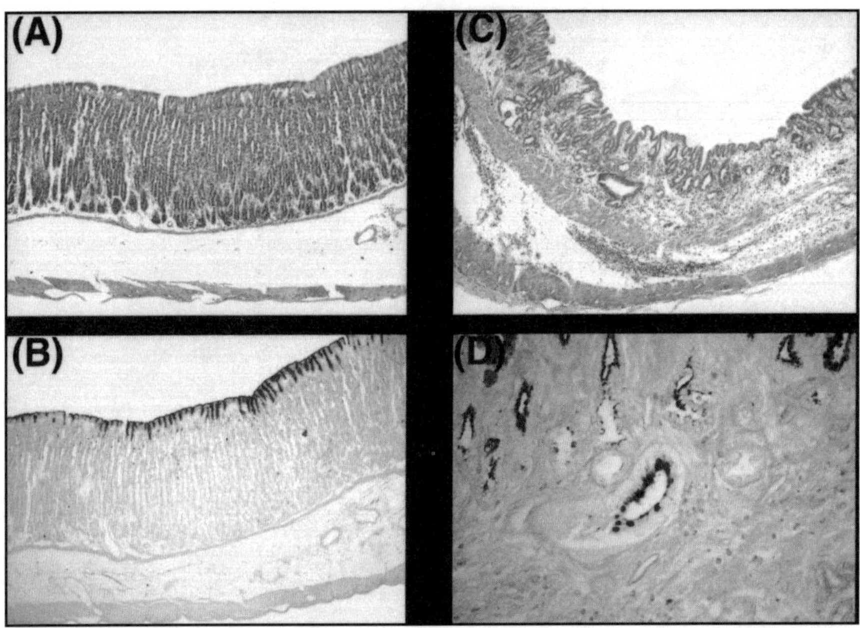

FIGURE 8. *Histological observation of M. gerbil gastric mucosa 21 months after* H. pylori *inoculation. Eradication of* H. pylori *with OME+CAM was performed beginning 4 (a, b) or 8 (c, d) months post-inoculation. Regardless of the timing of eradication, 21 months post-inoculation, the entire gastric mucosal architecture appeared to be normal, except for the presence of a few inflammatory cells. It is noteworthy that atrophy and intestinal metaplasia were observed (d) in the gastric mucosa of a M. gerbil that underwent eradication 8 months post-inoculation. [(a) ×50, (b) ×50, (c) ×50, (d) ×100].*

previous study demonstrated that repeated treatment of *H. pylori*-infected gerbils (3 months post-inoculation) with indomethacin prevented the development of gastric mucosal hyperplasia. Nontheless, indomethacin also induced one or two ulcers in the oxyntic mucosa at a prevalence of 5/6 gerbils. In addition, our previous study also confirmed that prostaglandin levels in the oxyntic mucosa of *H. pylori*-infected gerbils (3 months post-inoculation) significantly increased, in contrast to those of non-infected gerbils. It was hypothesized that over expression of endogenous prostaglandins in *H. pylori*-infected mucosa might be involved in the development of mucosal hyperplasia and hyperplastic polyps. In contrast, low expression of prostaglandins in *H. pylori*-infected mucosa might result in ulcer development in the oxyntic mucosa by an unelucidated mechanism.

In our unpublished data, we found that the serum gastrin levels in *H. pylori*-infected M. gerbils (6-month post-infection) significantly increased to 288.3 ± 23.7 pg/ml (vs 85.4 ± 6.4 pg/ml in the non-infected gerbils, n = 5 – 6). In this study, we also found a higher serum gastrin levels (approxi-

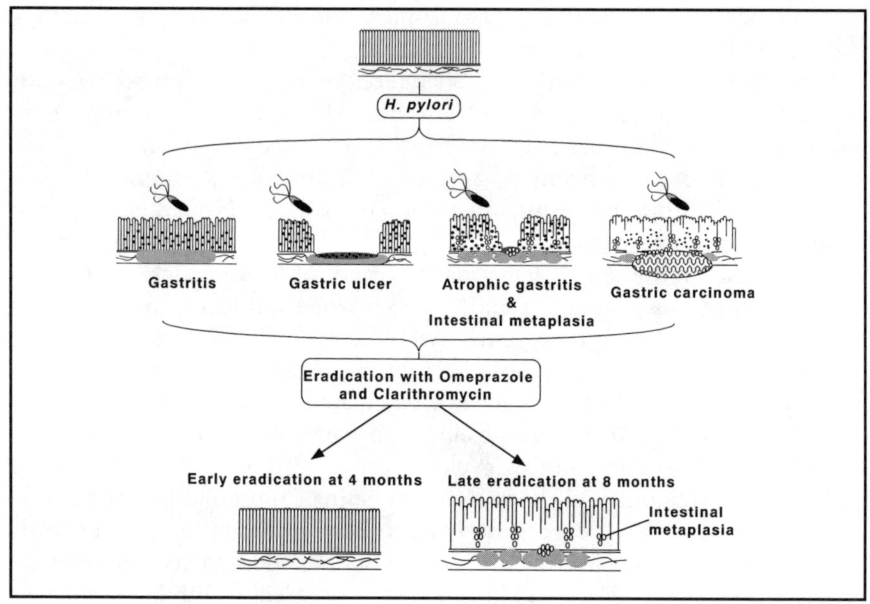

FIGURE 9. *Schematic illustration of pathological changes observed over the course of 24 months in M. gerbil gastric mucosa following* H. pylori *infection and pharmacologic* H. pylori *eradication at earlier and later timepoints.*

mately 260 to 300 pg/ml) in *H. pylori*-infected gerbils 21 and 24 month post-infection. These data suggest that such a high level of serum gastrin is involved in the development of hyperplastic polyp and ulceration. After the *H. pylori* eradication, the serum gastrin levels is reduced in most of the animals.

It should be noted that early *H. pylori* eradication executed 4–5 months post-inoculation, resulted in marked suppression of macro- and microscopic changes for up to 24 months. In contrast, late eradication executed 8–9 months post-inoculation, while successfully managing to prevent development of visible mucosal changes, could not prevent persistentence of gastric atrophy with intestinal metaplasia. We have previously demonstrated that despite potent *H. pylori* eradication 8–9 months post-inoculation, atrophic gastritis with intestinal metaplasia was observed in all animals 18 months post-inoculation. Furthermore, it was also demonstrated that gastric atrophy with intestinal metaplasia persisted for an additional 6 months, although at a slightly attenuated incidence (Figure 9). Such findings suggest that pharmacotherapy for *H. pylori* eradication 8 months after inoculation represents a timeframe too late to prevent pathological mucosal changes. As atrophic gastritis and intestinal metaplasia have typically been considered to represent the beginnings of intestinal/gastric adenocarcinoma (9, 10), early eradiation is recommended to ensure complete suppression of the potential development of gastric adenocarcinoma.

It has been reported that *H. pylori* infection in humans correlates with both intestinal and diffuse-type gastric cancer (16). Furthermore, in M. gerbils, *H. pylori* infection has been observed to enhance MNU and MNNG-induced gastric carcinogenesis, resulting in the development of both intestinal and diffuse-type gastric cancer (11, 12, 17). Nonetheless, in the present study, only well-differentiated intestinal-type adenocarcinoma was observed. Such a finding suggests that a variety of factors, such as *H. pylori* strain diversity, host immunity, and environmental influence, impacts upon carcinogenesis of diffuse-type gastric cancer.

The exact mechanisms underlying the progression to gastric carcinoma following *H. pylori* infection were not elucidated by the present study, but certain reports have suggested possible mechanisms. It has been reported that *H. pylori* infection induces cyclooxygenase-2 (COX-2) expression in both gastric carcinoma cell lines (18) and human intestinal-gastric adenocarcinoma (19). COX-2 expression has also been reported to correlate with lymphatic vessel invasion, lymph node metastasis, and advanced tumor stage in gastric cancer (20, 21). In addition, a COX-2 selective inhibitor reduced the proliferation of a COX-2-expressing human gastric cancer cell line, but failed to influence non-COX-2-expressing cell lines (22). Such reports suggest that COX-2 over-expression will undoubtedly be determined to be one factor implicated in gastric carcinogenesis.

In additional studies, it has been reported that *H. pylori* infection results in stimulation of mucosal reactive oxygen metabolite production (23). Such reactive metabolites react with ammonia derived from urease produced by *H. pylori,* leading to synthesis of monochloramines. Suzuki, et al. (24) demonstrated that monochloramines induce DNA damage in gastric cells. Recent studies (25–28) have also revealed that *H. pylori* infection in humans is associated with enhanced expression of iNOS in neutrophils and mononuclear cells. In addition, Mannick, et al. (29) reported that *H. pylori* infection is accompanied by formation of endogenous reactive nitrogen intermediates, which might conceivably contribute to DNA damage and apoptosis. In other words, such reactive nitrogen and monochloramine species contribute to carcinogenesis. In addition, our group recently demonstrated that *H. pylori* mixed with the cancer cell line MKN28 significantly increased the production of IL-8, which enhances neutrophil chemotaxis (30).

It has also been reported that *H. pylori* infection results in enhanced epithelial cell turnover rate (31). Peek, et al. (32) demonstrated alteration of gastric epithelial cell cycle events following *H. pylori* infection in M. gerbils. In the present study, hyperplastic polyps and submucosal hyperplasia were indeed observed in *H. pylori*-infected M. gerbils. Nonetheless, whether such an enhanced cell turnover rate is related with the mechanism underlying gastric carcinoid and adenocarcinoma pathogenesis remains undetermined. Rodent models for *H. pylori*-induced gastric carcinoma and therapy of *H. pylori*-associated gastric neoplasms have been reviewed by other authors (33, 34).

In conclusion, it was found that although early eradication of *H. pylori* clearly prevented development of visible and histological changes in M. gerbil stomachs 21 and 24 months post-inoculation, late eradication failed to prevent development of atrophic gastritis with intestinal metaplasia. Such results indicate that eradication timing plays a critical role in prevention of *H. pylori*-associated mucosal changes.

ACKNOWLEDGMENTS

We wish to thank CJ Hurt (John Hopkins University School of Medicine, USA) for a critical reading of the manuscript and K Nakajima, N Kataoka, K Kitagawa, and M Ooguma for their technical assistance.

REFERENCES

1. Danesh I. *Helicobacter pylori* infection and gastric cancer: systematic review of the epidemiological studies. *Aliment Pharmacol Ther* 1999;13:851–856.

2. Hang JQ, Sridhar S, Chen Y, Hunt RH. Meta-analysis of the relationship between *Helicobacter pylori* seropositivity and gastric cancer. *Gastroenterology* 1999;114:1169–1179.

3. Konturek PC, Bielanski W, Konturek SJ, Hahn EG. *Helicobacter pylori* associated gastric pathology. *J Physiol Pharmacol* 1999;50:695–710.

4. Uemura A, Okamoto S, Yamamoto S, Matsumura N, Yamaguchi S, Yamakido M, Taniyama K, Sasaki N, Schlemper RJ. *Helicobacter pylori* infection and the development of gastric cancer. *N Engl J Med* 2001;345:784–789.

5. Hirayama F, Takagi S, Kusuhara H, Iwao E, Yokoyama T, Ikeda Y. Induction of gastric ulcer and intestinal metaplasia in Mongolian gerbils infected with *Helicobacter pylori*. *J Gastroenterol* 1996;31:755–757.

6. Matsumoto S, Washizuka Y, Matsumoto Y, Tawara S, Ikeda F, Yokota Y, Karita M. Induction of ulceration and sever gastritis in Mongolian gerbil by *Helicobacter pylori* infection. *J Med Microbiol* 1997;46: 391–397.

7. Takahashi S, Keto Y, Fujita H, Muramatsu H, Nishino T, Okabe S. Pathological changes in the formation of *Helicobacter pylori*-induced gastric lesions in Mongolian gerbils. *Dig Dis Sci* 1998;43:754–765.

8. Keto Y, Takahashi S, Okabe S. Healing of *Helicobacter pylori*-induced gastric ulcers in Mongolian gerbils. Combined treatment with omeprazole and clarithromycin. *Dig Dis Sci* 1999;44:257–265.

9. Standtläder CT, Waterbor JW. Molecular epidemiology, pathogenesis and prevention of gastric cancer. *Carcinogenesis (Lond.)* 1999;20:2195–2208.

10. Schlemper RJ, Riddell RH, Kato Y, Borchard F, Cooper HS, et al. The Vienna classification of gastrointestinal epithelial neoplasia. *Gut* 2000;46:251–255.

11. Tatematsu M, Yamamoto M, Shimizu N, Yoshikawa A, Fukami H, Kaminishi M, Oohara T, Sugiyama A, Ikeno T. Induction of grandular stomach cancers in *Helicobacter pylori*-sensitive Mongolian gerbils treated with N-methyl-n-nitrosourea and N-methyl-N′-nitro-N-nitorosoguanidine in drinking water. *Jpn J Cancer Res* 1998;89:97–104.

12. Sugiyama A, Maruta F, Ikeno T, Ishida K, Kawasaki S, Katsuyama T, Shimizu N, Tatematsu M. *Helicobacter pylori* infection enhances N-methyl-N-nitrtosourea-induced stomach carcinogenesis in Mongolian gerbil. *Cancer Res* 1998;58:2067–2069.

13. Watanabe T, Tada M, Nagai H, Sasaki S, Nakano M. *Helicobacter pylori* infection induces gastric cancer in Mongolian gerbils. *Gastroenterology* 1998;115:642–648.

14. Keto Y, Ebata M, Okabe S. Gastric mucosal changes induced by long term infection with *Helicobacter pylori* in Mongolian gerbils: Effects of bacteria eradication. *J Physiol (Paris)* 2001;95:429–436.

15. Crabtree JE, Figura N. Mechanism of *Helicobacter-pylori*-induced mucosal damage. In: *Clinical Pharmacology and Therapy of* Helicobacter pylori *Infection*. Scarpignato and Porro GB, Ed. Progress in Basic Clin Pharmacol, Basel: Karger, 1999;11:21–43

16. Kikuchi S, Wada O, Nakajima T, Nishi T, Kobayashi O, Konishi T, Inada Y, and the Research Group on Prevention of Gastric Carcinoma among Young Adult. Serum anti-*Helicobacter pylori* antibody and gastric carcinoma among young adults. *Cancer* (Philia.) 1995;75:2789–2793.

17. Maruta F, Ota H, Genta RM, Sugiyama A, Tatematsu M, Katsuyama T, Kawasaki S. Role of N-methyl-N-nitrosourea in the induction of intestinal metaplasia and gastric adenocarcinoma in Mongolian gerbils infected with *Helicobacter pylori*. *Scand J Gastroenterol* 2001;36:283–290.

18. Romano M, Ricci V, Memoli A, Tuccillo C, Di Popolo A, Sommi P, Acquaviva AM, Del Vecchio Blanco C, Bruni CB, Zarrilli R. Helicobacter up-regulates cyclooxygenase-2 mRNA expression and prostaglandin E2 synthesis in MKN 28 gastric mucosal cells *in vitro*. *J Biol Chem* 1998;273:28560–28563.

19. Saukkonen K, Nieminen O, van Rees B, Vilkki S, Harkonen M, Juhola M, Mecklin JP, Sipponen P, Ristimaki A. Expression of cyclooxygenase-2 in dysplasia of the stomach and in intestinal-type gastric adenocarcinoma. *Clinical Cancer Research* 2001;7:1923–1931.

20. Murata H, Kawano S, Tsujii S, Tsujii M, Sawaoka H, Kimura Y, Shiozaki H, Hori M. Cyclooxygenase-2 overexpression enhances lymphatic invasion and metastasis in human gastric carcinoma. *Am J Gastroenterol* 1999;94:451–455.

21. Yamamoto H, Itoh F, Fukushima H, Hinoda Y, Imai K. Overexpression of cyclooxygenase-2 protein is less frequent in gastric cancers with microsatellite instability. *Int J Cancer* 1999;84:400–403.

22. Tsujii M, Kawano S, Sawaoka H, Takei Y, Kobayashi I, Nagano K, Fusamoto H, Kamada T. Evidence for involvement of cyclooxygenase-2 in proliferation of two gastrointestinal cancer cell lines. *Prostaglandins Leukot Essent Fatty Acids* 1996;55:179–183.

23. Davies GR, Simmonds NJ, Stevens TR, Sheaff MT, Banatvala N, Laurenson IF, Blake DR, Rampton DS. *Helicobacter pylori* stimulates antral mucosal reactive oxygen metabolite production *in vivo*. *Gut* 1994;35:179–185

24. Suzuki H, Mori M, Suzuki M, Sakurai K, Miura S, Ishii H. Extensive DNA damage induced by monochloramine in gastric cells. *Cancer Lett* 1997;115:243–248.

25. Sugiyama A, Maruta F, Ikeno T, Ishida K, Kawasaki S, Katsuyama T, Shimizu N, Tatematsu M. *Helicobacter pylori* infection enhances N-methyl-N-nitrosourea-induced stomach carcinogenesis in the Mongolian gerbil. *Cancer Res* 1998;58:2067–2069.

26. Rachmilewicz D, Karmeli F, Eliakim R, Stalnikowicz R, Ackerman Z, Amir G, Stamler JS. Enhanced gastric nitric oxide synthase activity in duodenal ulcer patients. *Gut* 1994;35:1394–1397.

27. Shapiro KB, Hotchkiss JH. Induction of nitric oxide synthesis in murine macrophages by *Helicobacter pylori*. *Cancer Lett* 1996;102:49–56.

28. Goto T, Haruma K, Kitadai Y, Ito M, Yoshihara M, Sumii K, Hayakawa N, Kajiyama G. Enhanced expression of inducible nitric oxide synthase and nitrotyrosine in gastric mucosa of gastric cancer patients. *Clin Cancer Res* 1999;5:1411–1415.

29. Mannick EE, Bravo LE, Zarama G, Realpe JL, Zhang XJ, Ruiz B, Fontham ETH, Mera R, Miller MJS, Correa P. Inducible nitric oxide synthase, nitrotyrosine, and apoptosis in *Helicobacter pylori* gastritis: effect of antibiotics and antioxidants. *Cancer Res* 1996;56:3228–3243.

30. Yamada H, Aihara T, Okabe S. A mechanism for *Helicobacter pylori* stimulation of interleukin-8 production in a gastric epithelial cell line (MKN 28): The role of mitogen-activated protein kinase and interleukin-1. *Biochemical Pharmacol* 2001;61:1595–604.

31. Yoshimura T, Shimoyama T, Tanaka M, Sasaki Y, Fukuda S, Munakata A. Gastric mucosal inflammation and epithelial cell turnover are associated with gastric cancer in patients with *Helicobacter pylori* infection. *J Clin Pathol* 2000;53:532–536.

32. Peek RM Jr, Wirth HP, Moss SF, Yang M, Abdalla AM, Tham KT, Zhang T, Tang LH, Modlin IM, Blaser MJ. *Helicobacter pylori* alters gastric epithelial cell cycle events and gastrin secretion in Mongolian gerbils. *Gastroenterology* 2000;118:48–59.

33. Fox JG. Rodent models for Helicobacter-induced gastric cancer. In: Hunt RH, Tytgat GNJ Ed. *Helicobacter pylori. Basic Mechanisms to Clinical Cure 2000*. Dordrecht: Kluwer Academic Publishers, 2000;489–505.

34. Meining A, Bayerdorffer E, Stolte M. Therapy of *Helicobacter pylori*-associated gastric neoplasms. In: *Clinical Pharmacology and Therapy of* Helicobacter pylori *Infection*. Scarpignato and Porro GB, Ed. Progress in Basic Clin Pharmacol, Basel: Karger, 1999;11:305–316

V.

Pancreatic Regulation

Gut-Brain Peptides in the New Millennium, edited by Y. Taché
CURE Foundation, Los Angeles, CA. © 2002

37

The Delta-to-Beta Cell Endocrine Axis Within the Islets of Langerhans

F. Charles Brunicardi, Stefan Moldovan, and Michael Norman
Michael E. DeBakey Department of Surgery, Baylor College of Medicine, Houston, TX

INTRODUCTION

In August of 1988, the Chairman of Surgery, Dr. Michael Zinner, invited me to interview with the Department of Surgery at UCLA. He told me that an outstanding aspect of joining the Department would be the opportunity to collaborate with CURE. Since my training included a three-year research fellowship in the laboratory of Dana K. Andersen studying pancreatic endocrine physiology, during which time I heard many stories about the legendary CURE, I was excited to visit. During that interview, I met John Walsh for the first time and remember most his brilliance. He knew more about the mechanisms I was interested in studying than anyone I had ever encountered. He offered full support of the CURE cores to help build a research program in pancreatic physiology and was also willing to serve as a mentor. In July of 1989, I was most fortunate to join the Department of Surgery at UCLA and begin a fruitful collaboration with CURE. Dr. Walsh kept his promise and fostered full support of the wonderful CURE cores: immunohistochemistry (Dr. Catia Sternini), antibody production (Helen Wong), radioimmunoassay (Dr. Seymour Levin) and microcirculation (Dr. Paul Guth). Most importantly, he served as a research mentor and always had answers to my many questions that helped direct the experiments to their next level.

It was during these years that we talked about the endocrine pancreas and how it functioned as a unit. By having access to the cores, a series of experiments were performed which enabled the testing of the hypothesis that there exists a delta-to-beta cell endocrine axis within the islets of Langerhans, which will be described in the following pages. These studies are dedicated to the memory of Dr. Walsh, who will always remain in my mind as one of the most brilliant and generous men.

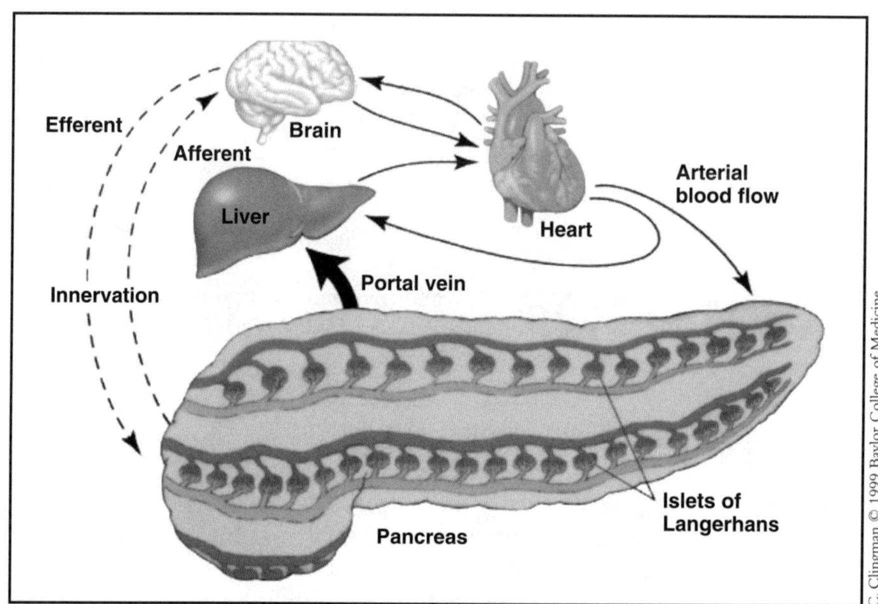

FIGURE 1. *The arterial milieu of hormones and nutrients is seen simultaneously by all islets and by the brain. In response to any change, the brain sends neural signals to the endocrine pancreas to alter both the islet microcirculation and the secretion of the islet cells. Flow to the endocrine pancreas and within the islets is optimized to expose the appropriate cell type required to respond to the changes in the arterial milieu. For example, low glucose would result in a shunting of blood away from the islets and would also shunt blood to the periphery of the islet where the alpha cells are located. High glucose would cause a shunting of blood to the islets and to the center of the islets where the beta cells are located. Within the islet, the islet cells also respond directly to the change in arterial concentrations of nutrients and hormones. Taken all together, the islets secrete the appropriate hormonal milieu into the portal vein, necessary for glucose homeokinesis.*

THE ENDOCRINE PANCREAS

There are approximately one million islets of Langerhans in the adult human pancreas. The islets range in size from 40–900uM and are located along different points of the pancreatic arterial tree with larger islets being located closer to the major arterioles and smaller islets being more deeply embedded into the parenchyma of the pancreas. The islets are perfused in parallel and simultaneously experience the systemic arterial hormonal milieu. The brain also receives the same arterial hormonal milieu and sends regulatory neural signals to the endocrine pancreas. Each islet contains approximately 2000 cells. There are four types of endocrine cells within an islet, alpha (A), beta (B), delta (D), and PP (F) cells which secrete more than 20 different hormones (1, 2). Traditionally, we think of the A, B, D and PP cells secreting glucagon, insulin, somatostatin, and pancreatic polypeptide, respectively, however, the hormonal milieu emanating from the endocrine pancreas is far more complex. Each islet has a complex neural supply and an intricate microcirculation that regulate hormone secretion from the cells via nitric oxide (3, 4). Furthermore, there is considerable cell-cell regulation within the islets, which is mediated by hormone secretion. The final product of these five regulatory mechanisms is a hormonal milieu which is secreted into the portal circulation and is largely responsible for glucose homeokinesis. This is the unifying hypothesis of the endocrine pancreas (Figure 1) (5).

In order to investigate intraislet regulatory mechanisms of the endocrine pancreas *in vitro*, isolated perfused human and rat pancreas models were used. The isolated perfused human pancreas model (IPHP) was conceptualized and developed in the laboratory of Dr. Andersen in 1983, and then established in my laboratory at CURE in 1989 (6, 7). I was fortunate to work with several outstanding surgical fellows during this time, Drs. Philip Watt, Robert Kleinman, Azmi Atiya, Stefan Moldovan, and Yie Ming Liu who helped perform many of the experiments. The scientific collaborators for this project were Drs. Ed Livingston, Ed Passaro, William Go, Tom Adrian, Catia Sternini, Gordon Ohning, Kent Lloyd, Roberto DiGiorgio, Jeff Gornbein, Seymour Levin, Helen Wong, and John Walsh.

Human pancreata were procured with the help of the local procurement agency from heart beating organ donors. Following removal from the body, the pancreas was transported on ice to the laboratory in Viaspan solution. The body and tail of the pancreas was perfused via the splenic artery and effluent was collected from the splenic vein; the pancreatic duct was cannulated with an 18-gauge catheter. Anterograde perfusion of the pancreas was performed with a modified Krebs-bicarbonate buffer. Aliquots from the venous cannula were collected every 1–2 minutes; samples were immediately assayed for glucose and frozen at −20°C for subsequent radioimmunoassay of islet hormones. Mean perfusion time was 214 ± 42 minutes with a range from 0.5 to 9 hours.

Statistical analysis of intrapancreatic and interpancreatic variables on hormone secretion was performed. The influence of preoperative donor factors, such as age, blood glucose, hospital days, positive CMV serology, blood transfusion, and smoking, on mean insulin secretion over time from the pancreas preparation was analyzed using multiple regression analysis. The most interesting finding from this analysis was that a faster decay of insulin secretion over time was seen from pancreata procured from donors with a history of smoking. No other donor variables achieved statistical significance with respect to their effect on insulin secretion (8).

Ratios of the concentrations of four major hormones in the venous effluent of the IPHP were analyzed and compared to ratios seen in portal venous and peripheral blood drawn from the organ donors and to peripheral

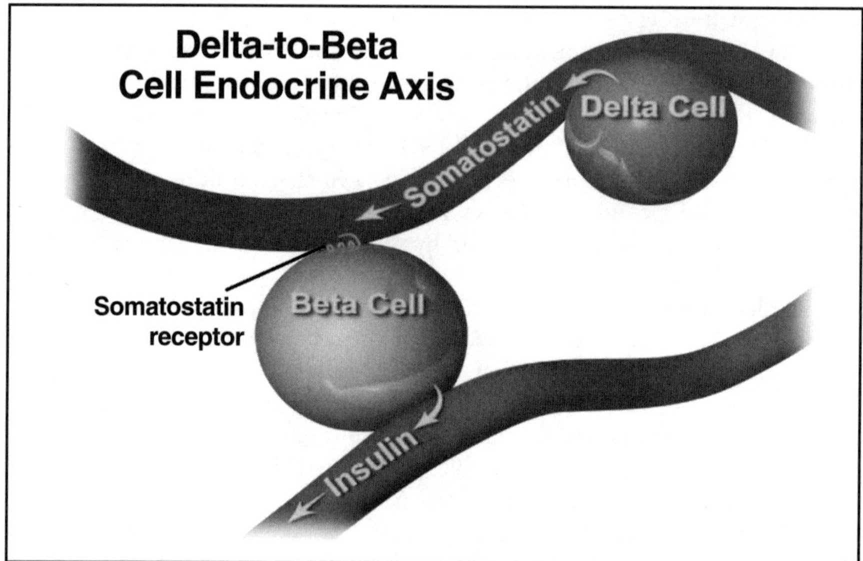

FIGURE 2. *In this model, intraislet somatostatin has an important role in the regulation of insulin secretion. Intraislet somatostatin, released from the delta cell into the islet microcirculation, reaches the beta cell via the capillaries, and binds to somatostatin receptors on the beta cell to inhibit insulin secretion.*

blood of healthy volunteers. Historic controls of hormone levels taken from published series were also analyzed. It was interesting to note that the circulating ratios of insulin, C-peptide, glucagon and pancreatic polypeptide are nearly equimolar in healthy volunteers and in the historic controls. This observation suggests that the endocrine pancreas secretes a hormonal milieu that results in equimolar circulating levels of its major hormones. However, the ratio of hormones were markedly altered in the portal vein and peripheral vein of heart beating, brain dead, cadaver donors, and were further altered in the venous effluent from the IPHP. These observations suggested that the hormonal milieu secreted from the human pancreas is altered by brain death and pancreatic denervation (9).

Comparisons of the responses of insulin, glucagon, pancreatic polypeptide and somatostatin responses to different stimuli led to the hypothesis that hormonal regulation of islet cell secretion was occurring within the islet. For example, high glucose resulted in stimulation of insulin and somatostatin secretion and inhibition of glucagon and pancreatic polypeptide secretion (5, 9, 11). In analyzing these responses, we hypothesized that glucagon and pancreatic polypeptide were inhibited by either (1) a direct effect of high glucose on the alpha and PP cells, (2) an indirect effect of intraislet insulin on these cells, or (3) an indirect of intraislet somatostatin on these cells. Therefore, antibodies to somatostatin, glucagon, and insulin were infused into the IPHP to immunoneutralize the respective hormones and hormonal responses in the venous effluent were examined. The results were striking and differed from previously published reports (12, 13).

The most striking results were found with the infusion of a potent monoclonal somatostatin antibody, which was developed by Helen Wong and Dr. John Walsh. During infusion of the antibody into the IPHP, insulin and glucagon were stimulated at both high and low glucose perfusions, but no significant change in pancreatic polypeptide was seen. This suggested that intraislet somatostatin is an inhibitory regulator of insulin and glucagon secretion, but not pancreatic polypeptide secretion. A series of experiments followed in the IPHP supporting the hypothesis that intraislet somatostatin inhibits insulin secretion both at high and low glucose concentrations and that the effect is mediated within the islet capillaries (14, 15, 16).

In the perfused rat pancreas, somatostatin antibody infusion resulted in the augmentation of second phase, but not first phase, insulin secretion (17, 18). Pancreatic polypeptide secretion was stimulated in the rat model. This suggested that in the rat pancreas, intraislet somatostatin inhibits second phase insulin secretion and pancreatic polypeptide secretion (19). These observations support the hypothesis that intraislet somatostatin is an endocrine regulator of islet hormone secretion in the rat pancreas (Figure 2).

In another experiment, a polyclonal insulin antibody (INS-Ab) was infused into the IPHP. Since INS-Ab interferes with the measurement of insulin, but not C-peptide, B cell secretion was measured by C-peptide response. Infusion of INS-Ab into the human pancreas stimulated C-peptide secretion, which support the hypothesis that intraislet insulin inhibits B cell secretion. However, it is possible that alterations in intraislet somatostatin caused the increase in C-peptide secretion, since somatostatin secretion was suppressed during the infusion of INS-Ab. Infusion of INS-Ab resulted in an increase in glucagon secretion and this response could have been secondary to the fall in somatostatin secretion (20).

In summary, two plausible forms of cellular communication might be occurring within the islet. The B cell secretory product could be directly inhibiting both B cell and A cell secretion. Alternatively, there exists regulatory feedback loops between A and D cells and the B and D cells, in which intraislet somatostatin is the mediator.

Infusion of glucagon antibody (GN-Ab) into the IPHP resulted in significant stimulation of insulin and pancreatic polypeptide secretion, whereas somatostatin secretion was inhibited (20). As above, these results suggest that either the A cell secretory product directly inhibits B and PP cell secretion, or the effect was due to the fall in somatostatin secretion.

In summary, these studies in the perfused human and rat pancreas models support the concept of a dynamic relationship between the different cell types within the islet. There appears to be remarkable cellular communication within the islet that is regulated by alterations in hormone secretion. The hormone responses seen in these studies support the hypothesis of regulatory feedback loops within the islet, which are mediated by intraislet somatostatin. In this hypothesis, the delta cell secretes somatostatin, which inhibits insulin secretion from the beta cells, glucagon secretion from the alpha cells, and PP secretion from the PP cells. Immunohistochemistry studies of human islets performed in the laboratory of Dr. Catia Sternini support this hypothesis: delta cells were seen scattered throughout the islets (15). This hypothesis is juxtaposed to the current dogma that the delta cells have no role within the islets, that intraislet somatostatin is secreted and exits the islet without influencing the other islet cells (12, 13).

IN VIVO MICROSCOPY OF THE ENDOCRINE PANCREAS

In order to support this hypothesis, microcirculation studies were performed using *in vivo* microscopy techniques in the laboratory of Dr. Paul Guth at CURE. The collaborators were Drs. Paul Guth, Ed Livingston, Harold Wayland, Robert McCusky, Stefan Moldovan and Dr. Liu. Using 20× *in vivo* microscopy, both rat and mouse islet microcirculations were studied using *in vivo* microscopy studies with intravital stains and fluorescent microsphere injections. Once an islet was identified in the pancreatic circulation, patterns of blood flow were examined and recorded under both light and fluorescent microscopy using intravenous and/or intraarterial infusions of fluorescent markers (FITC-labeled red cells, FITC-albumin, FITC-somatostatin antibodies and fluorescent microspheres). All video images were analyzed in real time and in slow motion. The passage of FITC-albumin and FITC-antibodies in real time moved as a wave across the islet from the afferent to the efferent pole (20, 21). The observation of polar flow suggests that all cell types of one hemisphere are perfused before the flow reaches the cells of the opposite hemisphere, i.e. all cell types of one hemisphere could potentially influence the cell types located in the other hemisphere. For example, somatostatin secreted from D cells in one hemisphere could influence insulin secretion of B cells and glucagon secretion from A cells of the other hemisphere. Any given cell type could also influence its own cell type, insulin secreted from B cells in one hemisphere could influence insulin secretion of B cells of the other hemisphere. The limitation of *in vivo* microscopy is that the images are viewed and analyzed in two dimensions and that only one islet per pancreas is visualized, however analysis of multiple preps suggests that flow across the islet is polar.

Flow to an islet appeared to be regulated at two levels in both the rat and mouse pancreas. Sphincters at the feeding arteriole would stop flow to the entire islet approximately three times per minute, while the flow through

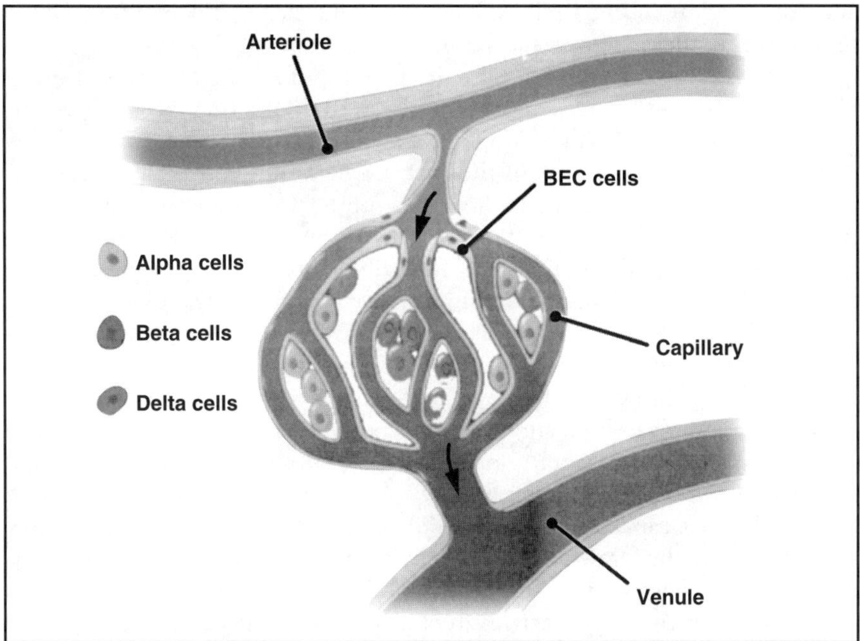

FIGURE 3. *Flow to the islets is regulated by external and internal gates, at the level of the feeding arteriole and islet capillaries, respectively. The external gates at the feeding arteriole control blood flow to the islet cell mass and pancreatic blood flow can be shunted way from or to the islets depending on the arterial concentration of hormones and nutrients. Internal gates (bulging endothelial cells) can direct flow within the islet to the appropriate endocrine cell type. Alpha cells are located in the periphery and beta cells are located in the center of the islet. The pattern of blood flow within the islet appears to proceed from one pole of the islet to the other, suggesting that cells in one hemisphere could potentially influence cells located in the other hemisphere.*

the parent arteriole was constant. These regulatory sphincters, or "external gates", are regulated by nitric oxide (20, 21). The presence of external gates is supported by the studies of Jansson and Hellerstrom (22, 23). Using the static microsphere technique in a rat model, it was demonstrated that glucose administration almost doubled the total blood flow to the islet mass. During hyperglycemia, the islet received 85% more blood than in basal condition by a mechanism that was mediated by a cholinergic mechanism. These studies suggest that within the pancreas, blood is shunted to the islets during hyperglycemia via a cholinergic mechanism (22, 23).

"Internal gates" regulate flow within the islet. In 1968, Dr. McCuskey reported contractile endothelial cells that bulge within the islet capillaries and intermittently occlude flow (bulging endothelial cells or BEC cells) (24). In a recent visit to his laboratory, an islet capillary was visualized using 100X *in vivo* microscopy of the mouse pancreas. An endothelial cell was seen to swell and occlude flow in the capillary. The cell would then shrink and flow would resume. Thus, there appeared to be internal gates regulating flow.

The studies performed in Dr. Guth's lab supported the presence of internal regulatory units in rat and mouse islets (20, 21). Using 20× *in vivo* microscopy, blood flow would stop in one portion of the islet, while flow continued in other portions of the islet. Utilizing fluorescent microspheres and other fluorescent markers, flow was noted to randomly stop and go within selected capillaries of the islet, while flow continued unimpeded in other capillaries of the same islet. These observations support the presence of internal gates regulating flow within the capillaries of the islet.

The effect of hyperglycemia on capillary flow within a single islet was investigated using *in vivo* microscopy of the mouse pancreas; under fluorescent light a bolus of FITC–albumin was injected retrogradely through a carotid catheter during baseline and hyperglycemic conditions. During hyperglycemia, there was a significant shortening of the FITC–albumin bolus transit time through the capillary network, suggesting an increase in blood flow in the islet capillary during hyperglycemia. The increase in blood flow was ablated in the presence of a nitric oxide synthase inhibitor. We concluded that hyperglycemia increases blood flow within the capillary of a mouse islet and that this mechanism is regulated by nitric oxide (21).

In summary of these experiments, each islet has a complex microcirculation, which resembles a glomerulus. Flow to the islets appears to be regulated by external and flow within the islet is polar and is regulated by internal gates. These gates are regulated in part by neural mechanisms and nitric oxide (25).

Based upon these observations, it was hypothesized that the microcirculation itself serves as a regulatory agent for islet hormone secretion (Figure 3) (5). In this hypothesis, changes in arterial concentrations of nutrients and hormones are recognized simultaneously by all islets of the endocrine pancreas and by the central nervous system, thus there might be two levels of response. At one level of response, the central nervous system sends neural signals to the endocrine pancreas to alter the microcirculation, which is regulated by internal and external gates. One of the final regulators of the gates is nitric oxide. Flow to the endocrine pancreas and within the islets is optimized to expose the appropriate cell type required to respond to the changes in the arterial milieu. The other level of response is within the islet. The islet cells respond directly to the change in arterial concentrations of nutrients and hormones. For example, an increase in arterial glucose would be sensed by the endocrine pancreas and the brain simultaneously, resulting in two tiers of response. The central nervous system sends a cholinergic signal to the endocrine pancreas, which is mediated by nitric oxide. Both external gates, which shunt blood flow to the entire endocrine pancreas, and internal gates, which shunt flow to B cells in the core of the islet and away from A cells in the mantle, are opened. In addition, B cells and A cells respond directly to the increase in capillary glucose and these responses are locally modified by hormonal feedback loops and nitric oxide. The two tiered response results in two-phased insulin secretion and a decrease in glucagon secretion.

Many of these studies of endocrine pancreatic physiology would not have been possible without the generosity and mentorship of Dr. John Walsh and the collegial atmosphere of CURE. Looking back, working with Dr. John Walsh was one of the highlights of my career and I will forever owe him a great debt of gratitude.

ACKNOWLEDGMENTS

This work was funded by NIH/NIDDK Grant, DK46441-08.

REFERENCES

1. Orci L. The microanatomy of the islets of Langerhans. *Metabolism* 1976;25:1303–1313.
2. Anderson DK and Brunicardi FC. Pancreatic Anatomy and Physiology. In *Surgery: Scientific Principles and Practice.* Edited by Greenfield L, J.B. Lippincott, 1993;775–791.
3. Brunicardi FC, Shavelle M, Anderson DK. Neural regulation of the endocrine pancreas. *Int J Pancreat* 1995;18 (3), 177–195.
4. Atiya A, Cohen G, Ignarro L, Brunicardi FC. Nitric oxide regulates insulin secretion in the isolated perfused human pancreas via a cholinergic mechanism. *Surgery* 1996;120(2):322–327.
5. Moldovan S, Brunicardi FC. Endocrine pancreas: summary of observations generated by surgical fellows. *World J Surg* 2001;25(4):468–473.
6. Brunicardi FC, Goulet RJ, Sun YS, Berlin SA, Elahi D, Anderson DK. Neural and hormonal regulation of insulin and glucagon secretion in the isolated perfused human pancreas. *Surg Forum* 1984;35:214–217.
7. Brunicardi FC, Druck P, Seymour N, Sun YS, Elahi D, Anderson DK. Selective neurohormonal interactions in islet cell secretion in the isolated perfused human pancreas. *J Surg Res* 1990;48:273–278.
8. Todd K, Kleinman R, Millis M, Brunicardi FC. The influence of preoperative donor factors on the performance of the isolated perfused human pancreas. *J Surg Res* 1994;56(2):141–145.
9. Brunicardi FC, Dyen L, Brostrom L, Kleinman R, Colonna J, Gelabert H, Gingerich R. The circulating hormonal milieu of the endocrine pancreas in healthy individuals, organ donors, and the isolated perfused human pancreas. *Pancreas* 2000;21(2):203–211.
10. Brunicardi FC, Sun YS, Druck P, Goulet RJ, Elahi D, Andersen DK. Splanchnic neural and regulation of insulin and glucagon secretion in the isolated perfused human pancreas. *Am J Surg* 1987;153:34–40.
11. Brunicardi FC, Druck P, Sun Y, Elahi D, Gingerich R, Anderson, DK. Regulation of pancreatic polypeptide secretion in the isolated perfused human pancreas. *Am J Surg* 1988;155:63–69.
12. Stagner JI, Samols E, Bonner-Weir S. B-A-D pancreatic islet cellular perfusion in dogs. *Diabetes* 1988;41:1715–1721.
13. Stagner JI, Samols E. The vascular order of perfusion in the human pancreas. *Diabetes* 1992;41:93–97.
14. Kleinman R, Ohning G, Wong H, Watt P, Walsh J, Brunicardi FC. A regulatory role of intraislet somatostatin on insulin secretion to in the isolated perfused human pancreas. *Pancreas* 1994;9(2), 172–178.
15. Kleinman R, Gingerich R, Wong H, Walsh J, Lloyd K, Ohning G, DeGiorgio R, Sternini C, Brunicardi FC. Use of the Fab fragment for immunoneutralization of somatostatin in the isolated perfused human pancreas. *Am J Surg* 1994;167:114–119.
16. Kleinman R, Gingerich R, Ohning G, Wong H, Olthoff K, Walsh J, Brunicardi FC. The influence of somatostatin on glucagon and pancreatic polypeptide secretion in the isolated perfused human pancreas. *Int J Pancreat* 1995;18:51–57.

17. Kleinman RM, Gingerich R, Ohning G, Bradley JC, Wong H, Livingston EH, Walsh J, Brunicardi FC. Intraislet regulation of pancreatic polypeptide secretion in the isolated perfused rat pancreas. *Pancreas* 1997;15(4):384–391.

18. Brunicardi FC, Wen D, Bradley JC, Elahi D, Miller CC, Hanks J. The effect of intraislet somatostatin immunoneutralization on insulin secretion in the isolated perfused rat pancreas. *Int J Surg Invest* 2000; 1(5):381–388.

19. Brunicardi FC, Kleinman R, Moldovan S, Nguyen TL, Watt P, Walsh J, Gingerich R. Immunoneutralization of somatostatin, insulin, and glucagon causes alterations in islet cell secretion in the isolated perfused human pancreas. *Pancreas* 2001;23(3):302–308.

20. Liu Y, Guth PH, Kaneko K, Livingston EH, Brunicardi FC. Dynamic *in vivo* observation of rat islet microcirculation. *Pancreas* 1993;8:15–21.

21. Moldovan S, Livingston E, Zhang RS, Kleinman R, Guth P, Brunicardi FC. Glucose induced islet hyperemia is mediated by nitric oxide. *Am J Surg* 1996;171:16–20.

22. Jansson L and Hellerstrom C. Stimulation by glucose of the blood flow to the pancreatic islets of the rat. *Diabetologia* 1983;25:45–50.

23. Jansson L and Hellerstrom C. Glucose induced changes in pancreatic islet blood flow mediated by central nervous system. *Am J Physiol* 1986;251:E644–E647.

24. McCuskey RT, Chapman TM. Microscopy of the living pancreas in situ. *Am J Anat* 1969;126: 395–406.

25. Brunicardi FC, Stagner J, Bonner-Weir S, Wayland H, Kleinman R, Livingston E, Guth P, Menger M, McCuskey R, Intaglietta M, Charles A, Ashley S, Cheung A, Ipp E, Gilman S, Howard T, Passaro E. Microcirculation of the islets of langerhans. Long Beach Veterans Administration Regional Medical Education Center Symposium. *Diabetes* 1996;45(4):385–392.

Gut-Brain Peptides in the New Millennium, edited by Y. Taché
CURE Foundation, Los Angeles, CA. © 2002

38

Expectation of Pancreatic Physiological Responses from CCK$_B$ Receptor Occupation in its Natural Environment

Sophie Julien, Jean Lainé, and Jean Morisset
Department of Medicine, Faculty of Medicine, University of Sherbrooke
Sherbrooke, Quebec, Canada

INTRODUCTION

The physiological regulation of multiple organs of the digestive tract of most mammals, including human, involves the interaction of various hormones and neurotransmitters with their specific receptors; most of them belong to the super family of guanine nucleotide-binding protein-coupled receptors. Among these, those of the cholecystokinin (CCK) family got our attention because of the major controversies reported in the literature regarding their distribution, localization, biochemical characteristics and physiological functions. This chapter, in memory of Dr. John Walsh, will focus on the CCK$_B$ subtype, the most controversial. Indeed, because of Dr. Walsh's generous gift of specific CCK$_B$ receptor antibodies, we were able to clearly localize and characterize this receptor in the pancreas of different species. In light of these data, we sincerely hope, in the near future, to clarify some of its physiological roles.

The CCK receptor family is composed of two subtypes: the pancreatic receptors, named "CCK$_A$ receptors" and the brain receptors named "CCK$_B$ receptors". This initial classification resulted from distinct pharmacological features in their ability to recognize CCK and gastrin (1). This classification was later confirmed when cloning of the CCK$_A$ receptor from pancreas and that of the CCK$_B$ receptor from stomach and brain were achieved (2–4). As summarized by Wank (5), the CCK$_A$ receptors are mostly found on pancreatic acini, pancreatic islets, gastric mucosa, gallbladder, muscles of the stomach and intestine, selected area of the central and peripheral nervous system and on some neoplastic cells. The CCK$_B$ subtype is mainly distributed throughout the CNS, on the gastric mucosa and numerous neoplastic cells of the GI tract origin.

In 1997, it was reported that in man, the CCK$_B$ receptor protein had not been identified; in canine pancreas, its proportion was estimated at 20%;

very few CCK_B receptor exists in guinea pig while the rat and mouse pancreas express only the CCK_A subtype (6). Ever since, this picture has greatly evolved. However, so far, no clear pancreatic biological functions have been ascribed to this CCK_B receptor. To fill up this gap in our knowledge, three main strategies were elaborated: the generation of transgenic mice expressing the CCK_B/gastrin receptors in pancreatic acinar cells where no one has yet established, in any species, that this subtype exists on these cells (7); the transfection of the CCK_B receptor in cells known to be free of the protein (8) and finally, the generation of CCK_B knockout mice (9). It is mandatory to identify the cell types within different tissues in which this CCK_B receptor is expressed. Indeed, detailed knowledge about its expression is important to fully characterize the physiological roles of CCK and gastrin. Receptor presence in a particular tissue or cell can thus be established biochemically, pharmacologically, functionally, immunohistologically at the level of the receptor protein or its gene.

In this chapter, we will review 1) The cellular and tissue localization of the CCK_B receptor; 2) The properties of the native and transfected CCK_B receptor, 3) The expression of this receptor on pancreatic cancer cells, 4) The importance of the CCK_B receptor knockout mice to assess the role of this receptor, and 5) The known physiological and potential biological actions in response to this receptor's occupation by CCK and gastrin. Finally, we will outline our present understanding of the potential roles for this CCK_B receptor in the pancreas.

Localization of the CCK_B Receptor

In the human pancreas, binding of ^{125}I-BH-CCK-8 evaluated by storage phosphor autoradiography was diffusely distributed and bound to the CCK_B subtype as established by displacement studies with the CCK_B receptor antagonist L-365,260 (10). More recently, in human fetal and adult pancreas, the CCK_B/gastrin receptor was localized by confocal microscopy and immunohistochemistry in islet cells, and more precisely in islet glucagon producing cells. In this study, specificity of the reaction was not confirmed by pre-incubation of the primary antibody with the corresponding peptide antigen (11). As described previously (12), our data indicate however that the human fetal and adult pancreas (Figure 1) express quite specifically the CCK_B receptor in the islet somatostatin cells as established by immunofluorescence from serial sections of pancreatic tissue. It is important to point out that in this case, identification of the CCK_B receptor by Western Blot was completely blocked by preincubation of the antibody with its antigen (Figure 1).

In the cynomolgus monkey, Miller, et al. established by RT-PCR and ribonuclease protection assay that their cloned CCK_B receptor was highly ex-

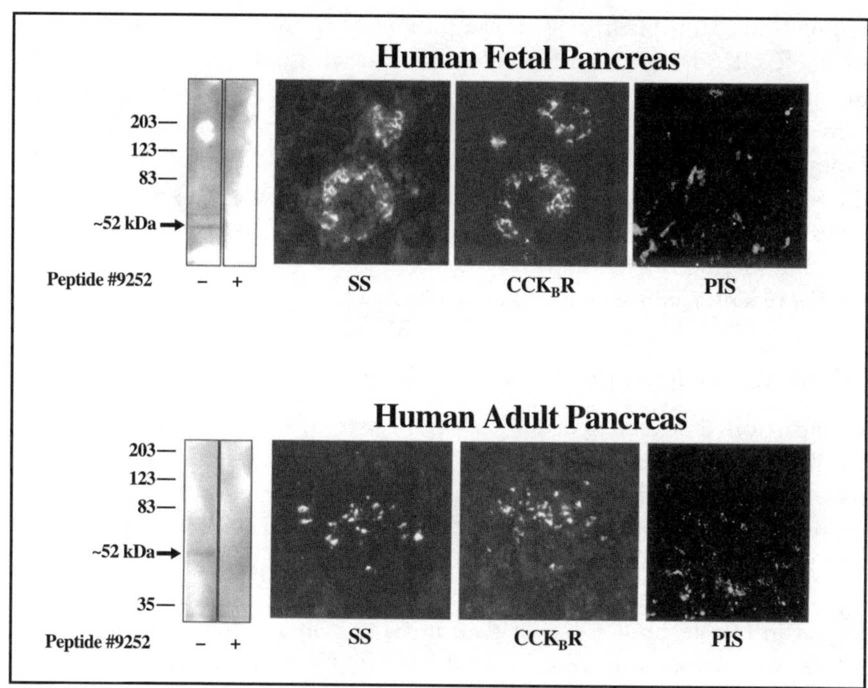

FIGURE 1. Colocalization of somatostatin and the CCK$_B$ receptor in human islets of Langerhans. *Western blots and indirect immunofluorescence of somatostatin (SS) and CCK$_B$ receptor from fetal and adult human pancreas. Polyclonal antibodies 9262 and 9252 with their respective peptide were used to identify and localize the CCK$_B$ receptor along with anti-somatostatin R21-B3 from Dr. Orci. Techniques are described in reference 12. PIS: preimmune serum.*

pressed in brain and stomach but undetectable in gallbladder and pancreas (13); they did not look, however, for the protein. In the pig pancreas (14), contrary to what was previously observed in human (11), the CCK$_A$ receptor not the CCK$_B$ subtype, co-localizes with glucagon in the islets α cells as evaluated by immunohistochemistry. In this study however, the expression of the CCK$_B$ receptor gene was not evaluated. In the CCK$_B$/gastrin receptor (Elas CCK$_B$) transgenic-mice, receptor autoradiography after binding of ^{125}I-BH-sulfated gastrin indicated a diffusely and homogeneously distributed CCK$_B$ receptor throughout the pancreatic gland and its absence on the pancreatic section of the wild type mice, suggesting specific localization of this transfected CCK$_B$ receptor on acinar cells (7). In the rat fetal and adult pancreas, our data localized the CCK$_B$ receptor on islets somatostatin delta cells (12), a finding which could not be reproduced recently by others. Indeed, Rooman, et al. (15) found by immunohistochemistry that all epithelial cells from rat fetal E17-18 pancreas were labeled for the CCK$_B$ receptor, but this labeling totally disappeared two days later and postnatally. However, they claimed that after birth, cells in the periphery of the islets became positive for the CCK_B receptor with a colocalization with glucagon without showing any data. In that study, the CCK_B receptor was also found on duct-like cells five days after duct ligature, a feature not found in normal pancreas. From all these data, confusion still exists regarding the localization of the CCK_B receptor in the pancreas in many species. In order to solve these discrepancies, colocalization and functional studies will have to be performed to really ascribe a specific physiological response to the occupation of this CCK_B receptor in a specific tissue and/or cell.

Properties of Recombinant and Natively Expressed CCK_B Receptor

Comparisons between biochemical properties of the native or transfected CCK_B receptor were established to determine whether this receptor subtype preserves its fundamental characteristics. When the human CCK_B receptor transfected in COS cells (16) was compared with that present on GH3 cells and cortical brain membranes known to express the CCK_B subtype (17), the affinity of the receptor for ^{125}I-BH-CCK-8S was much higher in transfected COS cells than in GH3 cells and brain membranes by 10 to 40 fold in displacement studies with CCK-8S. Similar differences were also observed with pentagastrin. Three to 10-fold differences were also obtained when L-365,260 was used to displace CCK-8S binding. A similar higher affinity for CCK was observed in Elas CCK_B transgenic mice (7). Indeed, binding of [Thr^{28},Ahy^{31}]CCK-(25-33) to pancreatic acini in the presence of a CCK_A receptor antagonist to neutralize the endogenous CCK_A receptor led to a K_D value of 0.95 nM, almost comparable to the K_D of 0.45 nM found on wild type mice pancreatic acini with CCK_A receptors on their acinar cells. An evaluation of the binding parameters of ^3H-PD140376, a CCK_B receptor antagonist, to the rat pancreatic cancer cells AR42J and to the guinea pig gastric membrane indicated that Ki obtained from displacement studies by the agonists CCK8S, G17-2, pentagastrin and the antagonist L-365,260 were comparable in the nM range (18). Finally, the CCK_B/gastrin receptors characterized on guinea pig pancreatic acini resemble those previously reported on gastric gland, mouse colon cancer cells, canine fundic somatostatin-releasing cells, isolated parietal cells, rabbit gastric mucosal cells and rat mucosal membranes in having an affinity for gastrin-17-1 and CCK-8 in the nanomolar range (19). It seems, therefore, that the CCK_B receptor present in its natural environment exhibits similar biochemical characteristics whether it is expressed in normal cells or in various cancer cells. However, transfection of the receptor in different cell types or in mice increased its affinity for gastrin and CCK, its natural agonists.

The Expression of CCK_B Receptor on Pancreatic Cancer Cells

Higher mammalian species can express CCK A and B receptors. Although doubts still exist about CCK_B cellular distribution and physiological relevance, the pancreatic cancer cells on the contrary do not seem to exhibit such uncertainty. Our data and those of Rooman, et al. clearly showed that CCK_B receptor expression remained undetected on exocrine acinar and on ductal cells of human, rat, mouse and pig pancreas (12, 15). On the contrary, all the rat (18) or human (20, 21) pancreatic cancer cells of ductal origin specifically exhibit the CCK_B receptor with comparable high affinity in the nM range for CCK-8S and gastrin-17S and for the CCK_B receptor antagonist L-365,260. These studies include the AR42J cells (18), the MIA-PaCa-2 cells (20) as well as the PANC-1, MDA-Panc-28, MDA-Amp-7, Capan 1 and BxPC-3 cells (21). In all these cells, except for some strains of AR42J cells, there was no binding with radiolabeled CCK_A receptor antagonist. In such pancreatic cancer, the CCK_B receptor could serve as a marker of dedifferentiation, as being an ubiquitous component of human pancreatic cancers. Such dedifferentiation does not appear in cells already expressing the CCK_B receptor. Indeed, in the African rodent Mastomys natalensis, the gastric ECL cells expressing the CCK_B receptor see its expression slightly increased in experimental ECL gastric carcinoid tumors (22). Recent data however suggest that a new type of CCK receptor, the CCK-c receptor, C for cancer, different from the CCK_B subtype, could be specifically expressed in human pancreatic cancer cells (23) and be responsible for their growth (24). This is an interesting new finding which needs further investigation to substantiate its true identity against that of the yet uncloned glycine-extended gastrin receptor (25).

Importance of CCK_B Receptor Knockout Mice to Estimate the Role of the CCK_B Receptor

Generation of the CCK_B receptor knockout mice has been so far limited, and the influence of its deletion was first studied in the stomach (9). Indeed, Nagata, et al. first reported that homozygous mice exhibited atrophy of the gastric mucosa due to a decrease in parietal and chromogranin A-positive entero-chromaffin-like cells in the presence of severe hypergastrinemia. These results were later confirmed by Langhans, et al. (26) with additional information that in these knockout animals, the gastric G cells were significantly increased by 53% and the somatostatin D cells reduced by 43%. In the pancreas of the CCK_B receptor knockout mice produced by Nagata, et al. (9), Miyasaka, et al. (27) clearly showed that the CCK_B receptor had no role in the control of pancreas growth, exocrine enzyme and bile secretion in adult mice, thus supporting our previous observation that this receptor subtype was not localized on pancreatic acinar cells (12). In gene therapy performed with an antisense oligonucleotide to the CCK-c receptor, growth of BxPC-3 pancreatic cancer cells in athymic nude mice and of the same cells transfected with the antisense cDNA was significantly reduced by 75 and 65%, respectively, indicating that this CCK-c receptor is involved in growth regulation of these specific cells (24).

Biological and Physiological Responses from the CCK$_B$ Receptor Occupation

At this point, we have to differentiate between what this receptor can do versus what it really does physiologically in its natural environment. One of the typical physiological responses of CCK$_B$ receptor occupation remains the absence of a classical inhibitory effect at high agonist concentrations seen following CCK$_A$ receptor stimulation: a plateau curve is rather observed. Such plateau type responses were seen *in vitro* (28) and *in vivo* (29) on HCl secretion following CCK-8, G17 or pentagastrin stimulation. In AR42J cells, thymidine incorporation into DNA in response to G17 also presented a plateau between 0.1 nM and 100 nM (25). In GH$_3$ cells naturally expressing the CCK$_B$ receptor, stimulation by CCK-8S and pentagastrin led to polyphosphoinositide turnover and Ca^{2+} mobilization in a dose-dependent manner with CCK-8S being 3 to 4 fold more potent (30). In human pancreatic cancer MIA-PaCa-2 cells, occupation of the natural CCK$_B$ receptor also led to increased Ins (1, 4, 5) P3 formation, Ca^{2+} mobilization, activation of specific PKC isoforms and cell proliferation in response to 1nM CCK-8S (20). Among all the studies on the effects of CCK$_B$ receptor occupation in its natural environment, those of Saillan-Barreau, et al. on glucagon secretion from purified human islets remains the most surprising (11). Indeed, they showed that glucagon secretion in response to CCK and gastrin in the presence of a CCK$_A$ receptor antagonist was maximal at a concentration of 30 pM of both agonists, along with secretion inhibition at agonist concentrations above 0.1 nM, a typical CCK$_A$ response. One can also question the presence of such a CCK$_A$ receptor antagonist, and wonder if its addition could not distort a normal CCK$_B$ dose-response. Furthermore, one should ask why two different species, man and pig, quite comparable in their gut physiology, would bear two different types of CCK receptors on their glucagon cells: the human with the B receptor (11) and the pig with the A type (14).

The presence of the CCK$_B$ receptor in a foreign environment can lead to some typical CCK$_B$ physiological responses. When rat CCK$_B$ receptor is transfected into CHO and Swiss 3T3 cells (8), receptor activation in both cell lines caused comparable specific second messengers production such as phosphoinositide hydrolysis and arachidonate release but opposite effects on growth parameters evaluated by thymidine incorporation into DNA, cell numbers and colonies formation. These opposite effects on growth remain unexplained. Activation of the CCK$_B$ receptors transfected into NIH3T3 fibroblasts also resulted in phosphoinositides hydrolysis, thymidine incorporation, tyrosine phosphorylation of p125-[FAK], activation of mitogen-activated protein kinase and induction of the early-responsive genes c-fos, c-myc and c-jun (31). These data stress that a foreign receptor transfected into cells with the proper intracellular equipment can respond to the intrinsic properties of this receptor.

The worst scenario to study the physiological properties of the CCK$_B$ receptor seems to be the preparation of a transgenic mouse expressing the CCK$_B$/gastrin receptor in the *exocrine* pancreas already equipped with the CCK$_A$ subtype (7). Such gene manipulation led to the expression of a CCK$_B$ transfected receptor with a K$_D$ of 0.95 nM for CCK established in the presence of a CCK$_A$ receptor antagonist, a value almost equal to the K$_D$ of 0.47 nM found for the natural CCK$_A$ receptor in the wild type mouse. Furthermore, this transfected receptor had more affinity for gastrin than for CCK, an unusual feature not found in tissue normally expressing this CCK$_B$ receptor (9) or in pancreatic cancer cells (20). Another strange observation resulting from such a transfection deals with the effects of gastrin on pancreatic protein synthesis (32). Indeed, gastrin increased p70^{S6k} activity, a kinase whose substrate is the S6 ribosomal protein, an important element in the regulation of protein synthesis and cell proliferation, at a maximal concentration of 1 nM with an inhibition at 100 nM. However, the incorporation of ^{35}S-methionine into protein, a result of p70^{S6k} activation, was maximal at 30 pM gastrin with a significant decrease below control values at 100 nM: this remains an unexplained and puzzling observation from two events linked together and stimulated maximally at such huge different gastrin concentrations. With the same model, it was recently shown that over-expression of the CCK$_B$ receptor in murine pancreatic acinar cells led to pancreas proliferation, transdifferentiation of acinar cells and neoplasia, a phenomenon usually originating from pancreatic ductal cells (33). Data from this transgenic CCK$_B$ receptor mice model clearly show what *occupation of this receptor can do* in an abnormal location in comparison with what *it really does physiologically in its natural environment.*

Potential Physiological Role of the CCK$_B$ Receptor in Pancreas

We have recently demonstrated by immunofluorescence and Western blotting that the pancreas of human, pig, mouse and rat (12) clearly possess the CCK$_B$ receptor in their islets of Langerhans with a specific location on the somatostatin delta cells. This finding was recently confirmed in rabbit, dog, calf, horse and deer pancreas (unpublished data).

Such a location for the CCK_B receptor on pancreatic delta cells, established by immunofluorescence with a specific CCK_B receptor antibody is not unanimous since our observation has been recently challenged (11, 15). Furthermore, questions have been raised about the pancreatic distribution because CCK_B receptor transcripts could not be detected in rat islets cells (34). In the stomach, location of the CCK_B receptor on somatostatin cells is also controversial. Indeed, Helander (35) has demonstrated by immunofluorescence the presence of CCK_B receptors on the somatostatin delta cells of the dog and guinea pig oxyntic and antral mucosae, a finding recently confirmed in the rat stomach with the same antibody (12). Roche, however, suggested that somatostatin release from stomach D-cells could be induced following CCK_A receptor occupation (36). Finally, the importance of the CCK_B receptor in maintaining the delta cell population and its somatostatin content is still debatable from the following observations: the stomach expression of somatostatin mRNA remained stable following CCKBR gene disruption (9) while its overexpression in naturally occurring CCK_A receptor gene knockout rats did not change the number of somatostatin cells in the pylorus area (37). However, in CCK_B knockout mice, the gastric somatostatin D cells were significantly reduced (26).

Supported by the earlier finding of Soll, et al. (38) that somatostatin release from canine fundic mucosal cells in short term culture was almost equally stimulated by CCK-8 and gastrin-17, a typical CCK_B receptor response, we pursued our studies on the implication of the CCK_B receptors on pancreatic metabolism of somatostatin in the islets delta cells.

Our initial approach was to establish in colocalization studies that the CCK receptor subtypes present on pancreatic cells from isolated islets were similar to those previously identified on pieces of pancreatic tissue using the same antibodies. As shown on Figure 2a, the CCK_A receptor antibody recognized the CCK_A receptor on insulin beta cells (Figure 2b) with a perfect match (Figure 2c). Binding of the CCK_A receptor antibody to its CCK_A receptor protein was totally inhibited by preincubation with its peptide antigen (Figure 2d). This leaves a clear recognition of the insulin beta cells (Figures 2e, 2f). Preincubation of insulin antibody with insulin (Figure 2h) eliminated β cells recognition; however, the CCK_A receptor antibody identified the CCK_A receptor on β cells (Figures 2g, 2i). Similarly, the CCK_B receptor (Figure 2j) colocalized with somatostatin (SST) in delta cells (Figure 2k) with a perfect match (Figure 2l). Binding of the CCK_B receptor antibody to its receptor protein was totally prevented by preincubation with its peptide antigen (Figure 2m), whereas the SST delta cells were perfectly identified with the SST antibody (Figures 2n, o). We were able to neutralize SST antibody binding to SST cells on slides of pancreatic tissue by SST, an observation not yet confirmed on isolated islets. Now that we have confirmed in the isolated rat pancreatic islets, the colo-

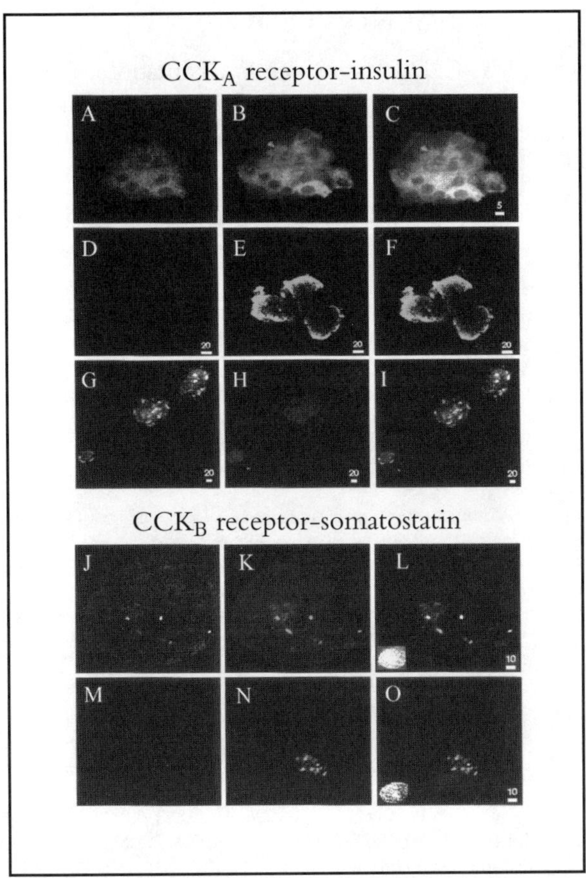

FIGURE 2. Colocalization by confocal microscopy of CCK$_A$ and CCK$_B$ receptors with insulin and somatostatin, respectively, in freshly purified rat islets of Langerhans. *The islets were fixed in 4% paraformaldehyde saturated in Na Borohydride 2 mg ml^{-1} and permeabilized in PBS 1X, 0.1% Triton X-100, 7% Normal goat or mouse sera. For these studies, the following antibodies and hormones were used. The CCK$_B$ receptor antibody 9262 (12) was used at 1:1500, somatostatin Barbar antibody at 1:100 and the CCK$_B$ peptide antigen at 40 µg ml^{-1}. The CCK$_A$ receptor antibody 1122 (39) was used at 1:200, insulin antibody (Santa Cruz) at 1:50, the CCK$_A$ peptide antigen and porcine insulin (Lilly) at 40 µg ml^{-1}. The primary antibodies were incubated overnight at 4°C. As secondary antibodies, 1h at room temperture, the following were used at 1 µg ml^{-1}: CCK$_A$, CCK$_B$ goat anti-rabbit 488 Alexa Fluor; SS rabbit anti-goat 546 Alexa Fluor; Insulin goat anti-mouse 546 Alexa Fluor.*

calization of CCK$_A$ receptor insulin in the β cells and of CCK$_B$ receptor-SST in the δ cells as previously shown on pieces of pancreatic tissue with the same antibodies (12, 39), we can safely initiate studies on these purified islets to document physiological responses from occupation of these CCK$_B$ receptors on the δ cells.

ACKNOWLEDGMENTS

We wish to thank Mrs C. Ducharme and S. Choufani for their secretarial and technical assistance, respectively. This research was supported by grant GP6369 from the Natural Sciences and Engineering Research Council of Canada.

REFERENCES

1. Silvente-Poirot S, Dufresne M, Vaysse N, Fourmy D. The peripheral cholecystokinin receptors. *Eur J Biochem* 1993;215:513–529.

2. Wank SA, Harkins RT, Jensen RT, Shapira H, DeWeerth A, Slattery T. Purification, molecular cloning and functional expression of the cholecystokinin receptor from rat pancreas. *Proc Natl Acad Sci USA* 1992;89:3125–3129.

3. Wank SA, Pisegna JR, DeWeerth A. Brain and gastrointestinal cholecystokinin receptor family: structure and functional expression. *Proc Natl Acad Sci USA* 1992;89:8691–8695.

4. Kopin AS, Lee YM, McBride EW, Miller LJ, Lu M, Lin HY, Kolakowski LF, Beinborn M. Expression cloning and characterization of the canine parietal cell gastrin receptor. *Proc Natl Acad Sci USA* 1992;89:3605–3609.

5. Wank SA. G protein-coupled receptors in gastrointestinal physiology 1. CCK receptors: an exemplary family. *Am J Physiol* 1998;274:G607-G613.

6. Philippe C, Lhoste EF, Dufresne M, Moroder L, Corring T, Fourmy D. Pharmacological and biochemical evidence for the simultaneous expression of CCK_B/gastrin and CCK_A receptors in the pig pancreas. *Brit J Pharmacol* 1997;120:447–454.

7. Saillan-Barreau C, Clerc P, Adato M, Escrieut C, Vaysse N, Fourmy D, Dufresne M. Transgenic CCK_B/gastrin receptor mediates murine exocrine pancreatic secretion. *Gastroenterology* 1998;115:988–996.

8. Detjen K, Yule D, Tseng M-J, Williams JA, Logsdon CD. CCK-B receptors produce similar signals but have opposite growth effects in CHO and Swiss 3T3 cells. *Am J Physiol* 1997;273:C1449–C1457.

9. Nagata A, Ito M, Iwata N, Kuno J, Takano H, Minowa O, Chihara K, Matsui T, Noda T. G protein-coupled cholecystokinin-B/gastrin receptors are responsible for physiological cell growth of the stomach mucosa *in vivo*. *Proc Natl Acad Sci USA* 1996; 93: 11825–11830.

10. Tang C, Biemond I, Lamers CBHW. Cholecystokinin receptors in human pancreas and gallbladder muscle: a comparative study. *Gastroenterology* 1996;111:1621–1626.

11. Saillan-Barreau C, Dufresne M, Clerc P, Sanchez D, Corominola H, Moriscot C, Guy-Crotte O, Escrieut C, Vaysse N, Gomis R, Tarasova N, Fourmy D. Evidence for a functional role of the cholecystokinin-B/gastrin receptor in the human fetal and adult pancreas. *Diabetes* 1999;48:2015–2021.

12. Morisset J, Wong H, Walsh JH, Lainé J, Bourassa J. Pancreatic CCK_B receptors: their potential roles in somatostatin release and δ cell proliferation. *Am J Physiol* 2000;279:G148–G156.

13. Holicky EL, Hadac EM, Ding X-Q, Miller LJ. Molecular characterization and organ distribution of type A and B cholecystokinin receptors in cynomolgus monkey. *Am J Physiol* 2001;281:G507–G514.

14. Schweiger M, Erhard MH, Amselgruber WM. Cell-specific localization of the cholecystokinin$_A$ receptor in porcine pancreas. *Anat Histol Embryol* 2000;29:357–361.

15. Rooman I, Lardon J, Flamez D, Schuit F, Bouwens L. Mitogenic effect of gastrin and expression of gastrin receptors in duct-like cells of rat pancreas. *Gastroenterology* 2001:121:940–949.

16. Denyer J, Gray J, Wong M, Stolz M, Tate S. Molecular and pharmacological characterization of the human CCK_B receptor. *Eur J Pharmacol* 1994;268:29–41.

17. Smith AJ, Patel S, Freedman SB. Characterization of CCK_B receptors on GH_3 pituitary cells: receptor activation is linked to Ca^{2+} mobilization. *Eur J Pharmacol* 1994:267:215–223.

18. Pinnock RD, Suman-Chauhan N, Daum P, Hill DR, Woodruff GN. The cholecystokinin-induced increase in intracellular calcium in AR42J cells is mediated by CCK_B receptors linked to interval calcium stores. *Neuropeptides* 1994;27:175–183.

19. Yu D-H, Noguchi M, Zhou Z-C, Villanueva ML, Gardner JD, Jensen RT. Characterization of gastrin receptors on guinea pig pancreatic acini. *Am J Physiol* 1987;253:G793–G801.

20. Kaufmann R, Schafberg H, Rudroff C, Henklein P, Nowak G. Cholecystokinin B-type receptor signaling is involved in human pancreatic cancer cell growth. *Neuropeptides* 1997;31:573–583.

21. Palmer Smith J, Liu G, Soundararajan V, McLaughlin PJ, Zagon IS. Identification and characterization of CCK-B/gastrin receptors in human pancreatic cancer cell lines. *Am J Physiol* 1994;266:R277–R283.

22. Kolby L, Wangberg B, Ahlman H, Modlin IM, Theodorsson E, Nilsson O. Altered influence of CCK-B/gastrin receptors on HDC expression in ECL cells after neoplastic transformation. *Regul Peptides* 1999;85:115–123.

23. Martenis M, Smith JP, Ballard E, Verderame MF, Zagon IS. Identification of the CCK-C receptor in human pancreatic cancer cells and tissues. *Gastroenterology* 2000;118:A645.

24. Smith JP, Verderame MF, Martenis M, Stanley WB, Zagon IS. Gene therapy with knock-out of the CCK-C gene decreases growth of human pancreatic cancer. *Pancreas* 2001;23:461.

25. Seva C, Dickinson CJ, Yamada T. Growth promoting effects of glycine-extended progastrin. *Science* 1994;265:410–412.

26. Langhans N, Rindi G, Chiu M, Rehfeld JF, Ardman B, Beinborn M, Kopin AS. Abnormal gastric histology and decreased acid production in cholecystokinin-B/gastrin receptor-deficient mice. *Gastroenterology* 1997;112:280–286.

27. Miyasaka K, Shinozaki H, Suzuki S, Sato Y, Kanai S, Masuda M, Jimi A, Nagata A, Matsui T, Noda T, Kono A, Funakoshi A. Disruption of cholecystokinin (CCK)-B receptor gene did not modify bile or pancreatic secretion or pancreatic growth: a study in CCK-B receptor gene knockout mice. *Pancreas* 1999;19:114–118.

28. Soll AH, Amirian DA, Thomas LP, Reedy TJ, Elashoff JD. Gastrin receptors on isolated canine parietal cells. *J Clin Invest* 1984;73:1434–1447.

29. Solomon TE. Trophic effects of pentagastrin on gastrointestinal tract in fed and fasted rats. *Gastroenterology* 1986;91:108–116.

30. Smith AJ, Freedman SB. CCK-B receptor-mediated stimulation of polyphosphoinositide turnover in GH$_3$ pituitary cells in response to cholecystokinin and pentagastrin. *Life Sciences* 1996;58:883–895.

31. Ito M, Iwata N, Taniguchi T, Murayama T, Chihara K, Matsui T. Functional characterization of two cholecystokinin-B/gastrin receptor isoforms: a preferential splice donor site in the human receptor gene. *Cell Growth Differentiation* 1994;5:1127–1135.

32. Desbois C, Le Huerou-Luron I, Dufresne M, Estival A, Clerc P, Romé V, Clémente F, Guilloteau P, Fourmy D. The CCK$_B$/gastrin receptor is coupled to the regulation of enzyme secretion, protein synthesis and p76 S6 kinase activity in acinar cells from Elas CCK$_B$ transgenic mice. *Eur J Biochem* 1999;266:1003–1010.

33. Clerc P, Leung-Theung-Long S, Bouisson M, Wang TC, Dockray GJ, Vaysse N, Pradayrol L, Fourmy D, Dufresne M. Overexpression of CCK2/gastrin receptors in the murine pancreas results in proliferation, transdifferentiation of acinar cells and neoplasia. *Pancreatology* 2001;1:143.

34. Karlsson S, Sundler F, Ahren B. CCK receptor subtype in insulin-producing cells: a combined functional and in situ hybridization study in rat islets and a rat insulinoma cell line. *Regul Peptides* 1998;78:95–103.

35. Helander HF, Wong H, Poorkhalkali N, Walsh JH. Immunohistochemical localization of gastrin/CCK-B receptors in the dog and guinea pig stomach. *Acta Physiol Scand* 1997;159:313–320.

36. Roche S, Gusdinar T, Bali JP, Magous R. Gastrin and CCK receptors on histamine and somatostatin-containing cells from rabbit fundic mucosa. *Biochem Pharmacol* 1991;42:765–770.

37. Miyasaka K, Kanai S, Ohta M, Jimi A, Kono A, Funakoshi A. Overexpression of cholecystokinin-B/gastrin receptor gene in the stomach of naturally occurring cholecystokinin-A receptor gene knockout rats. *Digestion* 1998:59:26–32.

38. Soll AH, Amirian DA, Park J, Elashoff JD, Yamada T. Cholecystokinin potently releases somatostatin from canine fundic mucosal cells in short-term culture. *Am J Physiol* 1985;248:G569-G573.

39. Bourassa J, Lainé J, Kruse ML, Gagnon MC, Calvo E, Morisset J. Ontogeny and species differences in the pancreatic expression and localization of the CCK$_A$ receptors. *Biochem Biophys Res Commun* 1999;260:820–828.

Gut-Brain Peptides in the New Millennium, edited by Y. Taché
CURE Foundation, Los Angeles, CA. © 2002

39

Gut Peptide Receptors in Pancreatic Tumors

Cornelis B.H.W. Lamers and Izäk Biemond
Leiden University Medical Centre, Leiden, The Netherlands

Chengwei Tang
West China Hospital, Sichuan University, Sichuan, P.R. China

Ruud A. Woutersen
TNO Nutrition and Food Research Institute, Zeist, The Netherlands

G. Johan A. Offerhaus
University Medical Centre, Amsterdam, The Netherlands

INTRODUCTION

I have had the privilege to work with John Walsh at the Center for Ulcer Research and Education (CURE) in the years 1978 and 1979. My studies at that time were on two main topics: molecular heterogeneity of cholecystokinin and gastrin in plasma of humans and, together with Irvin Modlin, dog experiments on the effect of gut peptides on gastric acid secretion and circulating gastrointestinal hormones. New ideas, different views of accepted ideas, critical data analysis among others, brought up by John, were greatly stimulatory to my work and ideas. Furthermore, John had created an excellent scientific atmosphere in which his co-workers were not only stimulated by him but they also stimulated each others. Apart from the research we had a lot of fun in the "Visiting scientists office" which I shared with Joe Reeve, Arthur Shulkes, Tachi Yamada, Irvin Modlin, Pierre Poitras, S.K. Lam, Ian Taylor and others. Back in the Netherlands I conveyed the knowledge, experiences and ideas acquired in Los Angeles to my co-workers stimulating gut peptide research in my country. My wife and I consider the period that we spent with John, his co-workers and other people in Los Angeles as one of the best times in our lives.

Pancreatic cancer remains a major therapeutic challenge because of a very poor prognosis. Radiotherapy and chemotherapy are usually ineffective (1). Therefore, other therapeutic approaches for treatment of pancreatic tumors need to be explored.

TABLE 1. *Gut peptide receptors in normal pancreas of man, hamster and rat as visualized by storage phosphor autoradiography.*

Receptor	Human	Hamster	Rat
Cholecystokinin (CCK)	+ (B-type)[a]	+ (A-type)[a]	+ (A-type)[a]
Bombesin (BBS)	+	−	+
Secretin	+	+	+
Vasactive intestinal polypeptide (VIP)	−	+	+
Somatostatin (SST)	−	+	+

+ visualized

− not visualized

[a] predominant type CCK receptor

Various studies have demonstrated that the growth of normal and malignant pancreas may be regulated by gut peptides and growth factors (2–8). These findings suggest that new approaches to treatment of human pancreatic tumors might be based on hormonal manipulation using various peptide receptor agonists or antagonists (9). To develop hormonal therapy for pancreatic tumors, a better understanding of the characteristics of the peptide receptors in normal pancreas and pancreatic tumor is of great importance.

In this chapter studies on the presence and characteristics of receptors for gut peptides on pancreatic tumors, normal pancreatic tissue in humans and in experimental animal models of pancreatic carcinogenesis are presented. Storage phosphor autoradiography was used to visualize, quantify and characterize receptor binding of gut peptides on tissue sections.

In humans, both pancreatic adenocarcinoma and endocrine tumor tissues were studied and compared to normal pancreatic tissue. Two animal models were used: azaserine-treatment of rats and N-nitrosobis (2-oxopropyl) amine (BOP) treatment of hamsters. As in humans, receptor binding of gut peptides was studied in both (pre)neoplastic pancreatic lesions and normal control pancreas.

Visualization and Characterization of Gut Peptide Receptors on Tissue Sections

Receptor autoradiography visualizes radiolabelled peptide binding sites on tissue sections. Like its parent technique high affinity binding analysis, receptor autoradiography is well established as an essential and widely used research methodology. Receptor autoradiographs can easily distinguish the bound ligands on tissue sections from the ligands adhered to the slides and these can therefore present accurate results. Storage phosphor technique, which is a new approach to generating non-emulsion autoradiographs, has made it possible to visualize gut peptide receptors in tissue sections of the pancreas and pancreatic tumors. Furthermore, accurate quantification with storage phosphor autoradiography does not require multiple exposures as in the case with the film autoradiography (10).

Beside the advantages of storage phosphor autoradiography, the technique has the disadvantage of a slightly lower resolution compared to film autoradiography. The choice of the suitable imaging technique depends upon the aim of the experiment. If the study is to localize peptide binding on the cellular level or very fine lesions (< 2 mm), emulsion or film autoradiography is the technique of choice. Storage phosphor autoradiography is sufficient to provide satisfying images and quantitative analysis with considerable gain of time when visualization and characterization of gut peptide receptors in tissue sections are the aims of the study.

Receptors for Gut Peptides in Normal Pancreas

Receptors for CCK were found in the pancreas of rat, hamster and humans. In rat and hamster, the receptors appeared to be mainly of the A-type, whereas in human pancreas the CCK-B type receptors was predominant (Table 1). In normal rat pancreas autoradiography showed an uneven density of CCK-A receptors (11). The heterogeneous binding of CCK can be attributed to the variable expression of the CCK receptors with interconvertible affinity states (12,13). An uneven density of CCK-B receptors in the autoradiographs was shown in normal human pancreas (14). CCK-B receptors presented one affinity-binding site because only one radioligand was used in the study. Using three radiologands (^{125}I-CCK-8, [^{3}H]L-364,718 and [^{3}H]L-365,260) others showed that the CCK-B receptor, like the CCK-A receptor, exists in three different affinity states for CCK-8 (13). This ability to exist in multiple affinity states was taken as an intrinsic property of the CCK receptor molecule itself. Therefore, the uneven expression of CCK-B receptors probably also infers variable states of cellular metabolism.

Hitherto, the knowledge of CCK receptors in pancreas is from experiments on various species of animals. CCK-A receptors with high, low and very low affinity binding sites in rat pancreatic acini have been shown in several studies (15–16). Both CCK-A and CCK-B receptors were identified in pancreas of guinea pig or dog (17–19). However, there is little information on characteristics of CCK receptors in the human pancreas. We found that the human pancreas predominantly expresses CCK-B receptors (14). Besides CCK receptors, we could show that the normal rat pancreas contains receptors for bombesin (BBS), secretin, vasoactive intestinal peptide (VIP) and somatostatin (SST) (20). All types of receptors mentioned above, except the BBS receptor, were also visualized in normal pancreas of hamsters (21). Of the five types of receptors studied we were able to demonstrate receptors only for CCK, BBS and secretin in the normal human pancreas (22) (Table 1). The distinct characteristics and spectra of receptors for peptides in pancreata of humans and rodents suggest important differences between humans and laboratory animals.

Expression of Peptide Receptors in Pancreatic Ductal and Acinar (Pre)neoplastic Lesions of Animal Models

CCK has been considered an important entero-hormone affecting pancreatic carcinogenesis (23, 24). The trophic effect of CCK on putative preneoplastic lesions in azaserine-treated rats has been attributed to the interaction of CCK with its specific cellular receptors (18). An increasing expression of high-affinity CCK A-type receptors in the pancreas of azaserine-treated rats was confirmed in our studies. However, the high density binding for CCK was not always related to atypical acinar cell nodules possible because the CCK receptors in putative preneoplastic lesions were also present in a multiple interconvertible affinity status as in normal rat pancreas. In contrast, CCK receptors could not be demonstrated in ductal neoplasms of BOP-treated pancreas in hamsters. This observation does not support the hypothesis that CCK plays an important role in ductal pancreatic cancer. The opposite results in the two different animal models may be due to differences in species, histogenesis and carcinogens involved.

Until now the effects of BBS, SST, secretin and VIP on pancreatic carcinogenesis are inconsistent partly due to lack of extensive and detailed investigations (25, 26). However, studies by our group demonstrate a reduction or absence of these receptors in the neoplastic lesions of pancreata in both hamsters and rats with progress of carcinogenesis (20, 21) indicating that both acinar and ductal pancreatic adenocarcinomas have, to a large extent, lost the hormone-dependent characteristics of the original tissue (Table 2).

Expression of Peptide Receptors in Human Pancreatic Cancer

Although the information from animal models is helpful to understand the biology of pancreatic cancer, the discrepancy between species unavoidably results in gaps in the knowledge on human pancreatic cancer. Table 2 summarizes the results of our studies on the expression of gut peptide receptors between normal pancreas and pancreatic cancer in human (22, 27), hamsters (21) and rats (20). The samples from the different species were handled in the same way and the conditions of the receptor binding assay were identical for each peptide, allowing the comparison presented in Table 2.

CCK is trophic to the pancreas and stimulates proliferation of rat acinar cell tumors, leading to the speculation that CCK may be involved in the development of human pancreatic ductal cell cancer. However, stimulatory, inhibitory or no effects of CCK on growth of human pancreatic cancer cell

TABLE 2. *Alterations in expression of peptide receptors between pancreatic cancer and normal pancreas in various species*

Receptor	Human	Hamster	Rat
Cholecystokinin (CCK)	↓	↓	↑
Bombesin (BBS)	↓	–	↓
Secretin	↓	↓	↓
Vasoctive intestinal polypeptide (VIP)	↑	↓	↓
Somatostatin (SST)	↑	↓	↓

↑ increase; ↓ decrease; – no change from normal pancreas

lines or human pancreatic cancer xenografts in nude mice have been reported (28–30). Moreover, specific CCK binding in intact cells could not be demonstrated (31). This study does not provide support for an important role of CCK in pancreatic cancer of humans and is in line with the results of a clinical trial that failed to demonstrate any impact of MK-329, a CCK-A receptor antagonist on tumor progression, pain, or nutrition in patients with advanced pancreatic cancer (32).

Studies on the receptors for VIP and SST in normal human pancreas are lacking although a weak expression of the SST receptor mRNA has been found in normal human pancreas (33). It cannot completely be ruled out that the normal human pancreas expresses VIP and SST receptors at very low affinities or binding capacities which may be difficult to be identified by the methods used currently. However, using storage phosphor autoradiography an up-regulation of VIP and SST receptors in human pancreatic cancer in comparison with normal pancreas was demonstrated. The alterations of VIP and SST receptors between normal pancreas and pancreatic adenocarcinoma in humans are opposite to those found in rodents and may be important when designing hormonal therapy strategies for pancreatic cancer.

Five subtypes of SST receptor, SSTR-1 to SSTR-5, have been cloned and functionally characterized (34). Sequence comparisons of the SST receptor subtypes clearly reveal two subgroups of receptors in the SST receptor gene family. SSTR-1 and SSTR-4 share common characteristics that differ from those of the subgroup containing the subtype SSTR-2, SSTR-3 and SSTR-5, SST-28, and SST-14 are non-selective ligands for all SST receptor subtypes. Short synthetic SST analogues, however, such as octreotide (SMS 201-995), octastatin (RC-160) and lantreotide (BIM-23014) demonstrate specific binding only for the subgroup consisting of SSTR-2, SSTR-3 and SSTR-5 (35). It is worth noting that our studies show that human pancreatic cancer expressed the SST receptor subgroup consisting of SSTR-1 and SSTR-4 (27). This finding may stimulate further investigations in the development of new SST analogues for the diagnosis and treatment of pancreatic cancer.

As reported previously, the normal pancreas of the hamster expressed specific receptors for secretin. However, the affinity and binding capacity of secretin receptors dramatically decreased in pancreatic preneoplastic lesions and no specific secretin binding was detected in adenocarcinomas of the pancreas. The presence of secretin receptors was also visualized in normal human pancreas and in less than half of the pancreatic cancers studied. These differences of secretin receptor status between normal pancreas and pancreatic adenocarcinoma in humans are similar to those observed in hamsters. These results are in agreement with data from studies of human pancreatic cancer cell lines, which did not show any growth response to secretin (36). In addition, another study also questioned the role of secretin as a cocarcinogen in pancreatic cancer of BOP-treated hamsters (37).

The role of BBS on pancreatic cancer cell lines of humans or tumor growth in hamster models is controversial (7, 36, 38–41). The disappearance of BBS receptors in human pancreatic cancer and absence of BBS receptor in pancreatic (pre)neoplastic lesions of rodents do not favor a direct action of BBS on the growth of pancreatic cancer.

Expression of Peptide Receptors in Human Endocrine Tumors of the Pancreas

Although the provocation of gastrin release by secretin or BBS is used as a test in the diagnosis of gastrinoma (42), the physiological basis for the provocation has been debated (43,44). We showed that secretin and BBS receptors could be visualized in all primary gastrinomas studied. The findings provide evidence for a direct molecular action of these provocative peptides and suggest that the stimulating effect of secretin and BBS on dispersed gastrinoma cells or cultured gastrinoma cells may be mediated through their receptors on the cells.

Because of their growth inhibitory effects, SST and its analogues may be good candidates for use as endocrine agents in the treatment of pancreatic neoplasm. In contrast to adenocarcinoma of the pancreas, gastrinoma predominantly expressed the SST receptor subgroup consisting of SSTR-2, SSTR-3 and SSTR-5. This finding is in agreement with the results from *in vitro* ^{125}I-Tyr^3-octreotide binding assays in human gastrinomas (46) and *in vivo* scintigraphy with ^{111}In-DAPA-octreotide in patients with gastrinoma (47).

Like the results in most human pancreatic cancers, our studies revealed that gastrinoma and VIPoma contain VIP receptors (45). Thus, these tumors may also be imaged *in vivo* with radiolabelled VIP as has recently been shown for insulinoma (47). However, a mass in the pancreas demonstrated by scintigraphy with radiolabelled VIP does not allow differentiation between an exocrine or endocrine pancreatic tumor.

Gastrin has been reported to act as an positive, autocrine growth factor in colonic carcinoma (49). Autocrine growth stimulation by bombesin-like peptides has been suggested for small-cell lung carcinoma (50). However, such a stimulating loop has not been reported in endocrine tumors of the pancreas. We found that autocrine loops may exist in VIPomas but not in gastrinomas or somatostatinomas. Investigations into the way by which peptides act, may add to the knowledge of the possible hormone responsiveness of pancreatic endocrine tumors.

The information from other groups (51) and the current studies suggest an increased expression of receptors for EGF, SST and VIP in neoplastic tissues when compared to the normal pancreas. The up-regulated expression of these peptide receptors will stimulate studies on the pathophysiological role of these peptides in pancreatic carcinogenesis and growth and may be valuable in the diagnosis or treatment of pancreatic cancer. Although the non-selectivity and the short duration of the effect of gut peptides may hamper their clinical application, the development of long-acting peptide or nonpeptide hormonal agonists and antagonists with high specificity and selectivity for receptor subtypes involved in pancreatic cancer has promise of clinical usefulness.

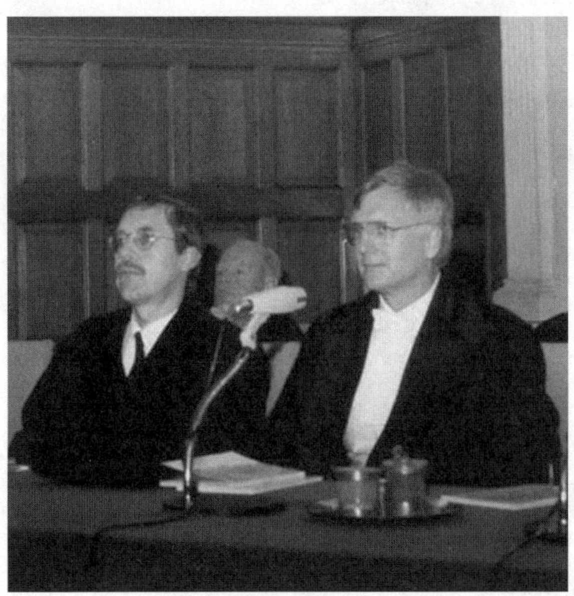

Drs. Cornelis Lamers and John Walsh at the PhD ceremony of Dr. Jan Kleibeuker in Groningen, The Netherlands, 1987.

REFERENCES

1. Williamson RCN. Pancreatic cancer: the greatest oncological challenge. *Br Med J* 1988;296:445–446.
2. Niederau C, Lüthen R, Heintges T. Effects of CCK on pancreatic function and morphology. *Ann NY Acad Sci* 1994;713:180–198.
3. Solomon TE, Vanier M, Morisset J. Cell site and time course of DNA synthesis in pancreas after caerulein and secretin. *Am J Physiol* 1983;245:G99–105.
4. Lehy T, Puccio F. Influence of bombesin on gastrointestinal and pancreatic cell growth in adult and suckling animals. *Ann NY Acad Sci* 1988;547:255–267.
5. Meijers M, van Garderen-Hoetmer A, Lamers CBHW, Rovati LC, Jansen JBMJ, Woutersen RA. Role of cholecystokinin in the development of BOP-induced pancreatic lesions in hamsters. *Carcinogenesis* 1990;11:2223–2226.
6. Edwards BF, Redding TW, Schally AV. The effect of gastrointestinal hormones on the incorporation of tritiated thymidine in the pancreatic adenocarcinoma cell line (WD PaCa). *Int J Pancreatol* 1989; 5:191–201.
7. Meijers M, van Garderen-Hoetmer A, Lamers CBHW, Rovati LC, Jansen JBMJ, Woutersen RA. Effect of bombesin on the development of N-nitrosobis(2-oxopropyl) amine-induced pancreatic lesions in hamsters. *Cancer Lett* 1991;59:45–50.
8. Robertson JFR, Watson SA, Hardcastle JD. Effect of gastrointestinal hormones and synthetic analogues on the growth of pancreatic cancer. *Int J Cancer* 1995;63:69–75.
9. Schally AV, Szepeshazi K, Qin Y, Halmos G, Ertl T, Groot K, Cai R-Z, Liebaw C, Poston GJ. Antitumor effects of analogs of somatostatin and antagonists of bombesin/GRP in experimental models of pancreatic cancer. *Int J Pancreatol* 1994;16:246–249.
10. Tang C, Biemond I, Lamers CBHW. Localization and quantification of cholecystokinin receptors in rat brain with storage phosphor autoradiography. *Biotechniques* 1995;18:886–889.
11. Tang C, Biemond I, Lamers CBHW. Visualization and characterization of CCK receptors in exocrine pancreas of rat with storage phosphor autoradiography. *Pancreas* 1996;13:311–315.
12. Blevins GT Jr, Williams JA. ATP induces two cholecystokinin binding affinity states in permeabilized rat pancreatic acini. *Am J Physiol* 1992;263:G44–51.
13. Huang S-C, Fortune KP, Wank SA, Kopin AS, Gardner JD. Multiple affinity states of different cholecystokinin receptors. *J Biol Chem* 1994;269: 26121–26126.
14. Tang C, Biemond I, Lamers CBHW. Cholecystokinin receptors in human pancreas and gallbladder muscle: a comparitive study. *Gastroenterology* 1996;111:1621–1626.
15. Talkad VD, Patto RJ, Metz DC, Turner RJ, Fortune KP, Bhat ST, Gardner JD. Characterization of the three different states of the cholecystokinin (CCK) receptor in pancreatic acini. *Biochimica et Biophysica Acta* 1994;1224:103–116.
16. Williams JA, Bailey AC, Roach E. Temperature dependence of high-affinity CCK receptor binding and CCK internalization in rat pancreatic acini. *Am J Physiol* 1988;254:G513–521.
17. Yu D-H, Huang SC, Wank SA, Mantey S, Gardner JD, Jensen RT. Pancreatic receptors for cholecystokinin: evidence for three receptor classes. *Am J Physiol* 1990;258:G86–95.
18. Yu D-H, Noguchi M, Zhou Z-C, Villanueva ML, Gardner JD, Jensen RT. Characterization of gastrin receptors on guinea pig pancreatic acini. *Am J Physiol* 1987;253:G793–801.
19. Fourmy D, Zahidi A, Fabre R, Guidet M, Pradayrol L, Ribet A. Receptors for cholecystokinin and gastrin peptides display specific binding properties and are structurally different in guinea-pig and dog pancreas. *Eur J Biochem* 1987;165:683–692.
20. Tang C, Biemond I, Appel MJ, Visser CJ, Wouterse RA, Lamers CBHW. Gut peptide receptors in pancreata of azaserine-treated and normal control rats. *Carcinogenesis* 1995;16:2951–2956.
21. Tang C, Biemond I, Appel MJ, Visser CJ, Woutersen RA, Lamers CBHW. Expression of receptors for gut peptides in pancreata of BOB-treated and control hamsters. *Carcinogenesis* 1996;17:2171–2175.
22. Tang C, Biemond I, Offerhaus GJ, Verspaget HW, Lamers CBHW. Expression of receptors for gut peptides in human pancreatic adenocarcinoma and tumor-free pancreas. *Br J Cancer* 1997;75:1467–1473.
23. Douglas BR, Woutersen RA, Jansen JBMJ, de Jong AJL, Rovati LC, Lamers CBHW. Influence of cholecystokinin antagonist on the effects of cholecystokinin and bombesin on azaserine-induced lesions in rat pancreas. *Gastroenterology* 1989;96:426–429.

24. Axelson J, Ihse I, Hakanson R. Pancreatic cancer: the role of cholecystokinin? *Scand J Gastroenterol* 1992;27:993–998.
25. Redding TW, Schally AV. Inhibition of growth of pancreatic carcinomas in animal models by analogues of hypothalamic hormones. *Proc Natl Acad Sci USA* 1984;81:248–252.
26. Meijers M, Woutersen RA, van Garderen-Hoetmer A, et al. Effects of sandostatin and castration on pancreatic carcinogenesis in rats and hamsters. *Int J Cancer* 1992;50:246–251.
27. Tang C, Biemond I, Verspager HW, Offerhaus GJ, Lamers CBHW. Expression of somatostatin receptors in human pancreatic tumor. *Pancreas* 1998;17:80–84.
28. Nio Y, Tsubono M, Morimoto H, et al. Loxiglumide (CR 1505), a cholecystokinin antagonist, specifically inhibits the growth of human pancreatic cancer lines xenografted into nude mice. *Cancer* 1993;72:3599–3606.
29. Smith JP, Solomon TE, Bagheri S, Kramer S. Cholecystokinin stimulates growth of human pancreatic adenocarcinomas SW-1990. *Dig Dis Sci* 1990;35:1377–1384.
30. Upp JR Jr, Sigh P, Townsend CM, Thompson JC. Predicting response to endocrine therapy in human pancreatic cancer with cholecystokinin receptors. *Gastroenterology* 1987;92:1677.
31. Herrington MK, Adrian TE. On the role of CCK in pancreatic cancer. *Int J Pancreatol* 1995;17:121–138.
32. Abbruzzese JL, Gholson CF, Daugherty K, et al. A pilot clinical trial of the cholecystokinin receptor antagonist MK-329 in patients with advanced pancreatic cancer. *Pancreas* 1992;7:165–171.
33. Buscail L, Delesque N, Estève J-P, et al. Stimulation of tyrosine phosphatase and inhibition of cell proliferation by somatostatin analogues: mediation by human somatostatin receptor subtypes SSTR1 and SSTR2. *Proc Natl Acad Sci USA* 1994;91:2315–2319.
34. Bruns C, Weckbecker G, Raulf F, et al. Molecular pharmacology of somatostatin-receptor subtypes. *Ann NY Acad Sci* 1994;733:138–146.
35. Reisine T, Bell GI. Molecular biology of somatostatin receptors. *Endocrine Rev* 1995;16:427–442.
36. Liehr RM, Melnykovych G, Solomon TE. Growth effects of regulatory peptides on human pancreatic cancer line PANC-1 and MIA PaCa-2. *Gastroenterology* 1990;98:1666–1674.
37. Howatson AG, Carter DC. Pancreatic carcinogenesis: effect of secretin in the hamster-nitrosamine model. *J Natl Cancer Inst* 1987;78:101–105.
38. Alexander RW, Upp JR Jr, Poston GJ, Townsend CM Jr, Singh P, Thompson JC. Bombesin inhibits growth of human pancreatic adenocarcinoma in nude mice. *Pancreas* 1988;3:297–302.
39. Qin Y, Ertl T, Cai R-Z, Halmos G, Schally AV. Inhibitory effect of bombesin receptor antagonist RC-3095 on the growth of human pancreatic cancer cells *in vivo* and *in vitro. Cancer Res* 1994;54:1035–1041.
40. Szepeshazi K, Schally AV, Cai R-Z, Radulovic S, Milovanovic S, Szoke B. Inhibitory effect of bombesin/gastrin releasing peptide antagonist RC-3095 and high dose of somatostatin analogue RC-160 on nitrosamine-induced pancreatic cancers in hamsters. *Cancer Res* 1991;51:5980–5986.
41. Szepeshazi K, Schally AV, Groot K, Halmos G. Effect of bombesin, gastrin-releasing peptide (GRP)(14-27) and bombesin/GRP receptor antagonist RC-3095 on growth of nitrosamine-induced pancreatic cancers in hamsters. *Int J Cancer* 1993;54: 282–289.
42. Jensen RT, Garner JD. Gastrinoma. In: *The Pancreas: Biology, Pathobiology, and Disease.* Go VLW, et al., Eds. New York: Raven Press, 1993:931–978.
43. Chiba T, Yamatani Y, Yamaguchi A, et al. Mechanism for increase of gastrin release by secretin in Zollinger-Ellison syndrome. *Gastroenterology* 1989;96:1439–1444.
44. Brady CE, Utts SJ, Hyatt JR, Dev J. Secretin provocation: gastrin results in various clinical situation. *Am J Gastroenterol* 1988;83:130–135.
45. Tang C, Biemond I, Lamers CBHW. Expression of pepetide receptors in human endocrine tumors of the pancreas. *Gut* 1997;40:267–271.
46. Reubi J-C, Häcki WH, Lamberts SWJ. Hormone-producing gastrointestinal tumors contain a high density of somatostatin receptors. *J Clin Endocrinol Metab* 1987;65:1127–1134.
47. Scherübl H, Bäder M, Fett U, et al. Somatostatin-receptor imaging of neuroendocrine gastroenteropancreatic tumors. *Gastroenterology* 1993;105:1705–1709.
48. Virgolini I, Raderer M, Kurtaran A, et al. Vasoactive intestinal peptide-receptor imaging for the localization of intestinal adenocarcinomas and endocrine tumors. *N Engl J Med* 1994;331:1116–1121.

49. Hoosein NM, Kiener PA, Curry RC, Brattain MG. Evidence for autocrine growth stimulation of cultured colon tumor cells by a gastrin/cholecystokinin-like peptide. *Experimental Cell Res* 1990;186:15–21.

50. Layton JE, Scanlon DB, Soveny C, Morstyn G. Effects of bombesin antagonists on the growth of small cell lung cancer cells *in vitro. Cancer Res* 1988;48:4783–4789.

51. Korc M, Meltzer P, Trent J. Enhanced expression of epidermal growth factor receptor correlates with alterations of chromosome 7 in human pancreatic cancer. *Proc Natl Acad Sci USA* 1986;83:5141–5144.

Gut-Brain Peptides in the New Millennium, edited by Y. Taché
CURE Foundation, Los Angeles, CA. © 2002

40

Neurohormonal Control of Pancreatic Exocrine Secretion: Role of Muscarinic M1 Receptors

Manfred V. Singer and Elke Niebergall-Roth
*Department of Medicine II, Gastroenterology and Hepatology, University Hospital
of Heidelberg at Mannheim, Mannheim, Germany*

INTRODUCTION

Pancreatic exocrine secretion is controlled by two fundamental mechanisms: neural (in particular vagal) and hormonal pathways. Efferent vagal impulses act on the exocrine pancreas via pancreatic ganglia, where the impulses are modulated and modified, and terminate via postganglionic fibers at the acinar cells. Acinar muscarinic receptors of the subtype M1 play an important role for the mediation of the stimulatory vagal influences on pancreatic exocrine secretion. In dogs, a potentiative interaction exists between the two most important mediators of the pancreatic exocrine response to intraduodenal stimuli, efferent vagal impulses and cholecystokinin (CCK). In contrast to humans and rats, in which all action of CCK on pancreatic enzyme output is vagally mediated, CCK acts in dogs in part as a classical humoral factor independent of the cholinergic system. Although several peptides found in pancreatic nerve cell bodies or fibers can stimulate or inhibit pancreatic exocrine secretion, their physiological importance in the neural control of the exocrine pancreas needs to be further evaluated.

The pancreatic secretory response to intestinal nutrients is mediated by a complex interplay of neural and humoral mediators. The extrinsic parasympathetic (vagal) innervation of the pancreas plays a major role in the control of pancreatic exocrine secretion. Apart from the gastrointestinal tract, the pancreas is the only peripheral organ that has a significant intrinsic nerve plexus. This chapter reports functional findings regarding the cholinergic control of pancreatic exocrine secretion and possible sites of interaction between cholinergic nerves and other neural and hormonal mediators.

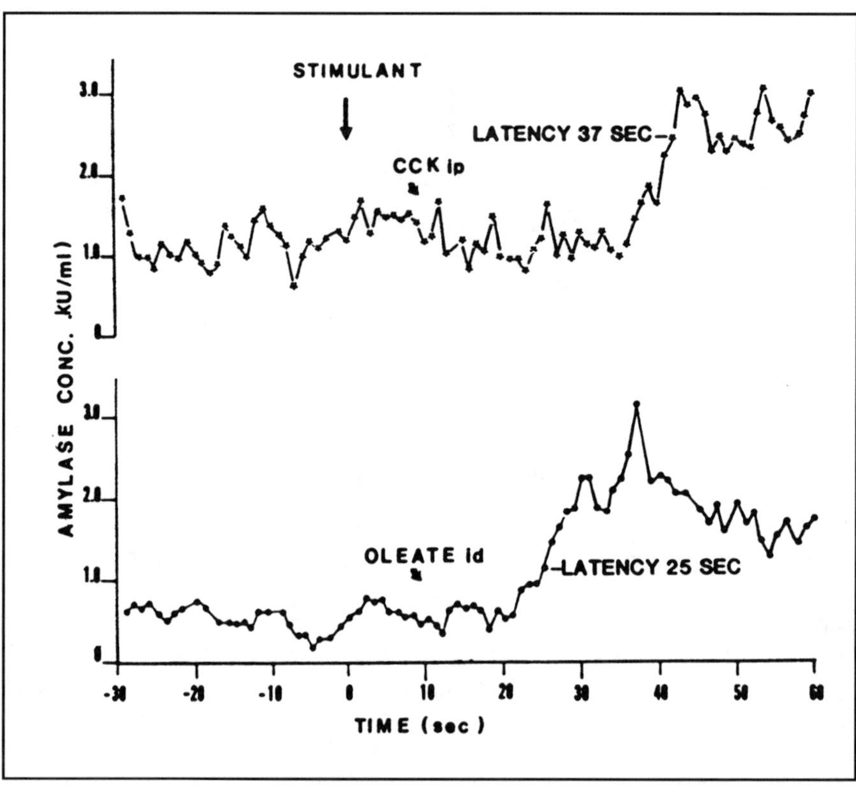

FIGURE 1. *Latency of pancreatic amylase response to intraduodenal injection of 1 mmol of sodium oleate or intraportal injection of 0.66 U/kg of CCK in representative experiments in the same dog. Adapted from Singer, et al. (3).*

CHOLINERGIC CONTROL OF PANCREATIC EXOCRINE SECRETION

There is strong support for the hypothesis that intrapancreatic postganglionic neurons regulate both enzyme and bicarbonate secretion. These neurons are activated by central input on the pancreatic ganglia during the cephalic phase and by vagovagal reflexes initiated by gastric and intestinal mediators released in response to a meal. Acetylcholine released by these neurons acts directly on muscarinic receptors on acinar cells (and presumably duct cells) to elicit secretion (1).

Role of the Vagus Nerves

Several studies have shown that the pancreatic enzyme response to intestinal perfusion with amino acids, peptides and fatty acids, and to a meal is strongly inhibited by atropine (2–6) and vagotomy (3, 6, 7). Experimental evidence for an enteropancreatic reflex has come from studies on the latency of pancreatic enzyme response, i.e., the time required to measure a significant increase in pancreatic enzyme output after a rapid intraduodenal bolus application of tryptophan or sodium oleate compared with intraportal injection of cholecystokinin (CCK) (3). In this study performed in dogs, even the shortest possible circulation time for a maximal dose of CCK (> 30 s) was significantly longer than the observed latency of amylase response to the intestinal nutrients (< 20 s) (Figure 1). Furthermore, truncal vagotomy and atropine both increased the latency to the intestinal stimulants by 10-fold but had no effect on the latency to intraportal CCK. Thus it was concluded that, at least in dogs, a cholinergic, vagovagal enteropancreatic reflex mediates the early pancreatic enzyme response to intestinal stimulants. Studies on the latency of the pancreatic fluid secretory response suggest that the early pancreatic fluid response to intestinal tryptophan or sodium oleate is also mediated, at least in part, via a vagovagal, cholinergic enteropancreatic reflex (8).

Follow-up studies performing stepwise extrinsic denervation of the pancreas ruled out possible splanchnic pathways of enteropancreatic reflexes (6). Celiac and superior mesenteric ganglionectomy did not alter the pancreatic protein response to intestinal tryptophan. Atropine significantly reduced the pancreatic protein response to low loads of tryptophan before but not after truncal vagotomy. These data suggest that, in dogs, the pancreatic protein response to intestinal tryptophan is, at least in part, mediated by long, cholinergic enteropancreatic reflexes with both afferent and efferent limb carried by the vagus nerves (6). Histochemical examinations demonstrated that in the rat there are enteric neurons that project to the pancreatic ganglia, thus providing anatomical evidence for these enteropancreatic reflexes (9).

Studies on the effect of truncal vagotomy or atropine on the pancreatic secretory response to different loads of intestinal nutrients have shown that vagal enteropancreatic reflexes are the major mediators of the pancreatic secretory response to low loads of intestinal stimulants, (4,6) whereas hormones mediate the secretory response particularly to high loads of intestinal stimuli (7, 10).

Role of M1 Receptors

Since at least three pharmacologically distinct subtypes (M1, M2, M3) of the muscarinic receptor do exist, the question emerged, which subtype is responsible for the vagal cholinergic control of pancreatic exocrine secretion. Based upon studies in which the M3 receptors were pharmacologically blocked, the M3 receptor was considered as the typical muscarinic receptor of the acinar cell (11–14). *In vivo* studies in humans and dogs, however, revealed a physiological role of M1 receptors in the control of pancreatic bicarbonate and enzyme secretion (15–17). More recently, analysis of the rat

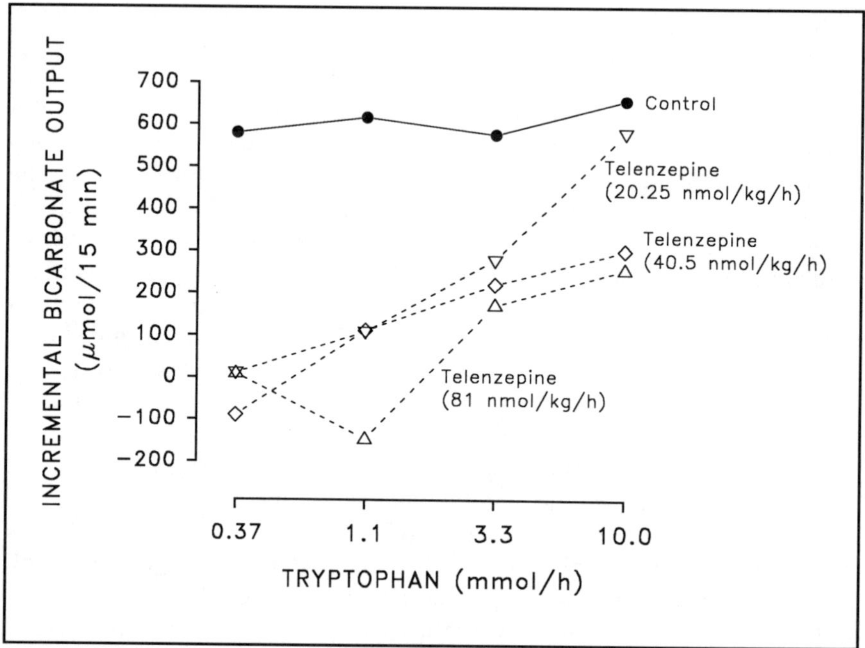

FIGURE 2. *Effect of different doses of telenzepine on the incremental pancreatic bicarbonate response to graded loads of intraduodenal tryptophan. Results are means of 6 dogs. Data are adapted from Niebergall-Roth, et al. (10).*

acinar cell muscarinic receptor by polymerase chain reaction revealed expression of both M1 and M3 subtypes (18). In addition, pharmacological blockade of M1 receptors caused a significantly greater inhibition of amylase secretion in isolated pancreatic acinar cells than blockade of the M3 receptors (18). To further estimate the role of M1 receptors in the control of pancreatic exocrine secretion, we have conducted in conscious dogs a series of studies to examine pancreatic exocrine secretion during selective M1 blockade by the M1 receptor antagonist telenzepine (19) under several study conditions.

M1 Receptors and Pancreatic Bicarbonate Secretion

Telenzepine significantly decreased the pancreatic bicarbonate response to intraduodenal tryptophan in conscious dogs up to total abolition (7, 10, 16) (Figure 2). Thus, intraduodenal amino acids stimulate bicarbonate secretion in part via M1 receptors. This mechanism seems to play a major role in the mediation of the bicarbonate response to low loads of intraduodenal amino acids, since the inhibitory effect of telenzepine was greater when low loads of tryptophan were given (Figure 2).

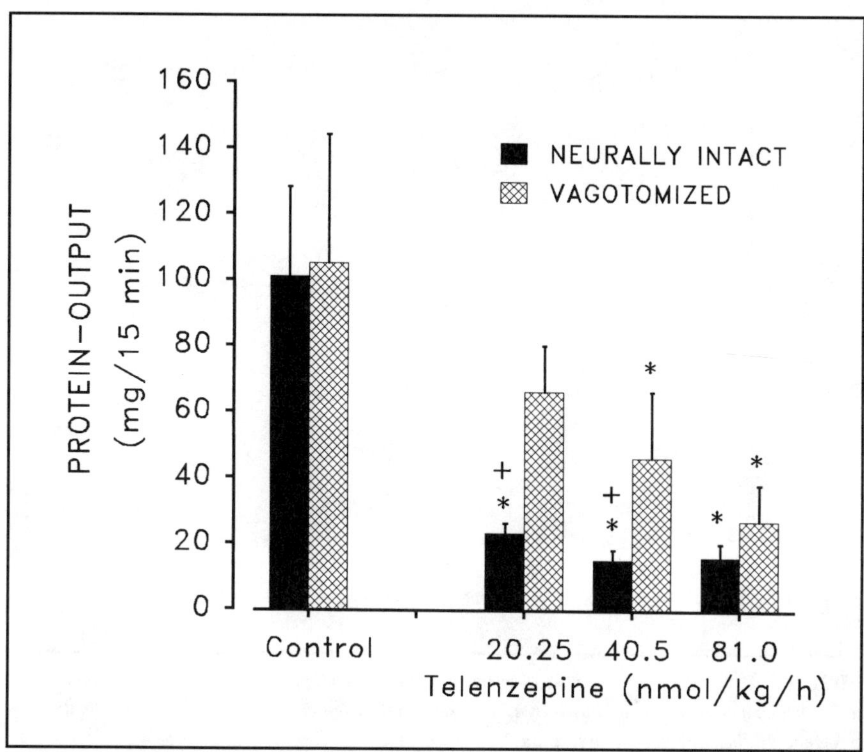

FIGURE 3. *Effect of different doses of telenzepine on pancreatic protein output during intravenous infusion of secretin (20.5 pmol/kg/h) in neurally intact and in truncally vagotomized dogs. Results are means ± SEM of 6 dogs. *p < 0.05 vs. control. + p < 0.05 before vs. after vagotomy. Data are adapted from Niebergall-Roth, et al. (7).*

M1 Receptors and Pancreatic Enzyme Secretion

During secretin infusion (to stimulate pancreatic fluid output), telenzepine significantly decreased canine pancreatic enzyme output by up to 85% (7, 20) (Figure 3). Since secretin does not stimulate pancreatic enzyme secretion in dogs (7, 16, 20), this finding suggests that M1 receptors are important mediators of basal pancreatic enzyme secretion. The observation that telenzepine still depresses basal enzyme output after truncal vagotomy (7) (Figure 3) suggests that the basal cholinergic tone of the pancreas does not significantly depend on the integrity of the vagus nerves but can be mainly ascribed to the intrinsic cholinergic nerves.

The pancreatic protein response to intraduodenal tryptophan was dose-dependently inhibited by telenzepine up to total abolition (7, 16, 20) (Figure 4). This inhibition was more pronounced when low loads of tryptophan were given, indicating that low loads of intraduodenal amino acids stimulate

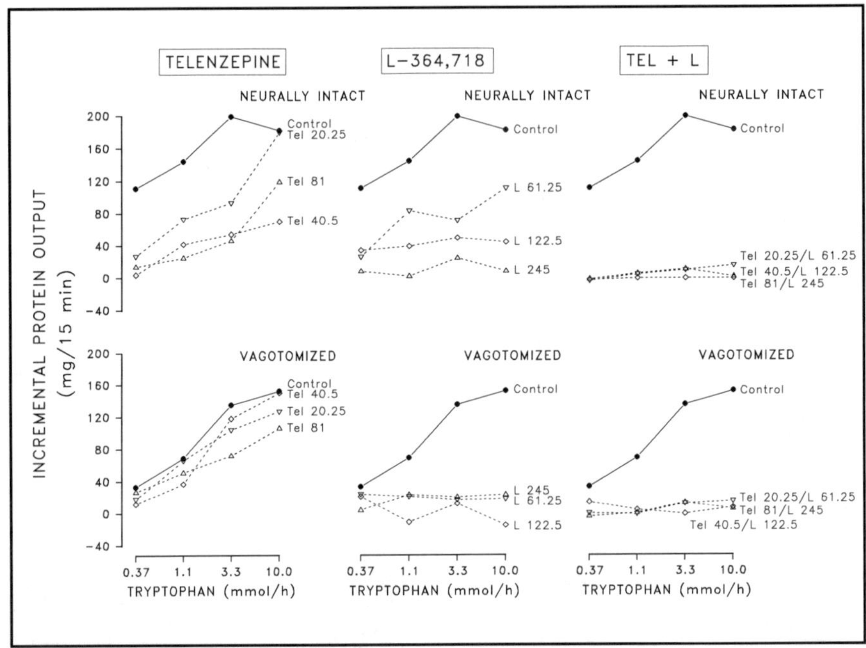

FIGURE 4. *Effect of different doses of telenzepine (Tel; nmol/kg/h iv.), L-364,718 (L; nmol/kg/h iv.) or both antagonists on the incremental pancreatic protein response to graded loads of intraduodenal tryptophan in neurally intact and in truncally vagotomized dogs. Results are means of six dogs. Data are adapted from Niebergall-Roth, et al. (7).*

pancreatic enzyme output predominantly by cholinergic mechanisms involving M1 receptors. However, telenzepine had no effect on tryptophan stimulated pancreatic protein output in vagotomized dogs (7) (Figure 4). Furthermore, telenzepine increased the latency of amylase response to rapid intraduodenal bolus injection of tryptophan or oleate by more than 10-fold (Table 1), indicating that enteropancreatic reflexes stimulate pancreatic enzyme secretion via activation of M1 receptors (21). These findings support the hypothesis that intraduodenal amino and fatty acids initiate an enteropancreatic reflex (3) that activates intrapancreatic postganglionic neurons ending on acinar M1 receptors.

NEUROHORMONAL INTERACTIONS

Besides cholinergic nerves, the hormone CCK is considered as the most important mediator of postprandial pancreatic exocrine secretion, particularly pancreatic enzyme output. To investigate possible interactions between cholinergic M1 receptors and CCK, we have studied the effects of telen-

TABLE 1. *Effect of telenzepine and L-364,718 on latency (in sec., unless otherwise stated) of pancreatic amylase response to intravenous (iv.) and intraduodenal (id.) stimulants.*

	Caerulein (7.4 pmol/kg iv)	L-Tryptophan (1 mmol id)	Sodium oleate (3 mmol id)
Control	28 ± 4	17 ± 7[#]	16 ± 5[#]
Telenzepine, 81 nmol/kg iv	30 ± 5	178 ± 116[*#]	208 ± 121[*#]
L-364,718, 245 nmol/kg iv	> 10 min.	> 10 min.	> 10 min.

Data are means ± SEM of 6 dogs. [*] p < 0.05 vs. control; [#] p < 0.05 vs. caerulein. Intravenous: iv; intraduodenal: id. Data are adapted from Niebergall-Roth et al. (21).

zepine in dogs during blockade of CCK-A-receptors by L-364,718 (MK-329, devazepide) (22).

Exogenous stimulation of the pancreatic protein output with the CCK analogue caerulein is not affected by telenzepine (7, 20) (Figure 5). This is in accordance with the observation that in dogs neither atropine nor vagotomy had any significant effect on pancreatic secretory response to exogenous CCK or caerulein (2, 6, 23). In addition, L-364,718 depressed the canine pancreatic protein response to tryptophan irrespective of the integrity of the vagus nerves (7) (Figure 4). Thus, endogenously released CCK controls canine pancreatic enzyme output at least in part by a pathway that does not involve M1 receptors, probably as a classical humoral factor acting at acinar CCK receptors. This mechanism, however, seems to represent a species particularity. In humans, the stimulatory effect of physiological doses of exogenous CCK or caerulein was almost completely inhibited by atropine (24, 25), suggesting that exogenous CCK at physiologic concentrations stimulates pancreatic enzyme output by interaction with the cholinergic system. In rats it was demonstated that the stimulatory action of exogenous CCK in a physiologic dose on pancreatic secretion is mainly mediated via capsaicin-sensitive vagal sensory afferents originating from the gastroduodenal mucosa (26).

Besides the action of CCK as a classical humoral factor, in dogs also experimental evidence exists for an interaction between the cholinergic system and the hormone CCK. The inhibition of the pancreatic protein response to intraduodenal tryptophan caused by a combination of telenzepine and L-364,718 was significantly greater than the sum of the inhibitory effects of each antagonist when given alone. In particular, the combination of the two antagonists in very low doses that had no significant effects on protein output when given separately, totally abolished the protein response when given together (7) (Figure 4). This finding indicates that in dogs—in addition to directs effects of CCK on the pancreatic acinar cell—a mechanism of potentiative interaction exists between cholinergic

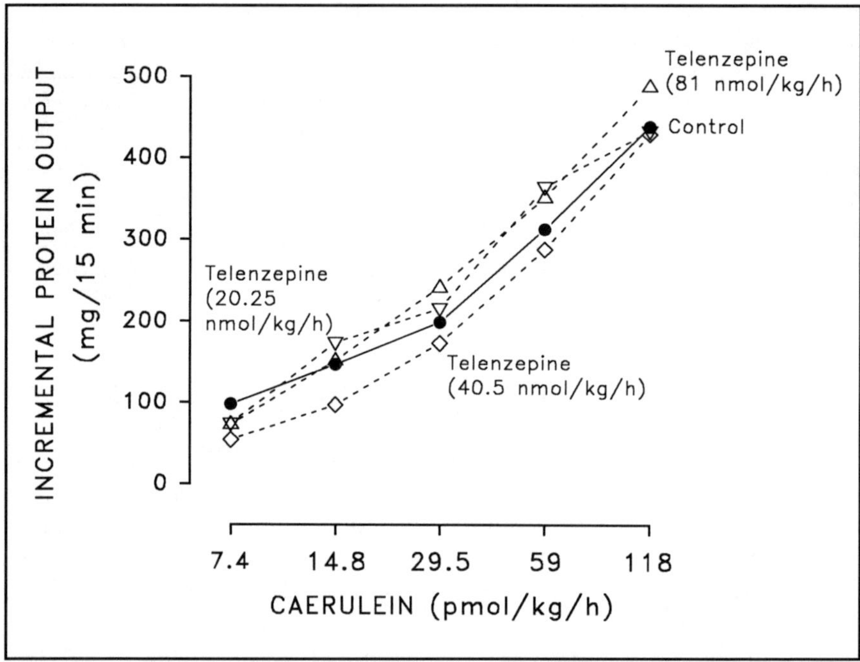

FIGURE 5. *Effect of different doses of telenzepine on the incremental pancreatic protein response to graded doses of intravenous caerulein. Results are means of 6 dogs. Data are adapted from Niebergall-Roth et al. (20).*

nerves ending on M1 receptors and CCK. Furthermore, L-364,718 was shown to interrupt the enteropancreatic reflex mediating the early amylase response to intraduodenal bolus application of tryptophan and oleate (21), indicating that the activation of (possibly vagal) CCK receptors is essential to run this reflex.

The question, where the interaction between the cholinergic system and CCK in the dog occurs, still needs to be answered. Firstly, CCK and cholinergic nerves may interact at the level of the acinar cell in as much a threshold of cholinergic input conditions the pancreatic secretory response of the acinar cell to hormonal acting CCK. However, this hypothesis is incompatible with the observation, that in dogs neither vagotomy, nor atropine, nor telenzepine alters the pancreatic protein response to exogenous CCK or caerulein in dogs (2, 6, 7, 23). Secondly, CCK may activate cholinergic vagal neurons and thus modulate the intrapancreatic neurons. An anatomical basis is provided by the discovery of type A receptors for CCK on afferent vagal fibers (27).

An intriguing hypothesis that integrates both—humoral and vagal—pathways of CCK in the dog was provided by Grossman (cited in 28). Intraduodenal infusion of nutrients would release CCK from endocrine cells of the

TABLE 2. *Non-adrenergic non-cholinergic neurotransmitters present in the pancreas and their effects on pancreatic exocrine secretion*

Stimulatory neurotransmitters	*Inhibitory neurotransmitters*
Nitric oxide (NO)	Serotonin (5-HT)
Serotonin (5-HT)	Calcitonin gene related peptide (CGRP)
Vasoactive intestinal polypeptide (VIP)	Enkephalines
Pituitary adenylate cyclase activating polypeptide (PACAP)	Galanin
Gastrin releasing polypeptide (GRP)	Neuropeptide Y (NPY)

duodenum. When low loads of nutrients were infused, only small amounts of CCK would be released, that would not reach the circulating blood but would diffuse across the intracellular space to the nervous CCK receptor and initiate a vago-vagal reflex. When high loads of nutrients were given, greater amounts of CCK would be released from the intestinal endocrine cells and discharged into the bloodstream and could thus stimulate pancreatic protein output by acting at the acinar CCK receptor. The higher treshold for hormonal than for nervous stimulation by CCK would explain the observation that in dogs L-364,718 inhibited the protein reponse to low and high amounts of intraduodenal nutrients, whereas telenzenzepine was mainly effective for inhibiting the response to low amounts of nutrients (7, 16, 20) (Figure 4). Furthermore, this mechanism would account for the finding that L-364,718 inhibits the pancreatic protein response even to low loads of intestinal amino acids, that do not cause measurable elevation of plasma CCK (7).

INTERACTIONS BETWEEN CHOLINERGIC AND NONCHOLINERGIC NERVES

Although several neurotransmitters found in pancreatic nerves do stimulate or inhibit pancreatic exocrine secretion under distinct experimental conditions (Table 2), the physiological significance of most of them are to be further evaluated. The most likely candidates are nitric oxide, serotonin and the neuropeptides vasoactive intestinal polypeptide, pituitary adenylate cyclase activating polypeptide and gastrin releasing polypeptide (29). Experimental evidence exists that nitrergic, serotonergic and GRP-containing nerves modulate the cholinergic control of pancreatic exocrine secretion.

Nitric oxide (NO)

In conscious dogs, the inhibitory effect of the NO synthase inhibitor N^G-nitro-L-arginine (L-NNA) on pancreatic exocrine secretion was most pronounced after vagal stimulation of the pancreas by sham feeding (30) or 2-Deoxy-D-glucose induced neuroglycopenia (31, 32). These findings suggest that the regulatory effect of NO on pancreatic secretion is related to a vagal pathway.

Serotonin (5-HT)

The axons of the serotonergic enteropancreatic neurons appear to form inhibitory axo-axonic synapses in the pancreas (33). 5-HT inhibits veratridine-mediated amylase secretion; this effect was blocked by the 5-HT$_{1P}$ receptor antagonist 5-HTP-DP. This observation suggests that serotonergic nerves inhibit pancreatic enzyme secretion via presynaptic 5-HT$_{1P}$ receptors on cholinergic neurons (33).

Gastrin releasing polypeptide (GRP)

GRP strongly stimulates pancreatic bicarbonate and enzyme output (34, 35). In the isolated perfused porcine pancreas, atropine inhibited the enzyme response to GRP, suggesting that acetylcholine somehow sensitizes the acinar cell to the effects of GRP. Another possibility is that, in addition to acting directly at the acinar bombesin/GRP receptor, GRP-containing nerves modulate pancreatic exocrine secretion through stimulation of acetycholine release from postganglionic cholinergic fibers. This hypothesis is supported by the findings that tetrodotoxin inhibited GRP stimulated amylase release in rat pancreatic lobules (35) and that bombesin, the amphibian counterpart of GRP, had no effect on enzyme output from dog pancreatic acini (36).

FUTURE RESEARCH PERSPECTIVES

Despite increasing knowledge about the function of pancreatic innervation several unanswered questions still remain. The study of the effects of M3 receptor antagonists *in vivo* could clarify the physiological role of acinar M3 receptors. The relative contribution of M1 and M3 receptors to the cholinergic control of pancreatic exocrine secretion is another intriguing question and could be answered by the comparison of the effects of M1 and M3 receptor antagonists under distinct experimental conditions.

Now that neurochemical investigations have revealed a number of peptides and other neuroactive substances in the nerve cell populations of the pancreas, subsequent studies should investigate the physiological significance of these substances as neurotransmitters of these cells. Further studies revealing the nature of the enteric stimuli that selectively activate either the excitatory or the inhibitory components of the enteropancreatic innervation will provide a deeper insight into the function of this system. In addition, further investigation of interaction pathways between these neurotransmitters could contribute to the understanding of the integration and/or summation of vagal, sympathetic, enteric and intrinsic pancreatic signals.

Finally, attention should be given to the role of the pancreatic innervation in pathophysiological processes such as acute and chronic pancreatitis. Future studies are necessary to establish whether and how pancreatic neurotransmission is altered or disrupted under pathophysiological conditions. A more comprehensive perspective of the neural mechanisms associated with such processes will lead to a better understanding of pancreatic disease.

ACKNOWLEDGMENTS

The experimental research by the authors reported in this chapter was supported by grants from the Deutsche Forschungsgemeinschaft (Si 228/7) and the Forschungsfonds of the Faculty for Clinical Medicine Mannheim of the University of Heidelberg, Germany (45/96; 16/97; 15/98).

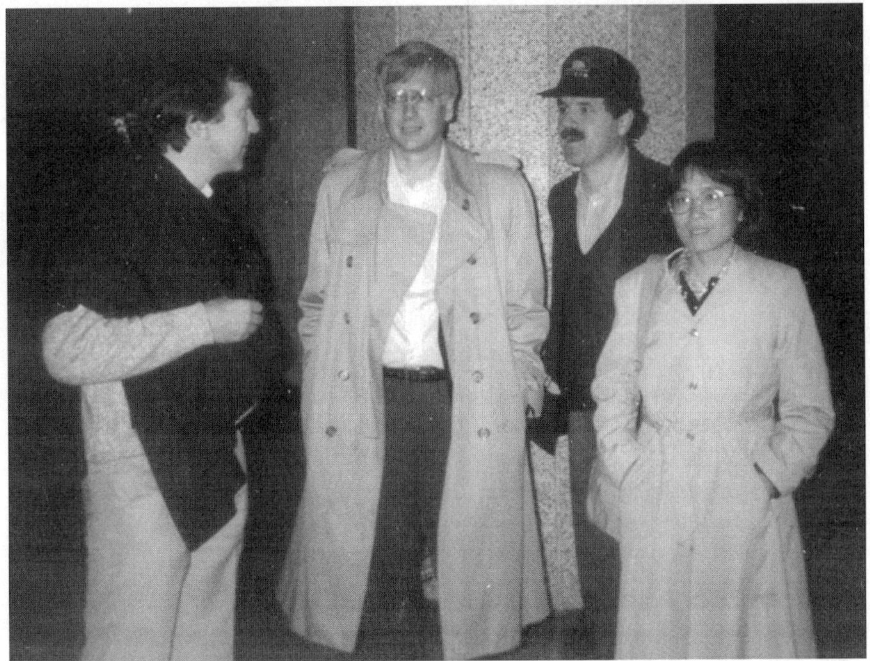

This picture was taken during Beijing International Conference on Brain-Gut Peptides, November, 1988. From left to right: G. Dockray, JH Walsh, MV Singer, Hong Yang.

REFERENCES

1. Solomon, TE. Control of exocrine pancreatic secretion. In: *Physiology of the Gastrointestinal Tract*, LR Johnson (ed). New York, Raven, 1994;1499–1529.
2. Singer MV, Solomon TE, Grossman MI. Effect of atropine and vagotomy on secretion from intact and transplanted pancreas in dog. *Am J Physiol* 1980;238:G18–G22.
3. Singer MV, Solomon TE, Wood J, Grossman MI. Latency of pancreatic enzyme response to intraduodenal stimulants. *Am J Physiol* 1980;238:G23–G29.
4. Vazquez-Echarri J, Baumgärtner D, Singer MV. Dose-reponse effects of atropine on pancreatic secretory response to intestinal tryptophan in dogs. *Am J Physiol* 1986;251:G847–G851.
5. Bozkurt T, Adler G, Koop I, Arnold R. Effect of atropine on intestinal phase of pancreatic secretion in man. *Digestion* 1988;41:108–115.
6. Singer MV, Niebel W, Jansen JBMJ, Hoffmeister D, Gotthold S, Goebell H, Lamers CBHW. Pancreatic secretory response to intravenous caerulein and intraduodenal tryptophan: Studies before and after stepwise removal of the extrinsic nerves of the pancreas in dogs. *Gastroenterology* 1989;96:925–934.
7. Niebergall-Roth E, Teyssen S, Wetzel D, Hartel M, Beglinger C, Riepl RL, Singer MV. Effects of telenzepine and L-364,718 on canine pancreatic secretion before and after vagotomy. *Am J Physiol* 1997;272:G1550–G1559.
8. Singer MV. Latency of pancreatic fluid secretory response to intestinal stimulants in the dog. *J Physiol (Lond)* 1983;339:75–85.
9. Kirchgessner AL, Liu M-T, Gershon MD. In situ identification and visualization of neurons that mediate enteric and enteropancreatic reflexes. *J Comp Neurol* 1990;371:270–286.
10. Niebergall-Roth E, Teyssen S, Hartel M, Beglinger C, Riepl RL, Singer MV. Pancreatic bicarbonate response to intraduodenal tryptophan in dogs. *Int J Pancreatol* 1998;23:31–39.
11. Louie DS, Owyang C. Muscarinic receptor subtypes on rat pancreatic acini: secretion and binding studies. *Am J Physiol* 1986;251:G275–G279.
12. Iwatsuki K, Horiuchi H, Yonekura H, Homma N, Haruta K, Chiba S. Suptypes of muscarinic receptors in pancreatic exocrine secretion in anesthetized dogs. *Pancreas* 1989;4:339–345.
13. Van Zwam AJ, Willems PH, Rodriguez de Miranda JF, de Pont JJ, van Ginneken CA. Binding characteristics of the muscarinic receptor subtype in rabbit pancreas. *J Recept Res* 1990;10:119–135.
14. Kato M, Ohkuma S, Kataoka K, Kashima K, Kuriyama K. Characterization of muscarinic receptor subtypes on rat pancreatic acini: Pharmacological identification by secretory responses and binding studies. *Digestion* 1992;52:194–203.
15. Singer MV, Teyssen S, Küppers U. Influence of the M1-receptor antagonists telenzepine and pirenzepine on pancreatic secretory response to intraduodenal tryptophan in dogs. *Digestion* 1991;48:34–42.
16. Teyssen S, Niebergall E, Chari ST, Singer MV. Comparison of two dose-response techniques to study the pancreatic secretory respopnse to intraduodenal tryptophan in the absence and in the presence of the M1-receptor antagonist telenzepine. *Pancreas* 1995;10:368–373.
17. Nelson DK, Malfertheiner P, Dahmen G, Dominguez-Munoz JE, Pieramico O, Adler G. Regulation of exocrine and endocrine pancreas via M1-muscarinic pathways. In: *Gastrointestinal Tract and Endocrine System*, MV Singer, R Ziegler, G Rohr (eds). Dordrecht, Kluwer, 1995;570–574.
18. Schmid SW, Modlin IM, Tang LH, Stoch A, Rhee S, Nathanson MH, Scheele GA, Gorelick FS. Telenzepine-sensitive muscarinic receptors on rat pancreatic acinar cells. *Am J Physiol* 1998;274:G734–G741.
19. Eltze M, Gönne S, Riedel R, Schlotke B, Schudt C, Simon WA, 1985: Pharmacological evidence for selective inhibition of gastric acid secreton by telenzepine, a new antimuscarinergic drug. *Eur J Pharmacol* 1985;112:211–224.
20. Niebergall-Roth E, Teyssen S, Singer MV. Blockade of M1 receptors has different effects on endogenously and exogenously stimulated pancreatic protein output in dogs. In: *Neurogastroenterology. From the Basics to the Clinics*, MV Singer, H-J Krammer (Eds). Dordrecht, Kluwer, 2000;389–393.
21. Niebergall-Roth E, Teyssen S, Singer MV. Effects of M1 and CCK antagonists on latency of pancreatic amylase response to intestinal stimulants. *Am J Physiol* 2000;279:G411–G416.

22. Chang RSL, Lotti VJ. Biochemical and pharmacological characterization of an extremely potent and selective nonpeptide cholecystokinin antagonist. *Proc Natl Acad Sci USA* 1986;83:4923–4926.

23. Vazquez-Echarri J, Baumgärtner D, Singer MV. Dose-response effects of atropine on pancreatic secretory response to intravenous caerulein in dogs. *Pancreas* 1986;1:341–346.

24. Adler G, Beglinger C, Braun U, Reinshagen M, Koop I, Schafmayer A, Rovati L, Arnold R. Interaction of the cholinergic system and cholecystokinin in the regulation of endogenous and exogenous stimulation of pancreatic secretion in humans. *Gastroenterology* 1991;100:537–543.

25. Soudah HC, Lu Y, Hasler WL, Owyang C. Cholecystokinin at physiological levels evokes pancreatic enzyme secretion via a cholinergic pathway. *Am J Physiol* 1992;263,G102–G107.

26. Li Y, Owyang C. Vagal efferent pathway mediates physiological action of cholecystokinin on pancreatic enzyme secretion. *J Clin Invest* 1993;92:418–424.

27. Dockray GJ. Vagally mediated actions of CCK. In: *Cholecystokinin Antagonists in Gastroenterology,* G Adler, C Beglinger (eds). Berlin, Springer, 1991;56–62.

28. Singer MV. Neurohormonal control of pancreatic enzyme secretion in animals. In: *The Pancreas: Biology, Pathobiology, and Diseases,* VLW Go (Ed). New York, Raven, 1993;425–448.

29. Chey WY, Chang T-M. Neural hormonal regulation of exocrine pancreatic secretion. *Pancreatology* 2001;1:320–335.

30. Konturek SJ, Bilski J, Konturek PK, Cieskowski M, Pawlik W. Role of endogenous nitric oxide in the control of canine pancreatic secretion and blood flow. *Gastroenterology* 1993;104:896–902.

31. Bilski J, Konturek SJ. Role of nitric oxide in the control of pancreatic secretion. In: *Biology of the Pancreas in Growing Animals,* S G Pierzynowsky, R Zabielski (eds). Amsterdam, Elsevier, 1999;93–212.

32. Niebergall-Roth E, Teyssen S, Singer MV. Inhibition of nitric oxide synthase has different effects on intestinally, hormonally and vagally stimulated pancreatic enzyme output in dogs. In: *Neurogastroenterology. From the Basics to the Clinics,* MV Singer, H-J Krammer (eds). Dordrecht, Kluwer, 2000;15–324.

33. Kirchgessner AL and Gershon MD. Presynaptic inhibition by serotonin of nerve mediated secretion of pancreatic amylase. *Am J Physiol* 1995;268:G339–G345.

34. Knuhtsen S, Holst JJ, Jensen SL, Knigge U, Nielsen OV. Gastrin-releasing peptide: Effect on exocrine secretion and release from isolated perfused porcine pancreas. *Am J Physiol* 1985;248:G281–G286.

35. Flowe KM, Welling TH, Mullholland WM. Gastrin-releasing peptide stimulation of amylase release from rat pancreatic lobules involves intrapancreatic neurons. *Pancreas* 1994;9:513–517.

36. Bommelaer G, Rozental G, Bernier C, Vaysse N, Ribet A. Action of secretagogues on amylase release from the dog pancreatic acini. *Digestion* 1981;21:248–254.

VI.

Clinical Research

Gut-Brain Peptides in the New Millennium, edited by Y. Taché
CURE Foundation, Los Angeles, CA. © 2002

41

Gastric Physiology in Human Subjects: The Clinical End of Translational Research

Gordon V. Ohning
*CURE/Digestive Diseases Research Center, UCLA Division of Digestive Diseases
Department of Medicine and VA Greater Los Angeles Healthcare System
Los Angeles, CA*

INTRODUCTION

One of my early experiences at CURE was to follow Dr. John Walsh into Room 209 of the CURE Clinic, where human acid secretion studies were performed. As I rounded the door, I was met by the sight of two human subjects seated in large reclining chairs with Anderson tubes coming out of their noses, the mechanical whirl of pumps circulating gastric fluid in and out of the tubing in order to measure and control the intragastric pH, and watching Bona Syntik rushing from subject-to-subject and machine-to-machine, checking the flow in the tubing, scrutinizing the LED displays on the pH titrators, and maneuvering the subjects in their chairs in order to orchestrate this controlled chaos. When I commented later on the astonishing pace of Bona's work, Dr. Walsh simply chuckled and said that it was actually an easy day for Bona as she usually had four subjects going at the same time.

Although the late Dr. John Walsh was internationally renowned for his basic research and knowledge of gastrointestinal physiology and hormones, his early career was heavily invested in clinical research. In the first decade of his career, approximately 50% of his publications were on clinical research topics. Dr. Walsh continued this important contribution throughout his career. He was a member of several clinical research organizations, including the American Federation for Clinical Research and both the Western and American Societies for Clinical Investigation as well as serving on many advisory committees for pharmaceutical companies engaged in clinical studies. Dr. Walsh was recognized by the American Gastroenterological Association (AGA) with the Joseph B. Kirsner Award for Clinical Research in Gastroenterology in 1993 for his substantial contributions to clinical research in gastroenterology.

Several years ago, I noted that the first publication in Dr. Walsh's bibliography was entitled *Hypernatremia complicating sodium sulfate therapy for hypercalcemic crisis* (15). When I commented that this seemed like an odd subject for a gastroenterologist to study, Dr. Walsh told me that he was initially interested in endocrinology during his training, but had been exposed to the neuroendocrine tumors of the pancreas while working with Dr. Sleisenger during his residency (41, 42). His subsequent military service as an EIS officer at the National Communicable Disease Center of the National Institutes of Health and as a consultant in Hepatitis for the Blood Bank Department led to his introduction to the technique of radioimmunoassay (RIA) as a method for detection of the Australian Antigen in screening blood products for Hepatitis B (43, 44). After his service commitment, he continued his medical research training at the Veterans Administration Hospital in Bronx, New York in the laboratory of Drs. R. Yalow and S. Berson. His interest in gastroenterology resurfaced after joining the late Dr. Morton Grossman's laboratory at the suggestion of his then-mentors Drs. R. Yalow and S. Berson. His primary interests at the time had been in radioimmunoassay of hormones and it seemed like a good idea to apply this technique to a hormone called gastrin for which a radioimmunoassay had recently been developed (46). After a while, the gastrointestinal tract just seemed like another way to study endocrinology and, as Dr. Walsh put it, he was simply a life-long endocrinologist who happened to study gastroenterology in his spare time.

Radioimmunoassay

The ability to measure tissue concentrations and circulating levels of gastrointestinal peptides added an important tool for studying the regulation of gastrointestinal physiology, particularly gastric acid secretion. Dr. Walsh applied his expertise in radioimmunoassay of gastrin in both human and animal studies. Early studies in canine animal models demonstrated the stimulatory effects of feeding, vagal tone, and insulin-induced hypoglycemia on gastrin release (9, 36, 39) and subsequent studies in human subjects demonstrated similar pathways of regulation (10, 12, 45). This validation of animal models by human clinical investigation was an important and continuing theme of Dr. Walsh's research programs and defined the concept of what is now called translational research. The value of research findings was measured not only by its inherent merit, but also by its ability to better understand the regulation and pathophysiology in humans.

One clinical condition that became particularly important in understanding the physiological and pathophysiological role of gastrin was Zollinger-Ellison syndrome (ZES). The altered regulation of gastrin release in ZES patients in response to secretin and calcium was identified (17, 27) and resulted in more reliable methods of confirming the diagnosis in patients suspected of having ZES (16). Use of radioimmunoassay in conjunction with fractionation techniques allowed for measurement of gastrin molecular forms in the serum and tissue of ZES patients and demonstrated that gastrin-34 was the predominant circulating form, while gastrin-17 was the major component in tumor tissue (11). Additional forms of gastrin, particularly the N-terminal 1-13 fragment of gastrin-17, were identified. Subsequent development of region-specific antisera for molecular forms of gastrin would detect the variation of even a single amino acid substitution and allow for rapid identification and measurement without the need for further separation methods (28).

Peptic ulcer disease was an area of intense interest in the 1970s due to the considerable morbidity and mortality associated with active disease. Medical treatments were not entirely satisfactory in the pre-*Helicobactor pylori* era and surgical treatment was commonly employed to control complications. Measurement of circulating gastrin in the post-surgical patient (Billroth II) with early recurrent peptic disease was invaluable in excluding ZES or isolated retained antrum as an etiology (37). The regulation of circulating gastrin levels was studied in peptic ulcer patients during basal or meal stimulation in an effort to identify a pathophysiologic role for gastrin or its molecular forms (1, 5, 40). Although many of these effects were later correlated with active Helicobacter pylori infection (14, 34) and not exclusively due to the presence of duodenal ulcer (18), the information concerning the regulation of gastrin release added to our understanding of the regulation of gastric physiology.

The ever-increasing list of gastrointestinal peptide hormones was substantially expanded in the 1970s and 1980s. The development of specific antibodies and RIA allowed for their characterization in a fashion similar to that employed for gastrin (4, 6, 20, 23, 32, 35). The physiology and pathophysiology of these gastrointestinal peptides are described in other chapters within this text and will not be reviewed here in detail. The radioimmunoassay techniques that were mastered and championed by Dr. John Walsh have played a critical role in the characterization of these peptides. Further, the ability to reliably measure both circulating and tissue levels has helped define their roles in normal and disease-altered human physiology.

Gastric Acid Secretion

The regulation of gastric acid secretion was of substantial interest in the earlier studies of peptic ulcer disease (33, 38) and remains of importance in controlling peptic disorders such as gastroesophageal reflux disease in the post-*Helicobacter pylori* era. The ability to accurately and reproducibly measure gastric acid output in human subjects continues to play an important role in the evaluation of effective medical treatments for controlling gastric acidity (8, 22, 26). Measurement of basal acid output (BAO) after fasting and maximum acid output (MAO) in response to a secretagogue, such as pentagastrin, can be used to characterize gastric acid secretion in humans. Continuous measurement of intragastric pH has been used to study gastric acidity; however, this provides only an estimate of actual gastric acid output. The ability to measure meal-stimulated gastric acid output in animal models (9, 39) led to an interest in perfecting a similar technique in human subjects.

In 1973, Drs. Fordtran and Walsh published their seminal paper describing a reproducible technique for measuring net gastric acid secretion in human subjects (13). The method employed intubation of the stomach with a Levin tube for sampling gastric contents to measure pH modified by the attachment of a small diameter polyvinyl tube for instilling sodium bicarbonate buffer. Gastric pH was maintained at a predetermined value by infusing sodium bicarbonate buffer. The net gastric acid output was calculated from the amount of buffer required per unit time. The response to a standard meal was tested and reproducible results were obtained when the intragastric pH was maintained at 5.5. The use of pH 6.0 or higher resulted in erroneous overestimation of acid secretion due to high CO_2 content at this pH range. This early system was complicated by the inability to continuously monitor pH and the lack of a pH controlled titration device. The buffer infusion rate was controlled by manually adjusting an infusion pump in response to manual pH measurements obtained approximately every 3 minutes. Further, the lack of continuous sampling required innovative methods of mixing the gastric contents, including shaking the subject and frequent changes in body position. Subsequent modifications of this method have included the use of a dual lumen Anderson tube, continuous sampling of gastric contents by use of a piston pump to improve both sampling and mixing of gastric contents, use of improved pH titration equipment with continuous monitoring and correction of gastric pH, and use of liquid (typically 8%) peptone rather than solid (albeit well chewed) food (19, 26) resulting in improved precision of the data and less wear-and-tear on both the subjects and the study personnel.

The measurement of gastric acid output in human subjects was used to determine both the regulation of gastric acid secretion (2, 21, 30) and the optimum therapeutic regimen for anti-secretory treatments (3, 7). As with gastrin RIA, the initial studies focused on patients with peptic ulcer disease or ZES. The intragastric titration method could be easily modified with respect to the pH at which gastric contents were maintained (25, 29) and the contents of the meal (24, 31), which provided tremendous flexibility in the experimental design.

Future Directions

Shortly before his untimely death, Dr. Walsh presented an overview of the achievements in the study of acid secretion over the past 3 decades highlighting the improved knowledge concerning the regulatory mechanisms involved in the cephalic, gastric, and intestinal phases of acid secretion. These included the recognition of non-cholinergic pathways and the importance of TRH in the cephalic phase, the confirmation of histamine in the inter-mediation of the gastrin effect, the discovery of H-2 receptors and H-K-ATPase as both important regulators and even more important drug targets, and the role of CCK and neural inhibition during the intestinal phase of acid secretion.

Dr. Walsh identified several key areas for continued investigations, includ-ing the role of PACAP and parietal cell M3 receptors in cephalic stimula-tion of acid secretion, the mechanism by which food causes the release of gastrin, and the emerging roles of inhibitory peptides in the regulation of acid secretion. As for clinical areas of relevance, he believed that peptic ulcer disease would remain an important clinical entity despite the eradication ef-forts for *Helicobactor pylori*. Further, the increasing prevalence of gastro-esophageal reflux, Barrett's esophagus, and esophageal adenocarcinoma would require a continued focus on gastric acid secretion and the injurious effects of peptic secretion on the gastrointestinal mucosa. By his statements, Dr. Walsh recognized the continued importance of studying the regulation of acid secretion and gastric physiology.

SUMMARY

Dr. John Walsh was a strong proponent of using animal models and *in vitro* methods to compare and contrast the regulatory pathways for gastrointestinal physiology in humans. He recognized that translational research is a two way street: knowledge obtained from animal models and *in vitro* methods provide insight into the design of human studies while information about human physiology and disease drive the experiments in the animal and *in vitro* mod-els. It has been stated that translational research is a "bench to bedside" ap-proach. I think that Dr. Walsh extended this to be a "bench to bedside to bench and back" pathway. His abbreviated career is a rich testimonial to the successful application of this doctrine.

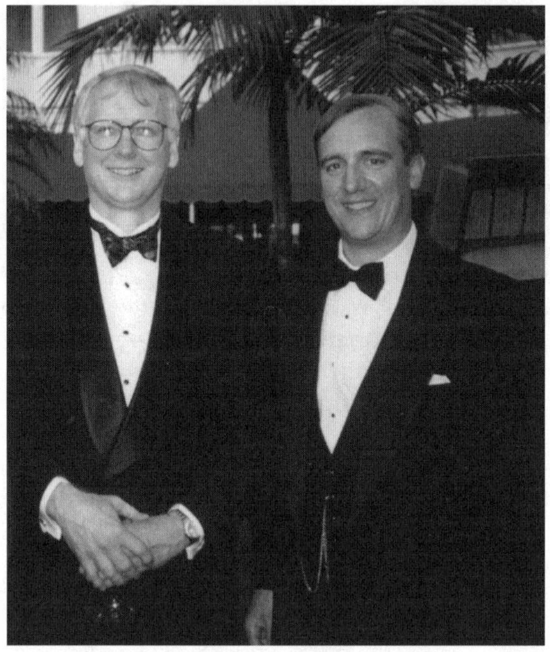

Attempt by the author to "blend" at Dr. Walsh's AGA Presidential Reception.

AMUSING ANECDOTE

Although Dr. Walsh was a superb scientist, he also excelled at being a human being. During my first year in his laboratory, John invited me to his house for Thanksgiving. Although I assumed this would be an informal affair in the manner of his world famous July 4th barbecues, it turned out to be a family gathering with only two non-family members present. John recognized that I had no plans or family in Los Angeles, so took it upon himself to make sure I was invited somewhere for the Holidays. During the course of the evening, the topic turned to the Civil War and I quickly realized that I was dining with a family that was steeped in Southern tradition. When asked if I had any ancestors whom had fought in the Civil War, I immediately replied "why, yes" and then successfully steered the conversation to another topic. Several years later, when John was preparing his "Chancellorsville" AGA Presidential address, we discussed this important Civil War battle at some length. At this point, John remembered our conversation of several years past and recalled that I had relatives who had fought in the Civil War. He then asked which unit they were in and where they had fought. I somewhat sheepishly replied "the Indiana 7th under General Sherman". After a brief moment of somewhat stunned silence, it suddenly dawned on John that my relative had fought on the "other" side. John then sort of half smiled and said "Oh, I thought you said your relatives fought for the South" to which I replied "No, you only asked if I had any relatives that fought, not which side they were on and I didn't think it was wise to offer this information unless I was directly asked."

REFERENCES

1. Azuma T, Magami Y, Habu Y, Kawai K, Taggart RT, Walsh JH. Carboxyl terminal glycine extended progastrin (gastrin-G) in gastric antral mucosa of patients with gastric or duodenal ulcer and in gastrinomas. *J Gastroenterol Hepatol* 1990;5:525–529.

2. Bieberdorf FA, Gray TK, Walsh JH, Fordtran JS. Effect of calcitonin on meal-stimulated gastric acid secretion and serum gastrin concentration. *Gastroenterology* 1974;66:343–346.

3. Bieberdorf FA, Walsh JH, Fordtran JS. Effect of optimum therapeutic dose of poldine on acid secretion, gastric acidity, gastric emptying, and serum gastrin concentration after a protein meal. *Gastroenterology* 1975;68:50–57.

4. Bilchik AJ, Hines OJ, Ashley SW, Adrian TE, Walsh J, Wong H, Liu CD, Zinner MJ, McFadden DW. Peptide YY immunoneutralization inhibits meal-induced absorption *in vivo. Surgery* 1994;116: 1153–1157.

5. Blair AJ, Feldman M, Barnett C, Walsh JH, Richardson CT. Detailed comparison of basal and food-stimulated gastric acid secretion rates and serum gastrin concentrations in duodenal ulcer patients and normal subjects. *J Clin Invest* 1987;79:582–587.

6. Bunnett NW, Reeve JRJ, Dimaline R, Shively JE, Hawke D, Walsh JH. The isolation and sequence analysis of vasoactive intestinal peptide from a ganglioneuroblastoma. *J Clin Endocrinol Metab* 1984;59:1133–1137.

7. Ciociola AA, Webb DD, Heath A, Walsh JH. Effects of ranitidine bismuth citrate on gastric acid secretion and gastrin release in subjects with and without *Helicobacter pylori* infection. *Aliment Pharmacol Ther* 1996;10: 905–912.

8. Ciociola AA, Webb DD, Heath A, Walsh JH. Effects of ranitidine bismuth citrate on gastric acid secretion and gastrin release in subjects with and without Helicobacter pylori infection. *Aliment Pharmacol Ther* 1996;10:905–912.

9. Csendes A, Walsh JH, Grossman MI. Effects of atropine and of antral acidification on gastrin release and acid secretion in response to insulin and feeding in dogs. Gastroenterology 1972;63:257–263.

10. Debas HT, Walsh JH, Grossman MI. After vagotomy atropine suppresses gastrin release by food. *Gastroenterology* 1976;70:1082–1084.

11. Dockray GJ, Walsh JH, Passaro EJ. Relative abundance of big and little gastrins in the tumours and blood of patients with the Zollinger Ellison syndrome. *Gut* 1975;16:353–358.

12. Farooq O and Walsh JH. Atropine enhances serum gastrin response to insulin in man. *Gastroenterology* 1975;68:662–666.

13. Fordtran JS and Walsh JH. Gastric acid secretion rate and buffer content of the stomach after eating. Results in normal subjects and in patients with duodenal ulcer. *J Clin Invest* 1973;52:645–657.

14. Graham DY, Opekun A, Lew GM, Klein PD, Walsh JH. Helicobacter pylori-associated exaggerated gastrin release in duodenal ulcer patients. The effect of bombesin infusion and urea ingestion. *Gastroenterology* 1991;100:1571–1575.

15. Heckman BA and Walsh JH. Hypernatremia complicating sodium sulfate therapy for hypercalcemic crisis. *N Engl J Med* 1967;276:1082–1083.

16. Isenberg JI, Walsh JH, Grossman MI. Zollinger-Ellison syndrome. *Gastroenterology* 1973;65:140–165.

17. Isenberg JI, Walsh JH, Passaro EJ, Moore EW, Grossman MI. Unusual effect of secretin on serum gastrin, serum calcium, and gastric acid secretion in a patient with suspected Zollinger-Ellison syndrome. *Gastroenterology* 1972;62:626–631.

18. Karnes WEJ, Ohning GV, Sytnik B, Kim SW, Walsh JH. Elevation of meal-stimulated gastrin release in subjects with *Helicobacter pylori* infection: reversal by low intragastric pH. *Rev Infect Dis* 1991;13 Suppl 8:S665–S670.

19. Karnes WEJ, Ohning GV, Sytnik B, Kim SW, Walsh JH. Elevation of meal-stimulated gastrin release in subjects with *Helicobacter pylori* infection: reversal by low intragastric pH. *Rev Infect Dis* 1991;13 Suppl 8:S665–70:S665–S670.

20. Kleibeuker JH, Eysselein VE, Maxwell VE, Walsh JH. Role of endogenous secretin in acid-induced inhibition of human gastric function. *J Clin Invest* 1984;73:526–532.

21. Levant JA, Walsh JH, Isenberg JI. Stimulation of gastric secretion and gastrin release by single oral doses of calcium carbonate in man. *N Engl J Med* 1973;289:555–558.

22. Lew EW, Pisegna JR, Starr JA, Soffer EF, Forsmark C, Modlin IM, Walsh JH, Beg M, Bochenek W, Metz DC. Intravenous pantoprazole rapidly controls gastric acid hypersecretion in patients with Zollinger-Ellison syndrome. *Gastroenterology* 2000;118:696–704.

23. Lloyd KC, Maxwell V, Ohning G, Walsh JH. Intestinal fat does not inhibit gastric function through a hormonal somatostatin mechanism in dogs. *Gastroenterology* 1992;103:1221–1228.

24. McArthur KE, Walsh JH, Richardson CT. Soy protein meals stimulate less gastric acid secretion and gastrin release than beef meals. *Gastroenterology* 1988;95:920–926.

25. Mogard MH, Maxwell V, Reedy TJ, Walsh JH. Gastric acidification inhibits meal-stimulated gastric acid secretion after prostaglandin synthesis inhibition by indomethacin in humans. *Gastroenterology* 1987;93:63–68.

26. Ohning GV, Barbuti RC, Kovacs TO, Sytnik B, Humphries TJ, Walsh JH. Rabeprazole produces rapid, potent, and long-acting inhibition of gastric acid secretion in subjects with Helicobacter pylori infection. *Aliment Pharmacol Ther* 2000;14:701–708.

27. Passaro EJ, Basso N, Walsh JH. Calcium challenge in the Zollinger-Ellison syndrome. *Surgery* 1972;72:60–67.

28. Rehfeld JF and Morley JS. Residue-specific radioimmunoanalysis: a novel analytical tool. Application to the C-terminus of CCK/gastrin peptides. *J Biochem Biophys Methods* 1983;7:161–170.

29. Richardson CT, Walsh JH, Hicks MI. The effect of cimetidine, a new histamine H2-receptor antagonist, on meal-stimulated acid secretion, serum gastrin, and gastric emptying in patients with duodenal ulcer. *Gastroenterology* 1976;71:19–23.

30. Richardson CT, Walsh JH, Hicks MI, Fordtran JS. Studies on the mechanisms of food-stimulated gastric acid secretion in normal human subjects. *J Clin Invest* 1976;58:623–631.

31. Schiller LR, Walsh JH, Feldman M. Distention-induced gastrin release: effects of luminal acidification and intravenous atropine. *Gastroenterology* 1980;78:912–917.

32. Shulkes A, Chick P, Wong H, Walsh JH. A radioimmunoassay for neurotensin in human plasma. *Clin Chim Acta* 1982;125:49–58.

33. Soll AH and Walsh JH. Regulation of gastric acid secretion. *Ann Rev Physiol* 1979;41:35–53.

34. Tarnasky PR, Kovacs TO, Sytnik B, Walsh JH. Asymptomatic H. pylori infection impairs pH inhibition of gastrin and acid secretion during second hour of peptone meal stimulation. *Dig Dis Sci* 1993;38:1681–1687.

35. Taylor IL, Solomon TE, Walsh JH, Grossman MI. Pancreatic polypeptide. Metabolism and effect on pancreatic secretion in dogs. *Gastroenterology* 1979;76:524–528.

36. Tepperman BL, Walsh JH, Preshaw RM. Effect of antral denervation on gastrin release by sham feeding and insulin hypoglycemia in dogs. *Gastroenterology* 1972;63:973–980.

37. Walsh JH. Clinical significance of gastrin radioimmunoassay. *Semin Nucl Med* 1975;5:247–254.

38. Walsh JH. Peptides as regulators of gastric acid secretion. *Ann Rev Physiol* 1988;50:41–63:41–63.

39. Walsh JH, Csendes A, Grossman MI. Effect of truncal vagotomy on gastrin release and Heidenhain pouch acid secretion in response to feeding in dogs. *Gastroenterology* 1972;63:593–600.

40. Walsh JH, Richardson CT, Fordtran JS. pH dependence of acid secretion and gastrin release in normal and ulcer subjects. *J Clin Invest* 1975;55:462–468.

41. Walsh JH and Sleisenger MH. Clinical syndromes associated with tumors of the pancreas. *Dis Mon* 1967;1–30.

42. Walsh JH and Sleisenger MH. Functioning tumors of the pancreas. *Med Times* 1968;96:890–901.

43. Walsh JH, Yalow R, Berson SA. Detection of Australia antigen and antibody by means of radioimmunoassay techniques. *J Infect Dis* 1970;121:550–554.
44. Walsh JH, Yalow RS, Berson SA. Radioimmunoassay of Australia antigen. *Vox Sang* 1970;19:217–224.
45. Walsh JH, Yalow RS, Berson SA. The effect of atropine on plasma gastrin response to feeding. *Gastroenterology* 1971;60:16–21.
46. Yalow RS and S.A. Berson SA. Radioimmunoassay of gastrin. *Gastroenterology* 1970;58:1–14.

Gut-Brain Peptides in the New Millennium, edited by Y. Taché
CURE Foundation, Los Angeles, CA. © 2002

42

Risk Factors and Recurrence of Ulcer Hemorrhage: Recommendations for Primary and Secondary Prevention

Thomas O.G. Kovacs and Dennis M. Jensen
CURE Digestive Disease Research Center
VA Greater Los Angeles Healthcare System
Los Angeles, CA

INTRODUCTION

John Walsh was keenly interested in the pathophysiologic mechanisms involved in peptic ulcer disease (PUD). His observations that patients with peptic ulcer disease had impaired acid and gastric secretion led to important advances in the understanding of the disease process (1, 2). With better awareness of the underlying pathophysiology came improved management of patients with both routine PUD and those with complicated ulcer disease, such as hemorrhage, perforation, and gastric outlet obstruction. At the Center for Ulcer Research and Education (CURE), a long-term follow-up of duodenal ulcer patients showed that 11% of patients had a complication during a 6-year study period (3). Complication rates were 2–7% per year for those without past complications and 5% for those with a prior complication. Elderly patients tended to have more complications and a more serious illness than younger patients with PUD. Since the mean age of the United States population is increasing, the number of patients with complicated ulcer disease will also increase. Therefore, the appropriate management and prevention of these complications will be important not only in the context of good patient care but also within the framework of health care utilization.

The purpose of this chapter is to review the risk factors contributing to ulcer hemorrhage and discuss the role of primary and secondary prevention. This review will focus on patients admitted with upper gastrointestinal (UGI) bleeding as a primary diagnosis and not those patients developing UGI hemorrhage while in the hospital for other medical or surgical conditions such as stress-related mucosal bleeding.

Peptic ulcer disease is the most common cause of acute UGI hemorrhage, accounting for about 50% of the cases (4). About 25% of ulcer patients bleed at some time during the course of their disease (5), with a greater portion of duodenal ulcer than gastric ulcer patients experiencing hemorrhage. In the United States there are about 150,000 hospitalizations per year for ulcer bleeding. The rate of ulcer hemorrhage is increasing in some groups such as the elderly and women.

RISK FACTORS

Helicobacter pylori and non-steroidal anti-inflammatory drugs (NSAIDs) account for the majority of peptic ulcers. However, while *Helicobacter pylori (Hp)* is the main etiology of uncomplicated ulcers, NSAIDs play a more critical role in complicated ulcers (6). The prevalence of *H. pylori* infection in patients with complicated ulcer disease is decreased. In one study, 93% of patients with non-bleeding duodenal ulcers were Hp positive in comparison to 71% of patients with bleeding duodenal ulcers (7). In CURE studies, Hp positive prevalence occurred in only 72% of bleeding duodenal ulcer patients and 79% of gastric ulcer patients (8).

The relation between *H. pylori* infection and NSAID use in ulcer pathogenesis is controversial. Intuitively, having both these risk factors for peptic ulcer disease would increase the likelihood of having an ulcer and subsequently, a complication such as bleeding. However, recent studies have provided conflicting results with some studies suggesting that *H. pylori* infection increases the risk for complications, while others suggest that *H. pylori* plays a protective role by increasing endogenous prostaglandin production. Kuyvenhaven et al. (9) evaluated the role of NSAID's and *H. pylori* in a Dutch population of bleeding ulcer patients. They reported that the relative risk for NSAID use was 8.2 and for *H. pylori*—only 1.2. When both NSAIDs and *H. pylori* were identified, no potentiation effect was noted (9). Henriksson et al. (10) also found that Hp infection and NSAID use were independent risk factors in 106 Swedish patients with active bleeding ulcers. Other authors studying bleeding ulcer patients found a two-fold increased risk of hemorrhage in *H. pylori* positive patients taking NSAID's. In elderly patients, one fourth of NSAID-related bleeding had *H. pylori* infection (11). These results conflict with other reports suggesting either an inverse relationship, i.e. a protective effect of *H. pylori* in NSAID users with gastric ulcer bleeding (12) or that *H. pylori* and NSAIDs act independently by different mechanisms in the elderly (13). Recent results have continued this conflicting trend. For example, in patients on chronic NSAID's with current or past ulcers, *H. pylori* eradication led to impaired healing of gastric ulcers and did not alter the rate of ulcer formation over 6 months (14). Chan et al. (15) however, showed that Hp eradication before NSAID use decreased the occurrence of NSAID associated ulcers in patients without prior NSAID exposure or ulcers. In a subsequent 6-month follow-up study in Hp positive patients requiring long-term NSAIDs, and who received either placebo or Hp eradication therapy, Chan et al. (16) found that the frequency of complicated ulcers was 4% in the eradicated group and 27% in the placebo group. In a meta-analysis, Huang et al. (17) found that PUD in NSAID-users occurred significantly more frequently in Hp-positive (42%) than Hp-negative (26%) patients. *H. pylori* infection and NSAID use increased the risk of ulcer bleeding by 1.79 times and 4.85 times, respectively. In the presence of both factors, the risk increased to 6.13-fold (17). These divergent findings suggest that patients without prior NSAID exposure differ from those who are already on these drugs.

After a single episode of ulcer hemorrhage and ulcer healing, the relative risk of recurrent ulcer hemorrhage during long term follow-up is 10–20 times that of the control population (18, 19) depending upon the number of risk factors. The risk factors (older age, NSAID use, and prior peptic ulcer) appear to be additive. For example, NSAID use and prior peptic ulcer disease resulted in a 17 times higher relative risk for ulcer hemorrhage than the control population (18). Ingestion of NSAIDs may cause either gastric or duodenal ulcers (20). Complications may develop shortly after starting NSAIDs and may be more frequent during the first month of treatment (21, 22). Overall, about 12–25% of patients on NSAIDs develop endoscopic ulcers within 3 months of continued use. The risk of ulcer bleeding is dose dependent and varies between different drugs (23). In a placebo-controlled trial comparing 300 mg or 1200 mg daily of aspirin for prophylaxis of transient ischemic attacks, the 1200 mg dose was found to have twice the relative risk of hemorrhage as the 300 mg dose. Nevertheless, the lower aspirin dose had statistically significantly higher relative risk of bleeding (7.7 times) than the group randomized to placebo (24). Even lower doses of aspirin have been associated with an increased risk of UGI bleeding and greater risks occurred when combined with other NSAIDs. Enteric coating did not reduce the risk (25). Use of low dose aspirin for cardiovascular and cerebrovascular prophylaxis has led to an increasing number of patients with iatrogenic UGI bleeding. Non-dose dependent differences in NSAID-associated UGI bleeding occur because of differences in selectivity between the constitutive cyclooxygenase (COX)-1 and inducible COX-2 enzymes. The anti-inflammatory effects of non-selective NSAIDs are mediated by COX-2 inhibition, whereas the damaging effects in the GI tract are caused mainly by COX-1 inhibition. Non-selective NSAIDs are associated with an increased risk of GI events (26). Ibuprofen has the lowest risk whereas, ketrolac and piroxicam have the greatest risks. The newer COX-2 inhibitors have increased GI safety compared to non-selective NSAIDs, since COX-2 inhibitors do not affect gastric mucosal prostaglandin synthesis and subsequently induce no (or less) gastroduodenal injury (27, 28). In CURE studies, aspirin or NSAID ingestion within 2 weeks of ulcer hemorrhage was identified as the main risk factor in

53% of duodenal and 61% of gastric ulcer patients (8, 29, 28), compared with about 30% of age-related non-bleeding ulcer patients (26, 28).

Corticosteroid use alone is not associated with an increased chance of complications such as ulceration or bleeding. However, concomitant steroid use with NSAID's doubles the risk of ulcer complications (22) compared with NSAID use alone, and increases by ten-fold the chance of upper gastrointestinal bleeding (31). Alcoholic beverages also increase the risk of acute UGI hemorrhage. In a Swedish-American study, alcohol ingestion increased the baseline incidence of acute UGI bleed by 3-fold from light (< once/ week) to heavy (> 21 drinks/week) drinking. In people using ethanol and either aspirin or ibuprofen, the risk of UGI hemorrhage was highest among heavy consumers of both alcohol and either of the two drugs (32).

Weil et al. (33) studied other risk factors for peptic ulcer hemorrhage in over 1,000 UGI bleed patients. Using logistic regression, oral anticoagulants (odds ratio, OR, 7.8) prior peptic ulcer (OR 3.8), treatment for heart failure (OR 5.9), oral corticosteroids (OR 2.7), treatment for diabetes (OR 3.1), and smoking (OR 1.6) were found to be independent risk factors (33). In CURE studies, about 10% of patients with bleeding ulcers had neither Hp infection nor NSAID use (8, 29, 30). A large Hong Kong study found a similar rate of non Hp, non NSAID bleeding ulcer (4.1–6.4%) (34). The underlying cause of the bleeding ulcer in these cases is unclear but may be related to acid secretion. The presence of acid is critical to ulcer formation (35). For example, in the Zollinger-Ellison syndrome, ulcers occur in almost every patient, while in pernicious anemia, benign ulcers are extremely rare. Although controversial, gastric acid hypersecretion is not necessary for hemorrhage in patients with peptic ulcers. No significant differences in secretory parameters such as basal, peak or meal stimulated acid output and parietal cell sensitivity have been noted among ulcer patients with and without bleeding (36, 37).

THERAPIES FOR LONG-TERM PREVENTION OF ULCER HEMORRHAGE

After the initial bleeding has stopped, further medical therapy is usually required since a 36% incidence of rebleeding over a mean 61 week period was reported in patients not taking maintenance medical therapy (38). Initially, we recommend potent acid suppression with a twice daily proton-pump inhibitor therapy. Subsequently, three separate approaches have been shown to decrease the incidence of recurrent ulcer hemorrhage: long-term maintenance acid suppression, eradication of *H. pylori,* and ulcer surgery. Patients should also be strongly encouraged to stop any aspirin and NSAID ingestion, which are independent risk factors for causing bleeding ulcers.

For patients with gastric ulcers complicated by GI bleeding, a follow-up endoscopy to document healing and lessen the possibility of missing a gastric cancer is appropriate. Follow-up endoscopy after a bleeding duodenal ulcer is controversial, but warranted to document ulcer healing prior to discontinuing therapy or changing to a maintenance regimen.

SECONDARY PREVENTION

Patients infected with *H. pylori* should receive optimal eradication therapy (39, 40). The diagnosis of *H. pylori* in the setting of acute ulcer bleeding deserves special attention. Although antral and body biopsies for rapid urease testing are standard practice (41), recent studies suggest that biopsy-based tests may be false-negative with UGI bleeding. One report comparing rapid urease test and a serological assay for *H. pylori* diagnosis in bleeding ulcer patients showed CLO-test sensitivity of about 60% (42). In another study of 181 consecutive patients with UGI bleeding, of whom 71% were *H. pylori* positive, antral biopsies were taken for rapid urease testing, histology, and culture, as well as a serologic assay. The outcome reported sensitivities of 41% (rapid urease test), 33% (histology) and 34% (culture) (43). Even combining the three tests achieved a sensitivity of only 48.8%. Lee et al. (44) described similar findings in bleeding duodenal ulcer patients biopsied during the initial endoscopy. Other diagnostic tests of *H. pylori* infection such as serology or urea breath test should be used in addition to endoscopic biopsy during acute UGI bleeding.

Studies have shown that eradication of *H. pylori* is associated with a marked decrease in ulcer recurrence in patients who have this infection as the only risk factor (39). Analysis of four randomized, double-blind, multicenter studies showed that in duodenal ulcer patients without prior hemorrhage, *H. pylori* eradication prevented ulcer-related hemorrhage for up to 1 year (45). Several trials have reported the effects of *H. pylori* eradication on preventing recurrent ulcer hemorrhage. Although the studies were limited by small sample size, short follow-up, absence of double-blinding or controlled protocol, and continuation of NSAID ingestion, the trends suggest that *H. pylori* eradication resulted in fewer symptomatic ulcer recurrences and decreased ulcer hemorrhages (46–49). A well-designed, randomized, prospective controlled trial of about 100 patients with duodenal ulcer bleeding with a mean follow-up of 52.8 months failed to show a significant reduction in bleeding recurrences in patients given anti-*H. pylori* therapy (50). These results highlight two important points: 1) treating patients with anti-*H. pylori* therapy does not guarantee absence of ulcer rebleeding; and 2) almost 60% of patients rebled more than 18 months after their prior bleeding episode, emphasizing the importance of long-term follow-up.

Although not usually necessary for uncomplicated ulcers, patients with ulcer bleeding should have the eradication of *H. pylori* confirmed 4-6 weeks after therapy to plan further long-term management (51). If still present, patients should be retreated (51). Currently available and accurate methods for confirming *H. pylori* eradication include urea breath testing, endoscopic biopsies for either rapid urease test or histology and detection of stool *H. pylori* antigen (52) as long as the patients are off treatment with proton pump inhibitors, high dose of H_2-receptor antagonists, antibiotics or bismuth-containing compounds. Currently, as described above, the effect of *H. pylori* on NSAID-associated ulcers and serious gastrointestinal complications is controversial. All ulcer patients should be tested and treated for *H. pylori,* independent of NSAID ingestion. For these patients with both *H. pylori* infection and NSAID use, the primary cause of ulceration and hemorrhage can not be ascertained, so we would recommend eradication of *H. pylori* and discontinuation of the NSAIDs. Alternatively, one could use a proton pump inhibitor (PPI) as co-therapy, if the NSAID or aspirin was continued (53).

As previously described, NSAIDs are an important cause of hemorrhage associated with peptic ulcer (26, 54, 55, 56). Cotherapies have been shown to reduce NSAID ulcers and prevent secondary recurrence of hemorrhage (57). Misoprostol decreases both DU and GU in patients taking NSAIDs (58) and significantly reduces serious gastrointestinal complications associated with NSAIDs (59). PPIs are more effective than standard dose H_2-receptor antagonists at preventing endoscopic gastric and duodenal ulcers (54). PPIs are also superior to twice daily misoprostol dosing at preventing NSAID-associated ulcers (60, 61). For patients with NSAID-associated ulcers, PPIs, H_2-receptor antagonists and misoprostol will heal ulcers if the NSAIDs are discontinued. If patients need to continue taking NSAIDs, proton pump inhibitors are the most effective at healing the ulcers (60, 61). Re-analysis of data from two trials suggested that PPIs were much less effective in gastric ulcer healing or in the prevention of ulcer relapse in patients with an NSAID ulcer (Hp negative) compared to patients with *H. pylori*-associated, NSAID ulcers (62). Further, the benefit observed in decreasing duodenal ulcer recurrence by PPIs may also have been influenced by the presence of a large number of *H. pylori* positive patients (62). After the ulcer has healed in the patient who must continue taking NSAID therapy, effective options for prophylaxis against ulcer recurrence are PPI or misoprostol or use of a COX-2 inhibitor (57). A recent study showed that lansoprazole was superior to placebo for the prevention of NSAID-induced gastric ulcers (in Hp-negative patients), but not superior to misoprostol (63). COX-2-inhibitors seem safer than traditional NSAIDs (64, 65, 66), although ulcers and associated complications such as bleeding have been reported following COX-2 inhibitor use (67, 68). The optimal use of COX-2 inhibitors in patients with prior NSAID-associated complication who require continued NSAID use, is unclear. Whether or not their use

TABLE 1. *CURE Epidemiologic Risk Factors and Long-Term Strategies for Prevention of Recurrent Ulcer Hemorrhage*

DU or GU	Prevalence (%)	Treatment Strategy
NSAID$^+$ Hp$^+$	42	Stop NSAIDs, eradicate Hp, PPI maintenance
NSAID$^-$ Hp$^+$	32	Eradicate H. pylori
NSAID$^+$ Hp$^-$	16	Stop NSAIDs, PPI maintenance
NSAID$^-$ Hp$^-$	10	PPI or H$_2$RA maintenance

Shown are CURE data of 422 patients with ulcer hemorrhage, prospectively studied. Gastric ulcers (GU) comprised 47% and duodenal ulcers (DU)—53%. *H. pylori* was determined by serology and one other test (biopsy or urea breath test).

NSAID+ is ingestion of one or more aspirin or NSAID tablets per day within 2 weeks of presentation with ulcer hemorrhage. Hp+ is positive evaluation for *H. pylori* infection.

PPI is a proton pump inhibitor.
H$_2$RA is histamine-2-receptor antagonist.

alone or with concomitant proton pump inhibitors is most beneficial and cost-effective remains to be determined.

For ulcer patients complicated by GI bleeding and without risk factors such as *H. pylori* or NSAID ingestion, maintenance acid suppression may be of benefit. Further, for a number of patients who continue to experience recurrent ulcer symptoms despite *H. pylori*-negative status, who require concurrent medication such as anticoagulants or who have severe comorbid conditions which increase their risk of recurrence or complications, potent acid suppression will maintain symptom relief and prevent ulcer recurrence. PPIs have been shown to be effective in maintenance therapy of both duodenal and gastric ulcers (69, 70). The long-term strategies for prevention of recurrent ulcer hemorrhage are summarized in Table 1.

PRIMARY PREVENTION

Several factors have been implicated in increasing the likelihood of NSAID-associated complications. These include past history of ulcer or GI complications, increasing age, high-dose NSAID, and steroid or anticoagulant use (57). In these high-risk patients, several different approaches have been tried to reduce NSAID-associated GI complications. When possible, non-NSAID analgesics use would prevent NSAID-associated side effects. Since both GI and non-GI toxicity is dose-dependent, the lowest effective dose, whether a selective or non-selective NSAID, should be used (71). Since some NSAIDs (such as nonacetylated salicylates) are associated with lower risk, these agents should be tried first. Co-therapy with PPIs or misoprostol should be considered. In endoscopic studies, PPIs and misoprostol were similarly effective in significantly reducing the occurrence of both duodenal and gastric ulcers (59, 61). To date, misoprostol is the only co-therapy that decreased clinical GI complications (59).

In comparison to usual NSAIDs, COX-2-specific inhibitors have also been shown to significantly reduce the occurrence of endoscopic ulcers and decrease upper GI complications. At present, the COX-2-specific inhibitors are much more expensive than traditional NSAIDs, and their cost-effectiveness has yet to be carefully evaluated. Thus, patients at high risk of NSAID-related complications should be considered for COX-2-specific therapy, while patients at low risk for adverse GI events should receive low dose, safer NSAIDs. For high risk patients requiring aspirin for cardiovascular prophylaxis, co-therapy with a PPI (not misoprostol) usually results in better compliance and fewer side effects (72). Whether or not patients at high risk on COX-2-specific inhibitors should receive co-therapy with a PPI is controversial.

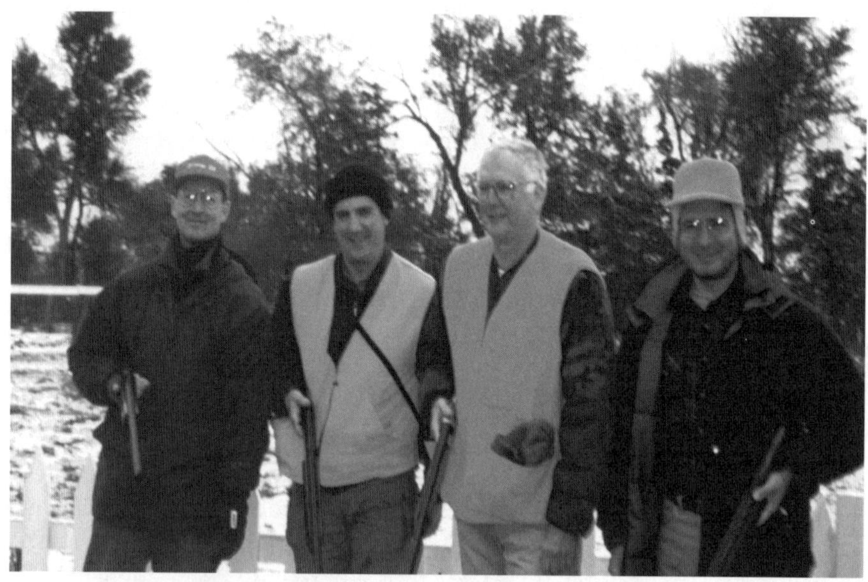

The CURE "Militia" (from right to left: Dean Jensen, Gordon Ohning, John Walsh, and Gus Machiocado) on an expedition to obtain pheasant gastrin in South Dakota, November, 1998.

REFERENCES

1. Walsh JH and Grossman M. Medical Progress: Gastrin. *N Engl J Med* 1975;292:1324–1332.

2. Walsh JH, Richardson L, Fordtran J. pH dependence of acid secretion and gastrin release in normal and ulcer patients. *J Clin Invest* 1975;55:462–469.

3. Elashoff JD, Van Deventer G, Reedy T, Ippoliti A, Samloff IM, Kurata J, Billings M, Isenberg M. Long-term follow-up of DU patients. *J Clin Gastroenterol* 1983;5:509–515.

4. Kovacs TOG and Jensen DM. Endoscopic control of gastroduodenal hemorrhage. *Ann Rev Med* 1987;38:267–277.

5. Bardhan KD. The presentation of peptic ulcer. In: *Diseases of the Gut and Pancreas.* Misiewicz JT, Pounder RE, Venables CU, eds. London:Blackwells, 1994;282–287.

6. Kovacs TOG and Jensen DM. Therapeutic endoscopy for upper gastrointestinal bleeding. In: *Gastrointestinal Emergencies,* Taylor MB, Gollan J, Peppercorn MA, et al, eds., 2nd ed. Baltimore, Williams & Williams, 1997:181–188.

7. Hosking SW, Yung MY, Chung SC, Li AK. Differing prevalence of Helicobacter in bleeding and non-bleeding ulcers (Abstract) *Gastroenterology* 1992;102 A85.

8. Jensen DM, You S, Pelayo E, Jensen ME. The prevalence of *H. pylori* and NSAID use in patients with severe ulcer hemorrhage and their potential role in recurrence of ulcer bleeding. *Gastroenterology* 1992;102 A90.

9. Kuyvenhaven JP, Veenendaal RA, Vandenbroucke JP. Peptic ulcer bleeding: interaction between non-steroidal anti-inflammatory drugs, *H. pylori* infection and the ABO blood group system. *Scan J Gastroenterol* 1999;34:1082–1086.

10. Henriksson AE, Edman A-C, Nilsson I, Bergqvist D, Wadstrom T. *Helicobacter pylori* and the relation to other risk factors in patients with acute bleeding peptic ulcer. *Scand J Gastroenterol* 1998;33: 1030–1033.

11. Aalykke C, Lauritsen JM, Hallas J, Reinholdt S, Krogfelt K, Lauritsen K. *H. pylori* and risk of ulcer bleeding among users of nonsteroidal anti-inflammatory drugs: a case-control study. *Gastroenterology* 1999;116:1305–1309.

12. Santolaria S, Lanos A, Benito R, Perez-Aisa M, Montoro M, Sainz R. *H. pylori* infection is a protective factor for bleeding Gus but not for bleeding Dus in NSAID users. *Aliment Pharmacol Ther* 1999;13:1511–1518.

13. Cullen DJE, Hawkey GM, Greenwood DC, Humphreys H, Shepherd V, Logan RF, Hawkey CJ. Peptic ulcer bleeding in the elderly: relative roles of *H. pylori* and non-steroidal anti-inflammatory drugs. *Gut* 1997;41:459–462.

14. Hawkey CJ, Tulassay Z, Szczepanski L, van Rensburg CJ, Filipowicz-Sosnowska A, Lanas A, Wason CM, Peacock RA, Gillon KR. Randomized controlled trial of *Helicobacter pylori* eradication in patients on non-steroidal anti-inflammatory drugs: HELP NSAIDs study. *Helicobacter* eradication for lesion prevention. *Lancet* 1998;352:1016–1021.

15. Chan FK, Sung JJ, Chung SC, To KF, Yung MY, Leung VK, Lee YT, Chan CS, Li EK, Woo J. Randomized trial of eradication of *Helicobacter pylori* before non-steroidal anti-inflammatory drug therapy to prevent peptic ulcers. *Lancet* 1997;350:975–979.

16. Chan FK, To KF, Wu CY, Yung MY, Leung WK, Kwok T, Hui Y, Chan HL, Chan CS, Hui E, Woo J, Sung JJ. Eradication of *Helicobacter pylori* and risk of peptic ulcers in patients starting long-term treatment with non-steroidal anti-inflammatory drugs: a randomized trial. *Lancet* 2002;359:9–13.

17. Huang J-Q, Snidhar S, Hunt RH. Role of *Helicobacter pylori* infection and non-steroidal anti-inflammatory drugs in peptic ulcer disease: a meta-analysis. *Lancet* 2002;359:14–22.

18. Rodriguez LAG and Jic KH. The risk of upper gastrointestinal bleeding and/or perforation associated with individual non-steroidal anti-inflammatory drugs. *Lancet* 1994;343:769–772.

19. McMahon AD, White G, Murray FE, McGilchrist MM, McDevitt DG, McDonald TM. New exposure to NSAIDs and hospitalization for upper gastrointestinal events and hemorrhage: a record-linkage study in the population of Tayride, Scotland. (Abstract) *Gastroenterology.* 1995;108:A164.

20. Kurata J and Abbey D. The effect of chronic aspirin use on duodenal and GU. *J Clin Gastroenterol* 1990;12:260–266.

21. Somerville K, Faulkner G, Langman M. Non-steroidal anti-inflammatory drugs and bleeding peptic ulcer. *Lancet* 1986;1:462–464.
22. Gabriel SE, Jaakkimainen L, Bombardier C. Risk for serious gastrointestinal complications related to use of non-steroidal anti-inflammatory drugs: a meta-analysis. *Ann Intern Med* 1991;115:787–796.
23. Henry D, Lim LL, Garcia Rodriguez LA, Perez Gutthann S, Carson JL, Griffin M, Savage R, Logan R, Moride Y, Hawkey C, Hill S, Fries JT. Variability in risk of gastrointestinal complications with individual non-steroidal anti-inflammatory drugs: results of a collaborative meta-analysis. *BMJ* 1996;312:1563–1566.
24. Griffin MR, Ray WA, Schaffner W. Nonsteroidal anti-inflammatory drug use and death from peptic ulcer in elderly persons. *Ann Intern Med* 1988;109:359–363.
25. Sorensen HT, Mellemkjaer L, Blot WJ, Nielsen GL, Steffensen FH, McLaughlin JK, Olsen JH. Risk of upper gastrointestinal bleeding associated with use of low-dose aspirin. *Am J Gastroenterol* 2000; 95:2218–2224.
26. Offman JJ, MacLean, Straus WL, Morton SC, Berger ML, Roth EA, Shekelle P. A meta-analysis of severe upper gastrointestinal complication of nonsteroidal antiinflammatory drugs. *J Rheumatol* 2002;29:804–812.
27. Bombardier C, Laine L, Reicin A Shapiro D, Burgos-Vargas R, Davis B, Day R, Ferraz MB, Hawkey CJ, Hochberg MC, Kvien TK, Schnitzer TJ . Comparison of upper gastrointestinal toxicity of rofecoxib and naproxen in patients with rheumatoid arthritis. VIGOR study group. *N Engl J Med* 2000;343:1520–1528.
28. Silverstein FE, Faich G, Goldstein JE Simon LS, Pincus T, Whelton A, Makuch R, Eisen G, Agrawal NM, Stenson WF, Burr AM, Zhao WW, Kent JD, Lefkowith JB, Verburg KM, Geis GS. Gastrointestinal toxicity with colecoxib vs non-steroidal anti-inflammatory drugs for osteoarthritis and rheumatoid arthritis: the CLASS study: A randomized controlled trial. Colecoxib Long-term Arthritis Safety Study. *JAMA* 2000;284:1247–1255.
29. Egan JV and Jensen DM. Long-term management of patients with bleeding ulcers. Rationale, results, and economic impact. *Gastrointest Endosc Clin N Am* 1991;1:367–386.
30. Jensen DM. Long term prevention of recurrent ulcer hemorrhage: Issues and insights. *Current Viewpoints on Digestive Health* 1995;2:1–14.
31. Piper JM, Ray WA, Daugherty JR, Griffin MR. Corticosteroid use and peptic ulcer disease: role of non-steroidal anti-inflammatory drugs. *Ann Intern Med* 1991;114:735–740.
32. Kaufman DW, Kelly JP, Wiholm BE, Laszlo A, Sheehan JE, Koff RS, Shapiro S. The risk of acute major upper gastrointestinal bleeding among users of aspirin and ibuprofen at various levels of alcohol consumption. *Am J Gastroenterol* 1999;94:3189–3196.
33. Weil J, Langman MJ, Wainwright P, Lawson DH, Rawlins M, Logan RF, Brown TP, Vessey MP, Murphy M, Colin-Jones DG. Peptic ulcer bleeding: assessing risk factors and interactions with non-steroidal anti-inflammatory drugs. *Gut* 2000;46:27–31.
34. Chan HL, Wu JC, Chan FK, Choi CL, Ching JY, Lee YT, Leung WK, Lau JY, Chung SC, Sung JJ. Is non-*Helicobacter pylori*, non-NSAID peptic ulcer a common cause of upper GI bleeding? A prospective study of 977 patients. *Gastrointest Endosc* 2001;53:438–442.
35. Kovacs TOG and Walsh JH. Standard Secretory Tests: Methodology. In: *Clinical Investigation of Gastric Function*. Scarpignato C and Bianchiporro G, eds. Front Gastrointest Res, Basel:Karger 1990;17:2–12.
36. Kovacs TOG, Sytnik B, Jensen DM, Walsh JH. A comparison of acid and gastric secretion in bleeding and non-bleeding DU patients. *Gastroenterology* 1991;100:A101.
37. Hui WM and Lam SK. Gastric acid secretion and parietal cell sensitivity in DU patients with stigmata of bleeding. *Gastroenterology* 1991;100:A87.
38. Jensen DM, Cheng S, Kovacs TOG, Randall G, Jensen ME, Reedy T, Frankl H, Machicado G, Smith J, Silpa M, Van Deventer G. A controlled study of ranitidine for the prevention of recurrent hemorrhage from duodenal ulcer. *N Engl J Med* 1994;330:382–386.
39. Walsh JH and Peterson WL. The treatment of *Helicobacter pylori* infection in the management of peptic ulcer disease. *N Engl J Med* 1995;333:984–991.
40. Fennerty BM, Kovacs TOG, Krause R, Haber M, Weissfeld A, Siepman N, Rose P. A comparison of 10 and 14 days of lansoprazole triple therapy for eradication of *Helicobacter pylori*. *Arch Intern Med* 1998;158:1651–1656.

41. Kovacs TOG and Kovacs SVB. The role of *Helicobacter pylori* in gastric disease. *Problems in General Surgery* 1997;14:25–36.

42. Lai KC, Hui WM, Lam SK. Bleeding ulcers have high false negative rates for antral *Helicobacter pylori* when tested with urease test. *Gastroenterology* 1996;110:A167.

43. Colin R. Czernichow P, Baty U, Touze I, Brazier F, Bretagne JF, Berkelmans I, Barthelemy P, Hemet J. Low sensitivity of the invasive tests for the detection of *Helicobacter pylori* infection in patients with bleeding ulcer. *Gastroenterol Clin Biol* 2000;94:31–35.

44. Lee JM, Breslin NP, Fallon C, O'Morain CA. Rapid urease tests lack sensitivity in *Helicobacter pylori* diagnosis when peptic ulcer disease presents with bleeding. *Am J Gastroenterol* 2000;95:1166–1170.

45. Sonnenberg A, Olson LA, Zhang J. The effect of antibiotic therapy on bleeding from duodenal ulcer. *Am J Gastroenterol* 1999;94:950–954.

46. Graham DY, Hepps KS, Ramirez FC, Lew GM, Saeed ZA. Treatment of *Helicobacter pylori* reduces the rate of rebleeding in peptic ulcer disease. *Scand J Gastroenterol* 1993;28:939–942.

47. Labenz J and Borsch G. Role of *Helicobacter pylori* eradication in the prevention of peptic ulcer bleeding relapse. *Digestion* 1994;55:19–23.

48. Rokkas T, Karameris A, Mavrogorgis A, Rallis E, Gannikas N. *H. pylori* eradication reduces the possibility of rebleeding in peptic ulcer disease. *Gastrointest Endosc* 1995;41:1–4.

49. Jasperson D, Koemer T, Schorr W, Brennenstuhl M, Raschka C, Hamar CH. *Helicobacter pylori* eradication reduces the rate of rebleeding in ulcer hemorrhage. *Gastrointest Endosc* 1995;41:5–7.

50. Lai KC, Hui WM, Wong W-M, Wong BC, Hu WH, Ching CK, Lam S. Treatment of *Helicobacter pylori* in patients with duodenal ulcer hemorrhage—a long-term randomized controlled study. *Am J Gastroenterol* 2000;95:2225–2232.

51. Howden CW and Hunt RH. Guidelines for the management of *Helicobacter pylori* infection. *Am J Gastroentrol* 1998;93:2330–2337.

52. Vaira D, Holton J, Menegatti M, Ricci C, Gatta L, Geminiani A, Miglioli M. Review article: invasive and non-invasive tests for *Helicobacter pylori* infection. *Aliment Pharmacol Ther* 2000;14 (Suppl 3):13–22.

53. Kovacs TOG and Walsh JH. Proton pump inhibitors in routine clinical practice. *Patient Care* 1999; 26–31.

54. Kovacs TOG and Soll AH. Peptic Ulcer Disease—Pathophysiology. In: *The Stomach*. Eds. Gustavson S, Kumar D, Graham D. Churchill Livingstone 1992;230–245.

55. Schoenfeld P, Kimmey MB, Schemian J, Bjorkman D, Laine L. Review article: non-steroidal anti-inflammatory drug-associated gastrointestinal complications: Guidelines for prevention and treatment. *Aliment Pharmacol Ther* 1999;13:1273–1285.

56. Wolfe MM, Lichtenstein DR, Singh G. Gastrointestinal toxicity of non-steroidal anti-inflammatory drugs. *N Engl J Med* 1999;340:1888–1899.

57. Laine L. Approaches to non-steroidal anti-inflammatory drug use in the high risk patient. *Gastroenterology* 2001;120:594–606.

58. Graham DY, White RH, Moreland LW, Schubert TT, Katz R, Jaszewski R, Tindall E, Triadafilopoulos G, Stromatt SC, Leoh LS. Duodenal and gastric ulcer prevention with misoprostol in arthritis patients taking NSAID's. *Ann Intern Med* 1993;119:257–262.

59. Silverstein F, Graham D, Senior J, Davies HW, Struthers BJ, Bittman RM, Geis GS. Misoprostol reduces serious gastrointestinal complications in patients with rheumatoid arthritis receiving nonsteroidal anti-inflammatory drugs. A randomized, double-bind, placebo-controlled trial. *Ann Intern Med* 1995; 123:241–249.

60. Yeomans ND, Tulassay Z, Juhasz L, Racz I, Howard JM, van Rensburg CJ, Swannell AJ, Hawkey CJ. A comparison of omeprazole with ranitidine for ulcers associated with non-steroidal anti-inflammatory drugs. *N Engl J Med* 1998;338:719–726.

61. Hawkey C, Karrasch JA, Szczepanski L, Walker DG, Barkun A, Swannell AJ, Yeomans ND. Omeprazole compared with misoprostol for ulcers associated with non-steroidal anti-inflammatory drugs. *N Engl J Med* 1998;338:727–734.

62. Graham D. Critical effect of *Helicobacter pylori* infection on the effectiveness of omeprazole for protection of gastric or duodenal ulcers among chronic NSAID users. *Helicobacter* 2002;7:1–8.

63. Graham DY, Agrawal NM, Campbell DR, Haber MM, Collis C, Lukasik NL, Huang B. Ulcer prevention in long-term users of non-steroidal anti-inflammatory drugs: Results of a double-blind, randomized, multicenter active and placebo-controlled study of misoprostol vs lansoprazole. *Arch Intern Med* 2002;162:169–175.

64. Feldman M and McMahon AT. Do cyclooxygenase-2 inhibitors provide benefits similar to those of traditional non-steroidal anti-inflammatory drugs, with less gastrointestinal toxicity. *Ann Intern Med* 2000;132:134–143.

65. Simon LS, Weaver AL, Graham DY, Kivitz AJ, Lipsky PE, Hubbard RC, Isakson PC, Verburg KM, Yu SS, Zhao WW, Geis GS. Anti-inflammatory and upper gastrointestinal effects of celecoxib in rheumatoid arthritis. *JAMA* 1999;282:1921–1928.

66. Bombardier C, Laine L, Reicin A, Shapiro D, Burgos-Vargas R, Davis B, Day R, Ferraz MB, Hawkey CJ, Hochberg MC, Kvien TK, and Schnitzer TJ. VIGOR Study Group. Comparison of upper gastrointestinal toxicity of rofecoxib and naproxen in patients with rheumatoid arthritis. *N Engl J Med* 2000;343:1520–1528.

67. Langman MJ, Jensen DM, Watson DJ, Harper SE, Zhao PL, Quan H, Bolognese JA, Simon TJ. Adverse upper gastrointestinal effects of rofecoxib compared with NSAID's. *JAMA* 1999;282:1929–1933.

68. Silverstein FE, Faich G, Goldenstein JL, Simon LS, Pincus T, Whelton A, Makuch R, Eisen G, Agrawal NM, Stenson WF, Burr AM, Zhao WW, Kent JD, Lefkowith JB, Verburg KM, Geis GS. Gastrointestinal toxicity with celecoxib vs nonsteroidal anti-inflammatory drugs for osteoarthritis and rheumatoid arthritis. The CLASS study: A randomized controlled trial. *JAMA* 2000;284:1247–1255.

69. Kovacs TOG, Campbell D, Richter J, Haber M, Jennings DE, Rose P. Double blind comparison of lansoprazole 15 mg, lansoprazole 30 mg and placebo as maintenance therapy in patients with healed duodenal ulcers resistant to H2-receptor antagonists. *Aliment Pharmacol Ther* 1999;13:959–967.

70. Kovacs TOG, Campbell D, Haber M, Rose P, Jennings DE, Richter J. Double-blind comparison of lansoprazole 15 mg, lansoprazole 30 mg and placebo in the maintenance of healed gastric ulcer. *Digestive Dis Sci* 1998;43:779–785.

71. Hawkey CJ. NSAID Toxicity: Where are we and how do we go forward? *J Rheumatol* 2002;29: 650–652.

72. Lanas AI. Current approaches to reducing gastrointestinal toxicity of low-dose aspirin. *Am J Med* 2001;110:705–735.

43

Clinical Effects of the Proton Pump Inhibitor in Relation to CYP2C19 Polymorphism

Mohamed Sagar[1,3] and Rein Seensalu[2,3]
*[1]Department of Medicine, Division of Gastroenterology
McMaster University Hamilton, Ontario, Canada*

[2]Departments of Medicine, St Görans Hospital

*[3]Departments of Medicine, Huddinge University Hospital, at Karolinska Institute
Stockholm, Sweden*

INTRODUCTION

The proton pump inhibitor omeprazole is hydroxylated in the liver by S-mephenytoin 4′-hydroxylase (*CYP2C19*) (1). This enzyme exhibits a genetic polymorphism with two determined phenotypes: extensive metabolizers (EMs) and poor metabolizers (PMs). According to the genotyping analysis of *CYP2C19*, PMs consist of three genotypes (m_1/m_1; *CYP2C19*2/*2*, m_1/m_2; *CYP2C19*2/*3* or m_2/m_2; *CYP2C19*3/*3*), while EMs include two genotypes, homozygous (wt/wt; *CYP2C19*1/*1*) and heterozygous (wt/m_1 or wt/m_2; *CYP2C19*1/*2* or **3*) EMs (2, 3). The enzyme is absent in 3% of whites and 12–20% of asians (4). In individuals with PM phenotype or genotype of *CYP2C19*, but also in heterozygous EMs, the plasma concentration-time curve of omeprazole is markedly increased, and pharmacodynamic effects of omeprazole assumed, on a theoretical basis, to be enhanced in them. Acid secretion in individuals with a PM status of *CYP2C19* who are undergoing omeprazole therapy is therefore expected to be more strongly inhibited than for those with homozygous EM status. Moreover, the inhibition of acid secretion caused by omeprazole is expected to enhance gastrin release from G cells in the antrum. Therefore, the genetic plymorphism of *CYP2C19* should be of a clinical concern in the treatment of acid-related disorders with proton pump inhibitors.

On the basis of this background, we have investigated the influence of *CYP2C19* genotype on the short and long-term effects of omeprazole treatment on intragastric acidity, and serum gastrin levels. Also, changes in the gastric mucosa morphology (assessed by plasma chromogranin A

(CGA), and serum pepsinogen I (PgI)) and serum vitamin B12 levels were examined.

MATERIAL AND METHODS

Subjects

Short-term Effects

Twenty-five white patients, with a mean age of 59 years, and with endo-scopically proven acid related disease participated in the study. Each patient received an oral dose of 20 mg omeprazole once daily in the morning for 8 days. Twenty-four hour-intragastric pH and AUC $_{4h}$ of serum gastrin were measured at day 0, and day 8. The influence of *H. pylori* status on intragastric acidity and gastrin levels was also monitored.

Long-term Effects

One hundred and eighty white patients with a mean age of 54 years, with acid related disorders were included in this part of the study. Of these, 108 patients were studied after their first dose of 20 mg omeprazole. The re-maining 72 patients had been treated continuously with 20 mg omeprazole once daily for more than one year (median 32 months). All studies were conducted in accordance with protocols approved by the Ethics Committee at Huddinge University Hospital.

Blood Analysis

The *CYP2C19* genotype was determined by the polymerase chain reaction (PCR) method, as originally described by de Morais, et al. (2, 3). Serum gas-trin (antibodies 4562, and 90184 were generously supplied by Professor Jens Rehfeld) and plasma CGA concentrations were determined by radioim-munoassay (5, 6). Serum concentrations of PgI were analyzed by a commer-cial enzyme linked immunosorbent assay (ELISA, Gastroset PGI, Orion Diagnostica, Espoo, Finland). Serum vitamin B12 levels were measured using an established technique (AutoDelfia, B12 kit, Wallac OY, Finland) employed for routine determination of vitamin B12. Finally, an in–house enzyme-linked immunosorbent assay (ELISA) was used to measure specific IgG and IgA *H. pylori* antibodies (7).

Intragastric pH Measurements

Intragastric pH was measured continuously with a glass electrode posi-tioned in the antral part of the stomach on day 0, and day 8 of treatment.

The position was confirmed by fluoroscopy. The electrode was connected to an ambulatory recorder (Digitrapper II, Synectics Medical, Sweden) and pH was registered, and stored every 4th second.

Statistics

Areas under the plasma concentration versus time curves (AUC) were calculated by the trapezoidal rule. Unpaired t-test, Wilcoxon signed rank test and Mann–Whitney U test, were used for statistical analysis whenever appropriate. p value of < 0.05 was considered significant.

RESULTS

CYP2C19 *Genotyping*

Of the 25 patients included in the short-term effects study, 11 were homozygous EMs (wt/wt), 12 were heterozygotes EMs (wt/mut) and 2 were PMs (mut/mut). Out of 180 patients included in the long-term effects study, 135 were wt/wt, 42 wt/mut and 3 were mut/mut.

Short-Term Study

Intragastric pH and Serum Gastrin

No significant differences in 24-hour intragastric pH were observed between the 3 groups on day 0 (Figure 1). After 8 days of omeprazole administration, omeprazole significantly increased the median 24-hour intragastric acidity in the heterozygous EM group compared to homozygous EM group (Figure 1). In the two PM patients the median pH was relatively high (5.7 and 6.6). *H. pylori* status had less influence than CYP2C19 on intragastric acidity.

As for intragastric acidity no significant differences in the gastrin AUC $_{4h}$ were observed between 3 groups on day 0. However, omeprazole increased meal stimulated plasma gastrin concentrations from day 0 to day 8 in both homozygous and heterozygous EMs by 16% and 157% respectively. On day 8 the mean gastrin AUC $_{4h}$ was significantly ($p < 0.001$) higher in the heterozygous EMs than in the homozygous EMs, (Table 1). In the two PMs the gastrin concentration increased by 2–3 fold from day 0 to day 8.

Within the heterozygous EMs group, gastrin concentration increased significantly ($p < 0.01$) in *H. pylori* positive compared with negative subgroup. No significant differences could be seen within the homozygous EMs *H. pylori* subgroups (*H. pylori* data not shown).

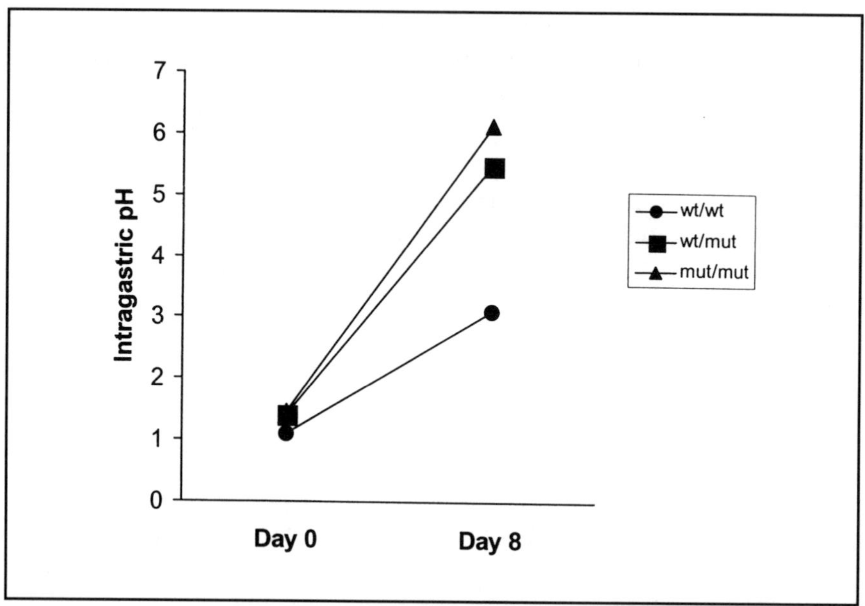

FIGURE 1. *Median 24-hour intragastric pH in the three* CYP2C19 *genotype groups before (day 0) and during (day 8) treatment with 20 mg omeprazole orally once daily.*

Long–Term Study

Effects of CYP2C19 Genotype on Gastric Secretory Parameters and Vitamin B12

Serum gastrin, PgI and plasma CGA were assessed in 180 patients with acid related disorder belonging to different *CYP2C19* genotype groups. In one hundred and eight patients, who received a single dose of 20 mg omeprazole, no differences in gastrin and CGA concentrations were found between heterozygous and homozygous EMs. In 72 patients treated for more than one year with omeprazole, serum gastrin and plasma CGA concentrations were higher (p = 0.0001) in the heterozygous compared to the homozygous EMs group (Table 2). In heterozygotes but not in the homozygotes EMs group, serum gastrin and plasma CGA concentrations were significantly (p < 0.0001) higher in patients on long-term treatment compared with those receiving one dose (Table 2). Serum PgI concentration was significantly (p = 0.04) lower in heterozygous compared with homozygous EMs group of patients (Table 2). In patients studied after the first dose, there was no significant difference in the mean serum vitamin B12 between heterozygous and homozygous EMs. However, in patients on long-term treatment, mean serum vitamin B12 levels were significantly lowered in

TABLE 1. *Area under the gastrin concentration vs time curve during 4 hours (AUC $_{4h}$) in the three genotype groups of patients with acid related disease on day 0 and after the eighth dose of 20 mg omeprazole.*

		AUC 4h (pM × h)		
Genotype	n	day 0	day 8	P (day 8 vs day 0)
wt/wt	11	103 ± 13	119 ± 19	ns
wt/mut	12	117 ± 14	301 ± 105★★★	0.002
mut/mut€	2	147; 134	333; 291	

Data expressed as mean (± SD)
Compared with wt/wt: ★★★p < 0.0001
€ Individual values given.

heterozygous compared with homozygous EMs (246 vs 305 pmol/L, p<0.01). Within the heterozygous group of patients, but not in the homozygous EMs, mean serum vitamin B12 was significantly lower in patients on long-term treatment compared with those receiving one dose (246 vs 350 pmol/L; p < 0.0001) (Figure 2). In the PM patient who was studied both after the first dose and after 15 months serum vitamin B12 decreased from 360 pmol/L to 178 pmol/L.

DISCUSSION

Our short-term study shows that the effect of omeprazole on intragastric pH significantly depends on *CYP2C19* genotype status, with higher pH not only in the PM group of patients, but also in the heterozygous EMs compared to the normal, homozygous EMs. According to the intragastric pH-profile over 24 hours, this difference seems to be due to a more effective inhibition of meal stimulated acid secretion by omeprazole in the heterozygous EMs and PMs. Some previous studies have reported considerable interindividual variability in the effect of omeprazole on acid secretion and gastrin concentrations in blood in healthy subjects (8) and in patients with peptic ulcer disease (9). The overall clinical effects of omeprazole on acid and gastrin secretion have generally been discussed in terms of mean or median effects for the whole study population without special consideration of individuals having profound divergent effects on acid secretion or marked hypergastrinemia after administration of normal daily doses of omeprazole (10). We have shown that the *CYP2C19* polymorphism, and thereby individual metabolic capacity, influences the efficacy of omeprazole. It has recently been suggested that it is necessary to take account of the *H. pylori* status of every subject or patient participating in investigations of gastroduodenal physiology or antisecretory drugs (11). Our results indicate that not

Sagar and Seensalu

TABLE 2. *Serum gastrin, plasma chromogranin A, and serum pepsinogen I concentrations in three CYP2C19 genotype groups of patients with acid related disorders both after the first dose and after long-term (> one year) treatment with 20 mg omeprazole once daily.*

	n		Gastrin(pmol/L)		Chromogranin A (nmol/L)		Pepsinogen I (µg/L)	
Genotype	First year	> one year	First dose	> one year	First dose	> one year	First dose	> one year
wt/wt	83	52	11.2 ± 0.8	14.7 ± 0.9	2.0 ± 0.1	2.5 ± 0.1	n/a	193 ± 12
wt/mut	23	19	12.3 ± 1.0	52 ± 7.6★#	2.2 ± 0.2	7.3 ± 1.3★#	n/a	147 ± 19§
mut/mut•	2	1	12.1	88	2.3	13.7	n/a	n/a

Data expressed as mean ± SE

★ p < 0.0001 compared with first dose

# p < 0.0001 compared with wt/wt

§p < 0.04 compared with wt/wt

• Individual values given

n/a, not available

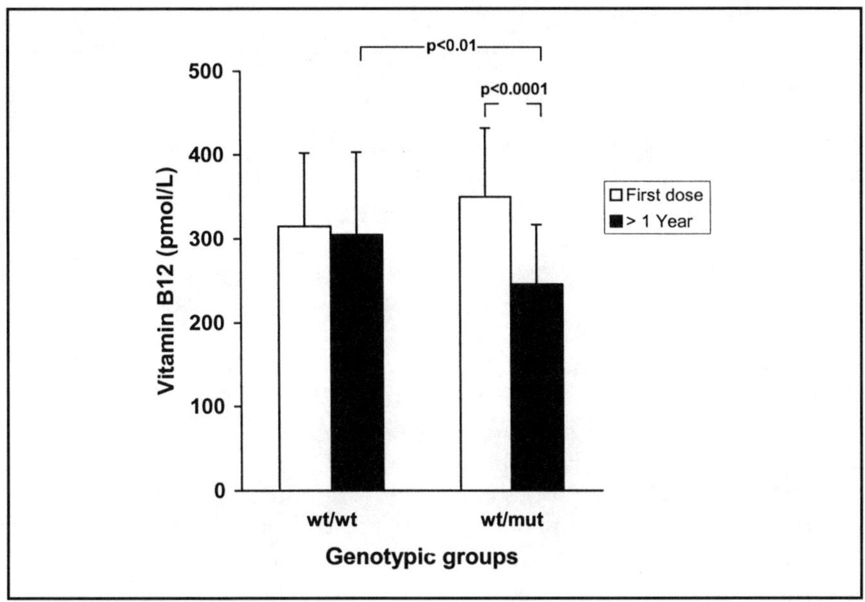

FIGURE 2. *Mean (SD) serum vitamin B12 levels in the wt/wt (n = 108) and wt/mut (n = 72) genotypic groups of patients after first dose and after long-term treatment with 20 mg omeprazole once daily.*

only *H. pylori* status, but also the *CYP2C19* genotype are significant factors to be determined in future studies with proton pump inhibitors (PPIs).

Another clinical observation of importance is the individual capacity to metabolize PPIs in relation to the eradication rates of *H. pylori* infection in different genotype groups of patients. Recent studies on *H. pylori* eradication shows that the rates of cure of *H. pylori* infection with omeprazole and amoxicillin depends on *CYP2C19* genotype patterns, with high eradication rates in the PMs, and heterozygous EMs groups of patients compared to homozygous EMs (12). A possible explanation is that the PMs, and heterozygous EMs were exposed to prolonged and potent inhibition of acid secretion resulting in higher intragastric pH. This may contribute to increase stability and availability of amoxicillin and result in a higher eradication rate of *H. pylori*.

In line with the relationship between *CYP2C19* polymorphism, and inhibition of intragastric acidity short-term treatment with omeprazole increases plasma gastrin concentrations significantly more in PMs, and in heterozygous EMs compared to patients with two functional *CYP2C19* alleles (homozygous EMs). Further, our results show that both the individual capacity to metabolize omeprazole and *H. pylori* status influence the magnitude of gastrin response during treatment with omeprazole, and most likely also during treatment by other PPIs. Several mechanisms have been suggested whereby *H. pylori* infection could increase plasma gastrin concentration in blood. Thus, hypergastrinemia associated with *H. pylori* infection results mainly from inhibition of antral somatostatin, thereby decreasing the paracrine inhibitory role of somatostatin on gastrin release from antral G-cells (13). *H. pylori* has also been shown to exert a direct effect on antral G-cells (14) and indirectly via an effect on mononuclear cells causing stimulation of gastrin release (15).

Much of the concern about hypergastrinemia during acid suppressive therapy has been focused on the trophic effect of gastrin on the enterochromaffin-like (ECL) cells located in the oxyntic mucosa of the stomach (16, 17). We have used CGA as an indicator for ECL-cell hyperplasia (18), and serum PgI, and gastrin (19) as indicators for atrophic gastritis of corpus mucosa. Our results show that compared to normal, homozygous EMs the heterozygous EMs and PMs groups of patients had significantly higher levels of circulating CGA and gastrin and lower serum PPI on long-term treatment with omeprazole. This indicates that patients may have more or less ECL-cell hyperplasia, and atrophic gastritis in relation to their metabolizing capacity of PPIs.

The present study shows also that serum vitamin B12 levels in patients on long-term treatment with omeprazole were affected by *CYP2C19* genotype with low serum vitamin B12 levels in heterozygous EMs and PMs groups. Since, release of vitamin B12 in the stomach is related to gastric acid and pepsin secretion (20), this finding is inconsistent with our short-term treatment results where we found profound and sustained acid inhibition in the heterozygous EMs and PMs group of patients. Our results may also explain the finding by Termanini and colleagues (21). They found a significant decrease in serum vitamin B12 in a small subgroup of patients with Zollinger–Ellison syndrome treated with omeprazole for 4.5 years. It can be speculated that the likelihood for patients to develop vitamin B12 deficiency increases during long-term treatment with PPIs in relation to the *CYP2C19* genotype and the magnitude of decreased metabolizing capacity.

In conclusion, our studies have shown that changes in intragastric pH, and serum gastrin concentration, together with indicators for morphological changes in the gastric mucosa and vitamin B12 levels are influenced by the *CYP2C19* genotype during omeprazole treatment. A fairly simple determination of *CYP2C19* genotype in patients considered for long-term treatment with omeprazole or other PPIs may enable an individual dose adjustment to maintain an adequate acid inhibition. Such adjustment may optimize the therapy, and at the same time minimize the risk for potentially negative consequences of profound acid inhibition.

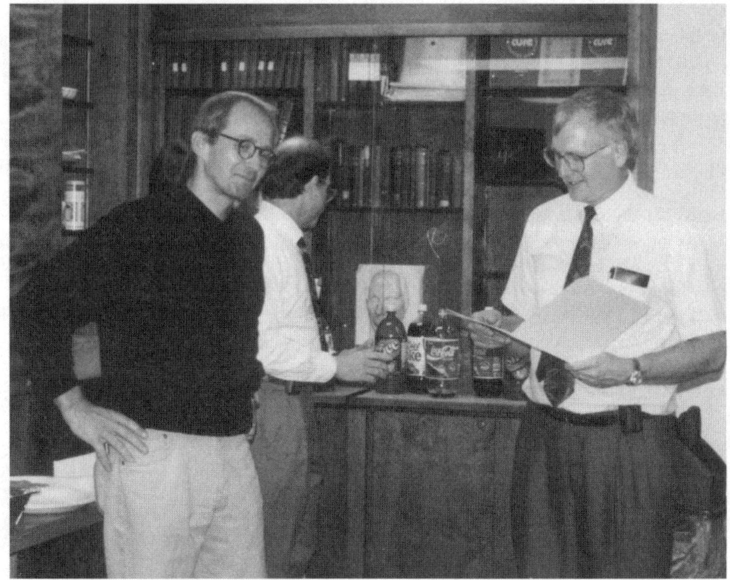

Rein Seensalu and John Walsh in the CURE Library at a farewell reception for Rein after nearly a two year stay at CURE.

ACKNOWLEDGMENTS

I have been privileged to have the opportunity to work with John who so unconditionally shared his immense knowledge with me and others at CURE. John was in many ways truly generous. My family and I miss him deeply.

REFERENCES

1. Regårdh CG. Pharmacokinetics and metabolism of omeprazole in man. *Scand J Gastroenterol* 1986;21 (suppl. 118):99–104.
2. de Morais SM, Wilkinson GR, Blaisdell J, Nakamura K, Meyer UA, Goldstein JA. The major genetic defect responsible for the polymorphism of S-mephenytoin metabolism in humans. *J Biol Chem* 1994;269:15419–15422.
3. de Morais SM, Wilkinson GR, Blaisdell J, Nakamura K, Meyer UA, Goldstein JA. Identification of a new genetic defect responsible for the polymorphism of (S)- mephenytoin metabolism in Japanese. *Mol Pharmacol* 1994;46:594–8.
4. Bertilsson L, Lou Y-Q, Du YL, Liu Y, Kuang TY, Liao XM, Wang KY, Reviriego J, Iselius L, Sjoqvist F. Pronounced differences between native Chinese and Swedish populations in the polymorphic hydroxylations of debrisoquin and S-mephenytoin. *Clin Pharmacol Ther* 1992;51:388–397.
5. Nilsson G. Increased plasma gastrin levels in connection with inhibition of gastric acid responses to sham feeding following bulbar perfusion with acid in dogs. *Scand J Gastroenterol* 1975;10:273–277.
6. Stridsberg M, Hellman U, Wilander E, Lundqvist G, Hellsing K, Öberg K. Fragments of chromogranin A are present in the urine of patients with carcinoid tumours: development of a specific radioimmunoassay for chromogranin A and its fragments. *J Endocrinol* 1993;139:329–37.

7. Granström M, Tindberg Y, Blennow M. Seroepidemiology of *Helicobacter pylori* infection in a cohort of children monitored from 6 months to 11 years of age. *J Clin Microbiol* 1997;35:468–470.

8. Sharma B, Axelson M, Pounder RP, Lundborg P, Ohman M, Santana A, Talbot M, Cederberg C. Acid secretory capacity and plasma gastrin concentration after administration of omeprazole to normal subjects. *Aliment Pharmacol Ther* 1987;1:67–76.

9. Savarino V, Mela GS, Zentilin P, Cutela P, Mele MR, Vigneri S, Celle G. Variability in individual response to various doses of omeprazole, implications for antiulcer therapy. *Dig Dis Sci* 1994;39: 161–168.

10. Lamberts R, Creutzfeldt W, Stråber HG, Brunner G and Solcia E. Long-term omeprazole therapy in peptic ulcer disease: Gastrin, endocrine cell growth, and gastritis. *Gastroenterology* 1993;104:1356–70.

11. Pounder RE, Williams MP. The treatment of *Helicobacter pylori* infection. *Alimentary Pharmacol Ther* 1997;11 (supp 11):35–41.

12. Furuta T, Ohashi K, Kamata T, Takashima M, Kosuge K, Kawasaki T, Hanai H, Kubota T, Ishizaki T, Kaneko E. Effect of genetic differences in omeprazole metabolism on cure rates for *Helicobacter pylori* infection and peptic ulcer. *Ann Intern Med* 1998;129:1027–1030.

13. Moss SF, Legon S, Bishop AE, Polak JM, Calam J. Effect of *Helicobacter pylori* on gastric somatostatin in duodenal ulcer disease. *Lancet* 1992;340:930–932.

14. Lehmann FS, Golodner EH, Wang J, Chen MC, Avedian D, Calam J, Walsh JH, Dubinett S, Soll AH. Mononuclear cells and cytokines stimulate gastrin release from canine antral cells in primary culture. *Am J Physiology* 1996;270:G783–8.

15. Lehmann FS, Schiller N, Cover T, Hatch R, Seensalu R, Kato K, Walsh JH, Soll AH. *H. pylori* stimulates gastrin release from canine antral cells in primary culture. *Am J Physiology* 1998;274:G992–6

16. Lamberts R, Crutzfeldt W, Stöckmann F, Jacubaschke U, Brunner G. Long-term omeprazole treatment in man: effects on gastric endocrine cell populations. *Digestion* 1988;39:126–135.

17. Eissele R, Brunner G, Solcia E, Arnold R. Gastric mucosa during treatment with lanzoprazole: *Helicobacter pylori* is a risk factor for argyrophil cell hyperplasia. *Gastroenterology* 1997;112:707–717.

18. Sanduleanu S, De Bruine A, Stridsberg M, Jonkers D, Biemond I, Hameeteman W, Lundqvist G, Stockbrugger RW. Serum chromogranin A as a screening test for gastric enterochromaffin-like cell hyperplasia during acid-suppressive therapy. *Eur J Clin Invest* 2001;31:802–11.

19. Keiki M, Salmon IM, Varies K, Ihamäki T. Serum pepsinogen I and serum gastrin in the screening of sever atrophic corpus gastritis. *Scand J Gastroenterol* 1991;26 (suppl 186):109–16.

20. Herzlich B, Herbert V. The role of the pancreas in cobalamin (vitamin B12) absorption. *Am J Gastroenterol* 1984;79:489–93.

21. Termanini B, Gigril F, Sutliff VE, Yu F, Venzon D, Jensen RT. Effect of long-term gastric acid suppression therapy on serum vitamin B12 levels in patients with Zollinger-Ellison syndrome. *Am J Med* 1998;422–30.

Gut-Brain Peptides in the New Millennium, edited by Y. Taché
CURE Foundation, Los Angeles, CA. © 2002

44

Unravelling the Mystery of Functional GI Disorders

Emeran A. Mayer

CURE Neuroenteric Disease Program, UCLA Division of Digestive Diseases
Los Angeles, CA

INTRODUCTION

When I first came to visit the Center for Ulcer Research and Education (CURE) in 1979, it was as a medical resident enrolled in the Internal Medicine Residency Program of the University of British Columbia in Vancouver, B.C. I had traveled together with Dr. Haile Debas, a staff surgeon at the Vancouver General Hospital at the time, to interview with about 10 of CURE's key investigators to decide in whose laboratory I wanted to work for the next 2 years. CURE at the time was the Mecca of research and training in gastrointestinal (GI) physiology, and the list of CURE key investigators read like a list from the *Who's Who* in a wide range of fields ranging from GI motility and emptying, peptic ulcer disease, and gastroesophageal reflux disease. In contrast to peptic disorders of the upper GI tract, functional disorders still belonged to a twilight zone in Gastroenterology, lying somewhere between endless anecdotes of a few interested clinicians and the general perception that these disorders really could not be studied with rigorous scientific methods. I had been interested in interactions between mind/brain and the viscera since the time I entered medical school, and given the conceptualization of upper functional GI disorders as a problem of GI motility, I was looking for a mentor and a laboratory that would allow me to pursue my longstanding research interest with the cutting edge technology at CURE at the time. After 2 exhaustive days of interviews I decided to work with John Walsh on the *in vitro* regulation of smooth muscle by neuropeptides and with James Meyer on the physiology and pathophysiology of gastric emptying.

Looking back 20 years, functional GI disorders are no longer conceptualized as simple motility disorders of the gut, as they were in the days when John Walsh became my mentor. Furthermore, they have moved out of the twilight zone on the fringes of gastroenterology and have become targets of intense research. John Walsh's visionary guidance and support throughout my time at CURE has played a major role in helping me to become part of the effort not only to develop more realistic pathophysio-logic models, but also to develop one of the first animal models of these common GI disorders. The development of these models is the content of the current chapter.

OVERVIEW

Despite a recent surge in interest in the neurobiology and drug development of functional GI disorders, wide gaps remain in our knowledge of the etiology and pathophysiology of the most common functional GI syndromes, such as irritable bowel syndrome (IBS), functional dyspepsia and non-cardiac chest pain. However, while functional GI disorders continue to be defined by symptom criteria, significant progress in the mechanistic understanding of these syndromes has recently been made. Well designed epidemiological information has clearly implicated psychosocial stressors (1-4) and acute gastroenteric infections (4, 5) as common central and peripheral triggers of first symptom onset or exacerbation. Perceptual hypersensitivity to physiologic and experimental visceral stimuli ("visceral hypersensitivity") has emerged as an important component for symptom generation (6) which may interact with co-existing alterations in GI motility and in intestinal secretory function (Figure 1). Recent data also implicate alterations in autonomic (7) and neuroendocrine responses to visceral stimuli (8, 9).

Enhanced Perceptual Response to Visceral Stimuli

In the following, I have selected one of the characteristic pathophysiologic aspects of functional GI disorders, and will give a brief overview of the current understanding underlying the enhanced perceptual responses to visceral stimuli.

Following the initial description by Ritchie of increased visceral sensitivity in IBS patients (10), a large number of laboratories have confirmed the existence of altered visceral perception in IBS (reviewed in Naliboff et al., 1996 (11) and Whitehead and Palsson, 1998 (12)). The current evidence can best be summarized as follows: 1) When tested at baseline and especially when using an ascending series of distensions, IBS patients as a whole show lower discomfort thresholds, and greater intensity and unpleasantness ratings during rectal and sigmoid distension. While abnormal perceptual thresholds for discomfort are only seen in about 40-60% of patients, some degree of altered perception as evidenced by lower discomfort threshold, aberrant referral area, or reproduction of IBS symptoms by balloon distension, is seen in nearly all patients (13). 2) Following a repetitive stimulus, a subset of IBS pa-

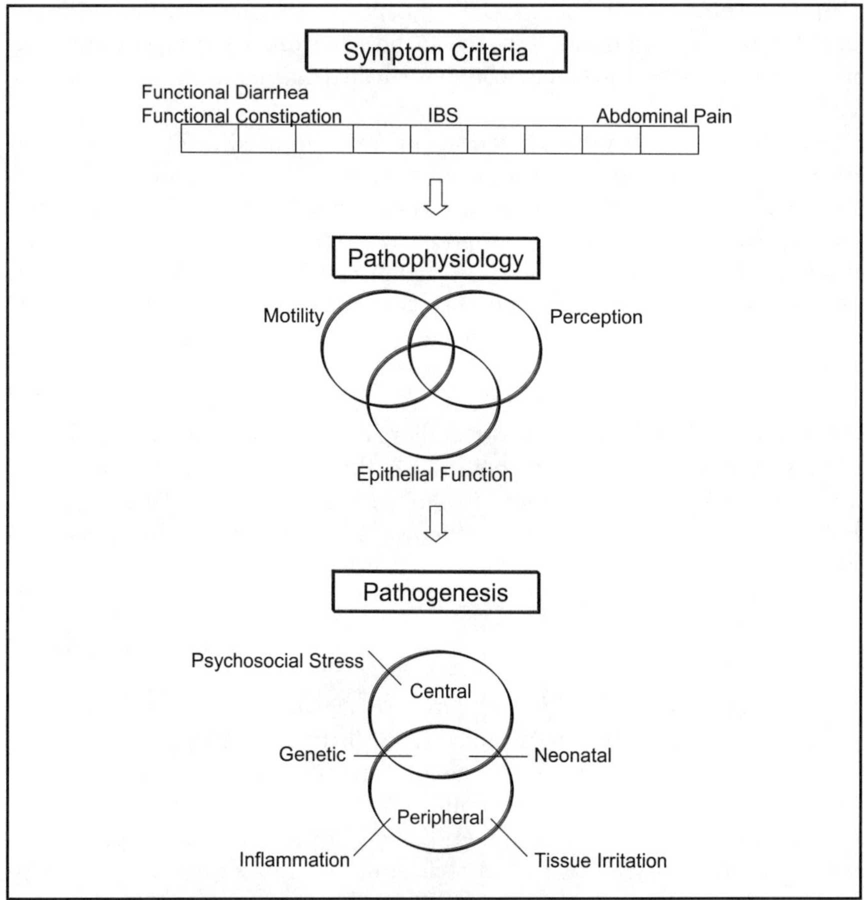

FIGURE 1. *Evolving concepts in functional GI disorders. Different constellations of symptoms are currently classified by the Rome II criteria into distinct syndromes (upper panel). Evolving pathophysiologic concepts incorporate alterations in GI motility, epithelial function and perception of visceral events as critical components resulting in IBS symptoms (middle panel). Several plausible pathogenetic mechanisms acting centrally or peripherally have been identified (lower panel). Pathophysiologic and pathogenetic concepts can be used to develop animal models.*

tients develop profound rectosigmoid hyperalgesia. 3) When exposed to a psychological (14) or physical stressor, such as food intake (15), IBS patients tend to show a greater increase in the subjective ratings of rectosigmoid distension compared to healthy controls. In general, while hypervigilance towards potentially aversive visceral stimuli is present in most IBS patients, alterations in the sensory perception of rectosigmoid distension are most pronounced in female patients with constipation-predominant bowel habit, and nearly absent in male patients with diarrhea-predominant bowel habit

(16). In summary, even though the concept of enhanced visceral sensitivity in IBS is strongly supported by clinical and experimental data, current techniques to quantify this perceptual abnormality are suboptimal and need to be improved.

Suggestive evidence for alterations in stress-induced modulation of viscerosomatic sensitivity comes from human and animal studies. IBS patients show cutaneous normo- or hypoalgesia combined with visceral hypersensitivity (17). A similar pattern was also seen in a recently described rat IBS model in response to an acute psychological stressor (18), and preliminary results suggest that central injection of corticotropin-releasing factor (CRF) can mimic stress-induced visceral hyperalgesia (19). Preliminary results using psychological laboratory stressors in healthy volunteers also suggest a stress-induced increase in colonic or rectosigmoid sensitivity to distension (20). Even though all published human studies are open to methodological criticism, they are consistent with reported findings in animals of a differential viscerosomatic pain modulation. It is of interest to note that patients with bulimia (who, in contrast to IBS patients, have a hyperactive hypothalamic-pituitary-adrenal (HPA) axis) show cutaneous hypoalgesia as well, which precedes symptom exacerbations (21).

Heterogeneity

Even though currently used symptom criteria implicitly assumes a homogenous disorder of "IBS," it is conceivable that the non-specific symptom complex of abdominal pain and discomfort associated with alterations in bowel habits reflects a heterogeneous group of disorders with different etiologies (e.g. peripheral vs. central etiologies), pathophysiologies (gut motor, sensory or secretory changes) and clinical presentations (diarrhea vs. constipation). One of the reasons for similar GI symptom expression may result from the fact that there are a limited number of perceptual (pain/discomfort) and behavioral (bowel movements) responses to gut stimulation, regardless if the stimuli are triggered centrally (autonomic) or intraluminally, and regardless of underlying mechanisms. This point is illustrated by another group of GI disorders previously referred to as the syndrome of chronic idiopathic intestinal pseudo-obstruction (22). While initially, the clinical syndrome (abdominal pain and discomfort associated with radiologic evidence for gut dilatation) was considered a homogeneous disorder of GI motility, it has since been demonstrated that a variety of different syndromes with different etiologies and different underlying pathophysiologies can produce identical symptoms (22). Further heterogeneity in clinical presentation of functional GI disorders may arise from the presence of various co-morbid disorders, such as affective disorders, fibromyalgia or interstitial cystitis. For example, the fact that such extraintestinal symptoms/syndromes are not seen in all patients suggests that they may not be a necessary element in the pathophysiology of IBS. Alternatively, there may be a non-specific core abnormality in IBS patients (vulnerability factor(s)), in the absence of which neither peripheral nor central factors may be able to trigger IBS symptoms.

Evolving IBS Models

Disease models (conceptual models and animal models) provide testable hypotheses essential for rational research into pathophysiologic mechanisms underlying IBS and other functional GI disorders. Without such models, the field of functional bowel research will lack credibility compared to other fields of gastroenterology, and progress in the area of drug development will continue to be hampered by lack of rational targets. Disease models can be assessed based on their face validity (how well the model resembles the clinical or pathophysiological characteristics of the clinical condition), construct validity, (how well the model is consistent with theoretical rationale) and their predictive validity (how well the model predicts treatment responses to specific drugs or non-pharmacologic interventions) (23). Throughout the chapter, we will discuss these models in terms of primary peripheral, primary central, and interacting central and peripheral pathogenetic mechanisms.

CONCEPTUAL IBS MODELS

Different conceptual models for IBS pathophysiology have been proposed to take into account the reported body of pathophysiologic and epidemiologic data. While traditional reductionistic models had focused primarily on isolated peripheral aspects of IBS, such as epithelial function ("mucous colitis"), GI motility ("spastic colon"), or a combination of both ("spastic colitis"), more recent conceptual models (visceral hypersensitivity (6)) and post-infective IBS (PI-IBS) (4, 5), have taken into account both peripheral and central dimensions of the disorder. Drossman first applied the concept of a biopsychosocial model to IBS, to accommodate the interacting role of genetic and biological factors with psychosocial and cognitive factors in the pathophysiology of IBS (24). Even though a significant improvement over the reductionistic models, the biopsychosocial model is based more on psychological and epidemiological aspects of the disease and, is therefore, limited in its ability to generate specific neurobiological hypotheses about etiology and pathophysiology. Valentino et al. have recently proposed a neurobiological model of IBS which is based primarily on mechanistic studies in animals (25). It has as its key component an altered responsiveness of pontine nuclei resulting in abnormal brain and gut responses to peripheral or central stimuli. Increased responsiveness of central noradrenergic (NA)

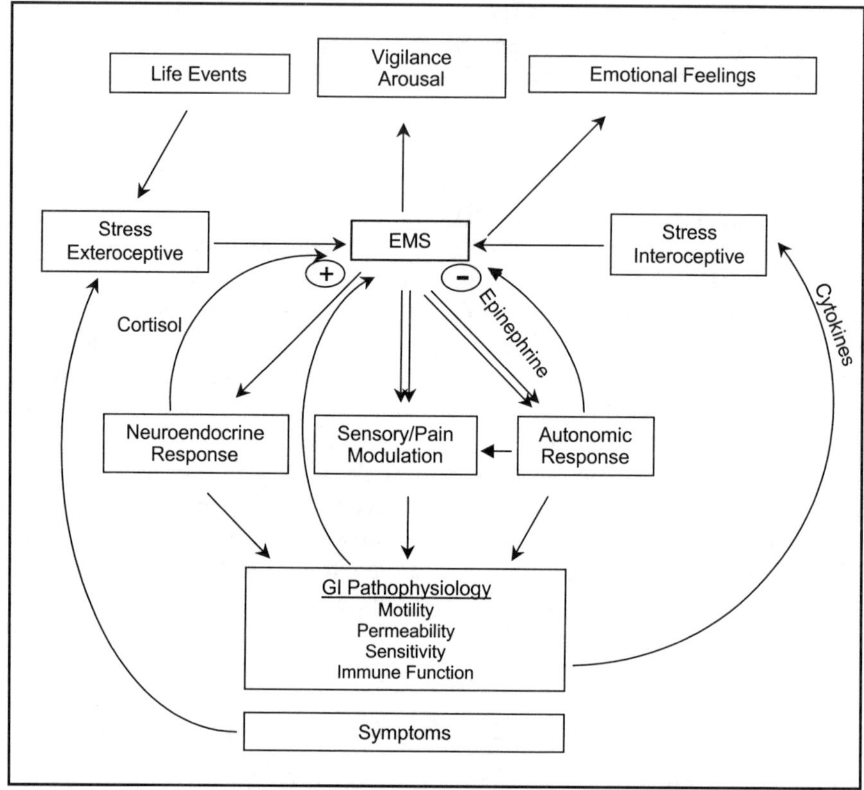

FIGURE 2a. *Enhanced stress responsiveness model of IBS (30). The central component of the model is the emotional motor system (EMS), a system of specific networks concerned with the induction of emotions (fear, anger, sadness, etc.) and the emotion-specific activation of parallel effector systems (107, 108). These effector systems ultimately modulate target cells in the gut, producing alterations in various GI functions. In addition, ascending effector systems from the EMS modulate cognitive functions such as attention and arousal, which in turn play a role in the perception of GI events. Modified from Mayer et al., 2001 (30).*

systems, in particular of the locus coeruleus (LC) complex (including Barrington's nucleus), has been implicated as a central mechanism in IBS by different investigators (reviewed in Mayer, 2000 (26)). This explains the wide variety of extraintestinal symptoms such as overlap with anxiety disorders, stress sensitization, and sleep disturbances.

Comprehensive Conceptual IBS Model Focusing on Central Mechanisms

Incorporating key concepts previously proposed in the psychiatric literature and applied to the area of functional GI disorders by Taché (27), Valentino

(25), Stam (28), and Lydiard (29), we have developed a comprehensive conceptual model which has been reported in detail elsewhere (26, 30). The key features of this model are summarized in Figure 2a.

The organism's response to different exteroceptive and interoceptive stressors is generated by a network comprised of integrative brain structures, in particular subnuclei of the hypothalamus (paraventricular nucleus, PVN), the amygdala complex and subregions of the periaqueductal grey (PAG). These structures receive input from visceral and somatic afferents, and from cortical structures, in particular the ventral subdivision of the anterior cingulate and the medial prefrontal (ventromedial and orbitofrontal) cortex (31, 32). This integrative network provides output to the pituitary and to pontomedullary nuclei, which in turn mediate the neuroendocrine, autonomic, and pain modulatory output to the body, respectively (Figure 2b). This central stress circuitry is under feedback control via ascending monoaminergic projections from brainstem nuclei, in particular serotonergic (raphe nuclei) and NA nuclei (including LC complex), and via circulating glucocorticoids, which exert an inhibitory control via central glucocorticoid receptors located in the medial prefrontal cortex and hippocampus. Positive feedback mediated by the modulatory effect of peripheral epinephrine on certain vagal afferent fibers projecting to the amygdala complex may also play a role in stress circuit regulation. The parallel outputs of this central circuitry ("emotional motor system", EMS) which is activated in response to various perturbations of the external or internal environment include responses of the autonomic nervous system, the HPA axis, endogenous pain modulatory systems, and ascending aminergic pathways which in turn modulate attention, vigilance and arousal (Figure 2a).

One important chemical mediator of the central stress response is CRF (and probably related, molecules such as urocortin and vasopressin) located in certain effector neurons of the PVN, the amygdala, and the LC complex (25). CRF secretion by PVN neurons is under positive feedback regulation by central NA pathways (including those originating from LC), thereby forming a bi-directional positive feedback loop between the CRF-NA systems (Figure 2c). Central injection of CRF can reproduce behavioral and physiologic responses similar to those seen in response to acute psychological stress (33, 34), and inhibition of CRF mediated responses by antagonists (27, 33), or in knock out animals, results in a decrease in the animals' response to stress (35, 36).

Enhanced Responsiveness of EMS

The responsiveness of the EMS is likely to be under partial genetic control and shows considerable plasticity in response to early life events (37) and to certain types of pathological stressors during adult life (38) (Figure 3). For example, studies in animals and humans have clearly demonstrated

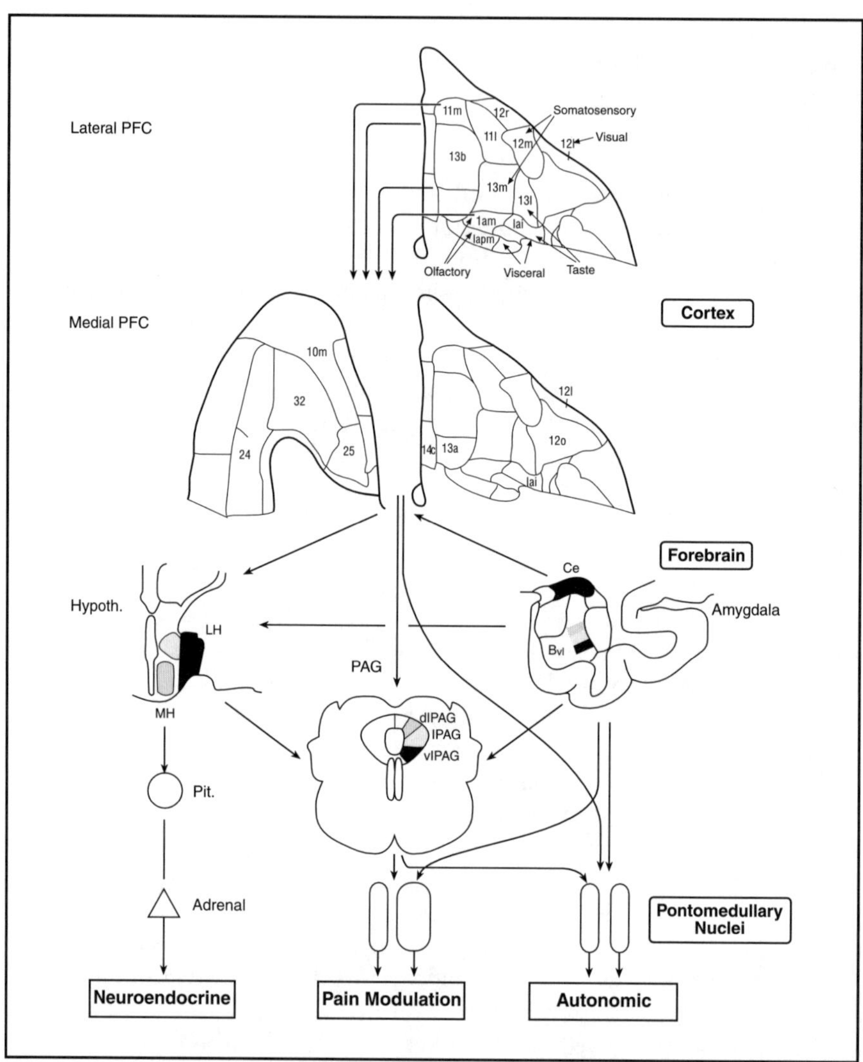

FIGURE 2b. *Enhanced stress responsiveness model of IBS (30). Basic functional neuroanatomy of the EMS. Medial prefrontal structures (ventromedial cortex, perigenual and infragenual cingulate cortex) receive input from lateral prefrontal cortex (PFC) where various sensory inputs are integrated. Output from medial PFC modulates integrative structures of the forebrain (amygdala, hypothalamus) and hindbrain (PAG). Output from these regions in turn projects to pontomedullary nuclei and to the pituitary gland. The integrated output occurs in terms of autonomic, neuroendocrine and pain modulatory responses to emotional stimuli and stressors (32, 75). PFC − prefrontal cortex; Hypoth. − Hypothalamus; LH − lateral hypothalamus; MH − medial hypothalamus; Ce − Central nucleus of amygdala; Bvl − basal ventrolateral nucleus of amygdala; dlPAG − dorsolateral PAG; lPAG − lateral PAG; vlPAG − ventrolateral PAG; Pit − pituitary. Modified from Bandler et al. (32). With permission from Mayer and Collins, 2002 (109).*

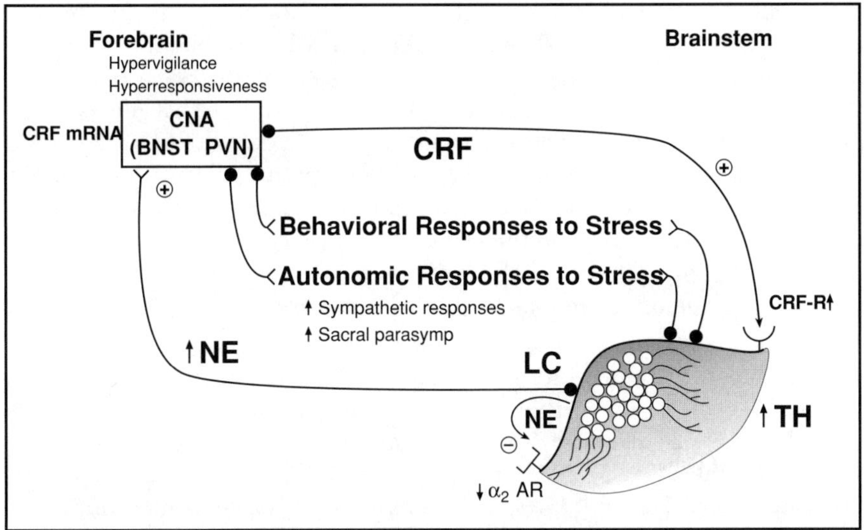

FIGURE 2c. *Enhanced stress responsiveness model of IBS (30). Upregulation of the bidirectional interactions between subcortical structures of EMS following neonatal stress. Projections of CRF-positive neurons from the central nucleus of the amygdala (CNA), from the bed nucleus of striae terminalis (BNST) and from the paraventricular nucleus (PVN) of the hypothalamus activated noradrenergic (NA) neurons of the locus coeruleus (LC). Norepinephrine (NE) containing neurons from the LC project to CRF neurons. Evidence for an upregulation of this system following neonatal stress has been provided (37). TH – tyrosine hydroxylase. Modified and with permission from Koob, 1999 (110).*

that certain types of pathological stress (e.g. stressors that permanently alter the gain of the stress response via persistent neuroplastic changes) can alter the responsiveness of feedback systems by downregulation of pre and/or postsynaptic receptors (adrenergic, serotonergic, dopaminergic, glucocorticoid receptors), and in the most severe forms by structural changes in certain brain regions, such as prefrontal cortex and hippocampus (reviewed in Mayer, 2000 (26)). These alterations could affect the individual output pathways of the EMS differentially and in different directions. For example, an increase or decrease in target-specific sympathetic and vagal outputs, up or down regulation of the HPA axis, and up or down regulation of perceptual sensitivity to visceral and somatic stimuli. Some of the best characterized alterations in this central adaptation to pathological stress are an increase in CRF synthesis and secretion (34), an increase in the activity and sensitivity of central NA systems (37, 39) (Figure 2c), and downregulation of glucocorticoid receptors (40) suggestive of an enhanced HPA response to stress. In contrast, an upregulation of glucocorticoid receptors has been postulated in patients with posttraumatic stress disorder (PTSD), resulting in an enhanced negative feedback control of cortisol and a blunted HPA response to stress

(41). Different mechanisms are likely responsible for alterations in different temporal domains of the HPA axis, such as diurnal variations and phasic responses to acute stress. As a consequence of these alterations in the central stress circuitry, secondary changes are likely to occur in spinal (dorsal horn neurons) and peripheral target cells (gut immune and epithelial cells, enteric nervous system, smooth muscle cells), including permeability changes of gut epithelium (42) and blood-brain barrier (43). Similar to the life long persistence of CNS changes, such peripheral changes may be of a permanent nature.

Validity of Enhanced EMS Responsiveness Model

The enhanced EMS responsiveness model provides plausible and testable explanations for the majority of reported clinical and pathophysiologic aspects of IBS. 1) Dysregulation of GI motility and secretion (44), 2) Enhanced perceptual responses to visceral stimuli and decreased responses to somatic stimuli (17), 3) Altered gut epithelial function, 4) Overlap with other functional GI syndromes, such as functional dyspepsia and noncardiac chest pain (45), 5) Comorbidity with affective disorders (46), 6) Stress-sensitivity (1–3), and 7) Presence of common extraintestinal symptoms, such as fatigue, decrease in libido and poor sleep (47, 48).

Conceptual IBS Model Focusing on Peripheral Mechanisms

Putative Role of Inflammation

Based on results from animal studies, low grade inflammation or immune activation may be a basis for altered motility, and/or afferent and epithelial function of the gut, analogous to reported changes in asthma (49). Several recent histological observations in IBS patients prompt further consideration of a possible inflammatory component in IBS pathophysiology. Several independent studies demonstrated increased mast cell numbers in the muscularis externa of the colon (50), and the ileal and colonic mucosa (51, 52). A selected group of patients with severe IBS were found to have a significant infiltrate of lymphocytes in the myenteric plexus (53). While the extent to which these findings apply to the broader sector of less severe IBS patients remains to be determined, other observations exist to support a role for low grade inflammation in IBS. Increased cellularity of the colonic mucosa and lamina propria of IBS patients has been documented in unselected IBS patients using semi-quantitative microscopy (54).

Post-Infective IBS

It has long been recognized that IBS-like symptoms may develop in patients recovering from enteric infection (55). In a review of several hundred IBS

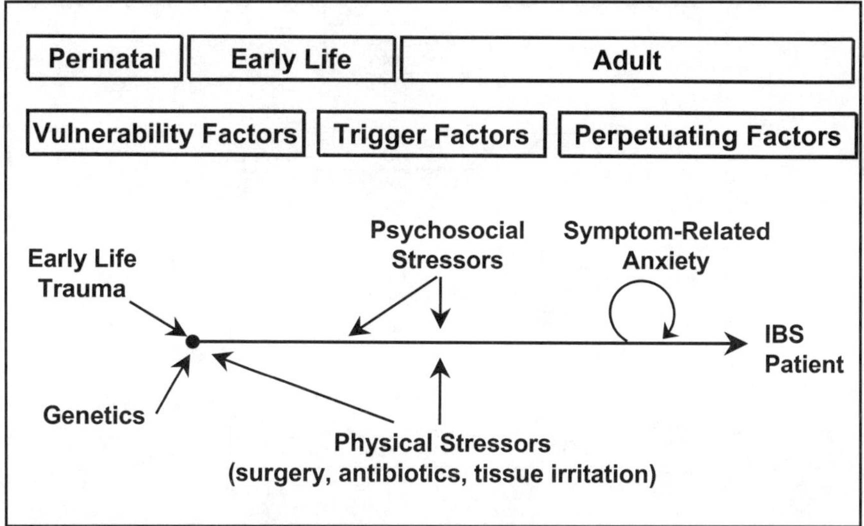

FIGURE 3. *Putative role of psychological and physical stressors on IBS symptom development and severity. Different types of stressors play distinct pathogenetic roles in the development of chronic IBS symptoms. Vulnerability factors for the development of enhanced stress responsiveness in adult life include genetic factors (111), and the quality of the early life environment (84). Psychological trauma occurring early in life (in humans: first decade) can result in permanent neuroplastic changes in the EMS (112, 113) increasing the vulnerability of the individual to stressors later in life. Physical stressors in the early life period may also result in permanent changes in pain systems. Trigger factors for the first development of IBS symptoms in the predisposed individual include certain psychosocial stressors as well as physical stressors (e.g. gut infection). Perpetuating factors include, but are not limited to symptom-related anxiety which may play a major role in chronicity of symptoms, even in the absence of other psychosocial stressors (30). With permission from Mayer and Collins, 2002 (109).*

patients, Chaudhary and Truelove found that approximately one third of these patients gave a history of an acute illness suggestive of acute gastroenteritis at the onset of their chronic IBS (56) and coined the term "Post-Infective IBS." More recent studies have monitored the development of IBS symptoms in patients recovering from proven bacterial gastroenteritis 3–12 months previously. IBS-like symptoms were present in 7–30% of patients (5, 57–59). Reported risk factors for the development of PI-IBS include female gender, and the presence of sustained psychosocial stressors around the time of infection. PI-IBS is not restricted to a particular organism and has been documented with a variety of bacterial infections (*Salmonella, Campylobacter* and *E. coli*) as well as parasitic infection (60), while the role of acute viral gastroenteritis in PI-IBS is unknown.

Studies on function and tissue in PI-IBS patients have shown changes in intestinal motility and epithelial function, but no convincing evidence for the presence of enhanced perceptual responses to visceral stimuli. There is

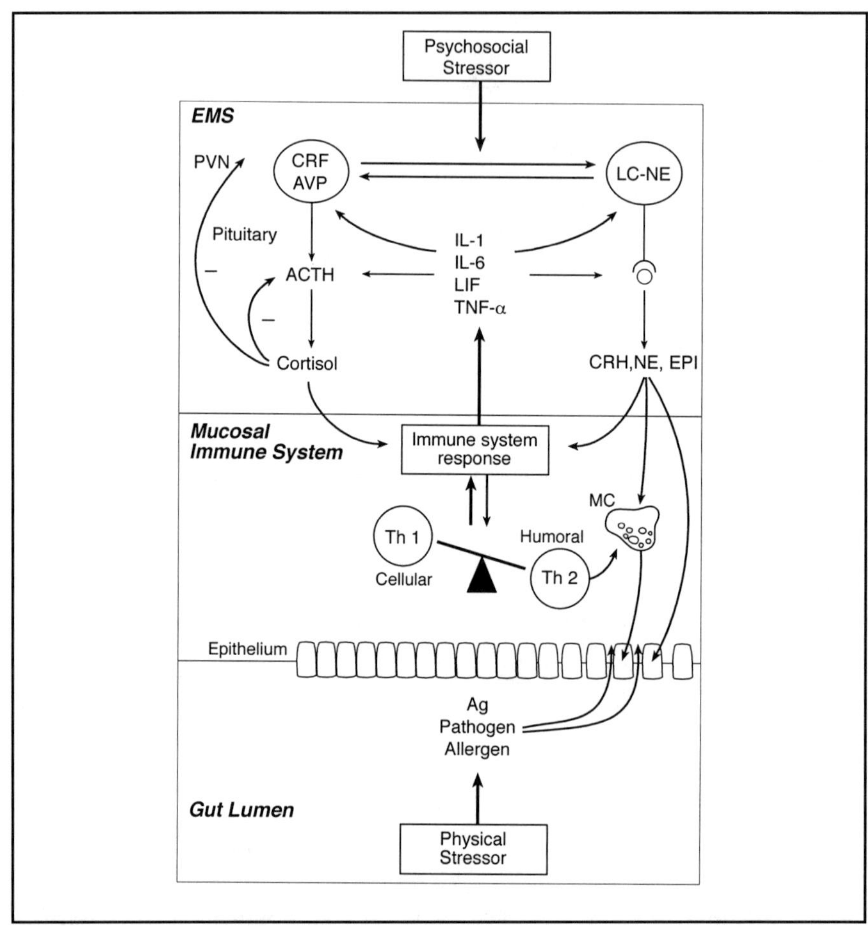

FIGURE 4. *Putative bidirectional brain-gut interactions involved in modulating responsiveness of organism to CNS- and gut-directed stressors. Psychosocial stressors activate stress circuits within the EMS and the resulting peripheral output in the form of neuroendocrine (cortisol), CRF and autonomic (norepinephrine (NE), epinephrine) responses shift the mucosal immune system towards a T_H2 response (increased mast cells, iNOS expression) (68, 114). Autonomic responses can also directly or indirectly modulate gut permeability, thereby changing the access of luminal factors (antigens, bacteria) to the gut immune system. Luminal factors (physical stressors) modulate gut immune function, and immune products from the gut such as cytokines and chemokines can modulate the responsiveness of the EMS (114). Temporal properties of the stressor and age to the animal at stress exposure are important determinants of type of neuroimmune interaction. Modified from Elenkov and Chrousos, 1999 (68). With permission from Mayer and Collins, 2002 (109).*

also histological evidence for alterations in mucosal immune function in PI-IBS, including an increased expression of IL-1β mRNA (61), increased cellularity of the lamina propria and an increase in CD3+ve lymphocytes (4).

However, since increased cellularity of the colonic mucosa and lamina propria has been reported in *unselected* IBS patients as well (54), it remains to be determined if altered gut immune function is a general characteristic of IBS patients, possibly related to an inability to efficiently down-regulate a mucosal inflammatory response (62). The implication of stressful life events in the development of PI-IBS suggests a convergence of central and peripheral mechanisms in the expression of this syndrome.

Relationship Between Central and Peripheral Models

Every conceptual model has to take into account that events within the CNS or in the GI tract do not occur in isolation, but that both systems interact with each other both under normal conditions and particularly during perturbations of homeostasis. As shown in Figure 4, psychosocial stressors may modulate the immune response of the gut to an infectious organism (4) as suggested by observations in PI-IBS, and gut directed physical stressors, including GI infections, may modulate the responsiveness of central stress circuits via pro-inflammatory cytokines (63, 64). A series of observations support bi-directional interactions between the CNS and the immune system, which may also be relevant for the pathophysiology of functional GI disorders.

Neuroimmune Interactions: Brain to Gut

Mast cell degranulation in the gut occurs in response to psychological stress (65, 66) and can even result from Pavlovian conditioning (67). Mast cell products released in the gut (such as proteases or histamine) have the potential of activating and/or sensitizing visceral afferent fibers even though a direct demonstration of pain or hyperalgesia resulting from release of mast cell products has not been demonstrated in humans. In analogy to neuroimmune interactions in other parts of the immune system, altered outputs of central stress circuits in terms of HPA axis and sympathetic and sympathoadrenal responses (described under comprehensive model above and summarized in Figure 1a), may have profound influences on the gut immune system, including cellularity, mast cell numbers, cytokine profiles and T_H1/T_H2 balance (68, 69). In the rat, enhanced stress responsiveness can be associated with increased permeability of the intestine, altering the access of luminal organisms and antigens to the gut immune system and thereby increasing susceptibility to inflammatory triggers in the gut lumen (65). Based on the existing, largely preliminary reports in poorly classified IBS patients, one can speculate that variations in the activity of HPA axis and SNS may play a role in producing subsets of IBS patients with increased cellular infiltrate (4, 54), increased mast cells (50–52) and either increases in proinflammatory markers (61, 70), or suppression of T_H1 cytokines with a shift in the

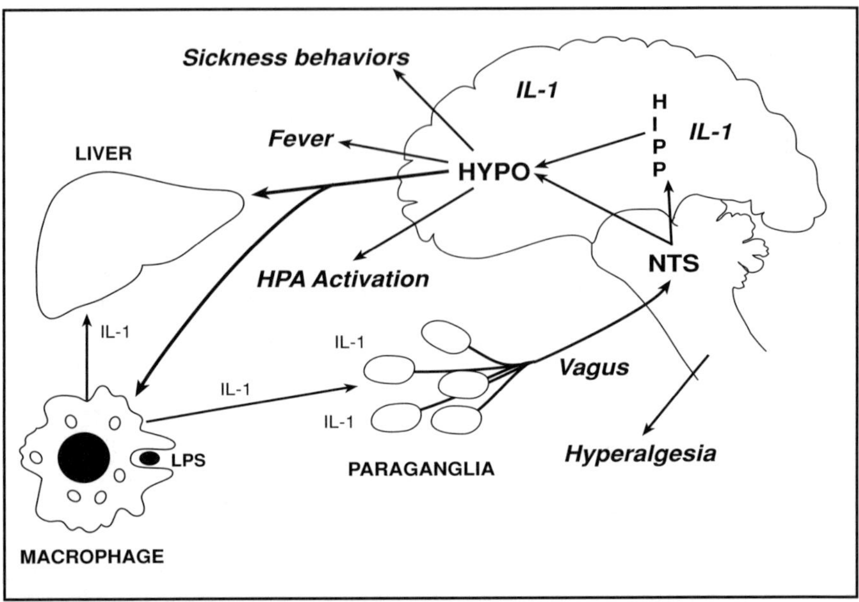

FIGURE 5. *Interactions between proinflammatory cytokines, vagal afferent nerves and central stress circuits. HYPO – hypothalamus; HIPP – hippocampus; LPS – lipopolysaccharide; NTS – nucleus tractus solitarius; IL-1 – interleukin 1. For details, see text. With permission from Maier and Watkins, 1998 (63).*

T_H1/T_H2 balance (71). Further studies are needed to determine a) in which IBS patient subsets mucosal immune alterations are found and b) what role, if any these mucosal changes play in IBS symptoms.

Neuroimmune Interactions: Gut to Brain

Immune cell products including different cytokines and chemokines released in the gut may have profound influences on the responsiveness of central stress circuits including gene expression of CRF and vasopressin. Figure 5 shows a schematic based on the extensive work of S. Maier and L. Watkins on the involvement of proinflammatory cytokines, in particular IL–1, in bi-directional brain-body interactions and involving the afferent vagus nerve as an important mechanism of GI tract (liver) to brain signaling (63). The proposed model implicates activation of paraganglion cells located in the liver by IL–1, resulting in release of paracrine substances from these cells signaling to peripheral terminals of the hepatic branch of the vagus nerve. Increased vagal afferent input to the brain results in activation of glial cells to produce IL-1, thereby causing an increase in central IL-1. Immune cell products signaling to the CNS via the vagus nerve play a major role in the pathogenesis of a symptom complex including hyperalgesia, fever, anorexia and taste aversion ("sickness syndrome"). While acute peripheral inflammation may be associated with an upregulation of central stress responsiveness, chronic inflammatory processes such as rheumatoid arthritis or ulcerative colitis may be associated with a downregulation. Even though it is currently not known if similar mechanisms exist for activation of other branches of the vagus nerve by cytokines, a fundamentally different role of the celiac branch of the vagus nerve has been reported by Jänig, et al. These fibers appear to exert a tonic, anti-inflammatory and antinociceptive function (72).

Even though it is too early to implicate altered neuroimmune interactions within the brain gut axis as mechanisms involved in the pathophysiology of functional GI disorders, one may speculate about possible scenarios of how such interactions could be involved.

Animal Models of IBS

Animal models can be assessed based on their face validity, i.e. how well the animal model resembles the human conditions in terms of etiology, behavioral features and underlying biology. Even though high face validity of an animal model for the entire syndrome is desirable, it is not essential. An example of an animal model with high face validity for interstitial cystitis, a condition frequently associated with IBS, develops spontaneously in the cat (73). However, given some of the unique clinical features of IBS patients (for example cognitive and behavioral features) it is unlikely for any animal model to reach perfect face validity. However, an animal model which adequately models specific aspects of the syndrome (target organ and/or tissue dysfunction), such as stress-induced visceral hyperalgesia, stress-induced motility changes in upper and lower GI tract, or postinfectious mucosal changes (increase in enterochromaffin cells, increased intestinal permeability) would be of significant benefit, in particular if such limited models showed good predictive validity.

Existing animal models can be divided into two broad categories: those which are *initiated* by central (psychosocial stressor, trauma) and those by peripheral perturbations of homeostasis (gut inflammation, infection, surgery, bacterial overgrowth). These categories can be further subdivided based on the age during which the animal has been exposed to the stressor, for example during the peri- and neonatal stage, or as an adult. Regardless of the mode and time of initiation, it is likely that responses of both peripheral and central elements of the brain gut axis will be altered in the fully expressed model. In addition to creating changes in the animal, an important aspect of animal models is the way responses are elicited. For example, assessment of read outs may be normal under baseline conditions, but only show abnormalities after the animal has been exposed to a particular psychological or inflammatory stressor. Also, the pattern of responses may vary depending on the nature of the stressor. For example, animals may show normal responses to interoceptive stressors (inflammation, hemorrhage) but abnormal responses to exteroceptive (psychological) stressors. Animals may show abnormal behavioral responses in one situation (open field) and abnormal autonomic responses to a different stressor (prod shock) (74).

Centrally Initiated Models

Several central models with relevance for IBS have been adapted from the psychiatric literature. Even though all models discussed below were developed as animal models of common affective disorders (e.g. anxiety disorders and depression), the subsequent demonstration of alterations in brain gut axis in some of these models focused attention on their potential usefulness as IBS models. Furthermore, in view of the high comorbidity of IBS with anxiety disorders (46), these models have a high face validity. Centrally initiated models can be separated into those which are induced by environmental influences and those induced by genetic manipulations of the central stress responsiveness.

Alterations in CRF System Gene Expression Induced by Environmental Manipulations: Effects of Repeated or Developmental Stressors

Neonatal Psychosocial Stress Model

The quality of the early family environment can serve as a major source of stress vulnerability in later life. Individuals who are the victims of physically, emotionally or sexually abusive families are at considerably greater risk for anxiety disorders and depression in later life (reviewed in Kaufman et al. 2000 (75)). Other less dramatic influences in early life, such as cold and distant parent-child relationships, and divorce of the parents or death of the mother before age 10 have also been associated with such enhanced vulnerability later in life. The enhanced vulnerability is not limited to affective disorders, but extends to a greater risk of chronic illness in general, including a greater risk for development of IBS (76–78). It has been suggested that this influence of early life events is mediated in part by parental influences on the development of neural systems that underlie the expression of behavioral, autonomic and neuroendocrine responses to stress (79–83).

Validated animal models of aversive early life events include situations in which the normal mother-infant interaction is compromised. In the rodent, one of the major maternal behaviors that determines the quality of maternal care is the characteristic licking/grooming of the pups by the mother (84). Daily separation of the litter from their mothers for 180 min each day during postnatal days 4–18 will result in an alteration of maternal behavior, with significant reduced times of the licking/grooming behavior (37). This neonatal stress in form of compromised mother-infant interaction results in permanent changes in the CNS, which have been documented at the level of gene expression, neurochemistry, electrophysiology, and morphology. A key component of the model is the compromised ability to restrain the synthesis and release of CRF in response to acute psychological stressors (75) (see also Figure 2c). Neurocircuits affected by the neonatal maternal separation protocol include hypothalamic and extrahypothalamic CRF systems, and ascending monoaminergic systems (37). The increase in CRF and norepinephrine drive in maternally deprived rats is associated with a decrease in tone of the inhibitory GABA/benzodiazepine system. Studies by Caldji et al. have demonstrated that these changes in the $GABA_A$ receptor are associated with altered expression of alpha and gamma subunits and with decreased GABA binding (84).

These neurochemical changes are associated with enhanced fearfulness, increased HPA responsiveness to stressors and an increased risk of developing depression-like behaviors. Our group has recently demonstrated that maternally-separated rats show evidence for alterations in stress-induced visceral and somatic pain sensitivity consistent with compromised stress-induced engagement of opioid systems (18, 85, 86). Additionally, colonic motor function in response to stress is also enhanced in these animals. Preliminary results suggest that rats exposed to neonatal stress also demonstrate evidence for increased intestinal permeability (42) and that stress-induced visceral hyperalgesia is inhibited by central administration of a CRF antagonist (18).

The demonstration of enhanced anxiety-like behaviors, hypervigilance, increased vulnerability to anhedonia under stress, alterations in the HPA axis responsiveness, stress-induced visceral hyperalgesia and enhanced stress-induced colonic motility in adult animals give this model excellent face and construct validity. The increased prevalence of functional GI symptoms in patients with a history of early adverse life events (see above) further contributes to the similarity of animal model and human condition.

Posttraumatic Stress Disorder Model

In adult man and in animals, exposure to an uncontrollable stressor can induce an alteration in the behavioral, autonomic and neuroendocrine responses to future stressors. Depending on its intensity, either repeated or single exposure to the same stressor can produce long-lasting sensitization to a wide range of stimuli that are unrelated to the initial stressor (reviewed in Stam et al., 1997, 2000 (28, 74)). DSM-IV diagnostic criteria for PTSD state that the clinical syndrome must follow experiencing or witnessing events that involve actual or threatened death or serious injury, or a threat to the physical integrity of self or others (87). Increased prevalence of GI symptoms in PTSD has been reported in prisoners of war, Vietnam combat veterans and former hostages. The reported increase in IBS prevalence in women with sexual abuse is highest in those who were raped at gun point or perceived life threat, meeting PTSD criteria (88).

Validated animal models use daily sessions of brief electric footshock to induce a sensitized state (reviewed in Stam et al., 2000 (74)). Other interventions include social defeat by an aggressive conspecific (89), repeated administration of psychostimulants or repeated central injection of CRF (90). In addition to the considerable overlap of IBS with PTSD in patients, animal models of PTSD have demonstrated long lasting alterations in reactivity (both hypo- and hyperresponsiveness) of the EMS, including alterations in colonic motility responses (91), cardiovascular responses, neuroendocrine responses, and regional Fos-responsivity in the brain to stressors (reviewed in Stam et al., 2000 (74)). Preliminary evidence suggests that such animals also show increased visceral afferent responses to colonic distension (92). It is of interest, that in contrast to the autonomic and neuroendocrine sensitization observed in response to the acute stressor, behavioral responses of these animals were only seen in response to other types of stressors, such as the open field test or novel environments.

Mechanisms underlying the observed alterations in stress responsiveness in both animal models and PTSD patients, include enhanced responses of central CRF/vasopressin and NA responses (93), increased spinal CRF levels (39), altered HPA axis responses (41), preattentive CNS hyperresponsiveness (94), and altered responses of limbic brain regions, including amygdala, PVN, LC and frontal cortex (95).

Animal models of adult stress sensitization show good face validity (similarity to several features of IBS) and good construct validity (how well the model is consistent with the concept of enhanced stress responsiveness). The predictive validity of this animal model for drugs with therapeutic potential in IBS remains to be determined.

Effects of CRF System Gene Targeting on Stress-related Behaviors: Use of Transgenic Mice and Antisense Oligonucleotides

Both behaviorally induced animal models described above share the increased responsiveness of the reciprocally related central CRF and NA systems as a core pathophysiologic mechanism. In view of the well documented role of central (and possibly peripheral) CRF systems in modulation of stress-induced motility changes of the upper and lower GI tract, and the postulated role of CRF in stress-induced visceral hyperalgesia, one may speculate that not only animal models with behaviorally induced, but also those with genetically induced changes in the CRF system (CRF_1 and CRF_2 receptor, CRF binding protein, CRF) (reviewed in Bakshi and Kalin, 2000 (96)) might be useful models for IBS. For the same reasons, animals with genetic manipulations of the $GABA_A$ and the NA system may be useful models for increased stress responsiveness in IBS. However, key features of IBS, such as visceral hypersensitivity or stress-induced motility alterations have not been reported in any of these models.

Peripherally Initiated Models

The newborn gut may be exposed to a variety of factors resulting in mucosal inflammation and tissue irritation (6). These factors include but are not limited to inflammation resulting from food allergies, viral infections, and acid reflux, all of which are common in early life. In view of underdeveloped responses of the nervous system (HPA axis, endogenous pain inhibition systems), these insults may result in permanent neuroplastic alterations manifesting as altered pain and neuroendocrine response to visceral stimuli as adults. For example, in rats, neonatal glucocorticoid treatment (97) or low dose endotoxin (98) has permanent programming effects on endocrine as well as immune functioning in adult life.

Neonatal Inflammation

Based on the concept of neonatal sensitization, a rodent model was recently published by Al-Chaer et al. (99). Daily colon irritation was produced in the neonatal period (days 8-21) either in the form of daily noxious colorectal distension (CRD) (two 60 s distensions separated by 30 min at rest) or in the form of daily intracolonic injection of mustard oil. Behavioral pain responses to CRD were significantly increased in the neonatally irritated rats when assessed at postnatal week 5 and persisted up to postnatal week 12, while colon histologies were not different from controls. In addition, electrophysiologic recordings of individual dorsal horn neurons from segments L6-S1 showed increased responses at baseline as well as increased responses to CRD and to somatic stimuli applied to the same dermatome. These findings suggest that two different perturbations of the intestinal homeostasis in early life result in permanent sensitization of dorsal horn neurons receiving convergent input.

The model has good face validity since it mimics a key feature of the human condition, i.e. visceral hypersensitivity. It remains to be determined if IBS patients exhibit somatic hyperalgesia in the same dermatome that receives afferent input from the colon: some studies have demonstrated hypoalgesia (100), while others have demonstrated hyperalgesia (101). Even though no convincing longitudinal studies exist to demonstrate irritation of the gut in early life as a risk factor for later development of IBS, such a course of event is plausible at least in a subset of IBS (or chronic abdominal pain) patients. There is also good construct validity of the model: Visceral hyperalgesia secondary to long lasting or permanent sensitization of dorsal horn neurons is a plausible mechanism that could result in enhanced pain and autonomic responses to physiological visceral events.

Other Animal Models of IBS

Several other animal models have been reported which mimic certain features of IBS. Gue et al. have reported the development of stress-induced visceral hyperalgesia in normal male Wistar rats following restraint stress (102). Since no other intervention is required in these animals to produce enhanced stress responsiveness, this model may represent a *genetic* model of altered stress sensitivity. Chen et al. recently reported altered bowel habits in a mouse model with targeted deletion of the serotonin reuptake transporter (SERT), and have implicated a genetic alteration in SERT as a possible model for IBS (103). Collins' group reported rodent models which might be considered as models of PI-IBS (104).

FUTURE DIRECTIONS IN THE DEVELOPMENT OF ANIMAL MODELS

Improvement of Face and Construct Validity

In order to enhance the face and construct validity of existing animal models and the clinical condition, more work is required. For example, the relative contributions and the interactions between peripheral and central stressors need to be delineated. Carefully designed studies are required to determine the presence and nature of visceral hypersensitivity, motility alterations and autonomic dysregulation in all animal models. Ideally, assessment of these functional alterations in different models should be done with comparable experimental techniques. The existing model of PI-IBS utilizes a parasitic model whereas most clinical cases of PI-IBS follow bacterial infections with *Salmonella, Campylobacter* and *Shigella*. Thus, models of PI-IBS based on more common pathogens need to be developed.

On the other side, observations made in existing animal models will generate hypotheses to be tested in the human condition. For example, is there evidence for persistent central sensitization (as demonstrated in the neonatal colon irritation model) based on hyperalgesia to both visceral and somatic stimuli in IBS? Are alterations in gut immune function present in all IBS patients or only in certain subsets, such as PI-IBS? Are the alterations in immune function observed in animal models detectable in human intestinal biopsies?

Demonstration of Predictive Validity

Evidence for predictive validity of existing animal models is currently lacking (105). The demonstration of such predictive validity will be essential to accept or reject any of the conceptual and animal models. For example, the experience with the kappa agonist fedotozine which showed high efficacy in the acute rat CRD model, but failed to show therapeutic effects on IBS symptoms in humans suggests a lack of predictive validity of the acute CRD distension model, at least for certain drugs. Does pharmacological normalization of enhanced stress responsiveness (e.g. by a CRF_1 antagonist) normalize autonomic and sensory abnormalities in the neonatal separation model and effectively reduce IBS symptoms? Does selective normalization of altered immune function reverse PI-IBS as suggested by the animal model?

Species

Rats are clearly the best characterized species in terms of functional neuroanatomy, neurochemistry and behavior. A variety of different rat strains differ in terms of stress responsiveness, anxiety, and endogenous pain modulation systems. On the other hand, the availability of transgenic animals and knock out technologies clearly make the mouse an attractive alternative. Finally, in certain situations, rodents other than mice or rats (e.g. gerbil, guinea-pig) may be preferable, since some of their receptor systems (e.g. neurokinin receptors) are more similar to humans than those of rats and mice.

Sex

Even though the majority of published studies on rat models for visceral pain, stress, anxiety and depression deal with male animals, the clinical disorders corresponding to these animal models, including functional bowel disorders show a greater prevalence in women. Careful comparisons of differences in male and female animal models, under strict control for the estrous cycle are needed.

Acute vs. Chronic

IBS is a chronic disorder and models need to reflect this temporal dimension of the disorder. For example, models of visceral hyperalgesia induced by acute gut inflammation have minimal face, construct and predictive validity with the human disorder. However, in an established model with chronic pathophysiology, responses to acute perturbations of the internal (acute inflammation, irritation) or external environment (acute stressors) may be important.

Lessons from Other Systems

Much can be learned from other chronic conditions which bear similarities with IBS or that frequently co-occur with IBS (106). It is obvious from the above discussion of the central IBS models that considerable similarities exist with models of affective disorders. Other disorders with certain clinical similarities to functional GI disorders include migraine, interstitial cystitis and asthma, all of which were once considered to be purely psychosomatic in origin, and which are now well recognized disease entities with recognizable triggers, pathophysiological pathways and therapeutic targets. In each case interactions between outputs of the EMS, autonomic dysregulation of target cells in respective tissues (smooth muscle, immune cells), and alterations in pain perception can be identified.

SUMMARY AND CONCLUSIONS

During the past 20 years, the field of functional GI disorders has seen tremendous progress: from being an isoteric area within gastroenterology, dominated by descriptive and poorly controlled clinical, and mechanistic studies into GI motility, to a respectable GI subspeciality, with testable scientific hypotheses and animal models with high validity. Several investigators at CURE, including Helen Raybould, Yvette Taché and members of my own research group, notably Lin Chang and Bruce Naliboff have made significant contributions to this change. All of us owe in many ways our success in this endeavor to John Walsh, who recruited, mentored and supported many of us.

ACKNOWLEDGMENTS

The author would like to thank Drs. Lin Chang, Bruce Naliboff and Steve Collins, as well as the participants of the workshop Pathophysiological Models of Functional Gastrointestinal Disorders (106) for their valuable input, and Teresa Olivas for her outstanding editorial assistance in the preparation of the manuscript.

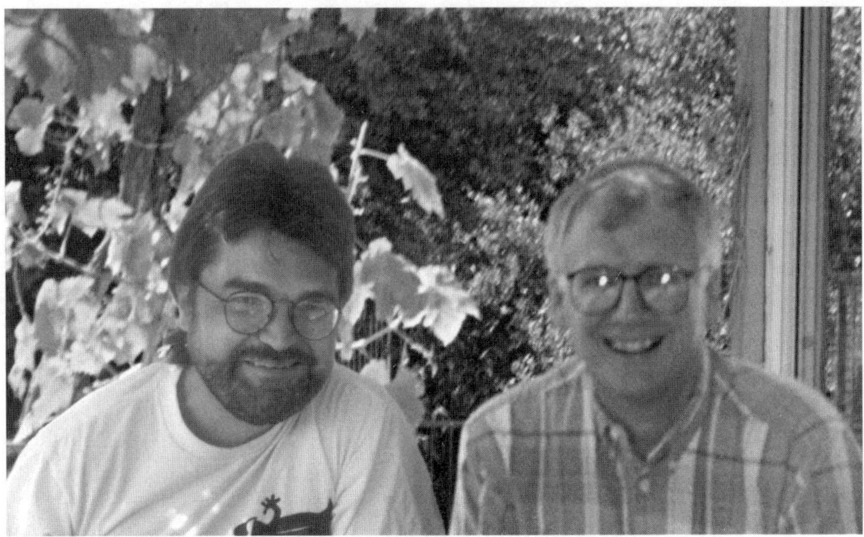

On a beautiful Sunday in the summer of 1998, we had John over for dinner at our house in Topanga. Left to right: Emeran Mayer and John Walsh.

REFERENCES

1. Bennett EJ, Tennant CC, Piesse C, Badcock CA, Kellow JE. Level of chronic life stress predicts clinical outcome in irritable bowel syndrome. *Gut* 1998;43:256–261.
2. Drossman DA, Sandler RS, McKee DC, Lovitz AJ. Bowel patterns among subjects not seeking health care. Use of a questionnaire to identify a population with bowel dysfunction. *Gastroenterology* 1982;83:529–534.
3. Whitehead WE, Crowell MD, Robinson JC, Heller BR, Schuster MM. Effects of stressful life events on bowel symptoms: subjects with irritable bowel syndrome compared with subjects without bowel dysfunction. *Gut* 1992;33:825–830.
4. Gwee KA. The role of psychological and biological factors in postinfective gut dysfunction. *Gut* 1999;44:400–406.
5. Gwee KA, Graham JC, McKendrick MW, Collins SM, Marshall JS, Walters SJ, Read NW. Psychometric scores and persistence of irritable bowel after infectious diarrhoea. *Lancet* 1996;347:150–153.
6. Mayer EA and Gebhart GF. Basic and clinical aspects of visceral hyperalgesia. *Gastroenterology* 1994;107:271–293.
7. Heitkemper M, Burr RL, Jarrett M, Hertig V, Lustyk MK, Bond EF. Evidence for autonomic nervous system imbalance in women with irritable bowel syndrome. *Dig Dis Sci* 1998;43:2093–2098.
8. Heitkemper M, Jarrett M, Cain K, Shaver J, Bond E, Woods NF, Walker E. Increased urine catecholamines and cortisol in women with irritable bowel syndrome. *Am J Gastroenterol* 1996;91: 906–913.
9. Munakata J, Mayer EA, Chang L, Schmulson M, Liu M, Tougas G, Kamath M, Naliboff B. Autonomic and neuroendocrine responses to recto-sigmoid stimulation. *Gastroenterology* 1998;114:808.
10. Ritchie J. Pain from distension of the pelvic colon by inflating a balloon in the irritable colon syndrome. *Gut* 1973;14:125–132.
11. Naliboff B and Mayer EA. Sensational developments in the irritable bowel. *Gut* 1996;39:770–771.
12. Whitehead WE and Palsson OS. Is rectal pain sensitivity a biological marker for irritable bowel syndrome: Psychological influences on pain perception. *Gastroenterology* 1998;115:1263–1271.

13. Mertz H, Naliboff B, Munakata J, Niazi N, Mayer EA. Altered rectal perception is a biological marker of patients with irritable bowel syndrome. *Gastroenterology* 1995;109:40–52.

14. Dickhaus B, Firooz N, Stains J, Fass R, Mayer EA, Naliboff BD. Psychological stress increases visceral sensitivity in patients with irritable bowel syndrome (IBS) but not controls. *Gastroenterology* 2001;120:A67.

15. Simrèn M, Abrahamsson H, Björnsson ES. An exaggerated sensory component of the gastrocolonic response in patients with irritable bowel syndrome. *Gut* 2001;48:20–27.

16. Chang L, Naliboff BD, Schmulson M, Lee OY, Olivas TI, Mayer EA. The role of gender and bowel habit predominance on visceral perception in IBS. *Gastroenterology* 2001;120:A755.

17. Naliboff BD, Chang L, Munakata J, Mayer EA. Towards an integrative model of irritable bowel syndrome. In: *The Biological Basis for Mind Body Interactions,* Mayer EA and Saper CB, eds. Amsterdam, Elsevier Science, 2000:413–423.

18. Coutinho SV, Miller JC, Plotsky PM, Mayer EA. Effect of perinatal stress on responses to colorectal distension in adult rats. *Soc Neurosci Abstr* 1999;25:687.

19. Cochrane SW, Gibson MS, Myers DA, Schulkin J, Rice KC, Gold PW, Greenwood-Van Meerveld B. Role of corticotropin-releasing factor-1 (CRF_1)-receptor mediated mechanisms in neural pathways modulating colonic hypersensitivity. *Gastroenterology* 2001;120:A7.

20. Delvaux MM. Stress and visceral perception. *Can J Gastroenterol* 1999;13(Suppl A):32A–36A.

21. Faris PL, Kim SW, Meller WH, Goodale RL, Hofbauer RD, Oakman SA, Howard LA, Stevens ER, Eckert ED, Hartman BK. Effect of ondansetron, a 5-HT_3 receptor antagonist, on the dynamic association between bulimic behaviors and pain thresholds. *Pain* 1998;77:297–303.

22. Schuffler MD. Chronic intestinal psuedo-obstruction. In: *Sleisenger's and Fordtran's Gastrointestinal and Liver Disease.* Feldman M, Scharschmidt BF, Sleizenger MH, eds. Philedelphia: WB Saunders, 1993;1820–1830.

23. Yadid G, Nakash R, Deri I, Tamar G, Kinor N, Gispan I, Zangen A. Elucidation of the neurobiology of depression: Insights from a novel genetic animal model. *Progr Neurobiol* 2000;62:353–378.

24. Drossman DA. Presidential address: Gastrointestinal illness and the biopsychosocial model. *Psychosom Med* 1998;60:258–267.

25. Valentino RJ, Miselis RR, Pavcovich LA. Pontine regulation of pelvic viscera: pharmacological target for pelvic visceral dysfunction. *Trends Pharmacol Sci* 1999;20:253–260.

26. Mayer EA. The neurobiology of stress and gastrointestinal disease. *Gut* 2000;47:861–869.

27. Tache Y, Martinez V, Million M, Rivier J. Corticotropin-releasing factor and the brain-gut motor response to stress. *Can J Gastroenterol* 1999;13:18A–25A.

28. Stam R, Akkermans LMA, Wiegant VM. Trauma and the gut: Interactions between stressful experience and intestinal function. *Gut* 1997;40:704–709.

29. Lydiard RB and Falsetti SA. Experience with anxiety and depression treatment studies: implication for designing Irritable Bowel Syndrome clinical trials. *Am J Med* 1999;107:65S–73S.

30. Mayer EA, Naliboff BD, Chang L, Coutinho SV. Stress and the gastrointestinal tract: V. Stress and irritable bowel syndrome. *Am J Physiol Gastrointest Liver Physiol* 2001;280:G519–G524.

31. López JF, Akil H, Watson SJ. Neural circuits mediating stress. *Biol Psychiatry* 1999;46:1461–1471.

32. Bandler R, Price JL, Keay KA. Brain mediation of active and passive emotional coping. In: *The Biological Basis for Mind Body Interactions.* Mayer EA and Saper CB, eds. Amsterdam. Elsevier Science, 2000:333–349.

33. Taché Y, Monnikes H, Bonaz B, Rivier J. Role of CRF in stress-related alterations of gastric and colonic motor function. *Ann NY Acad Sci* 1993;697:233–243.

34. Owens MJ and Nemeroff CB. The role of corticotropin-releasing factor in the pathophysiology of affective and anxiety disorders: laboratory and clinical studies. *Ciba Found Symp* 1993;172:296–316.

35. Timpl P, Spanagel R, Sillaber I, Kresse A, Reul JM, Stalla GK, Blanquet V, Steckler T, Holsboer F, Wurst W. Impaired stress response and reduced anxiety in mice lacking a functional corticotropin-releasing hormone receptor. *Nat Genet* 1998;19:162–166.

36. Smith GW, Aubry JM, Dellu F, Contarino A, Bilezikjian LM, Gold LH, Chen R, Marchuk Y, Hauser C, Bentley CA, Sawchenko PE, Koob GF, Vale W, Lee KF. Corticotropin releasing factor receptor 1-deficient mice display decreased anxiety, impaired stress response, and aberrant neuroendocrine development. *Neuron* 1998;20:1093–1102.

37. Ladd CO, Huot RL, Thrivikraman KV, Nemeroff CB, Meaney MJ, Plotsky P. Long-term behavioral and neuroendocrine adaptations to adverse early experience. In: *The Biological Basis for Mind Body Interactions.* Mayer EA, and Saper CB, eds., Amsterdam, Elsevier, 2000:81–103.

38. Fuchs E and Fluegge G. Modulation of binding sites for corticotropin-releasing hormone by chronic psychosocial stress. *Psychoneuroendocrinology* 1995;20:33–51.

39. Southwick SM, Bremner JD, Rasmusson A, Morgan III CA, Arnsten A, Charney DS. Role of nor-epinephrine in the pathophysiology and treatment of post-traumatic stress disorder. *Biol Psychiatry* 1999;46:1192–1204.

40. Sapolsky RM, Krey LC, McEwen BS. Stress down-regulates corticosterone receptors in a site-specific manner in the brain. *Endocrinology* 1984;114:287–292.

41. Yehuda R, Giller EL, Jr., Levengood RA, Southwick SM, Siever LJ. Hypothalamic-pituitary-adrenal functioning in post-traumatic stress disorder: Expanding the concept of the stress response spectrum. In: *Neurobiological and Clinical Consequences of Stress: From Normal Adaptation to Post-Traumatic Stress Disorder.* Friedman MJ, Charney DS, Deutch AY, eds. Philadelphia: Lippincott-Raven Publishers, 1995:351–366.

42. Soderholm JD, Yates DA, MacQueen G, Perdue M. Early maternal deprivation predisposes adult rats to colonic mucosal barrier dysfunction in response to mild stress. *Gastroenterology* 2001;120:A12.

43. Friedman A, Kaufer D, Shemer J, Hendler I, Soreq H, Tur-Kaspa I. Pyridostigmine brain penetration under stress enhances neuronal excitability and induces early immediate transcriptional response. *Nat Med* 1996;2:1382–1385.

44. Welgan P, Meshkinpour H, Beeler M. The effect of anger on colon motor and myoelectric activity in irritable bowel syndrome. *Gastroenterology* 1988;94:1150–1156.

45. Agreus L, Svärdsudd K, Nyren O, Tibblin G. Irritable bowel syndrome and dyspepsia in the general population: Overlap and lack of stability over time. *Gastroenterology* 1995;109:671–680.

46. Mayer EA, Craske MG, Naliboff BD. Depression, anxiety and the gastrointestinal system. *J Clin Psychiatry* 2001;62:28–36.

47. Fass R, Fullerton S, Tung S, Mayer EA. Sleep disturbances in clinic patients with functional bowel disorders. *Am J Gastroenterol* 2000;95:1195–2000.

48. Fass R, Fullerton S, Naliboff B, Hirsh T, Mayer EA. Sexual dysfunction in patients with irritable bowel syndrome and non-ucler dyspepsia. *Digestion* 1998;59:79–85.

49. Collins SM. Is the irritable gut an inflamed gut? *Scand J Gastroenterol Suppl* 1992;192:102–105.

50. Hiatt RB and Katz L. Mast cells in inflammatory conditions of the gastrointestinal tract. *Am J Gastroenterol* 1962;37:541–545.

51. Weston AP, Biddle WL, Bhatia PS, Miner PBJ. Terminal ileal mucosal mast cells in irritable bowel syndrome. *Dig Dis Sci* 1993;38:1590–1595.

52. Fallon PG, Smith P, Richardson EJ, Jones FJ, Faulkner HC, Van Snick J, Renauld JC, Grencis RK, Dunne DW. Expression of interleukin-9 leads to Th2 cytokine-dominated responses and fatal enteropathy in mice with chronic *Schistosoma mansoni* infections. *Infect Immun* 2000;68:6005–6011.

53. Tornblom H, Lindberg G, Nyberg B, Veress B, Inst K. Histopathological findings in the jejunum of patients with severe irritable bowel syndrome. *Gastroenterology* 2000;118:A140.

54. Salzmann JL, Peltier-Koch F, Bloch F, Petite JP, Camilleri JP. Methods in laboratory investigation: morphometric study of colonic biopsies: a new method of estimating inflammatory diseases. *Lab Invest* 1990;60:847–851.

55. Stewart GT. Post-dysenteric colitis. *BMJ* 1950;3:405–409.

56. Chaudhary NA and Truelove SC. The irritable bowel syndrome. *QJM* 1962;31:307–322.

57. McKendrick MW and Read NW. Irritable bowel syndrome—post *salmonella* infection. *J Infect* 1994;29:1–3.

58. McKendrick MW. Post *Salmonella* irritable bowel syndrome—5 year review. *J Infect* 1996;32:170–171.

59. Neal KR, Hebden J, Spiller R. Prevalence of gastrointestinal symptoms six months after bacterial gastroenteritis and risk factors for development of the irritable bowel syndrome: Postal survey of patients. *BMJ* 1997;314:779–782.

60. Munzer D and Eyad C. Spastic colitis and irritable bowel syndrome: Which expression is prevalent? (A review of 120 cases). *Trop Gastroenterol* 1992;13:27–35.

61. Gwee KA, Collins SM, Marshall JS, Underwood JE, Moochala SM, Read NW. Evidence of inflammatory pathogenesis in post-infectious irritable bowel syndrome. *Gastroenterology* 1998;114:758.

62. Chan J, Gonsalkorale WM, Perrey C, Previca V, Hajeer AH, Whorwell PJ, Hutchinson IV. Il-10 and Tgf-b genotypes in irritable bowel syndrome: Evidence to support an inflammatory component? *Gastroenterology* 2000;118:A184.

63. Maier SF and Watkins LR. Cytokines for psychologists: implications and bidirectional immune-to-brain communication for understanding behavior, mood, and cognition. *Psychol Rev* 1998;105: 83–107.

64. Kresse AE, Million M, Saperas E, Taché Y. Colitis induces CRF expression in hypothalamic magnocellular neurons and blunts CRF gene response to stress in rats. *Am J Physiol* 2001;281:G1203–G1213.

65. Söderholm JD, Perdue MH. Stress and the gastrointestinal tract II. Stress and intestinal barrier function. *Am J Physiol* 2001;280:G7–G13.

66. Santos J, Saperas E, Nogueiras C, Mourelle M, Antolìn M, Cadahia A, Malagelada JR. Release of mast cell mediators into the jejunum by cold pain stress in humans. *Gastroenterology* 1998;114:640–648.

67. MacQueen G, Marshall J, Perdue M, Siegel S, Bienenstock J. Pavlovian conditioning of rat mucosal mast cells to secrete mast cell protease II. *Science* 1989;243:83–85.

68. Elenkov IJ and Chrousos GP. Stress hormones, Th1/Th2 patterns, pro/anti-inflammatory cytokines and susceptibility to disease. *Trends Endocrinol Metab* 1999;10:359–368.

69. Elenkov IJ, Wilder RL, Chrousos GP, Vizi ES. The sympathetic nerve—an integrative interface between two supersystems: the brain and the immune system. *Pharmacol Rev* 2000;52:585–638.

70. O'Sullivan MA, Clayton N, Wong T, Bountra C, Buckley MM, O'Morain CA. Increased iNOS and nitrotyrosine expression in irritable bowel syndrome (IBS). *Gastroenterology* 2000;118:A702.

71. Chang L, Anton P, Elliott J, Reinholdt J, Taing P, Mayer EA. Decreased mucosal cytokines in diarrhea-predominant irritable bowel syndrome. *Gastroenterology* 2002, In Press.

72. Jänig W, Khasar SG, Levine JD, Miao FJP. The role of vagal visceral afferents in the control of nociception. In: *The Biological Basis for Mind Body Interactions.* Mayer EA and Saper CB, eds. Amsterdam, Elsevier Science, 2000:273–287.

73. Westropp JL and Buffington CAT. In vivo models of interstitial cystitis. *J Urol* 2002;167:694–702.

74. Stam R, Bruijnzeel AW, Wiegant VM. Long-lasting stress sensitization. *Eur J Pharmacol* 2000;405: 217–224.

75. Kaufman J, Plotsky PM, Nemeroff CB, Charney DS. Effects of early adverse experiences on brain structure and function: clinical implications. *Biol Psychiatry* 2000;48:778–790.

76. Hislop IG. Childhood deprivation: An antecedent of the irritable bowel syndrome. *Med J Aust* 1979;1:372–374.

77. Hill OW and Blendis L. Physical and psychological evaluation of non-organic abdominal pain. *Gut* 1967;8:221–229.

78. Lowman BC, Drossman DA, Cramer EM, McKee DC. Recollection of childhood events in adults with irritable bowel syndrome. *J Clin Gastroenterol* 1987;9:324–330.

79. Coplan JD, Andrews MW, Rosenblum LA, Owens MJ, Friedman S, Gorman JM, Nemeroff CB. Persistent elevations of cerebrospinal fluid concentrations of corticotropin-releasing factor in adult nonhuman primates exposed to early-life stressors: Implications for the pathophysiology of mood and anxiety disorders. *Proc Natl Acad Sci USA* 1996;93:1619–1623.

80. De Bellis M, Chrousos GP, Dorn LD, Burke L, Helmers K, Kling MA, Trickett PK, Putnam FW. Hypothalamic-pituitary-adrenal axis dysregulation in sexually abused girls. *J Clin Endocrinol Metabol* 1994;78:249–255.

81. Francis DD and Meaney MJ. Maternal care and the development of stress responses. *Curr Opin Neurobiol* 1999;9:128–134.

82. Heim C, Owens MJ, Plotsky PM, Nemeroff CB. The role of early adverse life events in the etiology of depression and post-traumatic stress disorder. Focus on corticotropin-releasing factor. *Ann NY Acad Sci* 1997;821:194–207.

83. Meaney MJ, Diorio J, Francis D, Widdowson J, LaPlante P, Caldji C, Seckl JR, Plotsky PM. Early environmental regulation of forebrain glucocorticoid receptor gene expression: implications for adrenocortical response to stress. *Dev Neurosci* 1996;18:49–72.

84. Caldji C, Diorio J, Meaney MJ. Variations in maternal care in infancy regulate the development of stress reactivity. *Biol Psychiatry* 2000;48:1164–1174.

85. Coutinho S, Sablad M, Miller J, Zhou H, Lam A, Bayati A, Plotsky P, Mayer EA. Neonatal maternal separation results in stress-induced visceral hyperalgesia in adult rats: A new model for IBS. *Gastroenterology* 2000;118:A637.

86. Coutinho SV, Sablad MR, Marvizon JC, Miller JC, Zhou H, Bayati AI, Plotsky PM, Mayer EA. Role of endogenous opiods in stress-induced visceral hyperalgesia in the rat. *Soc Neurosci Abstr* 2000; 26:2190.

87. American Psychiatric Association. *Diagnostic and Statistical Manual for the Mental Disorders (DSM-IV)*. Washington, D.C.: American Psychiatric Association, 1994.

88. Drossman DA, Leserman J, Nachman G, Li ZM, Gluck H, Toomey TC, Mitchell CM. Sexual and physical abuse in women with functional or organic gastrointestinal disorders. *Ann Intern Med* 1990;113:828–833.

89. Koolhaas JM, Hermann PM, Kemperman C, Bohus B, Van den Hoofdakker RH, Beersma DGM. Single social defeat in male rats induces a gradual but long lasting behavioural change: A model of depression? *Neurosci Res Comm* 1990;7:35–41.

90. Cador M, Cole BJ, Koob GF, Stinus L, Le Moal M. Central administration of corticotropin-releasing factor induces long-term sensitization to D-amphetamine. *Brain Res* 1993;606:181–186.

91. Stam R, Croiset G, Akkermans LM, Wiegant VM. Sensitization of the colonic response to novel stress after previous stressful experience. *Am J Physiol Regul Integr Comp Physiol* 1996;271:R1270–R1273.

92. Stam R, Bruijnzeel AW, Akkermans LMA, Wiegant VM. Long-term stress-induced sensitization of visceral afferent and cardiovascular responsivity in the rat. *Neurogastroenterol Motil* 2000;12:407.

93. Francis DD, Caldji C, Champagne F, Plotsky PM, Meaney MJ. The role of corticotropin-releasing factor-norepinephrine systems in mediating the effects of early experience on the development of behavioral and endocrine responses to stress. *Biol Psychiatry* 1999;46:1153–1166.

94. Neylan TC, Fletcher DJ, Lenoci M, McCallin K, Weiss DS, Schoenfeld FB, Marmar CR, Fein G. Sensory gating in chronic post-traumatic stress disorder: Reduced auditory P50 suppression in combat veterans. *Biol Psychiatry* 1999;46:1656–1664.

95. Bruijnzeel AW, Stam R, Compaan JC, Croiset G, Akkermans LM, Olivier B, Wiegant VM. Long-term sensitization of Fos-responsivity in the rat central nervous system after a single stressful experience. *Brain Res* 1999;819:15–22.

96. Bakshi VP and Kalin NH. Corticotropin-releasing hormone and animal models of anxiety: Gene-environment interactions. *Biol Psychiatry* 2000;48:1175–1198.

97. Bakker JM, Kavelaars A, Kamphuis PJ, Cobelens PM, Van Vugt HH, Van Bel F, Heijnen CJ. Neonatal dexamethasone treatment increases susceptibility to experimental autoimmune disease in adult rats. *J Immunol* 2000;165:5932–5937.

98. Shanks N, Windle RJ, Perks PA, Harbuz MS, Jessop DS, Ingram CD, Lightman SL. Early-life exposure to endotoxin alters hypothalamic-pituitary-adrenal function and predisposition to inflammation. *Proc Natl Acad Sci USA* 2000;97:5645–5650.

99. Al-Chaer ED, Kawasaki M, Pasricha PJ. A new model of chronic visceral hypersensitivity in adult rats induced by colon irritation during postnatal development. *Gastroenterology* 2000;119:1276–1285.

100. Chang L, Mayer EA, Johnson T, FitzGerald L, Naliboff B. Differences in somatic perception in female patients with irritable bowel syndrome with and without fibromyalgia. *Pain* 2000;84:297–307.

101. Verne GN, Robinson ME, Price DD. Hypersensitivity to visceral and cutaneous pain in the irritable bowel syndrome. *Pain* 2001;93:7–14.

102. Gue M, Del Rio-Lacheze C, Eutamene H, Theodorou V, Firoamonti J. Stress-induced hypersensitivity to rectal distension in rats: role of CRF and mast cells. *Neurogastroenterol Motil* 1997;9:271–279.

103. Chen JJ, Li Z, Pan H, Murphy DL, Tamir H, Koepsell H, Gershon MD. Maintenance of serotonin in the intestinal mucosa and ganglia of mice that lack the high-affinity serotonin transporter: Abnormal intestinal motility and the expression of cation transporters. *J Neurosci* 2001;21:6348–6361.

104. Collins SM, Piche T, Rampal P. The putative role of inflammation in the irritable bowel syndrome. *Gut* 2001;49:743–745.

105. Mayer EA. Some of the challenges in drug development for irritable bowel syndrome. *Gut* 2001;48:585–586.

106. Mayer EA, Collins SM, eds. *Evolving Pathophysiological Models of Functional GI Disorders: Implications for New Drug Development*. New York: Health Education Alliance, 2000.

107. Holstege G, Bandler R, Saper CB. The emotional motor system. In: *The Emotional Motor System.* Holstege G, Bandler R, Saper CB, eds., Amsterdam, Elsevier, 1996:3–6.

108. Nieuwenheuys R. The greater limbic system, the emotional motor system and the brain. In: *The Emotional Motor System.* Holstege G, Bandler R, Saper CB, eds., Amsterdam, Elsevier, 1996:627.

109. Mayer EA and Collins SM. Evolving pathophysiologic models of functional gastrointestinal disorders. *Gastroenterology* 2002, (in press).

110. Koob GF. Corticotropin-releasing factor, norepinephrine, and stress. *Biol Psychiatry* 1999;46: 1167–1180.

111. Eley TC and Plomin R. Genetic analysis of emotionality. *Curr Opin Neurobiol* 1997;7:279–284.

112. Heim C, Newport DJ, Heit S, Graham YP, Wilcox M, Bonsall R, Miller AH, Nemeroff CB. Pituitary-adrenal and autonomic responses to stress in women after sexual and physical abuse in childhood. *JAMA* 2000;284:592–597.

113. Heim C, Ehlert U, Hellhammer DH. The potential role of hypercortisolism in the pathophysiology of stress-related bodily disorders. *Psychoneuroendocrinology* 2000;25:1–35.

114. Chrousos GP. Stress, chronic inflammation, and emotional and physical well-being: Concurrent effects and chronic sequelae. *J Allergy Clin Immunol* 2000;106:S275–S291.

Index

Index

Note: *f* indicates figure citation; *t* indicates table citation.